Modulation of Oxidative Stress

Modulation of Oxidative Stress

Biochemical, Physiological and Pharmacological Aspects

Edited by

Luciano Saso
Department of Physiology and Pharmacology "Vittorio Erspamer", Sapienza University of Rome, Italy

Alessandro Giuffrè
Institute of Molecular Biology and Pathology, National Research Council, Rome Italy

Giuseppe Valacchi
University of Ferrara, Department of Environmental Sciences and Prevention, Ferrara, Italy; North Carolina State University, Animal Science Department, Plants for Human Health Institute, Kannapolis Research Campus, Kannapolis, NC, United States; Kyung Hee University, Department of Food and Nutrition, Seoul, South Korea

Mauro Maccarrone
University of L'Aquila, Department of Biotechnological and Applied Clinical Sciences, L'Aquila, Italy; European Center for Brain Research/IRCCS Santa Lucia Foundation, Laboratory of Lipid Neurochemistry, Rome, Italy

ELSEVIER

ACADEMIC PRESS
An imprint of Elsevier

Academic Press is an imprint of Elsevier
125 London Wall, London EC2Y 5AS, United Kingdom
525 B Street, Suite 1650, San Diego, CA 92101, United States
50 Hampshire Street, 5th Floor, Cambridge, MA 02139, United States
The Boulevard, Langford Lane, Kidlington, Oxford OX5 1GB, United Kingdom

ISBN: 978-0-443-19247-0

For information on all Academic Press publications visit our website at
https://www.elsevier.com/books-and-journals

Publisher: Andre G. Wolff
Acquisitions Editor: Andre G. Wolff
Editorial Project Manager: Pat Gonzalez
Production Project Manager: Omer Mukthar
Cover Designer: Mark Rogers

Typeset by TNQ Technologies

Contents

Contributors

Moussira Alameddine, Institute of Life Course and Medical Sciences, The MRC - Versus Arthritis Centre for Integrated Research into Musculoskeletal Ageing (CIMA), University of Liverpool, Liverpool, United Kingdom

Marcello Allegretti, R&D, Dompé farmaceutici S.p.A, L'Aquila, Italy

Laura Brandolini, R&D, Dompé farmaceutici S.p.A, L'Aquila, Italy

Lauren Byrd-Leotis, R&D, Dompé farmaceutici S.p.A, Milan, Italy

Vanessa Castelli, Department of Life, Health and Environmental Sciences, University of L'Aquila, L'Aquila, Italy

Carlo Cervellati, Department of Translational Medicine and for Romagna, University of Ferrara, Ferrara, Italy

Niki Chondrogianni, Institute of Chemical Biology, National Hellenic Research Foundation, Athens, Greece

Fabio Ciccarone, Department of Biology, University of Rome "Tor Vergata", Rome, Italy; IRCCS San Raffaele Roma, Rome, Italy

Annamaria Cimini, Department of Life, Health and Environmental Sciences, University of L'Aquila, L'Aquila, Italy; Sbarro Institute for Cancer Research and Molecular Medicine, Center for Biotechnology, Temple University, Philadelphia, PA, United States

Francesco Cimino, Department of Chemical, Biological, Pharmaceutical and Environmental Sciences, University of Messina, Messina, Italy

Maria Rosa Ciriolo, Department of Biology, University of Rome "Tor Vergata", Rome, Italy; IRCCS San Raffaele Roma, Rome, Italy

Valeria Cordone, Department of Environmental Sciences and Prevention, University of Ferrara, Ferrara, Italy

Zuzanna Cyske, Department of Molecular Biology, Faculty of Biology, University of Gdansk, Gdansk, Poland

Sergio Davinelli, Department of Medicine and Health Sciences "V. Tiberio", University of Molise, Campobasso, Italy

M. Rosário Domingues, Mass Spectrometry Centre, LAQV REQUIMTE, Department of Chemistry, Centre for Environmental and Marine Studies (CESAM), University of Aveiro, Santiago University Campus, Aveiro, Portugal

Ufuk Ersoy, Institute of Life Course and Medical Sciences, The MRC - Versus Arthritis Centre for Integrated Research into Musculoskeletal Ageing (CIMA), University of Liverpool, Liverpool, United Kingdom

Tânia Fernandes, CNC - Center for Neuroscience and Cell Biology, CIBB - Center for Innovative Biomedicine and Biotechnology, University of Coimbra, Coimbra, Portugal; IIIUC - Institute for Interdisciplinary Research, University of Coimbra, Coimbra, Portugal; CACC - Clinical Academic Center of Coimbra, Coimbra, Portugal; Faculty of Medicine, University of Coimbra, Coimbra, Portugal

Dalila G.F. Fernandes, Instituto de Tecnologia Química e Biológica António Xavier, NOVA University of Lisbon, Oeiras, Portugal

Federica Finetti, Department of Biotechnology, Chemistry and Pharmacy, University of Siena, Siena, Italy

Lidia Gaffke, Department of Molecular Biology, Faculty of Biology, University of Gdansk, Gdansk, Poland

Anna Gioran, Institute of Chemical Biology, National Hellenic Research Foundation, Athens, Greece

Alessandro Giuffrè, Institute of Molecular Biology and Pathology, National Research Council, Rome, Italy

Katarzyna Goljanek-Whysall, Institute of Life Course and Medical Sciences, The MRC - Versus Arthritis Centre for Integrated Research into Musculoskeletal Ageing (CIMA), University of Liverpool, Liverpool, United Kingdom; Department of Physiology, School of Medicine and REMEDI, CMNHS, NUI Galway, Galway, Ireland

Anna Grochot-Przeczek, Department of Medical Biotechnology, Faculty of Biochemistry, Biophysics and Biotechnology, Jagiellonian University, Krakow, Poland

Hideya Iwaki, Department of Gastroenterology, Tohoku University Graduate School of Medicine, Sendai, Japan; Department of Gene Expression Regulation, Institute of Development, Aging and Cancer, Tohoku University, Sendai, Japan

Malcolm J. Jackson, Institute of Life Course and Medical Sciences, The MRC - Versus Arthritis Centre for Integrated Research into Musculoskeletal Ageing (CIMA), University of Liverpool, Liverpool, United Kingdom

Alicja Jozkowicz, Department of Medical Biotechnology, Faculty of Biochemistry, Biophysics and Biotechnology, Jagiellonian University, Krakow, Poland

Ioannis Kanakis, Institute of Life Course and Medical Sciences, The MRC - Versus Arthritis Centre for Integrated Research into Musculoskeletal Ageing (CIMA), University of Liverpool, Liverpool, United Kingdom; Chester Medical School, Faculty of Medicine and Life Sciences, University of Chester, Chester, United Kingdom

Aleksandra Kopacz, Department of Medical Biotechnology, Faculty of Biochemistry, Biophysics and Biotechnology, Jagiellonian University, Krakow, Poland

Giuseppe Lazzarino, Department of Biomedical and Biotechnological Sciences, Division of Medical Biochemistry, University of Catania, Catania, Italy

Giacomo Lazzarino, UniCamillus—Saint Camillus International University of Health Sciences, Rome, Italy

José Lillo-Moya, Molecular and Clinical Pharmacology Program, Institute of Biomedical Sciences, Faculty of Medicine, University of Chile, Santiago, Chile

Renata Mangione, Institute of Biochemistry and Clinical Biochemistry, Catholic University of Rome, Rome, Italy

Alessandro Medoro, Department of Medicine and Health Sciences "V. Tiberio", University of Molise, Campobasso, Italy

Grzegorz Mincewicz, Department of Molecular Biology, Faculty of Biology, University of Gdansk, Gdansk, Poland

Paula I. Moreira, CNC - Center for Neuroscience and Cell Biology, CIBB - Center for Innovative Biomedicine and Biotechnology, University of Coimbra, Coimbra, Portugal; CACC - Clinical Academic Center of Coimbra, Coimbra, Portugal; Faculty of Medicine, University of Coimbra, Coimbra, Portugal

Hozumi Motohashi, Department of Gene Expression Regulation, Institute of Development, Aging and Cancer, Tohoku University, Sendai, Japan

Rubina Novelli, R&D, Dompé farmaceutici S.p.A, Milan, Italy

Eleni Panagiotidou, Institute of Chemical Biology, National Hellenic Research Foundation, Athens, Greece; Department of Biochemistry and Biotechnology, University of Thessaly, Larissa, Greece

Lucrezia Paradisi, Department of Biotechnology, Chemistry and Pharmacy, University of Siena, Siena, Italy

Alessandra Pecorelli, Department of Environmental Sciences and Prevention, University of Ferrara, Ferrara, Italy; Animal Science Department, Plants for Human Health Institute, North Carolina State University, Kannapolis Research Campus, Kannapolis, NC, United States; Department of Environmental Sciences, University of Ferrara, Ferrara, Italy

Mandy Jayne Peffers, Institute of Life Course and Medical Sciences, The MRC - Versus Arthritis Centre for Integrated Research into Musculoskeletal Ageing (CIMA), University of Liverpool, Liverpool, United Kingdom

Cláudia F. Pereira, CNC - Center for Neuroscience and Cell Biology, CIBB - Center for Innovative Biomedicine and Biotechnology, University of Coimbra, Coimbra, Portugal; CACC - Clinical Academic Center of Coimbra, Coimbra, Portugal; Faculty of Medicine, University of Coimbra, Coimbra, Portugal

Karolina Pierzynowska, Department of Molecular Biology, Faculty of Biology, University of Gdansk, Gdansk, Poland

Magdalena Podlacha, Department of Molecular Biology, Faculty of Biology, University of Gdansk, Gdansk, Poland

Estera Rintz, Department of Molecular Biology, Faculty of Biology, University of Gdansk, Gdansk, Poland

Ramón Rodrigo, Molecular and Clinical Pharmacology Program, Institute of Biomedical Sciences, Faculty of Medicine, University of Chile, Santiago, Chile

Catalina Rojas-Solé, Molecular and Clinical Pharmacology Program, Institute of Biomedical Sciences, Faculty of Medicine, University of Chile, Santiago, Chile

Antonella Saija, Department of Chemical, Biological, Pharmaceutical and Environmental Sciences, University of Messina, Messina, Italy

Giovanni Scapagnini, Department of Medicine and Health Sciences "V. Tiberio", University of Molise, Campobasso, Italy

E. Skrzydlewska, Department of Analytical Chemistry, Medical University of Bialystok, Bialystok, Poland

Antonio Speciale, Department of Chemical, Biological, Pharmaceutical and Environmental Sciences, University of Messina, Messina, Italy

Caroline Amy Staunton, Institute of Life Course and Medical Sciences, The MRC - Versus Arthritis Centre for Integrated Research into Musculoskeletal Ageing (CIMA), University of Liverpool, Liverpool, United Kingdom

Barbara Tavazzi, UniCamillus—Saint Camillus International University of Health Sciences, Rome, Italy

Lorenza Trabalzini, Department of Biotechnology, Chemistry and Pharmacy, University of Siena, Siena, Italy

W. Łuczaj, Department of Analytical Chemistry, Medical University of Bialystok, Bialystok, Poland

Giuseppe Valacchi, Department of Environmental Sciences and Prevention, University of Ferrara, Ferrara, Italy; Animal Science Department, Plants for Human Health Institute, North Carolina State University, Kannapolis Research Campus, Kannapolis, NC, United States; Department of Food and Nutrition, Kyung Hee University, Seoul, South Korea

Aphrodite Vasilaki, Institute of Life Course and Medical Sciences, The MRC - Versus Arthritis Centre for Integrated Research into Musculoskeletal Ageing (CIMA), University of Liverpool, Liverpool, United Kingdom

João B. Vicente, Instituto de Tecnologia Química e Biológica António Xavier, NOVA University of Lisbon, Oeiras, Portugal

Grzegorz Węgrzyn, Department of Molecular Biology, Faculty of Biology, University of Gdansk, Gdansk, Poland

P. Wójcik, Department of Analytical Chemistry, Medical University of Bialystok, Bialystok, Poland

N. Zarkovic, LabOS, Division of Molecular Medicine, Rudjer Boskovic Institute, Zagreb, Croatia

Karim Zuhra, University of Fribourg, Faculty of Science and Medicine, Department of Pharmacology, Fribourg, Switzerland

Preface

The redox state of healthy cells and tissues results from a balance between prooxidants and antioxidants, whereby the latter, either endogenously produced or achieved from the diet, counteract the oxidative effects of the former. It is now recognized that a condition known as oxidative stress (OS), determined by the inadequacy of the antioxidant defense systems, represents a common trait of largely diffused diseases.

In the last years, the detailed mechanisms and regulations of the cell response elements to OS have been unveiled, including activation of transcriptional regulators, enzymatic/nonenzymatic co-factors, and metabolites; this recalls the usefulness of collecting these contributions in a common context, that might be of help in defining a route to follow for the achievement of new tools for the diagnosis and contrast of these pathologies.

In this book, insights on both specific and shared elements of the OS-associated mechanisms involved in the pathogenesis of severe diseases are provided, that include neurodegenerations, cardiovascular disorders, chronic infections, and cancer. The molecular aspects related to genetic disorders accompanied by a chronic OS, such as the Rett syndrome (RTT), cerebral cavernous malformations (CCM) and the retinitis pigmentosa (RP), are addressed. The most relevant therapeutic strategies utilized for the treatment of the abovementioned defects and for ameliorate physiologic conditions in which a predisposition to inflammation is expected, such as ageing, are herein collected. Moreover, aspects related to the state of vulnerability of specific tissues (intestine, retina, reproductive system) to prooxidant insults are dissected, highlighting the mechanisms underlining the bioenergetics/metabolic default occurring in specific cell types extremely prone to accumulation of damages derived from a situation of a stable redox unbalance.

The volume is intended primarily addressed to researchers in the field with interests in specific aspects related to either OS biomarkers, regulative pathways related to OS or the molecular bases of the pathologies described, along with the opportunity to expand the knowledge respect to the wide scenario that includes the manifold OS areas. Moreover, young scientist and students in biochemical and pharmacological areas will have the opportunity to deepen, along the chapters of this book, the pivotal role played by the reactive species (RS), which include oxygen-, nitrogen-, and sulfur-derived compounds (ROS, RNS, and RSS, respectively) in eliciting a signaling action that, starting from mitochondrial level, may influence the redox homeostasis of the cell and contribute to the activation of a complex network of regulative pathways determining OS.

Through the studies on cell lines and animal models herein reported the authors describe available OS markers as promising for early diagnosis and reliable evaluation of a pathological course. Furthermore, the potential of natural or synthetic (last-generation) antioxidants as beneficial supplement to counteract OS-featured diseases is discussed in the frame of the recent clinical evidence showing how the upgrade from in vitro studies to in vivo pharmacological applications is not obvious, due to the complexity of the cellular machinery involved in the response to OS. Yet, thanks to the growing knowledge on the elements and factors promoting OS and on the cell stress-response mechanisms, emerging therapeutic markers, targets, and multitarget approaches are described as promising avenues for the early detection and treatment in the next future of widely diffused pathologies.

The book comprises 18 chapters written by outstanding scientists actively working in the field. A brief description of the addressed topics follows.

- The role of the proteasome as a fundamental component of the cell antioxidant apparatus is described by **Eleni Panagiotidou, Anna Gioran, and Niki Chondrogianni**. During ageing a gradual loss in efficiency of this large multienzymatic complex occurs, and impaired turnover of damaged proteins results in an overall default of cell proteostasis. The authors focus on how the proteasome dysfunction may contribute to the progression of pathologies such as Alzheimer's (AD), Parkinson's (PD), and Huntington's (HD) diseases, all characterized by an altered protein degradation. Recent studies on antioxidants (such as quercetin, curcumin, betulinic acid, and oleuropein) able to reinforce the proteasome function are described, as well as studies on master regulators of OS pathways/autophagy, like mTOR and sirtuins. The role of the nuclear factor (erythroid-derived-2)-like 2 (Nrf2) as a fundamental modulator of cell response to OS is addressed, particularly concerning its ability to promote the synthesis of most proteasomal subunits. The potential benefits of the administration of natural Nrf2 activators/modulators (sulforaphane, caprylic acid, *Ginkgo biloba* among others) in preventing/counteracting aging and neurodegenerative disorders are also discussed.

- The relevance of protein thiol modifications as basic chemical mediators of OS-related signaling is discussed by **Aleksandra Kopacz, Alicja Jozkowicz, and Anna Grochot-Przeczek.** The peculiar propensity of cysteines to undergo oxidation by pro-oxidants leads these amino acids to function as "redox switches". The various cysteine modifications are resumed, along with their effects on cell signaling. Some of the thiol post-translational modifications (PTMs), such as *S*-cyanylation and *S*-nitrosation (SNO), are described as relevant for disease progression, while persulfidation (-SSH), a reversible PTM, is rather involved in autophagy, inflammation, and cell death processes. At mitochondrial level, the relevance of *S*-glutathionylation in modulating the activity of metabolic enzymes is discussed, and the interplay between *S*-glutathionylation and nitric oxide-related modifications (mainly *S*-nitrosation) is addressed. The most relevant examples of regulatory protein thiol modifications, mostly in enzymes and transcription factors involved in the response to OS, are described, as the Nrf2 inhibitor KEAP1, which can undergo *S*-nitrosation, *S*-glutathionylation, or persulfidation to operate a tuned activation of Nrf2.
- The fundamental role played by NRF2 in maintaining the cell redox homeostasis is addressed by **Sergio Davinelli.** OS is dissected as a function of age, and its physio-pathological implications are linked to the accumulation of oxidative damage to macromolecules. The author reports literature evidence describing the correlation between an age-dependent decrease in Nrf2 expression/activity, a lowered expression of its target genes, decreased GSH levels, and increased accumulation of oxidation products. The relevant ways whereby Nrf2 activity influences the various aspects related to aging, including mitochondrial dysfunction and deregulation of nutrient sensing, are also discussed. The primary role of the KEAP1 inhibitor, and of its highly reactive cysteines, is here described in the context of the most validated model for Nrf2-KEAP1 regulatory mechanism (the "hinge and latch" model). The regulatory factors implicated in the tuning of Nrf2-mediated cell response to OS (phosphorylation events and interaction with stabilizing/activating factors) are described. Aspects related to the crosstalk between Nrf2 and NF-κB pathways are detailed in this chapter, highlighting the link between age-dependent decrease of the Nrf2-related gene expression and inflammation. The latest advances in the identification of (natural and synthetic) Nrf2 modulators, able to restore Nrf2activity, preserve cellular homeostasis, and counteract age-OS-inflammation dysfunctions are also presented, with a focus on those aimed at targeting KEAP1.
- The chapter by **Carlo Cervellati and Alessandra Pecorelli** focuses on the characterization of OS biomarkers and their application in the study of the molecular mechanisms involved in neurological diseases and in pharmacological treatments for therapeutic purposes. In the case of OS, RS-induced modifications of biomolecules can produce numerous different measurable products, including metabolites, genes, proteins, or miRNAs, that may be able to reveal a disease or a pathophysiological condition. Along the chapter, specific sections are presented to provide a classification of the available biomarkers based on structural properties and to detail the mechanisms of stress propagation and signaling alterations. The most representative examples of lipid peroxyl radicals and hydroperoxides generated from polyunsaturated fatty acid (PUFA) oxidation are also presented (F2-Isoprostanes (IsoPs), trans-4-hydroxy-2- nonenal (4-HNE), malondialdehyde (MDA), lipid hydroperoxides (LPO)), as well as markers of protein and nucleic acid oxidation, focusing on the correlation among the severity grade of the disease and the reversibility of the modification. The authors discuss the involvement of OS in the most widespread neurological diseases, like AD, vascular dementia, and PD, as well as molecules produced by oxidative damage that represent valuable diagnostic biomarkers. In this context, the aspects related to the reliability of the most utilized biomarkers for AD at different (pre- or postclinical) stages are discussed, also in consideration of possible bias due to inaccuracy of assays. The author addresses the difficulties encountered in validating quantitative methods for a given marker due to heterogeneity of controls (age, sex and other co-morbidities) and the broad specificity respect to diagnosis purposes for a given disease at early stage.

The chapter written by **Lorenza Trabalzini, Federica Finetti, and Lucrezia Paradisi** addresses aspects related to the cerebral cavernous malformations (CCM) disease. Mutations at the level of three genes—*CCM1/KRIT1*, *CCM2/MGC4607*, and *CCM3/PDCD10*—are responsible for heterogeneous phenotypes, that in their severe presentations may be associated to cerebrovascular lesions, seizures and intracerebral hemorrhage due to capillary malformation and endothelial barrier permeabilization. The authors describe studies on cellular and animal models, that illustrate the functions of the three CCM proteins and their multiple putative partners, overall supporting a complex regulatory network involved in adaptive responses to OS and inflammation. Several cellular processes are shown to be influenced through multiple interactions undertaken by the CCM proteins, among which cytoskeletal reorganization, cellular adhesion and migration, angiogenesis, and vascular permeability. The functional features of the KRIT1 protein are described in detail, with a particular focus on its antioxidant and cytoprotective role and ability to maintain mitochondrial homeostasis. OS-regulatory pathways influenced by loss of function of KRIT1, such as Nrf2, FOXO1, Sirt1, cJun/AP-1, Nd1-L/Rho/ROKI, are also addressed. Studies showing the association between altered autophagy and OS are outlined, also providing novel and promising options for the pharmacological treatment of CCM. In this context, the development of a combinatorial treatment able to target both oxidative and inflammatory states and autophagic dysfunction has emerged as a promising approach to overcome the problems related to this pathology.

In the chapter by **Ufuk Ersoy, Moussira Alameddine, Ioannis Kanakis, Caroline Amy Staunton, Mandy Peffers, Malcolm Jackson, Katarzyna Goljanek-Whysall, and Aphrodite Vasilaki,** the authors discuss studies that put in relation maternal nutrition, early life growth, and the risk of developing chronic disorders in later life. Alteration of redox homeostasis and OS in the onset of mitochondrial dysfunctions and an unfavorable growth environment at early developing stage turn to be responsible of the deleterious outcomes in later life, with epigenomic modifications as underlined mechanisms involved in these processes. Early life environment represents a complex mixture of elements that influence the different phases of the embryonic development; in this context, ROS fluctuations influence proliferation, differentiation, and apoptosis throughout embryogenesis. The ROS-mediated processes in embryogenesis depend on oxygen availability and energy demand, and the authors highlight how drastic redox impairment may result in permanent cell growth arrest and apoptosis. The authors discuss studies in animal models that highlight associations between the two extreme habits concerning maternal nutrition and the pathological predisposition of the offspring in late life: mother ipo-nutrition—offspring low birth weight (IUGR) was associated with type 2 diabetes and CVD, impaired glucose metabolism, hypertension, reduced mitochondrial number, and sarcopenia, whereas high weight at birth or exposure to intrauterine maternal obesity or diabetes was linked to insulin resistance, obesity, and heart hypertrophy in the adult offspring. It is outlined how redox-sensitive transcriptional factors (Nrf-2, Ref-1, HIF-1α, NF-κB, AP-1) are involved in the alteration of the gene transcription profile of the offspring, by altering the epigenetic landscape and affecting the late metabolic outcome. The authors outline the gender dependencies of the effects observed in adult age and dwell on the debated issue related to the efficacy of accelerated catch-up growth in case of maternal undernutrition.

Insights on the mitochondria-associated membranes (MAMs) functional role in association with oxidative stress and AD are reported in the chapter by **Tânia Fernandes, M. Rosário Domingues, Cláudia F. Pereira, and Paula I. Moreira**, where the authors highlight the relevance of the multiple cellular activities modulated by MAMs in fundamental processes such as energy metabolism, Ca^{2+} signaling, lipid synthesis and trafficking, ER stress response, inflammation, autophagy, and apoptosis. MAMs proteins such as PERK ERO1α, PDI, Nox4, and p66Shc are specifically mentioned in consideration of their functions related to the integration of ROS signal between ER and mitochondria. MAMs alterations are associated to disregulation of mitochondrial Ca^{2+} homeostasis and increased RS production, thus leading to OS. It is underlined how ROS-mediated lipid peroxidation, once propagated in MAMs, is responsible for the loss of the membrane permeability barrier function and constitutes a condition intimately associated to aging and diseases. Due to the high content of PUFAs and the high rate of O_2 utilization, the vulnerability to lipid peroxidation is of particular relevance at the central nervous system (CNS) level, and the association with the onset of neurodegenerative diseases is underlined. Key markers of oxidative stress (MDA, HNE) originating from ARA and DHA peroxidation are indicative of AD. A specific section deepens the incidence, diffusion, and factors linked to the onset of AD, both sporadic or familial, and the molecular pathways related to aberrant processing of key proteins, such as the amyloid-β (Aβ) precursor protein (APP); the newest therapeutic strategies for early detection of AD based on MAMs altered signals are highlighted. The authors focus on MAMs potential for the individuation of a therapeutic target for AD, pointing to the early outcome of MAMs alteration, and strengthen the idea that modulation of MAMs functions may reveal convenient to prevent or slowdown AD.

In the contribution by **Catalina Rojas-Solé, José Lillo-Moya, and Ramón Rodrigo**, a detailed description of the recent findings on the most notable OS biomarkers is presented, highlighting the predictive and pharmacological relevance of some specific compounds to be utilized to fight human diseases characterized by oxidative unbalance. After a description of the pathophysiological mechanisms of diseases associated to OS (cardiovascular, metabolic, neurodegenerative diseases, and cancer), recent research studies on the identification and validation of biomarkers as therapeutic targets of diseases are reported. Dedicated sections address the involvement of specific RS in cellular health and disease processes, with a description of the main enzymatic and non-enzymatic sources of ROS. It is described how available biomarkers for the so-called "redox diseases" allow to assess the progression or status of oxidative damage. Specific attention is paid to the Nrf2-ARE response axis, the main antioxidant enzymes (superoxide dismutase—SOD, catalase—CAT, glutathione peroxidase—GPx), and the vitamins and antioxidant metabolites (glutathione), contributing to the total antioxidant capacity of the plasma. The OS-mediated mechanisms underlying the onset and progression of classic disorders and relative biomarkers are examined. Hypertension and preeclampsia are described as conditions with high risk for cardiovascular default; ischemia-reperfusion injury (IRI), and acute renal failure (AKI) are also deepened, and the detrimental effect of the oxygen burst-mediated ROS production during reperfusion is discussed. Brain stroke is also described in light of the peculiar oxygen reliance and low antioxidant capacity of the brain and its consequent high susceptibility to oxidative damage. Lastly, the pathogenesis of sepsis is reported, with the vicious circle caused by an uncontrolled inflammation triggered by an infectious insult. Finally, the authors describe the specific biomarkers associated to the addressed dysfunctions and underline the use of antioxidants (MitoQ, ascorbic acid, NAC, vitamin C and E, selenium, NOS inhibitors and melatonin) as promising therapies.

In a further contribution, **José Lillo-Moya, Catalina Rojas-Solé and Ramón Rodrigo** discuss the main antioxidant elements and outline the major pathogenetic role of redox unbalance and OS in cardiovascular diseases. Pro-oxidant insults may arise from environmental factors and inadequate lifestyle, leading to OS and consequent accumulation of cardiovascular damage. Specific sections are dedicated to the description of the enzymatic and non-enzymatic components of the antioxidant system. The evidence that treatment of patients with vitamins C and D in combination led to improved recovery of blood pressure and cardiac function is promising. The cardioprotective function of dietary polyphenols is also outlined, highlighting the antiatherogenic/antithrombotic/anti-inflammatory effects induced by these compounds that are also Nrf2 activators, thus exerting an additional indirect antioxidant function. The available therapeutic interventions against cardiovascular diseases based on the modulation of antioxidant enzymatic activity and the reinforcement of the overall antioxidant components of the body are presented. The authors mention the side effect exerted by some pharmacological treatments, leading to toxic cardiomyopathy. The utilization of antioxidants such as N-acetylcysteine (NAC), carvedilol, or coenzyme Q_{10} to counteract these unfavorable effects is promising, supporting a multitarget approach to contrast OS in cardiovascular disease, also severe as heart failure.

In the chapter by **Fabio Ciccarone and Maria Rosa Ciriolo**, the authors describe the dysregulated mechanisms occurring in cancer cells, highlighting the role of ROS in the activation of metabolic pathways related to cell division and survival under stress conditions. The authors suggest anticancer strategies based on OS induction, by targeting Nrf2 or exploiting the cytotoxic action of reduced iron undergoing the Fenton reaction at high ascorbate concentration. The role of enzymatic source of ROS in cancer metabolic reprogramming is described, focusing on monoamine-oxidase MAOA, xanthine oxidase (XO), NADPH oxidase, cyclooxygenases, and lipoxygenases. The upregulation of enzymes involved in mitogenic or pro-survival processes, such as the promotion of angiogenesis (NOX1, 2, 4, and DUOX2), is also discussed. A wide section of the chapter focuses on the alteration of glucose metabolism in cancer. After presenting the Warburg effect, the authors describe the mechanisms related to the glycolytic switch and lactate accumulation occurring in cancerous cells and address the role of ROS in HIF-1α activation in the cancer hypoxic environment.

In the chapter by **Karim Zuhra, Dalila G. F. Fernandes, Alessandro Giuffrè, and João B. Vicente**, the authors describe the metabolic pathways related to the synthesis and breakdown of the "gasotransmitter" hydrogen sulfide (H_2S), a key element involved in cell redox homeostasis. Beside the food-derived polysulfides and vitamins and microbiota resident desulfurase, the authors describe endogenous enzymatic sources of H_2S, such as cystathionine β-synthase (CBS), cystathionine γ-lyase (CSE), 3-mercaptopyruvate sulfurtransferase (MST), and the selenium-binding protein 1 (SELENBP1). It is also described how mitochondria dispose of excess H_2S through specific enzymatic pathways. The chapter highlights that several human disease, such as Alzheimer (AD), Huntington (HD) disease, and atherosclerosis, are associated to disregulated metabolism of H_2S. Finally, it is remarked that the three gastrotransmitters (NO, CO, and H_2S) are intimately intertwined through a cross-regulative network occurring at transcriptional and post-translational levels, with important implications for human physiology and physiopathology.

In the contribution by **Hideya Iwaki and Hozumi Motohashi**, the intestinal structures are described in light of the unique cell environment, featured by limitations of oxygen supply and an instability of the redox homeostasis in relation of ROS and RNS fluxes derived from several physiological process, including immune response, proliferation, differentiation, and apoptosis. The connection between inflammatory bowel disease (IBD) and the expression of NADPH oxidases (NOX) and nitric oxide synthase (NOS) is also presented. The authors underline that environment-derived redox disturbance plays a significant role in idiopathic IBD, including environmental factors, dietary habits, lifestyle, and pollution. In addition, the intestinal antioxidant response is also described with special focus on glutathione (GSH/GSSG), cysteine (Cys-SH/Cys-SS-Cys), thioredoxin (Trx-SH/Trx-SS-Trx) and

KEAP1-Nrf2 regulatory axis. A detailed section is dedicated to the mucin protein family involved in mucus formation which plays a fundamental role to protect the intestinal tissue against xenobiotics and commensal bacteria. Finally, a session on the possible efficacy of drugs related to IBD treatment is also discussed including 5-aminosalicylic acid (5-ASA), steroids, immunosuppressive drugs, and monoclonal antibody drugs.

The chapter by **Francesco Cimino, Antonella Saija, and Antonio Speciale** focuses on the advantages offered by plant-based photodynamic techniques for the treatment of various pathologies. In particular, the potential benefit of natural photosensitizers (PS) in cancer therapy and microbial infections is addressed. Furthermore, the potential applications of plant-derived products in photodynamic therapy (PDT) for the treatment of cancer and infectious disease is also well presented and summarized. The aspects of noninvasiveness, nontoxicity, and short application time of the PDT method are highlighted. The key issues to take into account in order to increase the efficacy of PDT-induced cell death are also discussed (i.e., the concentration of molecular oxygen and the selective illumination of the target tissues, the PS adequacy based on its subcellular localization and bioavailability). The authors underline this last aspect as a main limitation of the PDT method, that may be overcome by a nanotechnology approach aimed to favor the selective accumulation of PS in target cells and tissues.

In the chapter by **Lidia Gaffke, Karolina Pierzynowska, Zuzanna Cyske, Estera Rintz, Magdalena Podlacha, Grzegorz Mincewicz, and Grzegorz Węgrzyn,** the biological properties of flavonoids, a wide class of natural plant metabolites endowed with antioxidant activity is described, and the aspect related to the potentiality of their utilization as therapeutic compounds to counteract a broad spectrum of human diseases including cancer, infectious diseases, and neurodegenerative disorders are discussed. The structural variability and the various functions exerted on animal cells are described, focusing on their redox modulatory and anti-inflammatory activity that emerge in the following properties: direct ROS scavenging, modulation of antioxidant enzymes, chelation of metal ions, inhibition of NAPDH oxidases, and increase of α-tocopheryl radicals and nitric oxide. The results of a wide number of studies asserting the efficacy of flavonoids in counteracting the invasion and proliferation of cancer cells and in the stimulation of autophagy and apoptosis is reported. An overview of the most promising compounds endowed with anticancer properties (such as apigenin, epigallocatechin-3-gallate, kaempferol, and quercetin) is provided, and the molecular targets at the level of regulatory pathways (mTOR, p53, NF-κB, MAPK, JAK/STAT, PI3K/AKT, and Wnt/β-catenin) in which different molecules are involved, are summarized. The involvement of flavonoids epigenetic regulations, miRNA/noncoding RNAs modulations or in the interplay with the microbiota aimed to preserve its protective anticancer function, underline the overall relevance of the various mechanism of action of flavonoids and strengthen the idea of their utilization in the treatment of infections, neurodegeneration and cancer. The recurrent discrepancies between the encouraging results obtained with flavonoids in vitro and in animal models respect to the negligibility of effective benefits emerged in clinical trials is discussed by the authors underlying the needs of further studies to clarify the therapeutic potentiality of this class of compounds.

In the chapter by **Valeria Cordone, Alessandra Pecorelli, and Giuseppe Valacchi,** the beneficial effects of omega-3 PUFAs is examined, focusing on their modulatory/anti-inflammatory properties and deepening their relevance in the context of the Rett syndrome (RTT), a multisystem disease with neurologic predominance. RTT is characterized by a postnatal developmental neurological regression accompanied by severe mental retardation, caused by a mutation in the X-linked gene for the methyl-CpG binding protein 2 (MeCP2), a ubiquitous epigenetic modulator with transcriptional and RNA/micro RNA processing activity. A detailed description of the altered metabolic pathways in RTT is provided, among which an unbalanced redox homeostasis associated to dysfunctional mitochondrial bioenergetics, alterations of cholesterol metabolism, and deregulated inflammasome response with the consequence of a chronic inflammation condition "OxInflammation." Hallmarks of the RTT disease are a low serum vitamin E levels and enhanced peroxidation damages; of relevance, RTT patient exhibit up-regulation of 15-lipoxygenase (ALOX15) involved in the oxidation of PUFA arachidonate. The most attractive interventions aimed at counteracting the onset and progression of RTT are described, based on gene therapy and genomic editing system CRISPR/Cas9. Natural-derived compounds (Trolox, a vitamin-E derivative, curcumin, coenzyme Q_{10}) whose properties may be beneficial in ameliorating the redox imbalance in RTT were described, by mentioning their supportive, nondefinitive effects. A wide section is dedicated to the description of the properties of n-3 PUFAs and to the promising evidence of a positive effect obtained through their supplementation to RTT patients. The authors also consider the unfavorable aspects related to excess of n-3 PUFAs in the body, mainly related to the suppression of cell response in case of pathogen infection.

In the chapter by **Vanessa Castelli, Lauren Byrd-Leotis, Rubina Novelli, Laura Brandolini, Annamaria Cimini, and Marcello Allegretti,** the peculiar features of the retina are described in consideration of the specific aerobic needs of the retinal cells and their exposure to photochemical reaction-derived ROS. The fluidity of the photoreceptors' membrane, reached by a high PUFA content, increase the cell vulnerability to light absorption, by inducing lipid peroxidation and oxidative stress; these events are associated to the production of HNE and MDA, expressing the level of damage to amino acids and proteins in retinal cells. The major degenerative diseases resulting from the accumulation of oxidative damage in the retinal tissue are described. These include: the diabetic retinopathy (DR), in which the chronic hyperglycemia lead to glucose-induced damage of the microvasculature, nerve, and retinal cells unable to modulate glucose transport; the retinitis pigmentosa (RP), which collect a number of inherited retinal degenerative diseases with different age of onset, whose progress leads to a gradual photoreceptor death with increased oxygen concentration exacerbating OS and culminating in vision loss; the multifactorial age-related macular degeneration (AMD), characterized by apoptosis of cone photoreceptors, determining a dysfunction in daily visual perception and color vision; and glaucoma, a degenerative defect in the retinal ganglion cells featured by increased intraocular pressure and progressive concentric damage and visual field defects. The described retinal degenerations are all featured by increased ROS level and onset of OS. Following diagnosis, antioxidant-based therapies (carotenoids and vitamin E) are applied to ameliorate the conditions of patients and delay the progression of the neurodegeneration. Studies reporting the effects exerted by sulfur-containing amino acids, methionine, cysteine, and their derivatives, endowed with antioxidant properties are described as new strategies to prevent and counteract the oxidative damage in the eye. The relevance of the nonproteinogenic sulfur β-amino acid taurine, abundantly expressed in photoreceptor cells, is deepened. The authors focus the discussion on results obtained in the treatment of retinal disorders with the antioxidant amino acids mentioned and NAC, thus highlighting their potential as supplement in therapies aimed at counteracting DR, RP, AMD, and glaucoma.

In the contribution by **Renata Mangione, Barbara Tavazzi, Giuseppe Lazzarino, and Giacomo Lazzarino**, the pathophysiological aspects related to male infertility, a multifactorial disease in which the contribution of oxidative stress is consolidated, are deepened. The main causes of infertility in human male patients are exposed by the authors, varying from genetic, pharmacological, environmental and lifestyle; these concur in the determination of different levels of functional alteration in the sperm cell. The role played by moderates ROS and RNS amounts in the modulation of the different aspects related to spermatozoa physiology are recalled, as these RS are involved in the differentiation, maturation, and acquisition of the fertilization capacity of the sperm cell and in the sperm-oocyte fusion. Of relevance, diet-derived antioxidant (polyphenols, α- γ-tocopherol, all-trans-retinoic acid/retinol, carotenoids) are actively transported and accumulated at the seminal plasma level, to sustain sperm cells for metabolic and antioxidant needs. Biochemical markers indicative of oxidative/nitrosative stress are found in seminal fluid of patients (MDA, 4-HNE, 8-OHdG, NO_2^-, and NO_3^-) and under these conditions the consequent mitochondrial impairment leads to alteration of the sperm cells structures, such as peroxidation of membranes PUFAs, fragmentation of mtDNA and altered expression/activity of metabolic enzymes. The trafficking/bioavailability and cross-mechanisms of action of low-molecular-weight antioxidant and vitamins are deepened, with focus on fat-soluble vitamins E (tocopherol), counteracting the damage occurring at the sperm membranes, and C (ascorbic acid) playing a crucial role in maintaining α-tocopherol in the reduced state. Among the low-molecular-weight antioxidants widely utilized to improve sperm quality/fertilization ability of patients N-acetylcysteine (NAC) action mechanism and effectiveness are addressed in detail. A conclusive discussion is opened by the authors on the efficacy of the antioxidant supplementations, underlining the discrepancies observed and the possible reasons of these outcomes. The authors express the needs of further case-control and longitudinal studies with more defined enrolling rules and administration protocols to achieve a more reliable data on the usefulness of antioxidant administration for the treatment of male infertility.

In the chapter by **P. Wójcik, W. Łuczaj, N. Zarkovic, and E. Skrzydlewska,** the features of the skin disease psoriasis are deepened. As a chronic immune-mediated inflammatory disease, psoriasis is caused by a combination of genetic and environmental factors that are also responsible for a different grade of severity in which over-inflammatory response is a crucial element that may involve other tissues than the skin.

The metabolic dysregulation of keratinocytes and the activation of proliferative and inflammatory response pathways, associated to neutrophils recruitment, are recalled by the authors that highlight the role of the transcription factors STAT3, NFkB, Foxp3, and HIF-1α in the pathogenesis.

Neutrophil-derived cytokine production determines RS unbalance and OS; in the plasma of patients with psoriasis, an increased activity of NADPH/xanthine oxidases and inducible nitric oxide synthase (iNOS) has been found, particularly in severe manifestations with cardiovascular complications (psoriatic arthritis). In parallel, a lower total antioxidant capacity has been detected in patients' blood cells, with a decreased vitamin C, E, β-carotene levels, paraoxonase, and SOD activity as well as decreased efficiency of glutathione and thioredoxin systems. Conflicting data are reported by the authors, concerning Nrf2 activation; the overall evidence of an increased level of its downstream product, the heme oxygenase 1 (HO-1) come in support to the Nrf2 involvement, but this is not of benefit for psoriatic patients due to the consequent production of proproliferative factors.

The authors underline the relevance of the alterations of the endocannabinoid system in the dysregulation of the cutaneous functions associated with the disease, and the recently unveiled role of the eicosanoids prostaglandin PGE2 in the development of psoriatic dermatitis. ROS-mediated peroxidation of PUFAs and alteration of lipoprotein metabolism have been associated with trans-epidermal barrier impairment in the keratinocytes of patients affected by psoriasis; the increased formation of advanced glycation products (AGEs) is responsible of the intensification of the immune reaction and the promotion of chronic inflammation, which contribute to the development of disease.

The antioxidants and anti-inflammatory compounds mostly utilized as therapy to ameliorate psoriasis are examined by the authors. Strategies based on the use of TNFα inhibitors and PPARγ modulators are deepened, and the advantage of UV phototherapy associated to topic/oral vitamin D analogs, omega-3 fatty acids, polyphenols and phytocannabinoid administration is discussed.

In virtue of its strong anti-inflammatory and antioxidant properties associated to the absence of psychoactive action, cannabidiol is described as a promising compound in therapy of psoriasis and of other diseases with robust inflammatory component.

We believe that this book will provide an important update on the aforementioned topics to young researchers in the field of redox biochemistry, physiology and pharmacology. Indeed, the theme is very complex (>350,000 articles in Pubmed) and evolved very much in the last decades from the study of radical scavengers to the modulation of cell pathways such as KEAP1/NRF2. The development of effective drugs capable of modulating oxidative stress in the diseases discussed in this book requires interdisciplinary research and a very close cooperation among biochemists, physiologists and pharmacologists.

We, the Editors, would like to thank very much all the Authors who contributed to this book, and other Colleagues who strictly collaborate with us on other scientific activities which made this publication possible such as the high level redox webinar series we coordinate (www.antiox.it). In particular we would like to thank very much Marzia Arese from Department of Biochemical Sciences "A. Rossi-Fanelli" of Sapienza University of Rome for cooperating very much with us for the preparation of this preface and Alessandro Leuti from Department of Medicine of the Campus Bio-Medico University of Rome for preparing the figure of the cover.

We would also like to thank Elsevier and in particular the Publisher André Gerhard Wolff and Senior Editorial Project Manager Patricia Gonzalez for the excellent assistance from the beginning to the end of this exciting project.

We wish all interested Colleagues a very pleasant and fruitful reading experience.

Luciano Saso, Alessandro Giuffrè,
Giuseppe Valacchi and Mauro Maccarrone

Chapter 1

Antioxidants as modulators of the ubiquitin–proteasome system against aging and proteinopathies

Eleni Panagiotidou[1,2,a], Anna Gioran[1,a] and Niki Chondrogianni[1]

[1]*Institute of Chemical Biology, National Hellenic Research Foundation, Athens, Greece;* [2]*Department of Biochemistry and Biotechnology, University of Thessaly, Larissa, Greece*

Introduction

Aging can be defined as the gradual, time-dependent decline of cell function and integrity that eventually mirrors the loss of the organismal function and integrity. Many theories have attempted to explain why organisms age, and although they may differ, there is some unanimity regarding the hallmarks of aging. These include genomic instability, telomere attrition, epigenetic alterations, deregulated nutrient sensing, mitochondrial dysfunction, cellular senescence, stem cell exhaustion, altered intercellular communication, and loss of proteostasis [1]. According to the World Health Organization (WHO), the number of people aged 60 years or older will more than double between 2015 and 2050, moving from 12% to 22% of the global population [2]. Although longer lifespans mean more opportunities to contribute to one's families and communities while pursuing further activities, the extent of these opportunities relies almost entirely on one factor: a person's health. In order to prolong the healthy and active years in human lives (the so-called healthspan), much research has focused on the identification of (mainly) preventive interventions, particularly through the identification/characterization of bioactive compounds that may facilitate this health extension. In fact, several human clinical trials testing bioactive compounds that affect aging-related pathways are underway [3]. Notably, the most recent development in the antiaging interventions is a group of compounds/drugs called senolytics. These compounds selectively target and eliminate senescent cells (lysis of senescent cells), thus alleviating the adverse effects that senescent cells have on their neighboring young cells. Although no results are yet available as these agents have just begun being tested for safety in humans, they currently represent one of the most promising antiaging interventions [4].

Proteinopathies entail the aggregation or amyloid fibril formation of proteins abundant in various tissues. Depending on the defective protein, proteinopathies may cause a wide range of pathologies involving individual diverse organs such as the brain, skeletal muscle, kidney, heart, lung, or multiple organs at the same time like in the case of multisystem proteinopathies [5]. Alzheimer's disease (AD) is one of the most common and largely studied age-related proteinopathy. AD is a form of dementia associated with changes in the cleavage of the amyloid precursor protein (APP) leading to the formation of the APP fragment beta-amyloid (Aβ) with aggregation-prone properties, as well as, enhanced levels of hyperphosphorylated tau protein that also forms aggregates. AD entails reduction in synaptic strength, synaptic loss, and neurodegeneration accompanied by metabolic, vascular, and inflammatory changes of the brain [6]. The very high incidence of AD in the population explains the intensive studies of AD in the past few decades. According to the WHO, 55 million people suffer from dementia at the moment, 60%–70% of which are attributed to AD [7]. Currently, AD and other dementias are the seventh leading cause of death globally [8]. The number of people affected by dementia is expected to rise to 78 million in 2030 and 139 million in 2050 [7].

Parkinson's disease (PD) is another age-related proteinopathy with high prevalence that represents the second most frequent neurodegenerative disorder after AD [9]. PD involves the progressive degeneration of dopaminergic neurons while the surviving neurons accumulate the

[a] These two authors contributed equally.

Modulation of Oxidative Stress. https://doi.org/10.1016/B978-0-443-19247-0.00007-2

defining neuropathological characteristics of the disease, namely Lewy bodies and Lewy neurites that are composed by abnormal protein inclusions mainly comprising aggregated alpha-synuclein [9]. The disease causes both motor symptoms including bradykinesia and resting tremor as well as non-motor symptoms like cognitive dysfunction and gastrointestinal symptoms [10]. Disability and death incidents due to PD are increasing faster than for any other neurological disorder. More specifically, the prevalence of PD has doubled in the past 25 years, while global estimates from 2019 showed that over 8.5 million individuals are afflicted by the disease [11].

Another group of neurodegenerative diseases that also belong to the family of proteinopathies are the so-called repeat expansion disorders. These are characterized by unstable repetitive simple sequence tracts dispersed throughout the human genome. Among the repeat expansion disorders with trinucleotide repeats in coding sequences, those with a repetition of a CAG triplet are the most common. The presence of repeated CAG triplets results into an elongated polyglutamine (polyQ) tract in the respective protein. Although polyQ diseases are not as prevalent as AD and PD, they represent a vast group of diseases, and they include widely studied diseases like Huntington's disease (HD) and spinocerebellar ataxias (SCAs) [12]. In the case of HD, the polyQ tract is located in the HTT gene while depending on the type of SCA the affected genes are ATXN1, ATXN2, ATXN3, etc. PolyQ diseases share some clinical features such as progressive motor disability and cognitive defects [13].

There are several common characteristics regarding the potential therapeutic or preventive schemes between age-related diseases and aging. For example, at the moment, there are no disease-modifying therapies for proteinopathies and all interventions remain palliative. Similarly, no one-size-fits all antiaging strategy is available. Most frequently, age-related diseases such as heart disease, stroke, and chronic lung disease [2] are treated upon onset and mostly symptomatically. A second common feature between many proteinopathies, and aging is the increased load of oxidative damage. In fact, there have been extensive studies on the potential merit of antioxidants as worthy antiaging strategies [14] or their benefits against the progression of proteinopathies like AD, PD [15], or polyQ diseases [16]. Thirdly, strong evidence suggests that activation of the proteasome, the main cellular proteolytic mechanism, may comprise an antiaging intervention as well as a therapeutic avenue against proteinopathies. Considering these three common features between therapeutic or preventive avenues regarding aging and proteinopathies, this chapter discusses the role of the proteasome in aging and proteinopathies with a special focus on proteasome modulation by antioxidant agents.

Proteasome in aging and proteinopathies

Ubiquitin–proteasome system structure and function

The proteasome is one of the main proteolytic mechanisms of the cell mediating the degradation of ~80% of the cellular proteins. It is a large multisubunit enzymatic complex that catalyzes the degradation of short-lived, misfolded, and damaged proteins in an ATP-dependent or independent manner [17,18]. It is found in the cytosol and nucleus, while it is also associated with the endoplasmic reticulum [19]. The main proteasome forms in eukaryotes are the so-called 20S core and the 26S and 30S complexes. The latter ones consist of the 20S core particle capped by one or two 19S regulatory particles, respectively (Fig. 1.1A). The 20S core particle is composed of 28 subunits 14 of which are α-type and 14 β-type. Of the latter, β1, β2, and β5 are the subunits carrying the catalytic activities of the proteasome; caspase-like (C-L), trypsin-like (T-L), and chymotrypsin-like (CT-L), respectively. The 20S core is responsible for the degradation of the substrates. The 20S proteasome can exist in an unbound form, and it is the main protease responsible for the degradation of oxidized proteins in an ATP- and ubiquitin-independent manner [20]. The 19S particle on the other hand is organized into two sub-complexes, the lid and the base, and it is responsible among others for the opening of the 20S gate. The base binds directly to the 20S particle, is composed of hexameric AAA-ATPases (Rpt1-6) and tetrameric non-ATPases Rpn1, Rpn2, Rpn10, and Rpn13, and is responsible for the unfolding of the substrates and their translocation to the 20S chamber [21]. The lid is composed of nine subunits (Rpn3, Rpn5-9, Rpn11, Rpn12, and Rpn15) and is necessary for the poly-ubiquitin chain binding and the deubiquitination of the substrate [22]. Proteasome-mediated protein degradation produces shorter peptides, mostly varying between 2 and 10 residues in size that can then be broken down into amino acids through amino- and carboxypeptidases [20].

Ubiquitin is a 76-amino acid protein that can be attached to protein substrates through a sophisticated three-step enzymatic process (Fig. 1.1B). In the first step, a ubiquitin-activating enzyme (E1) activates ubiquitin. In the second step, the ubiquitin is transferred from E1 onto the active site of a ubiquitin-conjugating enzyme (E2). In the third and final step, the E3 ubiquitin ligase transfers the ubiquitin for the E2 to a lysine residue of the substrate protein. Eukaryotes have only one or two types of E1 enzyme, 10–35 E2 enzymes, and even more E3 enzymes although their number is not yet defined. The combination of E2 and E3 enzymes dictates if the ubiquitin modification will include the addition of one

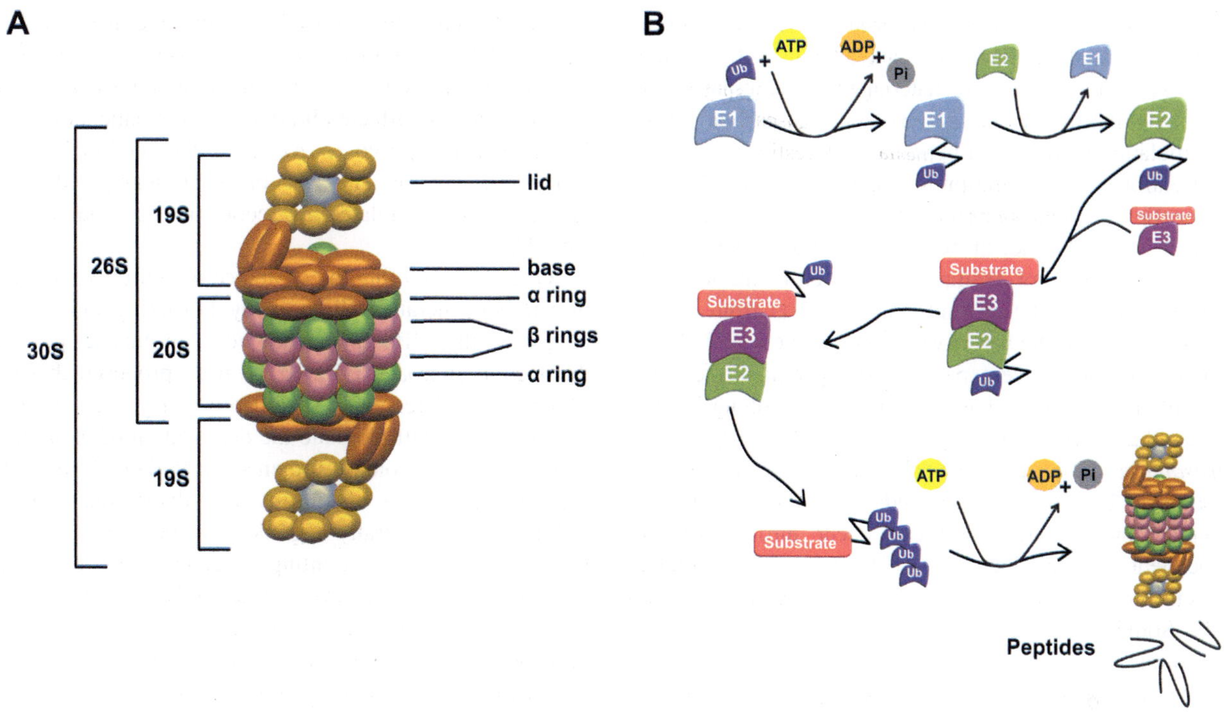

FIGURE 1.1 The main components of the UPS. (A) The 30S/26S proteasome consists of the 20S catalytic core and the 19S regulatory cap(s). Multiple α- and β-type subunits give rise to the α- and β-rings that are then organized in the 20S complex (see text for details). (B) Protein ubiquitination is an ATP-dependent process and occurs in distinct steps with the consecutive participation of E1, E2, and E3 ligases, resulting in the tagging of the protein substrate as a proteasome client.

ubiquitin (mono-ubiquitination) or of multiple ubiquitins (forming polyubiquitin chains). The standard form of ubiquitination is represented by the tetra-ubiquitination (at least four ubiquitin moieties on the substrate to be degraded) that is needed for protein recognition by the UPS system and subsequent degradation. Nevertheless, more recently, other forms of proteasomal targeting signals were also revealed such as mono-ubiquitination and multiple mono-ubiquitinations [23].

Briefly, once a protein has been appropriately ubiquitinated, it can be recognized by ubiquitin receptors and get shuttled to the 26S/30S proteasome for degradation. Ubiquitin receptors are known to be constituent proteasome subunits like the 19S subunits Rpn1, Rpn10, and Rpn13 or non-proteasomal ubiquitin-associated proteins. Before degradation, at least part of the ubiquitin chain is removed and rescued from degradation, while the released chain is further degraded into single ubiquitin molecules that can be reused. Then, the 19S cap translocates the substrate into the catalytic chamber of the 20S catalytic core while unfolding it. This process requires the opening of the gate formed by the N-terminal tails of the α-subunits, so that the substrate can further proceed into the proteolytic chamber. To complete the lifecycle of the proteasome, and although not entirely described, it has been shown that individual proteasome subunits can be degraded by the proteasome itself, while the entire 30S/26S proteasome is subjected to lysosomal degradation [24].

Proteasome involvement in aging

As already mentioned, the deterioration of the proteostatic mechanisms is one of the hallmarks of aging. Proteostatic mechanisms are responsible for the accurate synthesis and folding of proteins as well as their timely degradation. An interesting point that tethers aging with proteostasis is that several major pathways that determine lifespan also regulate parts of the proteostatic network [3]. In fact, several human clinical trials are testing compounds that affect aging-related pathways that, at the same time, are part of the proteostasis network. Among them, one can find rapamycin, a lifespan-extending compound that blocks the negative regulator of autophagy mTOR thereby enhancing autophagy, as well as compounds that activate sirtuins, proteins heavily involved in aging and metabolism [3]. The function and structure of the proteasome also undergo changes with aging, and it has long been considered a very interesting target to delay or reverse the consequences of aging.

Evidence from human and animal tissues indicates that the proteasome undergoes certain age-related alterations. Overall, in cells undergoing senescence as well as in aged rodents, nematodes, and flies, the activity of the proteasome declines without any strong evidence that the expression of the proteasome subunits is reduced (at least not in all models). This suggests that the proteasome may undergo posttranslational modifications that alter its activity. It is also likely that aggregated material that accumulates over time may inhibit the proteasome thus leading to further accumulation of damaged proteins [25].

Reinforcement of the proteasome with either chemical or genetic means has been shown to bestow organismal and cellular longevity and, in many cases, to delay age-related phenotypes [26]. For example, restoration of the levels of proteasomal catalytic subunits in fibroblasts from elderly donors decreased the severity of aging markers [27]. At the organismal level, overexpression of specific proteasome subunits in *C. elegans* has been shown to prolong its lifespan [28,29], while similar findings have been reported in *Drosophila* [30]. Proteasomal activities can also be modulated by various compounds in a direct or indirect manner. Indirect activation can occur through cAMP-dependent Protein kinase A (PKA), cGMP-dependent protein kinase G (PKG), and inhibition of deubiquitinases [31]. Some direct 20S proteasome activators (defined as structural proteasome activators since they promote stereochemical alterations in the 20S proteasome structure thus opening its α-gated channel) are chlorpromazines and dihydroquinazoles, among others, and several natural product-based activators such as betulinic acid and oleuropein [31], while we have recently identified a marine-derived compound, namely, 1R,3E,6R,7Z,11S,12S-dolabella-3,7,18-trien-6,17-olide (DBTO), as the first structural proteasome activator derived from the marine ecosystem [32]. Oleuropein was also shown to prolong the cellular lifespan of primary human fibroblasts [33], while DBTO was shown to promote cellular healthspan. The list of compounds that increase proteasome activity is long. However, the effects of these compounds may not always be restricted to the proteasome, and they may frequently have antioxidant or other beneficial effects independently of their effects on the proteasome. For example, quercetin, a plant-derived polyphenol, and its derivative quercetin caprylate have been shown to exert antioxidant effects but also to activate the proteasome and to prolong the cellular lifespan of primary human fibroblasts [34]. Nevertheless, seeking for compounds that activate the proteasome, with or without off-target beneficial effects, is considered a worthwhile approach in the antiaging field.

The proteasome in proteinopathies

Many lines of evidence suggest that aberrations in the proteasome may occur early enough in AD and PD to play a primary and direct role in the disease pathogenesis [35]. In support of this, the proteasome was found to have decreased activities in the hippocampi, the related limbic structures, and the inferior parietal lobes of AD patients [36]. Moreover, an inhibitory effect of tau-based paired helical filaments (PHFs) on the proteasome itself has been suggested [37]. Similarly, α- and β-type subunits of the proteasome as well as its enzymatic activities have been found reduced in affected brain regions of patients with PD [38–40]. As opposed to AD and PD, inhibition of the proteasome by mutant HTT or other aggregated polyQ proteins may be related to secondary neuronal damage [35,41].

Overall, promoting the clearance of neurotoxic proteins in neurodegenerative diseases by bolstering either autophagy or the UPS is considered a promising potential therapeutic approach [42]. It has been proposed that proteasome reinforcement specifically may be an ideal approach as it will facilitate the degradation of monomeric precursors of neurotoxic proteins, of oxidatively damaged proteins, as well as of "intrinsically disordered proteins" (IDPs) that are naturally degraded by the proteasome [43]. In support of this, mounting evidence from preclinical models implies that proteasome activation ameliorates several proteotoxic effects in various animal models of proteinopathies. Genetic activation of the proteasome in *C. elegans* has shown to counteract Aβ- and polyQ-mediated proteotoxicity [28,29]. Similar findings were recently reported for APP toxicity in mice [44]. Moreover, activation of the proteasome with natural compounds like quercetin, 18α-GA, or DBTO have been shown to delay Aβ-mediated toxicity in *C. elegans* [32,45,46].

Despite all the evidence favoring the concept of proteasome activation as a therapeutic strategy against proteinopathies, one should also consider the potential adverse effects of the possibly enhanced clearance of proteins unrelated to neurodegenerative pathways [47]. Nevertheless, this limitation could be circumvented with the use of PROTACs. PROTACs (proteolysis targeting chimeras) are chimeric molecules that can shuttle specific proteins to a ubiquitin ligase complex for targeted ubiquitination and degradation. Theoretically, PROTACs developed to target tau or Aβ for degradation could be used as a treatment in AD [48]. However, a limitation may also occur in this case; since both tau and Aβ have been shown to inhibit the proteasome, PROTACs may not be able to display their full potential [36]. Therefore, a combination of PROTACs with structural proteasome activators could theoretically be the ultimate solution. Structural proteasome activators can activate the 20S complex, which can recognize only oxidized proteins or IDPs, thus, few of the culprits of the various proteinopathies. However, if combined with PROTACs, specific proteins that need ubiquitination to be recognized would reach the 20S complex, which would be further activated due to the action of the structural activators.

Although the role of the proteasome in proteinopathies is at this point undisputable and strong preclinical evidence supports its activation as an attractive therapeutic target, there are still many gaps and controversies that need to be covered before proceeding to a complete therapeutic strategy.

Effects of cellular redox status on proteasome function

Several pathological conditions like AD, PD, and polyQ diseases as well as aging have been associated with elevated oxidative damage. Similarly, in these conditions, changes in the proteasome structure and function have been also observed [49]. This has led to the notion that oxidants or oxidative damage can affect the activity and/or conformation of the proteasome. This hypothesis has been validated by several studies showing that the proteasome structure and function can be affected by oxidative stress in both indirect and direct manner (Fig. 1.2).

With regard to the indirect regulation of the proteasome by oxidative stress, the nuclear factor (erythroid-derived-2)-like 2 (Nrf2)-dependent proteasome regulation has been revealed. Nrf2 is the main transcription factor that orchestrates the cellular response against oxidative stress. Under normal conditions, Nrf2 is bound to Keap1 (Kelch-like ECH associated protein 1), an intrinsic inhibitor of Nrf2. The Nrf2-Keap1 complex normally resides in the cytoplasm; it is ubiquitinated by an E3 ligase complex and degraded by the proteasome. However, under oxidative stress conditions, oxidative modifications on the cystein residues of Keap1 and the inactivation of the E3 ligase complex allow the dissociation of Nrf2 from Keap1 and its translocation and accumulation into the nucleus. Once in the nucleus and upon heterodimerization with other specific proteins, Nrf2 promotes the expression of several protective genes among which most of the proteasome subunits [50].

The proteasome has been found to be directly modified by oxidants with significant effects on its conformation and function. For example, under acute oxidative stress due to exposure to oxidants or mitochondrial defects, rapid disassembly of 30S/26S proteasomes into intact 20S and 19S particles occurs to allow the immediate ATP- and ubiquitin-independent degradation of oxidized proteins by the 20S particle [20,51]. It is suggested that oxidation of cysteine residues lies behind the observed proteasome disassembly, while reassembly in vivo and in vitro is possible upon reduction (i.e., treatment with antioxidants). Antioxidant treatment is also sufficient to restore the ubiquitin-dependent substrate degradation [51]. These findings were further supported by a study in yeast where S-glutathionylation of specific cysteine residues of the unbound 20S particle was shown to increase its effectiveness

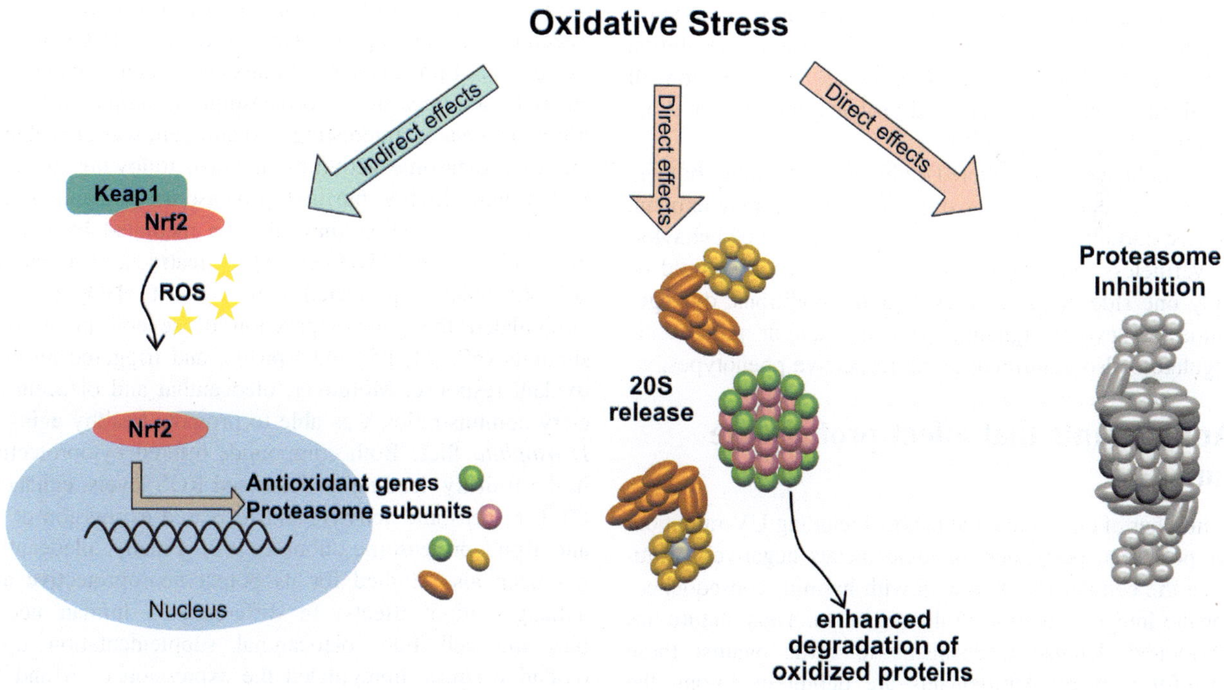

FIGURE 1.2 The cellular redox status can affect the proteasome function. Increased levels of oxidative stress can have two distinct outcomes on the function of the proteasome; activation or inhibition. Activation can occur in an indirect manner through the Nrf2-mediated enhanced expression of various proteasome subunits. Activation can also occur in a direct manner via posttranslational modifications of the proteasome that lead to the dissociation of the 19S regulatory particles from the 20S core, allowing the latter to degrade oxidized proteins or partially unfolded proteins (including IDPs) in an ATP- and ubiquitin-independent manner. Elevated oxidative stress may also lead to proteasome inactivation known to occur as a consequence of posttranslational modifications.

in the degradation of oxidized and partially unfolded proteins [52]. Several posttranslational modifications have been reported to occur in specific proteasome subunits upon oxidative stress like carbonylation, glycoxidation, and lipoxidation, but the exact effects of each one are not fully described yet [53]. It is likely that some have an activating effect, at least on the 20S proteasome, while some exhibit an inhibitory effect. For example, treatment with H_2O_2 or the oxidized form of glutathione (GSSG) of human lens epithelial cells inhibited all three proteasome activities [54]. Similarly in human neuroblastoma cells, the presence of an electrophile oxidant modified an ATPase of the 19S particle, resulting in significant reduction of the 26S proteasome activity [55].

Accumulation of oxidatively modified proteins is a characteristic of cellular aging while age-related or neurodegeneration-related cognitive impairment has been extensively linked with increased oxidative damage [56]. Examination of the AD brain has revealed several pathological hallmarks associated with oxidative damage. Although the source of free radicals is unclear (could be mitochondrial dysfunction, Aβ-mediated processes or even genetic factors), there is definitely a redox imbalance [57]. Importantly, the proteasome has been found to be affected by oxidative damage resulting in its inactivation in the brain of AD patients [58]. Similarly, in PD, it is suggested that the local and systemic oxidative damage by various free radicals may underlie the degeneration of dopaminergic neurons. The concomitant proteasome inhibition leads to a vicious cycle of constant accumulation of oxidized or otherwise damaged proteins thus further exacerbating the pathology [59].

Conclusively, the altered cellular redox status both in aging and neurodegenerative proteinopathies may explain, at least partially, the alterations of the proteasome behavior. Nevertheless, one should keep in mind that this could be only one side of the coin as in both conditions, dysregulation of several signaling pathways and/or proteostatic regulators also contribute to the respective phenotypes.

Antioxidants that affect proteasome function

A number of environmental factors including UV-radiation, air pollution, pesticides, or toxic metals negatively influence the cellular redox system with harmful consequences for the integral function of the organism. Thus, nature has developed defense mechanisms to battle against these harmful triggers. Antioxidants are definitely among the most precious allies against the redox imbalance and can be either naturally occurring, synthetic compounds or mineral elements from endogenous (metabolism) or exogenous (diet) sources. Given that the redox imbalance perturbates the proteome, the study of the relationship between antioxidants and proteostasis mechanisms attracts increased research interest. Here, we review antioxidant compounds that have been shown to affect the proteasome function during the progression of aging and aggregation-related disorders. We mainly refer to phenolic compounds that represent a large group of antioxidants. Phenolic compounds are subcategorized to phenols, phenolic acids, flavonoids, xanthones, stilbenes, and lignans. The rest of the groups include terpenoids, organosulfur compounds, carbohydrates, various extracts, and elements. Finally, we also report some antioxidants that have been shown to influence the proteasome function and thus to exhibit antiaging and antiaggregation properties, but nevertheless, their antioxidant effects have not been examined in the same studies. Table 1.1 summarizes the compounds mentioned in the chapter.

Phenolic compounds

Oleuropein, oleocanthal, and oleacein are phenolic compounds found in *Olea europaea* (olive tree). These compounds are well characterized for their antioxidant properties, including their ability to activate ROS-detoxifying enzymes [80]. Oleuropein treatment of human fibroblasts led to elongated cellular lifespan, lower levels of intracellular ROS, and reduced levels of oxidized proteins. These results have been suggested to be directly linked to the positive effects of oleuropein on proteasome function. Specifically, oleuropein was able to upregulate the expression of proteasome subunits and to enhance the three catalytic activities of the proteasome *in cellulo* in human fibroblast lysates. Interestingly, oleuropein was also able to induce proteasome activities in vitro, following its incubation with highly purified proteasome, indicating that proteasome activation may also be mediated by conformational changes [33]. Oleocanthal treatment of human BJ skin fibroblasts, protected cells against H_2O_2 toxicity, upregulated the gene expression of several proteasome subunits (α7, β4, β5, and Rpn11), and triggered an antioxidant response. Moreover, oleocanthal and oleacein dietary administration was able to promote healthy aging in *Drosophila* flies. Both compounds offered cytoprotection in the fruit fly, leading to decreased ROS levels, enhanced CT-L proteasome activity, and increased expression of β5 and Rpn7 proteasome subunits [60]. Finally, oleocanthal has been also studied for its potent neuroprotective and antiaggregation effects. In differentiated human neuroblastoma cell line, oleocanthal supplementation upon oxidative stress, upregulated the expression of β1and β4 proteasome subunits [61].

Curcumin is a flavonoid polyphenol that belongs to the group of curcuminoids. Curcumin has been extensively examined for its beneficial effects in health, which in many cases are attributed to its antioxidant activities [81]. More

TABLE 1.1 Summary of the reported antioxidant compounds that have been shown to induce proteasome activation and have been tested in cellular or organismal models of aging and/or proteinopathies.

Antioxidant compound	Model[a]	Aging/ cellular senescence[b]	Proteinopathies	Antioxidant response[c]	UPS		References
					Proteasome activity	Subunit regulation[d]	
Oleuropein	Human primary fibroblasts (IMR90, W138)	✓		↓ROS, ↓oxidized proteins	CT-L, C-L, and T-L	α7, β2, and Rpt4 (protein expression)	[33]
Oleocanthal	Human primary fibroblasts (BJ)					α7, β4, β5, and Rpn11 (gene expression)	[60]
	D. melanogaster	✓		↓ROS	CT-L	β5 and Rpn7 (Prosβ5 and Rpn7) (protein expression)	
	Human neuroblastoma cells (SH-SY5Y)					β1 and β4 (protein expression)	[61]
Oleacein	*D. melanogaster*	✓		↓ROS	CT-L	β5 and Rpn7 (Prosβ5 and Rpn7) (protein expression)	[60]
Curcumin	Rat dopaminergic cells (PC12)		PD	↓oxidized proteins	CT-L		[62]
Quercetin	Human primary fibroblasts (HFL1)	✓			CT-L	α7 and β5 (protein expression)	[34]
Isoquercitrin	Human neuroblastoma cells (SH-SY5Y)		AD	↓ROS	CT-L		[63]
Morin	Human neuroblastoma cells (SH-SY5Y)		AD	↓ROS	CT-L		[63]
Polyphenol digested metabolites	Yeast		PD	↑SOD1, ↑SOD2, ↑HAP4 ↓GSSG/GSH	Restored proteasome impairment		[64]
Puerarin	Human neuroblastoma cells (SH-SY5Y)		SCA	↓ROS, ↑SOD2	CT-L and C-L		[65]
Daidzein	Human neuroblastoma cells (SH-SY5Y)		SCA	↓ROS, ↑SOD2	CT-L and C-L		[65]

Continued

TABLE 1.1 Summary of the reported antioxidant compounds that have been shown to induce proteasome activation and have been tested in cellular or organismal models of aging and/or proteinopathies.—cont'd

Antioxidant compound	Model[a]	Aging/cellular senescence[b]	Proteinopathies	Antioxidant response[c]	UPS		References
					Proteasome activity	Subunit regulation[d]	
Tilidroside	*D. melanogaster*	✓		↓ROS, ↑*Trxr1*	CT-L	α7 and β5 (*Prosa7 and Prosb5*) (gene expression)	[66]
	Human primary fibroblasts (IMR90)				CT-L		
Chrysin	*C. elegans*		PD	↓ROS, ↑SOD	Proteasome activation		[67]
18α-GA	Human primary fibroblasts (HFL1)	✓		Nrf2	CT-L and T-L	α4, β1, β2 and β5	[68]
	C. elegans	✓		Nrf2	CT-L and T-L	α1-7, β5 and rpt6 (PAS1-7, PBS-5, RPT6) (protein expression)	[46]
	Human neuroblastoma cells (SH-SY5Y), murine primary neurons and *C. elegans*		AD	Nrf2			
Diosgenin	*N. guentheri*	✓		↓ROS, ↓protein oxidation, ↓lipid peroxidation, ↑CAT, ↑SOD, ↑GPX	CT-L		[69]
Sulforaphane	Murine neuroblastoma cells (Neuro2A)			↑NQO1, ↑γGGLr, ↑CAT	CT-L and C-L	β1, β2 and β5 (*Psmb6, Psmb6, Psmb5*) (gene and protein expression)	[70]
	Cells from HGPS patients	HGPS			CT-L		[71]
α-Lipoic acid	Normal human dermal fibroblasts (NHDF)	✓		↓ROS	CT-L		[72]
***Ginkgo biloba* extract**	Human embryonic kidney cells (HEK293)		HD		CT-L	β1, β2, and β5 (gene expression)	[73]

Myricetin	Fibroblast-like cell lines derived from monkey kidney tissue (Cos-7)		HD and SCA		Proteasome inhibition attenuated the antiaggregation effects		[74]
Guarana hydroalcohilic extract	*C. elegans*		AD	↓ROS, ↑SOD-3	CT-L		[75]
Carqueja hydroalcoholic extract	*C. elegans*		AD	↓ROS	CT-L		[76]
Trehalose	Human skin fibroblasts from HD patients		HD	↓ROS	CT-L		[77]
Fucoidan	*C. elegans*		AD	↓ROS	CT-L	β2 and β5 (*pbs-2* and *pbs-5*) (gene expression)	[78]
DBTO	Human primary fibroblasts (HFL1)				CT-L		[32]
	Human neuroblastoma cells (SH-SY5Y), *C. elegans*						
Zinc	Peripheral blood lymphocytes (elderly)	✓		↓oxidized proteins, ↑MSR	CT-L		[79]

[a]*Cellular or organismal models. If a model for a specific proteinopathy was used, the name of the pathology is presented in the "proteinopathies" column.*
[b]*Studies performed in aged cells or organisms or throughout the cellular or organismal lifespan and have shown extension of lifespan and/or healthspan.*
[c]*Antioxidant response (on top of the UPS induction) following treatment with oxidants or upon aging-associated oxidative stress or proteotoxicity-associated oxidative stress in models of proteinopathies.*
[d]*Name of the proteasome subunit. The approved names of the proteasome genes appear in all cases for consistency reasons while the nomenclature of the gene in the specific organismal model appears in parenthesis.*

specifically, it has been shown to exhibit anti-inflammatory, antioxidant, free radical scavenging, mitochondrial protecting, and iron-chelating effects. Studies have demonstrated the role of curcumin in proteinopathies such as AD and PD, and it has been proposed as a promising nutraceutical agent [82,83]. In the context of the proteasome, a recent study supported that curcumin and its synthetic polyphenolic compound, didemethylcurcumin, can either promote or suppress the proteasome activity in human neuroblastoma cells in a concentration-dependent manner [84]. In dopaminergic PC12 cells treated with the mitochondrial complex I inhibitor rotenone, a cell model of Parkinsonism, it has been observed that most of the identified carbonylated proteins are UPS components. Interestingly, curcumin treatment reduced the levels of oxidized proteins in rotenone-treated PC12 cells and promoted proteasome activation [62].

Quercetin is a flavonoid found in many products of a regular diet. Quercetin offers neuroprotection due to its ability to scavenge ROS, activate the Nrf2 signaling pathway, and improve mitochondria quality control [85]. Treatment of human HFL1 embryonic fibroblasts with quercetin resulted in antiaging and rejuvenating effects, increased resistance to H_2O_2 treatment, enhanced CT-L proteasome activity, and upregulated expression of β5 and α7 proteasome subunits [34]. Proteasome activation can also occur through isoquercitrin, one of the naturally occurring glucosides of quercetin. More specifically, isoquercitrin positively affected the CT-L proteasome activity and inhibited the ROS generation upon H_2O_2 treatment in human neuroblastoma cells expressing a mutated amyloid precursor protein. Similar results were reported for morin, a polyphenol with structural similarities with quercetin [63].

Regarding the group of polyphenols, (poly)phenol-digested metabolites (PDMs) have been reported to exert protective effects on PD through proteostasis regulation. PDMs can be obtained after in vitro gastrointestinal digestion of edible fruits (FPDMs) and leaves (LPDMs). PDMs from *Arbutus unedo* leaves were able to suppress the toxicity induced by alpha-synuclein expression in yeast and human cells, and this positive effect was attributed to the ability of PDMs to restore the proteasome activity. Furthermore, PDMs elevated *SOD1, SOD2,* and *HAP4* (a global regulator of mitochondrial electron transport) mRNA levels and reduced the oxidized to reduced glutathione ratio (GSSG/GSH), suggesting a reduction of oxidative stress. Similar results were obtained in human cells expressing alpha-synuclein where treatment with PDMs also protected the cells from oxidative stress and promoted their mitochondrial function [64].

Puerarin and daidzein belong to a class of compounds known as isoflavones. Both of them are active constituents of *Pueraria lobata* root and possess antioxidant activities [86]. Puerarin has been shown to promote cytoprotection in organismal and cellular PD models. In human neuroblastoma cells treated with MPP^+ (1-methyl-4-phenylpyridinium, a neurotoxin that inhibits mitochondrial complex I), puerarin administration attenuated the deregulation of the proteasome activity, and lowered the amount of alpha-synuclein and ubiquitin-conjugated proteins [87]. In cellular models of SCAs, puerarin and daidzein treatment reduced the ROS burden and enhanced the SOD2 protein levels. In the same cell line these isoflavones enhanced CT-L and C-L proteasome activities and promoted antiaggregation effects [65]. Similar results were obtained upon daidzein treatment of induced pluripotent stem cell lines from SCA3 patients [88].

Tilidroside is a glycosidic flavonoid found in several dietary plants. Tilidroside treatment of *Drosophila* flies reduced somatic tissue ROS burden, upregulated the mRNA levels of *Trxr1* (gene involved in the antioxidant response), and boosted proteasome function through elevation of the CT-L activity and upregulation of α7 and β5 subunits. These effects were accompanied by increased lifespan and healthspan. Enhanced proteasome activation and delayed progression of cellular senescence by tilidroside were also reported in normal human IMR90 fibroblasts [66].

Chrysin that belongs to the flavonoid family can be found in honey, propolis and in some passion flowers species like *Passiflora caerulea* and *Passiflora incarnata*. Chrysin was studied for its neuroprotective properties in *C. elegans* PD models. This study revealed that chrysin ameliorated the proteasome and superoxide dismutase activities and exerted antioxidative effects by reducing the ROS levels in 6-OHDA-(6-hydroxydopamine; a neurotoxin used to destroy dopaminergic and noradrenergic neurons and trigger PD-like symptoms in animal models)-treated nematodes [67].

Terpenoids

18α-Glycyrrhetinic acid (18α-GA) is a triterpenoid that has been shown to delay the replicative senescence of human primary fibroblasts and to extend the lifespan of *C. elegans*. In both cases, 18α-GA acted through the induction of Nrf2 (SKN-1; the ortholog in *C. elegans*) and promoted the proteasome assembly and activity. More specifically, in cells, 18α-GA enhanced the three proteolytic proteasome activities and upregulated the expression of β1, β2, β5, and α4 subunits, while in the nematode, 18α-GA enhanced the CT-L and T-L proteasome activities and elevated the protein expression levels of PBS-5, PAS-1-7, and RPT6 subunits that are orthologs of β5, α1-7 subunits, and Rpt6, respectively. Nrf2 and proteasome activation by 18α-GA resulted in cytoprotection, improvement of the phenotype of *C. elegans* AD models, and reduced Aβ toxicity in human neuroblastoma cells as well as in murine primary neurons [46,68].

Diosgenin is a phytosteroid sapogenin. It has been proposed to possess antioxidant and neuroprotective properties [89]. Recently, the antiaging effects of diosgenin were tested in the male killifish, *Nothobranchius guentheri*. Specifically, diosgenin extended the lifespan of the killifish, reduced ROS, protein oxidation and lipid peroxidation levels, and enhanced the activity of catalase, superoxide dismutase, and glutathione peroxidase antioxidant enzymes. Regarding the UPS, diosgenin enhanced and maintained higher CT-L activity levels over the lifetime of *N. guentheri* [69].

Organosulfurs

Nrf2 transcription factor can also be induced by the natural product sulforaphane, an isothiocyanate originally isolated from broccoli. The strong antioxidant activities of sulforaphane have beneficial impact on various models of aging and neurodegenerative disorders [90]. Many studies have attempted to reveal the mechanisms underlying the neuroprotective effects of sulforaphane [91]. In murine neuroblastoma Neuro2A cells, sulforaphane elevated the expression levels of *Psmb5, Psmb6*, and *Psmb7* subunits and the CT-L and C-L proteasome activities. In addition, sulforaphane enhanced the expression of antioxidant genes like *Nqo1*, regulatory chain of γGCL (*γGCLr*) and catalase, and protected Neuro2A cells against H_2O_2 cytotoxicity, while the cytoprotection was abolished upon proteasome inhibition [70]. Proteasome activation by sulforaphane has been reported to be mediated through the upregulation of Hsp27 [92]. In fibroblasts derived from patients with Hatchinson-Gilford progeria syndrome, a rare childhood premature aging disorder, treatment with sulforaphane enhanced progerin clearance, elevated the CT-L activity and increased the levels of Hsp27 [71]. Finally, sulforaphane-mediated Nrf2 activation was able to control self-renewal and pluripotency of human embryonic stem cells through the regulation of proteasome expression and activity [93].

a-Lipoic acid (ALA) is an organosulfur compound derived from caprylic acid, a naturally occurring medium-chain fatty acid. It is an Nrf2 inducer with antioxidant effects in various cell lines and organisms. ALA exerts its antioxidant activity through direct radical scavenging and interaction with other antioxidants and has been shown to positively affect lifespan in *C. elegans* and *Drosophila* [94,95]. Many studies report the beneficial effects of ALA on the progression of aging and neurodegeneration [96,97]. In normal human dermal fibroblasts, ALA decreased the percentage of ROS positive cells and carbonylated proteins following H_2O_2 treatment and promoted the CT-L proteasome activity leading to enhanced cell proliferation [72].

Crude extracts

The tree *Ginkgo biloba* is one of the oldest living plant species. The extract of *Ginkgo biloba* is commonly used in experimental and clinical studies related to neurodegenerative disorders. The neuroprotective effects of *Ginkgo biloba* extract are attributed to the strong antioxidant properties and its ability to trigger the Nrf2/ARE pathway [98,99]. *Ginkgo biloba* extract treatment of HEK293 cells expressing mHtt decreased the levels of polyQ aggregates, promoted CT-L activity, and elevated the transcript levels of β1, β2, and β5 subunits [73]. The *Ginkgo biloba* extract is composed of many phenolic acids and flavonoid compounds, including myricetin. Myricetin has been shown to exert neuroprotective and antioxidant properties [100]. The neuroprotective role of myricetin is mainly due to its antioxidant activities. Nevertheless, it was recently shown that the neuroprotective effects are also attributed to the capacity of myricetin to enhance protein quality control mechanisms. Specifically, treatment of Cos-7 cells with myricetin induced the levels of Hsp70 chaperone and E3 ubiquitin ligase E6-AP and decreased the aggregation of neurodegeneration-related proteins. The reduction in the protein aggregates was suggested to be proteasome-dependent since addition of MG132 proteasome inhibitor attenuated the observed antiaggregation effects [74].

Guarana (*Paullina cupana*) is widely used in the Brazilian beverage industry, and it is known for the stimulatory effects on the central nervous system. Compounds such as polyphenols, caffeine, and other methylxanthines are responsible for the antioxidant properties of guarana [101]. In *C. elegans* models of AD and PD, guarana hydroalcoholic extract (GHE) treatment alleviated the toxic phenotypes associated with protein misfolding and accumulation. In the case of the AD model, silencing of the *skn-1* (Nrf2) gene abolished the positive effects of GHE. In the same study, it was proposed that these positive effects may be attributed to both antioxidant effects and modulation of proteostasis. Specifically, GHE reduced ROS levels in wild type and AD *C. elegans* model, promoted the expression of the superoxide dismutase SOD-3 and the heat shock protein HSP-16.2, and elevated the CT-L proteasome activity [75].

Carqueja (*Baccharis trimera*) is a plant found in South America. Carqueja hydroalcoholic extract (CHE) has been shown to increase oxidative stress resistance in wild type *C. elegans* by reducing ROS levels. In the same study, CHE exhibited protective effects in an AD nematode model. More specifically, CHE enhanced the CT-L proteasome activity and upregulated *hsp-4* and *hsp-16.2* (heat shock genes that respond to protein misfolding and heat shock, respectively) gene expression [76].

Carbohydrates and zinc

Trehalose is a natural disaccharide able to affect the Nrf2 pathway [102]. In HD human skin fibroblasts, trehalose attenuated the ROS formation and huntingtin accumulation that resulted following proteasome inhibition. It was shown that trehalose was able to increase the CT-L activity even in the presence of the proteasome inhibitor epoxomicin [77]. Similar results were obtained by trehalose treatment of glial cultures from the striatum of HD mouse models [103].

Compounds derived from marine plants have been also proposed to be potent UPS modulators [104]. Fucoidan is a polysaccharide found in various species of brown algae. In a *C. elegans* AD model, fucoidan alleviated the paralysis phenotype mediated by Aβ and decreased Aβ deposition. Furthermore, fucoidan enhanced the CT-L activity, elevated the *pbs-2* and *pbs-5* gene expression, and exerted its antioxidant effects by reducing ROS and increasing hsp-16.2 expression in transgenic animals [78]. More recently, we have identified a compound derived from the brown alga *Dictyota mediterranea*, namely DBTO, as a structural proteasome activator. Continuous treatment of HFL1 human primary fibroblasts with DBTO throughout their cellular lifespan was shown to result in ameliorated healthspan. Ameliorated health status was also shown in wild type *C. elegans* under continuous exposure to DBTO. More importantly, treatment of various AD nematode models with DBTO resulted in enhanced protection against Aβ-induced proteotoxicity. This protective effect was also verified in human cells of neuronal origin challenged with exogenously added Aβ peptide. Although we did not observe differences in ROS levels, Nrf2 induction or SOD activity, one cannot rule out the possibility of induction of other antioxidant mechanisms [32].

Zinc is a chemical element implicated in many cellular pathways, and its deficiency has been associated with aging [105], while serum zinc levels have been shown to decrease with age [106]. In a population study in the elderly, it was revealed that zinc supplementation enhanced the CT-L and methionine sulfoxide reductase activities and eliminated the oxidized protein accumulation in peripheral blood lymphocytes [79].

Concluding remarks

As outlined in this chapter, in aging and neurodegenerative proteinopathies, the accompanying redox imbalance may inhibit proteasome function. Due to this inhibition, damaged proteins may escape degradation and accumulate thus further contributing to the oxidative damage (Fig. 1.3A). Some antioxidants may directly or indirectly

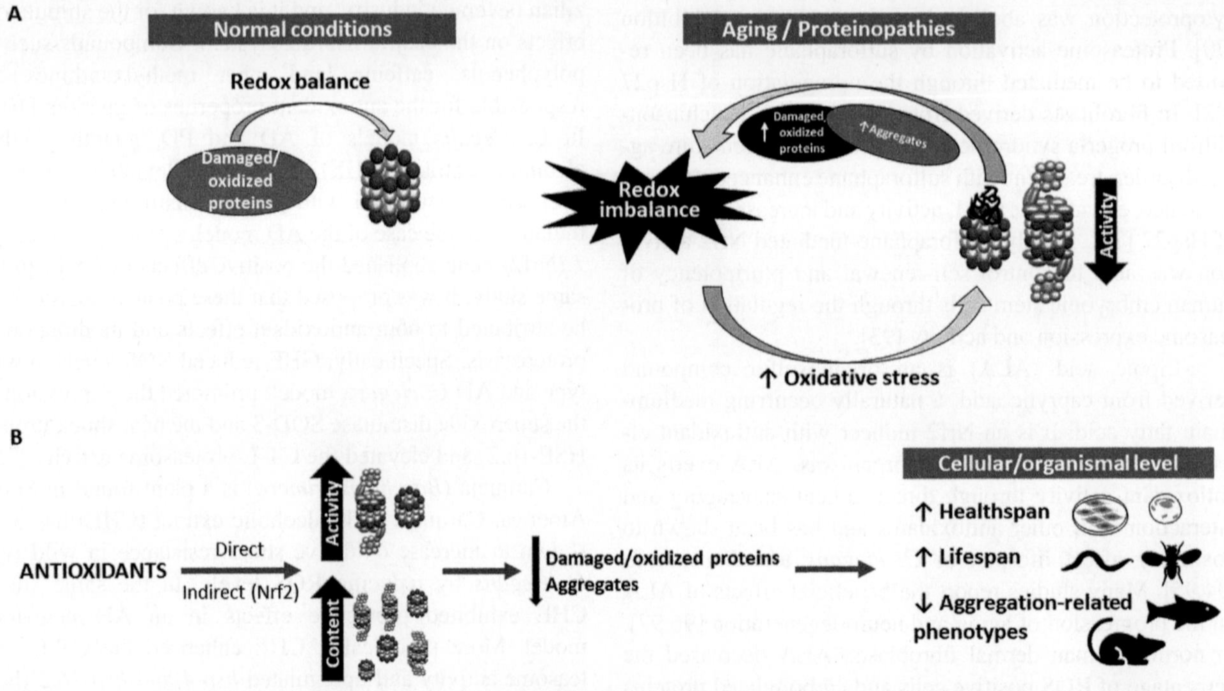

FIGURE 1.3 The proteasome deregulation upon oxidative stress in aging and proteinopathies and the protective effects of antioxidants. (A) Under normal conditions, oxidized proteins are removed in a 20S proteasome-dependent manner. Upon the progression of aging or proteinopathies, redox imbalance and decreased proteasome activity occur that establish a vicious cycle; the redox imbalance leads to enhanced ROS levels that negatively affect the activity and function of the proteasome. Moreover, enhanced levels of oxidized protein and aggregates further inhibit the 20S proteasome through allosteric impairment of the substrate gate. In turn, impairment of the 20S and 30S/26S proteasomes leads to elevated levels of oxidized proteins and aggregates, which negatively affect the redox balance. (B) Antioxidants can promote proteasome activation (in terms of activity and/or expression) in a direct or indirect manner (through the induction of the Nrf2 pathway) favoring the clearance of oxidized and aggregated proteins. The alliance between antioxidants and the proteasome has been shown to enhance the lifespan, promote healthspan and protect against proteotoxicity in several cellular and organismal models.

improve proteasomal function under these conditions leading to healthspan and lifespan extension as well as ameliorated phenotypes in models of various proteinopathies (Fig. 1.3B).

Numerous compounds have been tested for their antioxidant properties and their concomitant ability to promote proteasome activation in various contexts of both aging and proteinopathies. Despite this substantial effort, there is still an enormous need to decelerate the rate of aging that is an important risk factor for age-associated diseases and to develop disease-modifying therapies for proteinopathies.

Understanding the intricacies of proteostatic mechanisms and the effects of the cellular redox status on them is pivotal for the efficient design of new therapeutic compounds/strategies. Moreover, designing appropriate preclinical studies to identify bioactive compounds is highly important, although often neglected. For example, proteasome activators are frequently identified based on their capacity to enhance the proteasome-mediated degradation of small fluorogenic peptides in vitro. However, it has been suggested that this readout may lead to the discovery of activators that do not open the 20S gate widely enough for larger protein substrates like the ones associated with proteinopathies [107]. Similarly, the current general notion regarding antioxidants and their benefits is not what it used to be in the past. It is becoming clearer that the oxidative stress has specific signaling roles in the cell, and it is not only associated with adverse effects. Although increased oxidative stress may be part of several pathologies, the endogenous antioxidant defenses of the human body are carefully regulated. Consequently, large quantities of exogenous antioxidants may be ineffective or even harmful [108].

In conclusion, the reinforcement of the proteasome through the regulation of the cellular redox status is achievable. Although it presents particular interest as it opens a new avenue for proteasome manipulation through antioxidants that can be found in our diet, there is still much that needs to be understood before we can harness the full potential of this knowledge.

Acknowledgments

Research from N.C. lab is currently co-financed by the European Union and Greek national funds through the Operational Program Competitiveness, Entrepreneurship and Innovation, under the call "Research – Create – Innovate" (project code: T1EDK-00353 and T1EDK-01610), as well as under the call Special actions "Aquaculture – Industrial Materials – Open Innovation in Culture" (project code: T6UBΠ-00474, project acronym: ALGOSMETIC). EP received an HFRI PhD Fellowship grant (Fellowship Number: 1540) by the Hellenic Foundation for Research and Innovation (HFRI).

References

[1] López-Otín C, Blasco MA, Partridge L, Serrano M, Kroemer G. The hallmarks of aging. Cell 2013.

[2] WHO. 10 facts on ageing and health. 2017.

[3] Campisi J, Kapahi P, Lithgow GJ, Melov S, Newman JC, Verdin E. From discoveries in ageing research to therapeutics for healthy ageing. Nature July 2019;571(7764):183–92.

[4] Kirkland JL, Tchkonia T, Zhu Y, Niedernhofer LJ, Robbins PD. The clinical potential of senolytic drugs. J Am Geriatr Soc 2017;65(10):2297–301.

[5] Chiti F, Dobson CM. Protein misfolding, amyloid formation, and human disease: a summary of progress over the last decade. Annu Rev Biochem June 2017;86:27–68.

[6] Soria Lopez JA, González HM, Léger GC. Alzheimer's disease. Handb Clin Neurol 2019;167:231–55.

[7] WHO. Dementia. 2021.

[8] WHO. The top 10 causes of death. 2020.

[9] Lesage S, Brice A. Parkinson's disease: from monogenic forms to genetic susceptibility factors. Hum Mol Genet April 2009;18(R1):R48–59.

[10] Costa HN, Esteves AR, Empadinhas N, Cardoso SM. Parkinson's disease: a multisystem disorder. Neurosci Bull August 2022.

[11] WHO. Parkinson disease. 2022.

[12] Fourier A, Quadrio I. Proteinopathies associated to repeat expansion disorders. J Neural Transm February 2022;129(2):173–85.

[13] Bunting EL, Hamilton J, Tabrizi SJ. Polyglutamine diseases. Curr Opin Neurobiol February 2022;72:39–47.

[14] Dhanjal DS, Bhardwaj S, Sharma R, Bhardwaj K, Kumar D, Chopra C, et al. Plant fortification of the diet for anti-ageing effects: a review. Nutrients September 2020;12(10).

[15] Aborode AT, Pustake M, Awuah WA, Alwerdani M, Shah P, Yarlagadda R, et al. Targeting oxidative stress mechanisms to treat Alzheimer's and Parkinson's disease: a critical review. Oxid Med Cell Longev 2022;2022:7934442.

[16] Gkekas I, Gioran A, Boziki MK, Grigoriadis N, Chondrogianni N, Petrakis S. Oxidative stress and neurodegeneration: interconnected processes in PolyQ diseases. Antioxidants (Basel, Switzerland) September 2021;10(9).

[17] Ciechanover A, Stanhill A. The complexity of recognition of ubiquitinated substrates by the 26S proteasome. Biochim Biophys Acta Mol Cell Res 2014.

[18] Davies KJA. Degradation of oxidized proteins by the 20S proteasome. In: Biochimie; 2001.

[19] Enenkel C. Proteasome dynamics. Biochim Biophys Acta January 2014;1843(1):39–46.

[20] Raynes R, Pomatto LCD, Davies KJA. Degradation of oxidized proteins by the proteasome: distinguishing between the 20S, 26S, and immunoproteasome proteolytic pathways. Mol Aspects Med August 2016;50:41–55.

[21] Tomko RJJ, Hochstrasser M. Order of the proteasomal ATPases and eukaryotic proteasome assembly. Cell Biochem Biophys June 2011;60(1–2):13–20.

[22] Glickman MH, Rubin DM, Fu H, Larsen CN, Coux O, Wefes I, et al. Functional analysis of the proteasome regulatory particle. Mol Biol Rep April 1999;26(1–2):21–8.

[23] Livneh I, Kravtsova-Ivantsiv Y, Braten O, Kwon YT, Ciechanover A. Monoubiquitination joins polyubiquitination as an esteemed proteasomal targeting signal. Bioessays June 2017;39(6).

[24] Livneh I, Cohen-Kaplan V, Cohen-Rosenzweig C, Avni N, Ciechanover A. The life cycle of the 26S proteasome: from birth, through regulation and function, and onto its death. Cell Res August 2016;26(8):869–85.

[25] Stolzing A, Grune T. The proteasome and its function in the ageing process. Clin Exp Dermatol October 2001;26(7):566–72.

[26] Chondrogianni N, Sakellari M, Lefaki M, Papaevgeniou N, Gonos ES. Proteasome activation delays aging in vitro and in vivo. Free Radic Biol Med 2014.

[27] Hwang JS, Hwang JS, Chang I, Kim S. Age-associated decrease in proteasome content and activities in human dermal fibroblasts: restoration of normal level of proteasome subunits reduces aging markers in fibroblasts from elderly persons. J Gerontol A Biol Sci Med Sci May 2007;62(5):490–9.

[28] Chondrogianni N, Georgila K, Kourtis N, Tavernarakis N, Gonos ES. 20S proteasome activation promotes life span extension and resistance to proteotoxicity in *Caenorhabditis elegans*. FASEB J 2015.

[29] Vilchez D, Morantte I, Liu Z, Douglas PM, Merkwirth C, Rodrigues APC, et al. RPN-6 determines *C. elegans* longevity under proteotoxic stress conditions. Nature 2012.

[30] Nguyen NN, Rana A, Goldman C, Moore R, Tai J, Hong Y, et al. Proteasome β5 subunit overexpression improves proteostasis during aging and extends lifespan in *Drosophila melanogaster*. Sci Rep 2019.

[31] George DE, Tepe JJ. Advances in proteasome enhancement by small molecules. Biomolecules November 2021;11(12).

[32] Vasilopoulou MA, Gioran A, Theodoropoulou M, Koutsaviti A, Roussis V, Ioannou E, et al. Healthspan improvement and anti-aggregation effects induced by a marine-derived structural proteasome activator. Redox Biol October 2022;56:102462.

[33] Katsiki M, Chondrogianni N, Chinou I, Rivett AJ, Gonos ES. The olive constituent oleuropein exhibits proteasome stimulatory properties in vitro and confers life span extension of human embryonic fibroblasts. Rejuvenation Res 2007.

[34] Chondrogianni N, Kapeta S, Chinou I, Vassilatou K, Papassideri I, Gonos ES. Anti-ageing and rejuvenating effects of quercetin. Exp Gerontol 2010.

[35] Ciechanover A, Brundin P. The ubiquitin proteasome system in neurodegenerative diseases: sometimes the chicken, sometimes the egg. Neuron October 2003;40(2):427–46.

[36] Keller JN, Hanni KB, Markesbery WR. Impaired proteasome function in Alzheimer's disease. J Neurochem July 2000;75(1):436–9.

[37] Keck S, Nitsch R, Grune T, Ullrich O. Proteasome inhibition by paired helical filament-tau in brains of patients with Alzheimer's disease. J Neurochem 2003.

[38] McNaught KS, Jenner P. Proteasomal function is impaired in substantia nigra in Parkinson's disease. Neurosci Lett January 2001;297(3):191–4.

[39] McNaught KSP, Belizaire R, Jenner P, Olanow CW, Isacson O. Selective loss of 20S proteasome alpha-subunits in the substantia nigra pars compacta in Parkinson's disease. Neurosci Lett July 2002;326(3):155–8.

[40] Opattova A, Cente M, Novak M, Filipcik P. The ubiquitin proteasome system as a potential therapeutic target for treatment of neurodegenerative diseases. Gen Physiol Biophys October 2015;34(4):337–52.

[41] Fernández-Cruz I, Reynaud E. Proteasome subunits involved in neurodegenerative diseases. Arch Med Res January 2021;52(1):1–14.

[42] Boland B, Yu WH, Corti O, Mollereau B, Henriques A, Bezard E, et al. Promoting the clearance of neurotoxic proteins in neurodegenerative disorders of ageing. Nat Rev Drug Discov September 2018;17(9):660–88.

[43] Jones CL, Tepe JJ. Proteasome activation to combat proteotoxicity. Molecules August 2019;24(15).

[44] Chocron SE, Munkácsy E, Harper SK, Karpowicz P, Jiang N, Van Skike C, et al. Genetic and pharmacologic proteasome augmentation ameliorates Alzheimer's-like pathology in mouse and fly APP overexpression models. Sci Adv June 2022;8(23):eabk2252.

[45] Panagiotidou E, Chondrogianni N. We are what we eat: ubiquitin-proteasome system (UPS) modulation through dietary products. Adv Exp Med Biol 2020.

[46] Papaevgeniou N, Sakellari M, Jha S, Tavernarakis N, Holmberg CI, Gonos ES, et al. 18α-Glycyrrhetinic acid proteasome activator decelerates aging and Alzheimer's disease progression in *Caenorhabditis elegans* and neuronal cultures. Antioxid Redox Signal 2016.

[47] Engelender S, Stefanis L, Oddo S, Bellucci A. Can we treat neurodegenerative proteinopathies by enhancing protein degradation? Mov Disord July 2022;37(7):1346–59.

[48] Sakamoto KM, Kim KB, Kumagai A, Mercurio F, Crews CM, Deshaies RJ. Protacs: chimeric molecules that target proteins to the Skp1-Cullin-F box complex for ubiquitination and degradation. Proc Natl Acad Sci USA July 2001;98(15):8554–9.

[49] Lefaki M, Papaevgeniou N, Chondrogianni N. Redox regulation of proteasome function. Redox Biol 2017;13:452–8. https://doi.org/10.1016/j.redox.2017.07.005.

[50] Itoh K, Wakabayashi N, Katoh Y, Ishii T, Igarashi K, Engel JD, et al. Keap1 represses nuclear activation of antioxidant responsive elements by Nrf2 through binding to the amino-terminal Neh2 domain. Genes Dev January 1999;13(1):76–86.

[51] Livnat-Levanon N, Kevei É, Kleifeld O, Krutauz D, Segref A, Rinaldi T, et al. Reversible 26S proteasome disassembly upon mitochondrial stress. Cell Rep June 2014;7(5):1371–80.

[52] Silva GM, Netto LES, Simões V, Santos LFA, Gozzo FC, Demasi MAA, et al. Redox control of 20S proteasome gating. Antioxid Redox Signal June 2012;16(11):1183–94.

[53] Höhn TJA, Grune T. The proteasome and the degradation of oxidized proteins: part III-redox regulation of the proteasomal system. Redox Biol 2014;2:388–94.

[54] Petersen A, Carlsson T, Karlsson J-O, Zetterberg M. The proteasome and intracellular redox status: implications for apoptotic regulation in lens epithelial cells. Curr Eye Res October 2007;32(10):871–82.

[55] Ishii T, Sakurai T, Usami H, Uchida K. Oxidative modification of proteasome: identification of an oxidation-sensitive subunit in 26 S proteasome. Biochemistry October 2005;44(42):13893–901.

[56] Singh P, Barman B, Thakur MK. Oxidative stress-mediated memory impairment during aging and its therapeutic intervention by

natural bioactive compounds. Front Aging Neurosci 2022;14:944697.

[57] Smith MA, Rottkamp CA, Nunomura A, Raina AK, Perry G. Oxidative stress in Alzheimer's disease. Biochim Biophys Acta July 2000;1502(1):139–44.

[58] Cecarini V, Ding Q, Keller JN. Oxidative inactivation of the proteasome in Alzheimer's disease. Free Radic Res June 2007;41(6):673–80.

[59] Dorszewska J, Kowalska M, Prendecki M, Piekut T, Kozłowska J, Kozubski W. Oxidative stress factors in Parkinson's disease. Neural Regen Res July 2021;16(7):1383–91.

[60] Nikou T, Liaki V, Stathopoulos P, Sklirou AD, Tsakiri EN, Jakschitz T, et al. Comparison survey of EVOO polyphenols and exploration of healthy aging-promoting properties of oleocanthal and oleacein. Food Chem Toxicol March 2019;125:403–12.

[61] Giusti L, Angeloni C, Barbalace MC, Lacerenza S, Ciregia F, Ronci M, et al. A proteomic approach to uncover neuroprotective mechanisms of oleocanthal against oxidative stress. Int J Mol Sci 2018.

[62] Buratta S, Chiaradia E, Tognoloni A, Gambelunghe A, Meschini C, Palmieri L, et al. Effect of curcumin on protein damage induced by rotenone in dopaminergic PC12 cells. Int J Mol Sci April 2020;21(8).

[63] Carmona V, Martín-Aragón S, Goldberg J, Schubert D, Bermejo-Bescós P. Several targets involved in Alzheimer's disease amyloidogenesis are affected by morin and isoquercitrin. Nutr Neurosci August 2020;23(8):575–90.

[64] Macedo D, Jardim C, Figueira I, Almeida AF, McDougall GJ, Stewart D, et al. (Poly)phenol-digested metabolites modulate alpha-synuclein toxicity by regulating proteostasis. Sci Rep 2018.

[65] Chen I-C, Chang C-N, Chen W-L, Lin T-H, Chao C-Y, Lin C-H, et al. Targeting ubiquitin proteasome pathway with traditional Chinese medicine for treatment of spinocerebellar ataxia type 3. Am J Chin Med 2019;47(1):63–95.

[66] Chatzigeorgiou S, Thai QD, Tchoumtchoua J, Tallas K, Tsakiri EN, Papassideri I, et al. Isolation of natural products with anti-ageing activity from the fruits of *Platanus orientalis*. Phytomedicine 2017.

[67] Muhammad F, Liu Y, Wang N, Zhao L, Zhou Y, Yang H, et al. Anti-α-synuclein toxicity and anti-neurodegenerative role of chrysin in transgenic *Caenorhabditis elegans* models of Parkinson's disease. ACS Chem Neurosci February 2022;13(4):442–53.

[68] Kapeta S, Chondrogianni N, Gonos ES. Nuclear erythroid factor 2-mediated proteasome activation delays senescence in human fibroblasts. J Biol Chem 2010.

[69] Som S, Antony J, Dhanabal SP, Ponnusankar S. Neuroprotective role of Diosgenin, a NGF stimulator, against Aβ (1-42) induced neurotoxicity in animal model of Alzheimer's disease. Metab Brain Dis February 2022;37(2):359–72.

[70] Kwak MK, Cho JM, Huang B, Shin S, Kensler TW. Role of increased expression of the proteasome in the protective effects of sulforaphane against hydrogen peroxide-mediated cytotoxicity in murine neuroblastoma cells. Free Radic Biol Med 2007.

[71] Gabriel D, Roedl D, Gordon LB, Djabali K. Sulforaphane enhances progerin clearance in Hutchinson-Gilford progeria fibroblasts. Aging Cell 2015.

[72] Sikdar S, Papadopoulou M, Dubois J. Effect of-lipoic acid on proteasomal induction: protection against oxidative damage in human skin fibroblasts cell line NHDF. Pharmacol Pharm 2017;08(09):292–305.

[73] Stark M, Behl C. The *Ginkgo biloba* extract EGb 761 modulates proteasome activity and polyglutamine protein aggregation. Evid Based Complement Altern Med 2014.

[74] Joshi V, Mishra R, Upadhyay A, Amanullah A, Poluri KM, Singh S, et al. Polyphenolic flavonoid (Myricetin) upregulated proteasomal degradation mechanisms: eliminates neurodegenerative proteins aggregation. J Cell Physiol November 2019;234(11):20900–14.

[75] Boasquívis PF, Silva GMM, Paiva FA, Cavalcanti RM, Nunez CV, De Paula Oliveira R. Guarana (*Paullinia cupana*) extract protects *Caenorhabditis elegans* models for Alzheimer disease and Huntington disease through activation of antioxidant and protein degradation pathways. Oxid Med Cell Longev 2018.

[76] Paiva FA, Bonomo L de F, Boasquivis PF, de Paula ITBR, Guerra JF da C, Leal WM, et al. Carqueja (*Baccharis trimera*) protects against oxidative stress and β-amyloid-induced toxicity in *Caenorhabditis elegans*. Oxid Med Cell Longev 2015;2015:740162.

[77] Fernandez-Estevez MA, Casarejos MJ, Sendon JL, Caldentey JG, Ruiz C, Gomez A, et al. Trehalose reverses cell malfunction in fibroblasts from normal and Huntington's disease patients caused by proteosome inhibition. PLoS One 2014.

[78] Wang X, Yi K, Zhao Y. Fucoidan inhibits amyloid-β-induced toxicity in transgenic *Caenorhabditis elegans* by reducing the accumulation of amyloid-β and decreasing the production of reactive oxygen species. Food Funct January 2018;9(1):552–60.

[79] Cabreiro F, Perichon M, Jatje J, Malavolta M, Mocchegiani E, Friguet B, et al. Zinc supplementation in the elderly subjects: effect on oxidized protein degradation and repair systems in peripheral blood lymphocytes. Exp Gerontol 2008.

[80] Castejón ML, Montoya T, Alarcón-de-la-Lastra C, Sánchez-Hidalgo M. Potential protective role exerted by secoiridoids from *Olea europaea* L. In cancer, cardiovascular, neurodegenerative, aging-related, and immunoinflammatory diseases. Antioxidants February 2020;9(2).

[81] Pulido-Moran M, Moreno-Fernandez J, Ramirez-Tortosa C, Ramirez-Tortosa M. Curcumin and health. Molecules February 2016;21(3):264.

[82] Chen M, Du Z-Y, Zheng X, Li D-L, Zhou R-P, Zhang K. Use of curcumin in diagnosis, prevention, and treatment of Alzheimer's disease. Neural Regen Res April 2018;13(4):742–52.

[83] Nebrisi EE. Neuroprotective activities of curcumin in Parkinson's disease: a review of the literature. Int J Mol Sci October 2021;22(20).

[84] Khan TK, You Y, Nelson TJ, Kundu S, Pramanik SK, Das J. Modulation of proteasome activity by curcumin and didemethylcurcumin. J Biomol Struct Dyn April 2021:1–8.

[85] Islam MS, Quispe C, Hossain R, Islam MT, Al-Harrasi A, Al-Rawahi A, et al. Neuropharmacological effects of quercetin: a literature-based review. Front Pharmacol 2021;12:665031.

[86] Jin SE, Son YK, Min B-S, Jung HA, Choi JS. Anti-inflammatory and antioxidant activities of constituents isolated from Pueraria lobata roots. Arch Pharm Res (Seoul) May 2012;35(5):823–37.

[87] Cheng Y-F, Zhu G-Q, Wang M, Cheng H, Zhou A, Wang N, et al. Involvement of ubiquitin proteasome system in protective

mechanisms of Puerarin to MPP(+)-elicited apoptosis. Neurosci Res January 2009;63(1):52–8.
[88] Chen I-C, Chang K-H, Chen Y-J, Chen Y-C, Lee-Chen G-J, Chen C-M. Pueraria lobata and daidzein reduce cytotoxicity by enhancing ubiquitin-proteasome system function in SCA3-iPSC-derived neurons. Oxid Med Cell Longev 2019;2019:8130481.
[89] Gupta DD, Mishra S, Verma SS, Shekher A, Rai V, Awasthee N, et al. Evaluation of antioxidant, anti-inflammatory and anticancer activities of diosgenin enriched *Paris polyphylla* rhizome extract of Indian Himalayan landraces. J Ethnopharmacol April 2021;270:113842.
[90] Santín-Márquez R, Alarcón-Aguilar A, López-Diazguerrero NE, Chondrogianni N, Königsberg M. Sulforaphane—role in aging and neurodegeneration. GeroScience October 2019;41(5):655–70.
[91] Klomparens EA, Ding Y. The neuroprotective mechanisms and effects of sulforaphane. Brain Circ 2019;5(2):74–83.
[92] Gan N, Wu YC, Brunet M, Garrido C, Chung FL, Dai C, et al. Sulforaphane activates heat shock response and enhances proteasome activity through up-regulation of Hsp27. J Biol Chem 2010.
[93] Jang J, Wang Y, Kim HS, Lalli MA, Kosik KS. Nrf2, a regulator of the proteasome, controls self-renewal and pluripotency in human embryonic stem cells. Stem Cell 2014.
[94] Brown MK, Evans JL, Luo Y. Beneficial effects of natural antioxidants EGCG and alpha-lipoic acid on life span and age-dependent behavioral declines in *Caenorhabditis elegans*. Pharmacol Biochem Behav November 2006;85(3):620–8.
[95] Du G, Qiao Y, Zhuo Z, Zhou J, Li X, Liu Z, et al. Lipoic acid rejuvenates aged intestinal stem cells by preventing age-associated endosome reduction. EMBO Rep August 2020;21(8):e49583.
[96] Molz P, Schröder N. Potential therapeutic effects of lipoic acid on memory deficits related to aging and neurodegeneration. Front Pharmacol 2017;8:849.
[97] Kaur D, Behl T, Sehgal A, Singh S, Sharma N, Chigurupati S, et al. Decrypting the potential role of α-lipoic acid in Alzheimer's disease. Life Sci November 2021;284:119899.
[98] Liu H, Ye M, Guo H. An updated review of randomized clinical trials testing the improvement of cognitive function of *Ginkgo biloba* extract in healthy people and Alzheimer's patients. Front Pharmacol 2019;10:1688.
[99] Singh SK, Srivastav S, Castellani RJ, Plascencia-Villa G, Perry G. Neuroprotective and antioxidant effect of *Ginkgo biloba* extract against AD and other neurological disorders. Neurotherapeutics July 2019;16(3):666–74.
[100] Li J, Xiang H, Huang C, Lu J. Pharmacological actions of myricetin in the nervous system: a comprehensive review of preclinical studies in animals and cell models. Front Pharmacol 2021;12:797298.
[101] Torres EAFS, Pinaffi-Langley ACDC, Figueira MDS, Cordeiro KS, Negrão LD, Soares MJ, et al. Effects of the consumption of guarana on human health: a narrative review. Compr Rev Food Sci Food Saf January 2022;21(1):272–95.
[102] Mizunoe Y, Kobayashi M, Sudo Y, Watanabe S, Yasukawa H, Natori D, et al. Trehalose protects against oxidative stress by regulating the Keap1-Nrf2 and autophagy pathways. Redox Biol May 2018;15:115–24.
[103] Perucho J, Gómez A, Muñoz MP, de Yébenes JG, Mena MÁ, Casarejos MJ. Trehalose rescues glial cell dysfunction in striatal cultures from HD R6/1 mice at early postnatal development. Mol Cell Neurosci July 2016;74:128–45.
[104] Vasilopoulou MA, Ioannou E, Roussis V, Chondrogianni N. Modulation of the ubiquitin-proteasome system by marine natural products. Redox Biol May 2021;41:101897.
[105] Cabrera ÁJR. Zinc, aging, and immunosenescence: an overview. Pathobiol Aging Age-Relat Dis 2015.
[106] Wong CP, Magnusson KR, Sharpton TJ, Ho E. Effects of zinc status on age-related T cell dysfunction and chronic inflammation. Biometals April 2021;34(2):291–301.
[107] Trader DJ, Simanski S, Dickson P, Kodadek T. Establishment of a suite of assays that support the discovery of proteasome stimulators. Biochim Biophys Acta Gen Subj April 2017;1861(4):892–9.
[108] Halliwell B. The antioxidant paradox: less paradoxical now? Br J Clin Pharmacol March 2013;75(3):637–44.

Chapter 2

Cysteine thiol modifications—Oxidative (eu)stress perspective

Aleksandra Kopacz, Alicja Jozkowicz and Anna Grochot-Przeczek
Department of Medical Biotechnology, Faculty of Biochemistry, Biophysics and Biotechnology, Jagiellonian University, Krakow, Poland

Introduction

The unique chemical features of cysteines render them very susceptible to modification by oxidants [1]. The disulfide bond formation between thiols is a rapid, reversible reaction that predisposes them to act as redox switches [2,3]. Moreover, plenty of cysteine modifications exist and largely affect signal transduction, regulation of cellular processes, and disease progression [4]. They are also crucial for proper development [5]. The field of cysteine modification develops fast, with new posttranslational modifications (PTMs) being outlined, such as S-cyanylation [6]. However, their interplay with oxidative stress has not been elucidated yet. Here, we aim to reconcile the impact of thiol modification on the overall cellular redox status, indicate plausible determinants of the interplay, and order the available data in the context of oxidative injury. In this review, we will mainly focus on mammals; however, we will also try to outline the emerging concepts studied in bacteria, yeast, and plants.

Cysteines: The archetypal regulatory amino acid

Cysteine appearance correlates with the degree of organism complexity, reaching the maximal 2.26% in mammals. Still, it is significantly less than what could be statistically inferred [7]. The sulfur biochemistry of the thiol group offers cysteines distinctive and distinct features that allow them to perform various cell functions. A broad context of cysteine redox regulation and the propensity of cysteine-based redox regulators was recently shown using genetically engineered oximouse [8]. Cysteines are highly conserved in proteins, functioning as structural, catalytic, metal-binding, and redox-regulating components [9]. The highly polarizable sulfur atom can adopt 9 oxidation states (ranging from -2 to $+6$ [10]) due to the existence of vacant d-orbitals primed for bonding [11]. The most common are oxidation states are $-$II, $-$I, 0, +II and +IV (Fig. 2.1). The large atomic radius of the sulfur atom and the low dissociation energy of the thiol S—H bond renders cysteine thiol redox active. It can act as a strong nucleophile or reducing agent, whereas its equivalent disulfide can act as an electrophile or oxidizing agent [12]. Cysteine nucleophilicity is a property that may have been selected during evolution to offer points of protein control by oxidative stress pathways [13].

Most cytoplasmic protein thiols have pKa values above 8.0 and thus are protonated at physiological pH, rendering them nonreactive. Thiol groups of redox-sensitive cysteines exhibit significantly lower pKa values (ex. 3.5 in thiol transferase). These thiols are deprotonated, forming extremely reactive thiolate anions (RS-) at physiological pH. The lowering of pKa is triggered by the proximity of positively charged amino acids. This promotes the charge—charge interactions between thiolate anion and positively charged or aromatic side chains [2]. The pKa and ionization state of the thiol dictate the nucleophilicity of a cysteine residue [14], whereas the redox potential of a disulfide pair governs the oxidative capacity. Similarly, the redox potentials of cysteine residues can range from 470 to 90 mV. The proclivity for cysteine ionization and/or oxidation in the immediate environment is sensitive to changes in pH and reduction potential [15]. The median percentage of cysteine residue oxidation in the proteome is between 5% and 12%, which can be increased to >40% by adding oxidants [16]. Furthermore, the distribution of redox-active cysteines within a cell is not uniform, providing essential regulatory mechanisms (exhaustively reviewed in Ref. [15]). The key to this is the collaboration of the nonprotein thiols—glutathione (GSH) and coenzyme A (CoA) [17].

Modulation of Oxidative Stress. https://doi.org/10.1016/B978-0-443-19247-0.00005-9

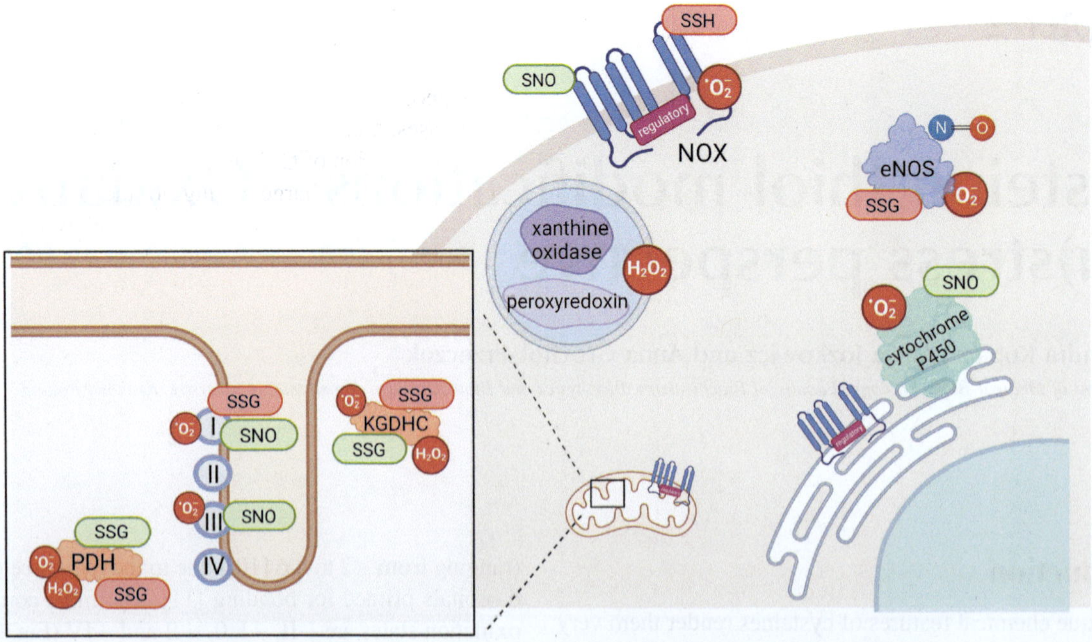

FIGURE 2.1 Modifications of cysteine—most common oxidation states of the sulfur atom.

The interplay between cysteine PTMs and oxidative stress—Protective or detrimental?

Upon each discovery, the significance of cysteine PTMs became a subject of discussion. It was proposed that S-nitrosation (SNO) could represent a mechanism of protection against further cysteine oxidation [18–21]. On the other hand, the same modification was associated with enhanced oxidative stress [22] and is considered labile [23] with a balance with other PTMs [24]. Moreover, SNO-prone cysteines do not overlap with the oxidation-prone residues [25], raising doubts about the real protection against oxidative stress. Inhibition of further oxidation could also be applied to harnessing the de novo endogenous production to maintain a fairly stable oxidation state of modifications. A way to reconcile all these proposed mechanisms is to understand the impact of cysteine PTMs on the activity of primary intracellular sources of ROS (Fig. 2.2).

The major ones are the mitochondrial proteins, producing approx. 90% ROS [26]. The two major sites for ROS generation are believed to be at sites of complex I and III, where large changes in the potential energy of the electrons, relative to the reduction of oxygen, occur. Experimental manipulations that augment the redox potential of site I generally increase the rate of ROS generation, lending credence to the notion that the redox potential of these reactive sites plays a role in free radical formation [26]. In pathological conditions, complex II may also be the source of ROS [27]. Moreover, mitochondrial enzymes α-ketoglutarate dehydrogenase (KGDHC) and pyruvate dehydrogenase (PDC) are also significant ROS producers and are thought to produce significantly more ROS than complex I [28]. In cytosol, ROS are produced by the family of NADPH oxidases (NOXes) [29,30], xanthine oxidase (XO) [31], cytochrome P450 oxidases [32], and uncoupled nitric oxide synthase (NOS) [33]. Some of these enzymes, NOS [33] and XO [34], only create ROS after being damaged by them. In contrast, NADPH oxidases produce ROS as their primary and sole function. Peroxisomes are also a significant source of ROS. In particular, peroxisomes produce H_2O_2 due to an abundance of O_2-consuming oxidases [35].

S-oxidation

Unusual oxidative thiol changes can often occur in eukaryotes, not accidently, as permanent ROS/RNS damage or experimental artifacts, but as standard alterations with fundamental sensing, signaling, feedback, and regulatory roles [36]. The first product of the oxidation of cysteine is sulfenic acid (Cys-SOH), most commonly induced by H_2O_2 [37], with proximal threonine being the specificity determinant [38]. Then it can be oxidized to sulfinic acid (Cys-SO_2H) and sulfonic acid (Cys-SO_3H). If not oxidized, sulfenics can either form disulfide bonds (inter- or intramolecular) assisting in protein folding [39] or can react with glutathione, leading to protein S-glutathionylation [40]. Chemically, only sulfenic acid was considered a reversible modification of thiol; however, in the experimental studies, neither DTT nor TCEP could reverse the oxidation [1]. However, upon the discovery of sulfiredoxin,

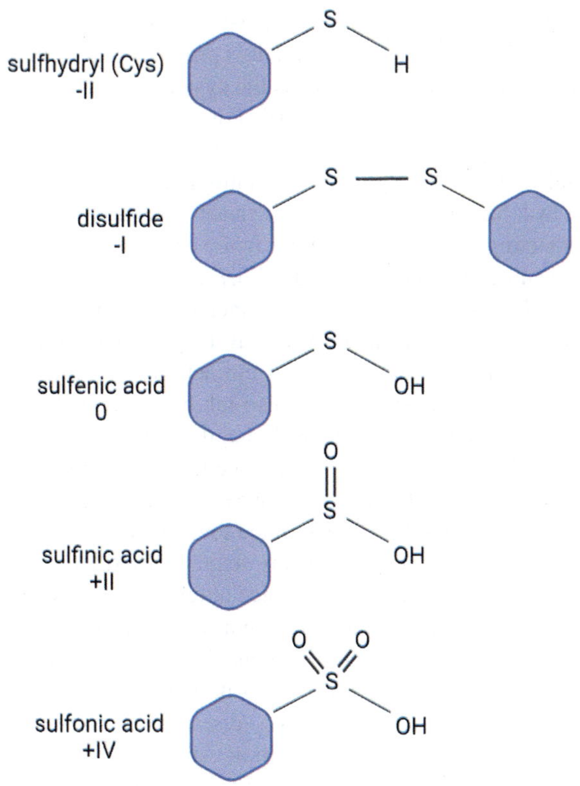

FIGURE 2.2 Cellular sources of reactive oxygen species (ROS). The mitochondrial electron transport chain is the primary source of ROS in cells. Mitochondrial proteins α-ketoglutarate dehydrogenase (KGDHC) and pyruvate dehydrogenase (PDC) also produce ROS. Among cytoplasmatic proteins, NADPH oxidases (NOXes), xanthine oxidase (XO), cytochrome P450 oxidases, uncouples nitric oxide synthase (NOS) are the most important. *SNO*, S-nitrosation; *SSG*, S-gluthationylation; *SSH*, persulfidation. *Green*, decrease in enzyme activity, *red*, increase in enzyme activity.

sulfinic acid was also proved to be reduced in an ATP-dependent manner [41]. Notably, cysteine modification by sulfonic acid is irreversible [37,42].

The impact of S-oxidation on ROS production by endogenous sources is mainly related to the facilitation of subsequent cysteine modification. The sensitivity to higher oxidation state species frequently prevents the collection of this transitory sulfenic SOH intermediate [43]. On the other hand, ROS production is crucial for cellular homeostasis. DUOX1- and NOX2-produced H_2O_2 impacts the cellular signaling through activating sulfenylation followed by other cysteine PTMs (S-glutathionylation) [44]. The hypertension models showed a similar mechanism for the NOX1 and NOX4 [45]. When considering the whole cellular redox status, NOX4-induced oxidation of unfolded protein response regulator IRE1α may be a counter-regulatory mechanism against oxidative stress [45].

S-glutathionylation

The subsequent S-glutathionylation process can occur spontaneously or with the action of glutathione S-transferases, most commonly glutathione S-transferase π [46]. The addition of GSH to a protein cysteine changes the protein size and charge owing to the addition of three amino acids and a glutamic acid moiety, resulting in structural and functional changes. It may also protect proteins from irreversible oxidation [47]. Under normal circumstances, deglutathionylation is catalyzed by glutaredoxins (GLRX), restoring the sulfhydryl groups to their natural form [48,49]. Therefore, assessment of redox status in the *Glrx*-knockout animals may give insights into the role of this modification in the maintenance of redox status. Deficiency in cytosolic and mitochondrial glutaredoxins, Glrx1 and Glrx2, respectively, differentially affect the cellular redox status. The lack of first leads to a higher level of oxidized glutathione in the hyperoxia-injured lung [50] or the appearance of atherosclerosis-related nitrotyrosine in aged females [51]. On the other hand, *Glrx2*-knockout mice do not show any difference in redox markers, superoxide level, lipid peroxidation, and antioxidative enzymes [52]. In a larger context, abnormalities in the protein S-glutathionylation have been observed in the airways of patients with asthma [53] or ischemic myocardium [54].

Mitochondrial matrix biochemical and redox characteristics enhance S-glutathionylation. There, the environment is strongly reducing and basic, which along with the significant level of glutathione (1–5 mM [GSH] and 0.01 mM [GSSG]), renders it a perfect compartment for the protein glutathionylation [40]. Protein S-glutathionylation links energy metabolism to redox signaling in mitochondria [55]. Key mitochondrial metabolic enzymes and ROS producers, PDC and KGDHC, may be regulated by S-glutathionylation in a dual way, dependent on electron transfer. During the forward electron transfer, the ROS production is attenuated, whereas S-glutathionylation during reverse electron transfer augments ROS from PDC and KGDHC [56]. Notably, this PTM also enhances the superoxide production from complex I [57,58] and is required for the function of complex II [59]. Interestingly, inhibition of S-glutathionylation of SDHA, a key component of complex II, has emerged as a promising therapeutic strategy in hematological malignancies [60]. Similarly, S-glutathionylation of the regulatory units enhances ROS production through NOX2 [61]. S-glutathionylation remains in a constant interplay with nitric oxide-related modifications, mainly S-nitrosation [62,63].

S-nitrosation

S-nitrosation is the modification of thiols by NO moiety. It is also called S-nitrosylation to underline that it is a posttranslational modification [64,65], though, from the chemical point of view, the correct reaction name is S-nitrosation. It is said to modulate most nitric oxide cellular functions and is considered chief among the modifications concerning the prevalence and demonstrated functions [66]. Interestingly, SNO is also a modulator of the activity of guanylate cyclase, a downstream regulator of NO activity [67]. While SNO modification seemed chemically driven throughout the years, it becomes clearer that it could also be enzymatically regulated. The mechanisms of de novo formation are not fully elucidated. Experimental data show that S-nitrosation does not occur through the direct addition of NO to thiol and in a hydrophobic environment. It was proposed that S-nitrosation occurs only after the initial reaction between NO and oxygen to form nitrogen dioxide [68]. Another possible mechanism requires the oxidation of NO to NO^+ through a single electron which cSNO synthases produce protein S-nitrosothiol by first conjugating NO^+ with thiol and then adding the product to the protein. Two different SNO synthases have been discovered so far: the hybrid cluster protein (HCP) serves as an SNO synthase in bacteria, whereas the mammalian one is hemoglobin, which uses nitrate as a substrate [69]. Also, KEAP1 has been postulated to be another SNO synthase. Still, the direct mechanism of how it could exert the enzymatic function has not been shown [70]. It was proposed that either transition metal like Fe^{3+} could bind to cysteine in KEAP1 in place of Zn^{2+} and oxidize NO or the reaction occurs with a thiyl radical as an intermediate [70]. Transnitrosylases are enzymes that transfer the SNO group from themselves to Cys residues on substrates to facilitate SNO-based signaling propagation. It has been determined that there is more than one transnitrosylase. GAPDH [71] and S100A9 [72] are two well-known examples.

Denitrosation is carried out by thioredoxin reductases and S-nitrosoglutathione reductase (GSNOR). Recently another mammalian denitrosating enzyme has been identified—AKR1A1. Both enzymes act on low-molecular-weight SNOs, which are in equilibrium with SNO proteins. While GSNOR acts on GSNO (S-nitrosoglutathione) in an NADH-dependent manner [73], ARK1A1 denitrosases SNO-CoA using NADPH [74]. Proteins can be directly denitrosated through the transfer of the SNO group to thioredoxin. The Trx/TrxR (thioredoxin/thioredoxin reductase) system also depends on NADPH [75]. Importantly, GSNOR is not only a denitrosase but also a key enzyme in formaldehyde metabolism [76], which may regulate cellular processes, especially DNA damage [77].

SNO pathological effects can be prolonged by oxidation [78,79], and on the other hand, it is proposed that, similarly to glutathionylation, it protects the cysteine residues against further oxidation [18,20,21,80]. For instance, it decreases the activity of NOXes through the regulation of the enzyme itself [81] or the regulatory subunits [82]. S-nitrosation of NOX4 has fundamental significance in endothelial cells, protecting them from apoptosis in the absence of NRF2, the critical cellular redox regulator [70]. Thereby, S-nitrosation may determine cellular fate, balancing between premature senescence and cellular death. It may also regulate the expression of NOX1 [83] and the activity of cytochrome P450 [84]. Similarly, it may also inhibit the mitochondrial respiratory chain subunits [85], mainly complex I [86–88]. Therefore, key ROS-producing cellular proteins can be inhibited by SNO. In accordance, the inspection of the redox status in GSNOR KO mice reveals that enhanced S-nitrosation does not trigger any feature of oxidative stress (Table 2.1). Moreover, these mice upregulate the protective and antioxidant pathways in response to liver injury [98].

Excessive S-nitrosation is considered as a fateful posttranslational modification due to its detrimental effect on various cellular processes, diseases (reviewed in Refs. [99,100]), and induction of premature aging [70,101,102]. In *C. elegans*, SNO has a regulatory role in the development through the regulation of miRNA through modification of Argonaut protein [103]. However, whether the exact mechanisms are present in mammals has not been elucidated. Accordingly, S-nitrosothiol signaling impacts liver development [98] and lymphocyte development at early stages in bone marrow in mice [104].

S-sulfenylation/persulfidation

Cysteine persulfidation (also known as sulfhydration or sulfuration) is a reversible posttranslational modification of protein cysteinyl thiols (-SH) to persulfides (-SSH), which increases cysteine reactivity [105]. The formation may occur via several routes, including reactions between hydrogen sulfide (or rather HS^-, anionic form is 4 times more abundant [105]), oxidized protein thiols, or reactions between inorganic polysulfides and protein [106]. The reaction may be facilitated if cysteine is in the form of a thiolate anion (which is the case for low-pKa cysteine residues at physiological pH), which then can undergo sulfenylation or S-glutathionylation [107], rendering persulfidation a readout of oxidant stress [108]. Notably, the moonlighting activity of cysteinyl—transfer RNA synthases (CARS) leads to the production of cysteine persulfides and translationally incorporates these into nascent polypeptide chains [109].

Persulfidation, like other cysteine redox changes, has emerged as a key method for fine-tuning protein function,

TABLE 2.1 Oxidative stress status in GSNOR KO mice.

General conditions	Oxidative stress markers in mouse models (GSNOR KO)	References
Hepatocarcinogenesis	No difference (in 8-oxo, GSSG) in the liver in the basal state	[89]
Hepatocarcinogenesis	Increases DCF DA-depicted ROS in response to complex II stimulants	[90]
Hypothermia	No difference and a significant decrease in DCF DA-depicted ROS DCF at 37 and 23°C, respectively. Less DCF at 23°C	[91]
Sepsis-induced myocardial depression	Higher level of hydroxynonenal in plasma	[92]
Cardiac arrest and resuscitation	A lower level of H_2O_2 upon CPR	[93]
Parkinson's disease and ALS	Decrease in DCF DA-measured ROS and protein carbonyls	[94]
Neuromuscular dysfunction	Less nitrotyrosines and more antioxidative proteins (NRF2, NQO1, catalase)	[95]
Preeclampsia	Higher ROS, NO, and HNE upon pregnancy	[96]
Bladder function	No difference in HNE	[97]

interaction, and localization in cells. This alteration has also been shown to have a critical role in regulating various redox-dependent biological processes, including autophagy, cellular metabolism, inflammation, cell cycle, and cell death in normal and pathological situations. It is also considered a way to increase H_2S activity and provide a protein-related context for the gasotransmitter [110]. The modification can be reversed by thioredoxin [111] and glutathione [112] systems. The new regulators, including thioredoxin-related proteins, are being unraveled [113]. Persulfidation can also be reversed by exogenous reducing agents like DTT or TCEP [114].

The stepwise oxidation of a persulfide group leads to the consecutive formation of perthiosulfenic acid, perthiosulfinic acid, and perthiosulfonic acid (-SSOH, -SSO_2H, and -SSO_3H, respectively) [115]. Interestingly, while irreversible oxidation of cysteine residues to sulfinic/sulfonic forms typically impairs protein function, persulfidation (CysSSH) protects cysteines from irreversible oxidative loss of function by the formation of $CysSSO_{1-3}H$ derivatives that can subsequently be reduced back to native thiols [113]. Interestingly, given the presence of these modifications on the key signaling proteins, it is proposed that it may represent a novel, as yet uncharacterized, event in redox-based signaling [116].

Persulfidation prevents irreversible cysteine overoxidation, preserving protein function [117]. Persulfidated MnSOD was more resistant to tyrosine nitration by peroxynitrite, suggesting the modification may act as a protective mechanism against enzyme nitration, a feature of many oxidative stress-related diseases [117]. While the impact of persulfidation on NOX activity in mammals is not elucidated, in plants, this modification increases the oxidative burst from NADPH oxidases [118]. Furthermore, hydropersulfides inhibit lipid peroxidation and cell death by scavenging radicals [119].

Modulation of cellular processes in response to oxidative stress

Thiol modifications regulate the cellular response to oxidative stress, ensuring cellular survival by enhancing protein degradation and inhibiting translation and cell cycle progression. This regulatory role was primarily outlined in the context of glutathionylation. This modification of actin and tubulin inhibits their polymerization, abrogating the formation of the mitotic spindle and resulting in arrested mitosis. Lastly, *S*-glutathionylation of 14-3-3ζ serves as a signal for caspase-dependent protein degradation under metabolic stress [120]. In the context of protein homeostasis, S-glutathionylation of cysteines on the α5 subunit enhances 20S proteasomal activity by further supporting ring opening [121], which stays in contrast to oxidative modifications promoting the disassembly of 26S proteasome during oxidative stress [122]. Furthermore, glutathionylation triggers the induction of chaperone activity of Hsc70 [123].

The impact on transcription factors achieves the broader cellular context of the regulatory function of thiol modifications. The hallmark cysteine-related regulation is KEAP1-dependent repression of NRF2. The modification of KEAP1 cysteines by S-nitrosation [124], S-glutathionylation [125], and persulfidation [126] results in the enhancement of NRF2 transcriptional activity. Redox-related mechanisms are essential for the NRF2 homologs: OxyR [127,128] and YAP1 [129].

Sulfenylation with concomitant S-glutathionylation p50 subunit of NFkB leads to the inhibition of DNA binding [130], and S-glutathionylation of IKK [131] may also achieve upstream regulation. Similarly, the transcriptional activity of c-Jun may also be inhibited by S-glutathionylation [132]. Many redox-related transcription factors (ex. Sp1) contain the zinc finger motif, where thiols directly respond to oxidative burden [133]. Moreover, H_2O_2-responsive peroxiredoxins can regulate the activity of FOXO3 and STAT3 [134,135], providing evidence for controlling many transcription factors, not only the typical oxidative stress ones [136].

Conclusions

The described modifications seem to have a mainly inhibitory impact on the ROS production in the cells, pointing out regulatory mechanisms aimed at fine-tuning ROS production to maintain the homeostatic cellular level (redox buffering capacity). Similarly, upon exogenous oxidants delivery, the level of modifications rises, which could decrease the intracellular/endogenous production. Accordingly, the knockout of specific enzymes triggers the general transcriptional pathways to restore proper balance. Thiol modifications should instead be considered as the indicator of increased redox status and compensatory mechanisms to maintain the appropriate balance.

Abbreviations

CoA	Coenzyme A
DTT	Dithiothreitol
GLRX	Glutaredoxin
GSH	Glutathione
GSNOR	S-nitrosoglutathione reductase
IRE1α	Inositol-requiring enzyme-1a
KEAP1	Kelch Like ECH Associated Protein 1
KGDHC	α-Ketoglutarate dehydrogenase
NADP	Nicotinamide adenine dinucleotide phosphate
NOS	Nitric oxide synthase
NOX	NADPH oxidase
NRF2	Transcription factor, nuclear factor erythroid 2−related factor
PDC	Pyruvate dehydrogenase
PTM	Posttranslational modification
RNS	Reactive nitrogen species
ROS	Reactive oxygen species
SNO	S-nitrosation
TCEP	Tris(2-carboxyethyl)phosphin
XO	Xanthine oxidase

Acknowledgments

AK is supported by National Science Center Preludium (grant no. 2019/35/N/NZ3/04230), AJ is supported by National Science Center Maestro (grant no. 2018/30/A/NZ3/00495). This work was supported by National Science Center Opus (grant no. 2021/43/B/NZ4/02130 to AGP). Figures were created with BioRender.com.

References

[1] Held JM, Gibson BW. Regulatory control or oxidative damage? Proteomic approaches to interrogate the role of cysteine oxidation status in biological processes. Mol Cell Proteomics 2012;11. https://doi.org/10.1074/mcp.R111.013037. R111.013037.

[2] Brandes N, Schmitt S, Jakob U. Thiol-based redox switches in eukaryotic proteins. Antioxid Redox Signal 2009;11:997−1014. https://doi.org/10.1089/ars.2008.2285.

[3] Baba SP, Bhatnagar A. Role of thiols in oxidative stress. Curr Opin Toxicol 2018;7:133−9. https://doi.org/10.1016/j.cotox.2018.03.005.

[4] Küküt A, Gelen V, Başer ÖF, Deveci HA, Karapehlivan M, Kükürt A, et al. Thiols: role in oxidative stress-related disorders. IntechOpen; 2021. https://doi.org/10.5772/intechopen.96682.

[5] Pimkova K, Jassinskaja M, Munita R, Ciesla M, Guzzi N, Cao Thi Ngoc P, et al. Quantitative analysis of redox proteome reveals oxidation-sensitive protein thiols acting in fundamental processes of developmental hematopoiesis. Redox Biol 2022;53:102343. https://doi.org/10.1016/j.redox.2022.102343.

[6] Pacher P. Cyanide emerges as an endogenous mammalian gasotransmitter. Proc Natl Acad Sci USA 2021;118. https://doi.org/10.1073/pnas.2108040118. e2108040118.

[7] Miseta A, Csutora P. Relationship between the occurrence of cysteine in proteins and the complexity of organisms. Mol Biol Evol 2000;17:1232−9. https://doi.org/10.1093/oxfordjournals.molbev.a026406.

[8] Xiao H, Jedrychowski MP, Schweppe DK, Huttlin EL, Yu Q, Heppner DE, et al. A quantitative tissue-specific landscape of protein redox regulation during aging. Cell 2020;180:968−983.e24. https://doi.org/10.1016/j.cell.2020.02.012.

[9] Poole LB. The basics of thiols and cysteines in redox biology and chemistry. Free Radic Biol Med 2015;0:148−57. https://doi.org/10.1016/j.freeradbiomed.2014.11.013.

[10] Alcock LJ, Perkins MV, Chalker JM. Chemical methods for mapping cysteine oxidation. Chem Soc Rev 2018;47:231−68. https://doi.org/10.1039/C7CS00607A.

[11] Kamada M, Hideshima T, Azuma J, Yamamoto I, Imamura M, Takahashi K. Occupied and unoccupied electronic structures of an L-cysteine film studied by core-absorption and resonant photoelectron spectroscopies. AIP Adv 2016;6:045306. https://doi.org/10.1063/1.4947072.

[12] Paulsen CE, Carroll KS. Cysteine-mediated redox signaling: chemistry, biology, and tools for discovery. Chem Rev 2013;113:4633−79. https://doi.org/10.1021/cr300163e.

[13] Weerapana E, Wang C, Simon GM, Richter F, Khare S, Dillon MBD, et al. Quantitative reactivity profiling predicts functional cysteines in proteomes. Nature 2010;468:790−5. https://doi.org/10.1038/nature09472.

[14] LoPachin R, Gavin T. Reactions of electrophiles with nucleophilic thiolate sites: relevance to pathophysiological mechanisms and remediation. Free Radic Res 2015;50:1−11. https://doi.org/10.3109/10715762.2015.1094184.

[15] Bak DW, Bechtel TJ, Falco JA, Weerapana E. Cysteine reactivity across the subcellular universe. Curr Opin Chem Biol 2019;48:96−105. https://doi.org/10.1016/j.cbpa.2018.11.002.

[16] Go Y-M, Jones DP. The redox proteome. J Biol Chem 2013;288:26512−20. https://doi.org/10.1074/jbc.R113.464131.

[17] Gout I. Coenzyme A, protein CoAlation and redox regulation in mammalian cells. Biochem Soc Trans 2018;46:721–8. https://doi.org/10.1042/BST20170506.

[18] Sun J, Steenbergen C, Murphy E. S-nitrosylation: NO-related redox signaling to protect against oxidative stress. Antioxid Redox Signal 2006;8:1693–705. https://doi.org/10.1089/ars.2006.8.1693.

[19] Evangelista AM, Kohr MJ, Murphy E. S-nitrosylation: specificity, occupancy, and interaction with other post-translational modifications. Antioxid Redox Signal 2013;19:1209–19. https://doi.org/10.1089/ars.2012.5056.

[20] Sun J, Murphy E. Protein S-nitrosylation and cardioprotection. Circ Res 2010;106:285–96. https://doi.org/10.1161/CIRCRESAHA.109.209452.

[21] Murphy E, Kohr M, Sun J, Nguyen T, Steenbergen C. S-nitrosylation: a radical way to protect the heart. J Mol Cell Cardiol 2011;52:568–77. https://doi.org/10.1016/j.yjmcc.2011.08.021.

[22] Fang J, Nakamura T, Cho D-H, Gu Z, Lipton SA. S-nitrosylation of peroxiredoxin 2 promotes oxidative stress-induced neuronal cell death in Parkinson's disease. Proc Natl Acad Sci USA 2007;104:18742–7. https://doi.org/10.1073/pnas.0705904104.

[23] Wolhuter K, Whitwell HJ, Switzer CH, Burgoyne JR, Timms JF, Eaton P. Evidence against stable protein S-nitrosylation as a widespread mechanism of post-translational regulation. Mol Cell 2018;69:438–450.e5. https://doi.org/10.1016/j.molcel.2017.12.019.

[24] Martínez-Ruiz A, Lamas S. Signalling by NO-induced protein S-nitrosylation and S-glutathionylation: convergences and divergences. Cardiovasc Res 2007;75:220–8. https://doi.org/10.1016/j.cardiores.2007.03.016.

[25] Go Y-M, Chandler JD, Jones DP. The cysteine proteome. Free Radic Biol Med 2015;84:227–45. https://doi.org/10.1016/j.freeradbiomed.2015.03.022.

[26] Balaban RS, Nemoto S, Finkel T. Mitochondria, oxidants, and aging. Cell 2005;120:483–95. https://doi.org/10.1016/j.cell.2005.02.001.

[27] Zorov DB, Juhaszova M, Sollott SJ. Mitochondrial reactive oxygen species (ROS) and ROS-induced ROS release. Physiol Rev 2014;94:909–50. https://doi.org/10.1152/physrev.00026.2013.

[28] Quinlan CL, Goncalves RLS, Hey-Mogensen M, Yadava N, Bunik VI, Brand MD. The 2-oxoacid dehydrogenase complexes in mitochondria can produce superoxide/hydrogen peroxide at much higher rates than complex I. J Biol Chem 2014;289:8312–25. https://doi.org/10.1074/jbc.M113.545301.

[29] Moghadam ZM, Henneke P, Kolter J. From flies to men: ROS and the NADPH oxidase in phagocytes. Front Cell Dev Biol 2021;9. https://www.frontiersin.org/articles/10.3389/fcell.2021.628991. [Accessed 5 October 2022].

[30] Laurindo FRM, Araujo TLS, Abrahão TB. Nox NADPH oxidases and the endoplasmic reticulum. Antioxid Redox Signal 2014;20:2755–75. https://doi.org/10.1089/ars.2013.5605.

[31] Harris CM, Sanders SA, Massey V. Role of the flavin midpoint potential and NAD binding in determining NAD versus oxygen reactivity of xanthine oxidoreductase. J Biol Chem 1999;274:4561–9. https://doi.org/10.1074/jbc.274.8.4561.

[32] Fleming I, Michaelis UR, Bredenkötter D, Fisslthaler B, Dehghani F, Brandes RP, et al. Endothelium-derived hyperpolarising factor synthase (Cytochrome P450 2C9) is a functionally significant source of reactive oxygen species in coronary arteries. Circ Res 2001;88:44–51. https://doi.org/10.1161/01.res.88.1.44.

[33] Vásquez-Vivar J, Kalyanaraman B, Martásek P, Hogg N, Masters BS, Karoui H, et al. Superoxide generation by endothelial nitric oxide synthase: the influence of cofactors. Proc Natl Acad Sci USA 1998;95:9220–5. https://doi.org/10.1073/pnas.95.16.9220.

[34] Zhang Z, Blake DR, Stevens CR, Kanczler JM, Winyard PG, Symons MC, et al. A reappraisal of xanthine dehydrogenase and oxidase in hypoxic reperfusion injury: the role of NADH as an electron donor. Free Radic Res 1998;28:151–64. https://doi.org/10.3109/10715769809065801.

[35] Sandalio LM, Rodríguez-Serrano M, Romero-Puertas MC, del Río LA. Role of peroxisomes as a source of reactive oxygen species (ROS) signaling molecules. Subcell Biochem 2013;69:231–55. https://doi.org/10.1007/978-94-007-6889-5_13.

[36] Giles GI, Nasim MJ, Ali W, Jacob C. The reactive sulfur species concept: 15 years on. Antioxidants (Basel) 2017;6:38. https://doi.org/10.3390/antiox6020038.

[37] Gupta V, Carroll KS. Sulfenic acid chemistry, detection and cellular lifetime. Biochim Biophys Acta Gen Subj 2014;1840:847–75. https://doi.org/10.1016/j.bbagen.2013.05.040.

[38] Salsbury FR, Knutson ST, Poole LB, Fetrow JS. Functional site profiling and electrostatic analysis of cysteines modifiable to cysteine sulfenic acid. Protein Sci 2008;17:299–312. https://doi.org/10.1110/ps.073096508.

[39] Rehder DS, Borges CR. Cysteine sulfenic acid as an intermediate in disulfide bond formation and nonenzymatic protein folding. Biochemistry 2010;49:7748–55. https://doi.org/10.1021/bi1008694.

[40] Mailloux RJ, McBride SL, Harper M-E. Unearthing the secrets of mitochondrial ROS and glutathione in bioenergetics. Trends Biochem Sci 2013;38:592–602. https://doi.org/10.1016/j.tibs.2013.09.001.

[41] Woo HA, Chae HZ, Hwang SC, Yang K-S, Kang SW, Kim K, Rhee SG. Reversing the inactivation of peroxiredoxins caused by cysteine sulfinic acid formation. Science 2003;300:653–6. https://doi.org/10.1126/science.1080273.

[42] Saurin AT, Neubert H, Brennan JP, Eaton P. Widespread sulfenic acid formation in tissues in response to hydrogen peroxide. Proc Natl Acad Sci USA 2004;101:17982–7. https://doi.org/10.1073/pnas.0404762101.

[43] Beedle AEM, Lynham S, Garcia-Manyes S. Protein S-sulfenylation is a fleeting molecular switch that regulates non-enzymatic oxidative folding. Nat Commun 2016;7:12490. https://doi.org/10.1038/ncomms12490.

[44] Heppner DE, Hristova M, Dustin CM, Danyal K, Habibovic A, van der Vliet A. The NADPH oxidases DUOX1 and NOX2 play distinct roles in redox regulation of epidermal growth factor receptor signaling. J Biol Chem 2016;291:23282–93. https://doi.org/10.1074/jbc.M116.749028.

[45] Camargo LL, Harvey AP, Rios FJ, Tsiropoulou S, de Oliveira Silva RDN, Cao Z, et al. Vascular Nox compartmentalisation, protein hyperoxidation and ER stress response in hypertension. Hypertension 2018;72:235–46. https://doi.org/10.1161/HYPERTENSIONAHA.118.10824.

[46] Townsend DM, Manevich Y, He L, Hutchens S, Pazoles CJ, Tew KD. Novel role for glutathione S-transferase π: regulator of

protein S-glutathionylation following oxidative and nitrosative stress**This work was supported, in whole or in part, by National Institutes of Health Grants CA08660 and CA117259. This work was also supported by the South Carolina Centers of Excellence program. The costs of publication of this article were defrayed in part by the payment of page charges. This article must therefore be hereby marked "advertisement" in accordance with 18 U.S.C. Section 1734 solely to indicate this fact. J Biol Chem 2009;284:436–45. https://doi.org/10.1074/jbc.M805586200.

[47] Hill BG, Bhatnagar A. Protein S-glutathiolation: redox-sensitive regulation of protein function. J Mol Cell Cardiol 2012;52:559–67. https://doi.org/10.1016/j.yjmcc.2011.07.009.

[48] Beer SM, Taylor ER, Brown SE, Dahm CC, Costa NJ, Runswick MJ, et al. Glutaredoxin 2 catalyses the reversible oxidation and glutathionylation of mitochondrial membrane thiol proteins: implications for mitochondrial redox regulation and antioxidant defense. J Biol Chem 2004;279:47939–51. https://doi.org/10.1074/jbc.M408011200.

[49] Matsui R, Ferran B, Oh A, Croteau D, Shao D, Han J, et al. Redox regulation via glutaredoxin-1 and protein S-glutathionylation. Antioxid Redox Signal 2020;32:677–700. https://doi.org/10.1089/ars.2019.7963.

[50] Liu X, Li K, Zhang F, Zhang Y, Deng C, Guo C. Ablation of glutaredoxin 1 promotes pulmonary angiogenesis and alveolar formation in hyperoxia-injured lungs by modifying HIF-1α stability and inhibiting the NF-κB pathway. Biochem Biophys Res Commun 2020;525:528–35. https://doi.org/10.1016/j.bbrc.2020.02.129.

[51] Ahn YJ, Wang L, Tavakoli S, Nguyen HN, Short JD, Asmis R. Glutaredoxin 1 controls monocyte reprogramming during nutrient stress and protects mice against obesity and atherosclerosis in a sex-specific manner. Nat Commun 2022;13:790. https://doi.org/10.1038/s41467-022-28433-2.

[52] Wohua Z, Weiming X. Glutaredoxin 2 (GRX2) deficiency exacerbates high fat diet (HFD)-induced insulin resistance, inflammation and mitochondrial dysfunction in brain injury: a mechanism involving GSK-3β. Biomed Pharmacother 2019;118:108940. https://doi.org/10.1016/j.biopha.2019.108940.

[53] Kuipers I, Louis R, Manise M, Dentener MA, Irvin CG, Janssen-Heininger YMW, et al. Increased glutaredoxin-1 and decreased protein S-glutathionylation in sputum of asthmatics. Eur Respir J 2013;41:469–72. https://doi.org/10.1183/09031936.00115212.

[54] Chen J, Chen C-L, Rawale S, Chen C-A, Zweier JL, Kaumaya PTP, et al. Peptide-based antibodies against glutathione-binding domains suppress superoxide production mediated by mitochondrial complex I. J Biol Chem 2010;285:3168–80. https://doi.org/10.1074/jbc.M109.056846.

[55] Mailloux RJ, Treberg JR. Protein S-glutathionlyation links energy metabolism to redox signaling in mitochondria. Redox Biol 2016;8:110–8. https://doi.org/10.1016/j.redox.2015.12.010.

[56] O'Brien M, Chalker J, Slade L, Gardiner D, Mailloux RJ. Protein S-glutathionylation alters superoxide/hydrogen peroxide emission from pyruvate dehydrogenase complex. Free Radic Biol Med 2017;106:302–14. https://doi.org/10.1016/j.freeradbiomed.2017.02.046.

[57] Kang PT, Zhang L, Chen C-L, Chen J, Green KB, Chen Y-R. Protein thiyl radical mediates S-glutathionylation of complex I. Free Radic Biol Med 2012;53:962–73. https://doi.org/10.1016/j.freeradbiomed.2012.05.025.

[58] Taylor ER, Hurrell F, Shannon RJ, Lin T-K, Hirst J, Murphy MP. Reversible glutathionylation of complex I increases mitochondrial superoxide formation. J Biol Chem 2003;278:19603–10. https://doi.org/10.1074/jbc.M209359200.

[59] Chen Y-R, Chen C-L, Pfeiffer DR, Zweier JL. Mitochondrial complex II in the post-ischemic heart: oxidative injury and the role of protein S-glutathionylation. J Biol Chem 2007;282:32640–54. https://doi.org/10.1074/jbc.M702294200.

[60] Jones CL, Stevens BM, D'Alessandro A, Culp-Hill R, Reisz JA, Pei S, et al. Cysteine depletion targets leukemia stem cells through inhibition of electron transport complex II. Blood 2019;134:389–94. https://doi.org/10.1182/blood.2019898114.

[61] Nagarkoti S, Dubey M, Awasthi D, Kumar V, Chandra T, Kumar S, et al. S-Glutathionylation of p47phox sustains superoxide generation in activated neutrophils. Biochim Biophys Acta Mol Cell Res 2018;1865:444–54. https://doi.org/10.1016/j.bbamcr.2017.11.014.

[62] Kalinina E, Novichkova M. Glutathione in protein redox modulation through S-glutathionylation and S-nitrosylation. Molecules 2021;26:435. https://doi.org/10.3390/molecules26020435.

[63] Belcastro E, Gaucher C, Corti A, Leroy P, Lartaud I, Pompella A. Regulation of protein function by S-nitrosation and S-glutathionylation: processes and targets in cardiovascular pathophysiology. Biol Chem 2017;398:1267–93. https://doi.org/10.1515/hsz-2017-0150.

[64] Stamler JS. Redox signaling: nitrosylation and related target interactions of nitric oxide. Cell 1994;78:931–6. https://doi.org/10.1016/0092-8674(94)90269-0.

[65] Stamler JS, Jaraki O, Osborne J, Simon DI, Keaney J, Vita J, et al. Nitric oxide circulates in mammalian plasma primarily as an S-nitroso adduct of serum albumin. Proc Natl Acad Sci USA 1992;89:7674–7. https://doi.org/10.1073/pnas.89.16.7674.

[66] Stomberski CT, Hess DT, Stamler J. Protein S-nitrosylation: determinants of specificity and enzymatic regulation of S-nitrosothiol-based signaling. Antioxid Redox Signal 2017. https://doi.org/10.1089/ars.2017.7403.

[67] Cui C, Wu C, Shu P, Liu T, Li H, Beuve A. Soluble guanylyl cyclase mediates noncanonical nitric oxide signaling by nitrosothiol transfer under oxidative stress. Redox Biol 2022;55:102425. https://doi.org/10.1016/j.redox.2022.102425.

[68] Keszler A, Zhang Y, Hogg N. Reaction between nitric oxide, glutathione, and oxygen in the presence and absence of protein: how are S-nitrosothiols formed? Free Radic Biol Med 2010;48:55–64. https://doi.org/10.1016/j.freeradbiomed.2009.10.026.

[69] Angelo M, Singel DJ, Stamler JS. An S-nitrosothiol (SNO) synthase function of hemoglobin that utilises nitrite as a substrate. Proc Natl Acad Sci USA 2006;103:8366–71. https://doi.org/10.1073/pnas.0600942103.

[70] Kopacz A, Klóska D, Proniewski B, Cysewski D, Personnic N, Piechota-Polańczyk A, et al. Keap1 controls protein S-nitrosation and apoptosis-senescence switch in endothelial cells. Redox Biol 2020;28:101304. https://doi.org/10.1016/j.redox.2019.101304.

[71] Kornberg MD, Sen N, Hara MR, Juluri KR, Nguyen JVK, Snowman AM, et al. GAPDH mediates nitrosylation of nuclear proteins. Nat Cell Biol 2010;12:1094–100. https://doi.org/10.1038/ncb2114.

[72] Jia J, Arif A, Terenzi F, Willard B, Plow EF, Hazen SL, et al. Target-selective protein S-nitrosylation by sequence motif

recognition. Cell 2014;159:623–34. https://doi.org/10.1016/j.cell.2014.09.032.

[73] Liu L, Hausladen A, Zeng M, Que L, Heitman J, Stamler JS. A metabolic enzyme for S-nitrosothiol conserved from bacteria to humans. Nature 2001;410:490–4. https://doi.org/10.1038/35068596.

[74] Stomberski CT, Anand P, Venetos NM, Hausladen A, Zhou H-L, Premont RT, et al. AKR1A1 is a novel mammalian S-nitroso-glutathione reductase. J Biol Chem 2019;294:18285–93. https://doi.org/10.1074/jbc.RA119.011067.

[75] Benhar M, Forrester MT, Hess DT, Stamler JS. Regulated protein denitrosylation by cytosolic and mitochondrial thioredoxins. Science 2008;320:1050–4. https://doi.org/10.1126/science.1158265.

[76] Burgos-Barragan G, Wit N, Meiser J, Dingler FA, Pietzke M, Mulderrig L, et al. Mammals divert endogenous genotoxic formaldehyde into one-carbon metabolism. Nature 2017;548:549–54. https://doi.org/10.1038/nature23481.

[77] Dingler FA, Wang M, Mu A, Millington CL, Oberbeck N, Watcham S, et al. Two aldehyde clearance systems are essential to prevent lethal formaldehyde accumulation in mice and humans. Mol Cell 2020;80:996–1012.e9. https://doi.org/10.1016/j.molcel.2020.10.012.

[78] Vanin AF. How is nitric oxide (NO) converted into nitrosonium cations (NO^+) in living organisms? (Based on the results of optical and EPR analyses of dinitrosyl iron complexes with thiol-containing ligands). Appl Magn Reson 2020;51:851–76. https://doi.org/10.1007/s00723-020-01270-6.

[79] Viner RI, Williams TD, Schöneich C. Peroxynitrite modification of protein thiols: oxidation, nitrosylation, and S-glutathiolation of functionally important cysteine residue(s) in the sarcoplasmic reticulum Ca-ATPase. Biochemistry 1999;38:12408–15. https://doi.org/10.1021/bi9909445.

[80] Chen Y-Y, Chu H-M, Pan K-T, Teng C-H, Wang D-L, Wang AH-J, et al. Cysteine S-nitrosylation protects protein-tyrosine phosphatase 1B against oxidation-induced permanent inactivation. J Biol Chem 2008;283:35265–72. https://doi.org/10.1074/jbc.M805287200.

[81] Qian J, Chen F, Kovalenkov Y, Pandey D, Moseley A, Foster M, et al. Nitric oxide reduces NADPH oxidase 5 (NOX5) activity by reversible S-nitrosylation. Free Radic Biol Med 2012;52:1806–19. https://doi.org/10.1016/j.freeradbiomed.2012.02.029.

[82] Selemidis S, Dusting GJ, Peshavariya H, Kemp-Harper BK, Drummond GR. Nitric oxide suppresses NADPH oxidase-dependent superoxide production by S-nitrosylation in human endothelial cells. Cardiovasc Res 2007;75:349–58. https://doi.org/10.1016/j.cardiores.2007.03.030.

[83] Plesková M, Beck K-F, Behrens MH, Huwiler A, Fichtlscherer B, Wingerter O, et al. Nitric oxide down-regulates the expression of the catalytic NADPH oxidase subunit Nox1 in rat renal mesangial cells. FASEB J 2006;20:139–41. https://doi.org/10.1096/fj.05-3791fje.

[84] Morgan ET, Skubic C, Lee C, Cokan KB, Rozman D. Regulation of cytochrome P450 enzyme activity and expression by nitric oxide in the context of inflammatory disease. Drug Metab Rev 2020;52:455–71. https://doi.org/10.1080/03602532.2020.1817061.

[85] Chang AHK, Sancheti H, Garcia J, Kaplowitz N, Cadenas E, Han D. Respiratory substrates regulate S-nitrosylation of mitochondrial proteins through a thiol-dependent pathway. Chem Res Toxicol 2014;27:794–804. https://doi.org/10.1021/tx400462r.

[86] Burwell LS, Nadtochiy SM, Tompkins AJ, Young S, Brookes PS. Direct evidence for S-nitrosation of mitochondrial complex I. Biochem J 2006;394:627–34. https://doi.org/10.1042/BJ20051435.

[87] Clementi E, Brown GC, Feelisch M, Moncada S. Persistent inhibition of cell respiration by nitric oxide: crucial role of S-nitrosylation of mitochondrial complex I and protective action of glutathione. Proc Natl Acad Sci USA 1998;95:7631–6. https://doi.org/10.1073/pnas.95.13.7631.

[88] Galkin A, Moncada S. S-nitrosation of mitochondrial complex I depends on its structural conformation. J Biol Chem 2007;282:37448–53. https://doi.org/10.1074/jbc.M707543200.

[89] Tang C-H, Wei W, Hanes MA, Liu L. Hepatocarcinogenesis driven by GSNOR deficiency is prevented by iNOS inhibition. Cancer Res 2013;73:2897–904. https://doi.org/10.1158/0008-5472.CAN-12-3980.

[90] Rizza S, Montagna C, Cardaci S, Maiani E, Di Giacomo G, Sanchez-Quiles V, et al. S-nitrosylation of the mitochondrial chaperone TRAP1 sensitises hepatocellular carcinoma cells to inhibitors of succinate dehydrogenase. Cancer Res 2016;76:4170–82. https://doi.org/10.1158/0008-5472.CAN-15-2637.

[91] Dulce RA, Mayo V, Rangel EB, Balkan W, Hare JM. Interaction between neuronal nitric oxide synthase signaling and temperature influences sarcoplasmic reticulum calcium leak. Circ Res 2015;116:46–55. https://doi.org/10.1161/CIRCRESAHA.116.305172.

[92] Lee JA, Kuchakulla M, Arora H, Kulandavelu S, Gonzalez E, Masterson TA, et al. Age induced nitroso-redox imbalance leads to subclinical hypogonadism in male mice. Front Endocrinol 2019;10. https://www.frontiersin.org/articles/10.3389/fendo.2019.00190. [Accessed 2 October 2022].

[93] Hayashida K, Bagchi A, Miyazaki Y, Hirai S, Seth D, Silverman MG, et al. Improvement in outcomes after cardiac arrest and resuscitation by inhibition of S-nitrosoglutathione reductase. Circulation 2019;139:815–27. https://doi.org/10.1161/CIRCULATIONAHA.117.032488.

[94] Rizza S, Cirotti C, Montagna C, Cardaci S, Consales C, Cozzolino M, et al. *S*-nitrosoglutathione reductase plays opposite roles in SH-SY5Y models of Parkinson's disease and amyotrophic lateral sclerosis. Mediat Inflamm 2015;2015:e536238. https://doi.org/10.1155/2015/536238.

[95] Montagna C, Di Giacomo G, Rizza S, Cardaci S, Ferraro E, Grumati P, et al. S-nitrosoglutathione reductase deficiency-induced S-nitrosylation results in neuromuscular dysfunction. Antioxid Redox Signal 2014;21:570–87. https://doi.org/10.1089/ars.2013.5696.

[96] Kulandavelu S, Dulce RA, Murray CI, Bellio MA, Fritsch J, Kanashiro-Takeuchi R, et al. S-nitrosoglutathione reductase deficiency causes aberrant placental S-nitrosylation and preeclampsia. J Am Heart Assoc 2022;11:e024008. https://doi.org/10.1161/JAHA.121.024008.

[97] Akakpo W, Musicki B, Burnett AL. cAMP-dependent regulation of RhoA/Rho-kinase attenuates detrusor overactivity in a novel mouse experimental model. BJU Int 2017;120:143–51. https://doi.org/10.1111/bju.13847.

[98] Cox AG, Saunders DC, Kelsey PB, Conway AA, Tesmenitsky Y, Marchini JF, et al. S-nitrosothiol signaling regulates liver development and improves outcome following toxic liver injury. Cell Rep 2014;6:56–69. https://doi.org/10.1016/j.celrep.2013.12.007.

[99] Rizza S, Filomeni G. Chronicles of a reductase: biochemistry, genetics and physio-pathological role of GSNOR. Free Radic Biol Med 2017;110:19–30. https://doi.org/10.1016/j.freeradbiomed.2017.05.014.

[100] Barnett SD, Buxton ILO. The role of S-nitrosoglutathione reductase (GSNOR) in human disease and therapy. Crit Rev Biochem Mol Biol 2017;52:340–54. https://doi.org/10.1080/10409238.2017.1304353.

[101] García-Ortiz A, Martín-Cofreces NB, Ibiza S, Ortega Á, Izquierdo-Álvarez A, Trullo A, et al. eNOS S-nitrosylates β-actin on Cys374 and regulates PKC-θ at the immune synapse by impairing actin binding to profilin-1. PLoS Biol 2017;15:e2000653. https://doi.org/10.1371/journal.pbio.2000653.

[102] Montagna C, Rizza S, Maiani E, Piredda L, Filomeni G, Cecconi F. To eat, or NOt to eat: S-nitrosylation signaling in autophagy. FEBS J 2016;283:3857–69. https://doi.org/10.1111/febs.13736.

[103] Seth P, Hsieh PN, Jamal S, Wang L, Gygi SP, Jain MK, et al. Regulation of microRNA machinery and development by interspecies S-nitrosylation. Cell 2019;176:1014–1025.e12. https://doi.org/10.1016/j.cell.2019.01.037.

[104] Yang Z, Wang Z-E, Doulias P-T, Wei W, Ischiropoulos H, Locksley RM, Liu L. Lymphocyte development requires S-nitrosoglutathione reductase. J Immunol 2010;185:6664–9. https://doi.org/10.4049/jimmunol.1000080.

[105] Paul BD, Snyder SH. H_2S signalling through protein sulfhydration and beyond. Nat Rev Mol Cell Biol 2012;13:499–507. https://doi.org/10.1038/nrm3391.

[106] Filipovic MR, Zivanovic J, Alvarez B, Banerjee R. Chemical biology of H_2S signaling through persulfidation. Chem Rev 2018;118:1253–337. https://doi.org/10.1021/acs.chemrev.7b00205.

[107] Finkel T. From sulfenylation to sulfhydration: what a thiolate needs to tolerate. Sci Signal 2012;5:pe10. https://doi.org/10.1126/scisignal.2002943.

[108] Wages PA, Lavrich KS, Zhang Z, Cheng W-Y, Corteselli E, Gold A, et al. Protein sulfenylation: a novel readout of environmental oxidant stress. Chem Res Toxicol 2015;28:2411–8. https://doi.org/10.1021/acs.chemrestox.5b00424.

[109] Akaike T, Ida T, Wei F-Y, Nishida M, Kumagai Y, Alam MM, et al. Cysteinyl-tRNA synthetase governs cysteine polysulfidation and mitochondrial bioenergetics. Nat Commun 2017;8:1177. https://doi.org/10.1038/s41467-017-01311-y.

[110] Ida T, Sawa T, Ihara H, Tsuchiya Y, Watanabe Y, Kumagai Y, et al. Reactive cysteine persulfides and S-polythiolation regulate oxidative stress and redox signaling. Proc Natl Acad Sci USA 2014;111:7606–11. https://doi.org/10.1073/pnas.1321232111.

[111] Krishnan N, Fu C, Pappin DJ, Tonks NK. H_2S-Induced sulfhydration of the phosphatase PTP1B and its role in the endoplasmic reticulum stress response. Sci Signal 2011;4:ra86. https://doi.org/10.1126/scisignal.2002329.

[112] Dóka É, Pader I, Bíró A, Johansson K, Cheng Q, Ballagó K, et al. A novel persulfide detection method reveals protein persulfide- and polysulfide-reducing functions of thioredoxin and glutathione systems. Sci Adv 2016;2:e1500968. https://doi.org/10.1126/sciadv.1500968.

[113] Dóka É, Ida T, Dagnell M, Abiko Y, Luong NC, Balog N, et al. Control of protein function through oxidation and reduction of persulfidated states. Sci Adv 2020;6:eaax8358. https://doi.org/10.1126/sciadv.aax8358.

[114] Wedmann R, Onderka C, Wei S, Szijártó IA, Miljkovic JL, Mitrovic A, et al. Improved tag-switch method reveals that thioredoxin acts as depersulfidase and controls the intracellular levels of protein persulfidation. Chem Sci 2016;7:3414–26. https://doi.org/10.1039/C5SC04818D.

[115] Ono K, Akaike T, Sawa T, Kumagai Y, Wink DA, Tantillo DJ, et al. Redox chemistry and chemical biology of H_2S, hydropersulfides, and derived species: implications of their possible biological activity and utility. Free Radic Biol Med 2014;77:82–94. https://doi.org/10.1016/j.freeradbiomed.2014.09.007.

[116] Heppner DE, Hristova M, Ida T, Mijuskovic A, Dustin CM, Bogdándi V, et al. Cysteine perthiosulfenic acid (Cys-SSOH): a novel intermediate in thiol-based redox signaling? Redox Biol 2018;14:379–85. https://doi.org/10.1016/j.redox.2017.10.006.

[117] Zivanovic J, Kouroussis E, Kohl JB, Adhikari B, Bursac B, Schott-Roux S, et al. Selective persulfide detection reveals evolutionarily conserved antiaging effects of S-sulfhydration. Cell Metab 2019;30:1152–1170.e13. https://doi.org/10.1016/j.cmet.2019.10.007.

[118] Shen J, Zhang J, Zhou M, Zhou H, Cui B, Gotor C, et al. Persulfidation-based modification of cysteine desulfhydrase and the NADPH oxidase RBOHD controls guard cell abscisic acid signaling. Plant Cell 2020;32. https://doi.org/10.1105/tpc.19.00826.tpc.00826.2019.

[119] Barayeu U, Schilling D, Eid M, Silva T, Schlicker L, Mitreska N, et al. Hydropersulfides inhibit lipid peroxidation and ferroptosis by scavenging radicals. Nat Chem Biol 2022:1–10. https://doi.org/10.1038/s41589-022-01145-w.

[120] Kim HS, Ullevig SL, Nguyen HN, Vanegas D, Asmis R. Redox regulation of 14-3-3ζ controls monocyte migration. Arterioscler Thromb Vasc Biol 2014;34:1514–21. https://doi.org/10.1161/ATVBAHA.114.303746.

[121] Silva GM, Netto LES, Simões V, Santos LFA, Gozzo FC, Demasi MAA, et al. Redox control of 20S proteasome gating. Antioxid Redox Signal 2012;16:1183–94. https://doi.org/10.1089/ars.2011.4210.

[122] Livnat-Levanon N, Kevei É, Kleifeld O, Krutauz D, Segref A, Rinaldi T, et al. Reversible 26S proteasome disassembly upon mitochondrial stress. Cell Rep 2014;7:1371–80. https://doi.org/10.1016/j.celrep.2014.04.030.

[123] Hoppe G, Chai Y-C, Crabb JW, Sears J. Protein s-glutathionylation in retinal pigment epithelium converts heat shock protein 70 to an active chaperone. Exp Eye Res 2004;78:1085–92. https://doi.org/10.1016/j.exer.2004.02.001.

[124] Um H-C, Jang J-H, Kim D-H, Lee C, Surh Y-J. Nitric oxide activates Nrf2 through S-nitrosylation of Keap1 in PC12 cells. Nitric Oxide 2011;25:161–8. https://doi.org/10.1016/j.niox.2011.06.001.

[125] Carvalho AN, Marques C, Guedes RC, Castro-Caldas M, Rodrigues E, van Horssen J, et al. S-glutathionylation of Keap1: a new role for glutathione S-transferase pi in neuronal protection. FEBS (Fed Eur Biochem Soc) Lett 2016;590:1455–66. https://doi.org/10.1002/1873-3468.12177.

[126] Tocmo R, Parkin K. S-1-propenylmercaptocysteine protects murine hepatocytes against oxidative stress via persulfidation of Keap1 and activation of Nrf2. Free Radic Biol Med 2019;143:164–75. https://doi.org/10.1016/j.freeradbiomed.2019.07.022.

[127] Hausladen A, Privalle CT, Keng T, DeAngelo J, Stamler JS. Nitrosative stress: activation of the transcription factor OxyR. Cell 1996;86:719–29. https://doi.org/10.1016/S0092-8674(00)80147-6.

[128] Seth D, Hausladen A, Stamler JS. Anaerobic transcription by OxyR: a novel paradigm for nitrosative stress. Antioxid Redox Signal 2020;32:803–16. https://doi.org/10.1089/ars.2019.7921.

[129] Delaunay A, Pflieger D, Barrault MB, Vinh J, Toledano MB. A thiol peroxidase is an H_2O_2 receptor and redox-transducer in gene activation. Cell 2002;111:471–81. https://doi.org/10.1016/s0092-8674(02)01048-6.

[130] Pineda-Molina E, Klatt P, Vázquez J, Marina A, García de Lacoba M, Pérez-Sala D, et al. Glutathionylation of the p50 subunit of NF-κB: a mechanism for redox-induced inhibition of DNA binding. Biochemistry 2001;40:14134–42. https://doi.org/10.1021/bi011459o.

[131] Reynaert NL, van der Vliet A, Guala AS, McGovern T, Hristova M, Pantano C, et al. Dynamic redox control of NF-kappaB through glutaredoxin-regulated S-glutathionylation of inhibitory kappaB kinase beta. Proc Natl Acad Sci USA 2006;103:13086–91. https://doi.org/10.1073/pnas.0603290103.

[132] Klatt P, Molina EP, de Lacoba MG, Padilla CA, Martínez-Galisteo E, Barcena J, Lamas S. Redox regulation of c-Jun DNA binding by reversible S-glutathiolation. FASEB J 1999;13:1481–90. https://doi.org/10.1096/fasebj.13.12.1481.

[133] Knoepfel L, Steinkühler C, Carrì MT, Rotilio G. Role of zinc-coordination and of the glutathione redox couple in the redox susceptibility of human transcription factor Sp1. Biochem Biophys Res Commun 1994;201:871–7. https://doi.org/10.1006/bbrc.1994.1782.

[134] Marinkovic D, Zhang X, Yalcin S, Luciano JP, Brugnara C, Huber T, Ghaffari S. Foxo3 is required for the regulation of oxidative stress in erythropoiesis. J Clin Invest 2007;117:2133–44. https://doi.org/10.1172/JCI31807.

[135] Grillo M, Palmer C, Holmes N, Sang F, Larner AC, Bhosale R, Shaw PE. Stat3 oxidation-dependent regulation of gene expression impacts on developmental processes and involves cooperation with Hif-1α. PLoS One 2020;15:e0244255. https://doi.org/10.1371/journal.pone.0244255.

[136] Hopkins BL, Neumann CA. Redoxins as gatekeepers of the transcriptional oxidative stress response. Redox Biol 2019;21:101104. https://doi.org/10.1016/j.redox.2019.101104.

Chapter 3

Regulation of NRF2 signaling pathway and the hallmarks of aging: An overview

Alessandro Medoro, Giovanni Scapagnini and Sergio Davinelli
Department of Medicine and Health Sciences "V. Tiberio", University of Molise, Campobasso, Italy

Introduction

Aging is an extraordinarily complicated process defined by a gradual loss of physiological abilities and adaptive capacities and an increase in the risk of illness and mortality. The incidence of age-related diseases has become the greatest health threat in the 21st century. Understanding the relationships between the processes of aging and age-related diseases is an important issue to improve the health of the aging population [1].

Oxidant stress increases across a variety of tissues in an age-dependent manner and plays a crucial role in the development of diverse chronic age-related diseases including cancer, neurodegeneration, and cardiovascular disease [2]. The oxidative stress theory of aging is based on the structural damage-based hypothesis that age-associated functional losses are due to the accumulation of oxidative damage to macromolecules (lipids, carbohydrates, DNA, and proteins). This damage is caused by many electrophilic molecules, principally the reactive oxygen species (ROS). Although the oxidative stress theory of aging has received criticism, it remains true that oxidant stress plays a significant role in the aging process [3]. Therefore, the imbalance caused by the accumulation of these species leads to oxidative stress and promotes disease when they are not effectively removed. This is particularly relevant in the context of aging, where the accumulation of oxidative stress is considered a key driving force that ultimately increases susceptibility to developing age-related pathologies. The overall redox, metabolic, and protein homeostasis of the cell are all impacted by the damage that ROS-induced free radicals cause to important intracellular components, which contributes to increased sensitivity [4].

Numerous endogenous antioxidant systems are in place to ensure that ROS are properly reduced, but the first line defense is represented by the nuclear factor erythroid 2-related factor 2 (NRF2)-Kelch-like ECH-associated protein 1 (KEAP1) signaling pathway. Oxidation–reduction mechanisms promoted by NRF2 transcriptional activity are vital regulators of cellular survival and homeostasis [5]. Nevertheless, only recent studies address NRF2 function in other contexts such as aging and lifespan regulation. Indicatives are examples of the involvement of the NRF2 homolog skinhead-1 (SKN-1) in *Caenorhabditis elegans* and the *Drosophila melanogaster* homolog CncC, in determining longevity. Genes involved in the oxidative stress response, including many orthologs of those regulated by mammalian NRF2, are upregulated by the activation of SKN-1 and CncC, significantly increasing longevity [6,7].

However, despite its ability to counteract biochemical alterations which are at the basis of aging, NRF2 activity and expression are reduced during aging. Evidence for this phenomenon was initially reported in a rat model showing a decline with age of basal levels of NRF2. Such NRF2 reduced function directly correlates with lower expression of its target genes, intracellular glutathione levels, and increased generation of oxidation products [6,8]. Indeed, it has been reported that aged mice show a loss in cellular redox capacity to those observed in NRF2-knockout (KO) mice [8,9].

Therefore, the failure of dynamical regulation of NRF2 expression and transcriptional activity may intensively contribute to the loss of cellular homeostasis. In this scenario, cells become more sensitive to functional alterations, driven by NRF2-mediated transcription reduction, which in turn promotes the aging phenotype. Accordingly, the relationship between NRF2 and aging is not limited to the reduction of oxidative stress. There is a number of key pathological features associated with aging, collectively called the "hallmarks of aging," that play an important role in driving age-related pathologies and to which reduction of

Modulation of Oxidative Stress. https://doi.org/10.1016/B978-0-443-19247-0.00004-7

NRF2 in aging cells massively contributes [2,10]. However, several synthetic and natural NRF2 modulators were studied with the scope to restore NRF2 activity during aging as a promising therapeutic approach for diverse age-related diseases [11].

NRF2 and KEAP1 structures and pathways

NRF2-KEAP1 pathway is a ubiquitous conserved antistress mechanism aimed to preserve cellular homeostasis, principally preventing a deregulated redox status induced by excessive production of reactive molecules, principally ROS, and detoxifying the organism from exogenous or endogenous harmful substances [12]. The importance of NRF2 in regulating antioxidant defense is underlined by an evolutionary basis. Indeed, it is highly conserved across vertebrates. Compared with human NRF2, mouse NRF2 has DNA and protein homology scores of 83.4% and 82.5%, respectively; rat NRF2, 84%, and 83%; cow NRF2, 91% and 89%; dog MRF2, 89.4% and 88.9%; chicken NRF2, 72% and 67% [13].

The prevailing model by which KEAP1 regulates NRF2 is the so-called "hinge and latch" model [14,15], where KEAP1 conformational changes are involved in catching and releasing NRF2. Nevertheless, KEAP1 is not simply an NRF2 intracellular inhibitor, but it can be considered the central hub for sensing endogenous and environmental oxidative and electrophilic stress in all vertebrates. The elaborate system involving KEAP1 thiol groups of specific cysteines is the primary transducer of redox signals within signaling proteins [16].

In detail, KEAP1 is a 69-kDa protein that shows some homology with actin-binding Kelch protein and acts as an NRF2 negative regulator. The human KEAP1 protein sequence contains 627 amino acid residues structured into five diverse domains: (1) the N-terminal region (NTR), (2) the Broad complex, Tramtrack, and Bric-a-Brac (BTB), (3) the linker intervening region (IVR), (4) Kelch domain, and (5) the C-terminal region (CTR) (Fig. 3.1). BTB domain is responsible for homodimerization and interaction with Cullin (Cul3)-based ubiquitin E3 ligase complex necessary for NFR2 ubiquitination. IVR-containing cysteine residues are sensitive to oxidation and nuclear export signal (NES) motifs. Kelch domain has six kelch repeats and multiple protein contact sites that mediate the binding of KEAP1 with NRF2 and cytoskeleton proteins. KEAP1 contains a total of 27 cysteine residues, and three of them (i.e., Cys151, Cys273, and Cys288) are highly reactive and susceptible to covalent modifications by ROS and other electrophiles, converting this protein in a redox sensor for endogenous and environmental oxidative signals [17].

NRF2 is a member of the cap "n" collar (CNC) subfamily of basic region leucine zipper (bZip) transcription factors. In humans, NRF2 protein is 605 amino acids long and contains seven highly conserved regions known as NRF2-ECH homology (Neh) domains (Fig. 3.1). Neh2 domain is an N-terminal regulatory domain and contains seven lysine residues that influence the ubiquitin conjugation and two peptide binding motifs (ETGE and DLG) that regulate NRF2 interaction with Kelch domain of KEAP1 [17,18]. Neh1 contains the CNC−bZIP domain, which regulates DNA-binding, and a nuclear localization signal (NLS) that is responsible for the nuclear translocation of NRF2, while Neh3, Neh4, and Neh5 are transactivation domains mediating the interaction of NRF2 with other coactivators [18−21]. Neh6 domain with serine-rich residues is a negative regulatory domain that binds to a β-transducin repeat-containing protein (β-TrCP) leading to an alternative pathway for NRF2 ubiquitination [22]. The

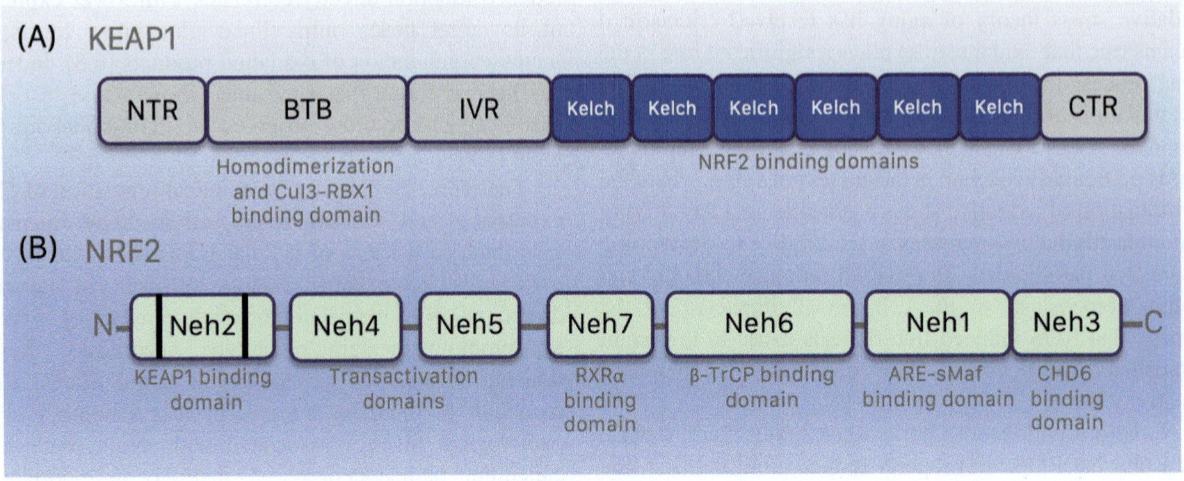

FIGURE 3.1 (A) Schematic structure of KEAP1 and (B) NRF2. NRF2 contains seven highly conserved domains (Neh1-Neh7). KEAP1 consists of five domains that include the l region (NTR), the BTB domain, the central linker domain called IVR, six Kelch domains, and the C-terminal region (CTR).

Neh7 domain inhibits the NRF2 signaling pathway by promoting the binding of NRF2 to the retinoic X receptor α (RXRα) [23].

As mentioned, the interaction between NRF2 and KEAP1 is necessary for the regulation of many pathways during physiological and stress conditions. Therefore, under basal conditions, NRF2 is a protein of low abundance in the cytoplasm with a limited half-life. Therefore, the binding between NRF2 and KEAP1 homodimer, in turn, involved in a complex with Cul3-RING box protein 1 (Rbx1) ubiquitin ligase, promotes a rapid turnover of NRF2 through polyubiquitination and proteasomal degradation [24] (Fig. 3.2). Instead, under cellular stress conditions, such as oxidative imbalance, oxidative/electrophilic modification of thiol residues of cysteines in KEAP1 induces a conformational change, disrupting the Cul3-Rbx1 ubiquitin ligase interaction required for NRF2 proteasomal degradation. This activation allows NRF2 translocation into the nucleus to initiate the transcription of genes, which contain the regulatory sequence known as antioxidant responsive element (ARE), encoding proteins with many different functions, including important enzymes with detoxifying and antioxidant roles [25,26].

NRF2 nuclear translocation is facilitated by the phosphorylation by protein kinase C delta type (PKCδ) [28] and AMP-activated protein kinase (AMPK) [27]. Karyopherin α1 (importin α5) and karyopherin β1 (importin β1) are responsible for NRF2 nuclear translocation through the nuclear pore complex [21].

For its transcriptional activity, NRF2 requires several binding partners, such as: (a) sMaf, fundamental dimeric co-activator that binds NRF2 allowing the recognition of ARE sequence in the target gene promoter region [28]; (b) CREB-binding protein (CBP)/p300 and SUMO-conjugating enzyme UBC9, which has respectively acetyltransferase and SUMOylation activity allowing promoter-specific DNA binding [18,20,29]; (c) chromodomain helicase DNA binding protein 6 (CHD6), a chromo-adenosine triphosphate (ATP)ase/helicase DNA binding protein that allows chromatin remodeling [19]; (d) the mediator, an evolutionarily conserved multiprotein complex essential for RNA polymerase II-driven transcription [30]; and (e) other transcription factors, such as Jun-D, c-Jun, and Jun-B, activating transcription factors 3 and 4 (ATF3, ATF4), receptor-associated coactivator 3 (RAC3), runt-related transcription

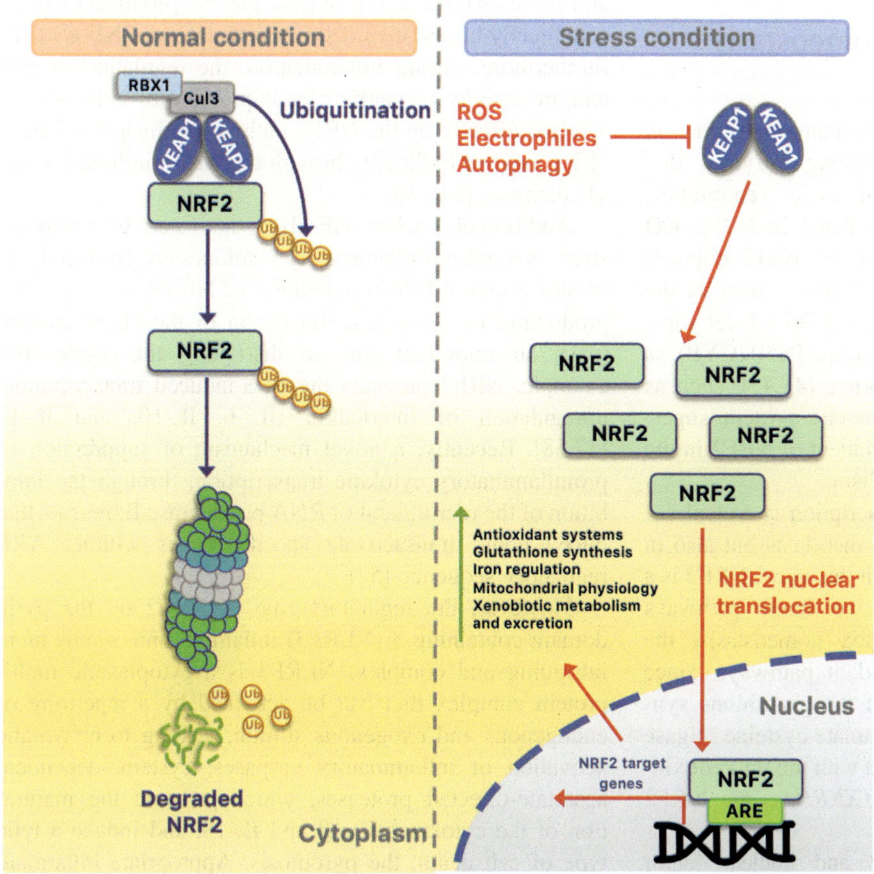

FIGURE 3.2 NRF2 pathways under normal and stress conditions. NRF2 is negatively regulated by KEAP1-Cul3-RBX1 complex under normal condition. De novo NRF2 protein levels increase following exposure of KEAP1 to ROS, electrophiles, or autophagy dysregulation, NRF2 translocates to the nucleus, binding the ARE to activate the transcription of its target genes.

factor 2 (Runx2), and Yin Yang 1 (YY1), able to increase NRF2 transcriptional activity [24,31].

However, emerging evidence has revealed several regulation mechanisms of NRF2 degradation that are independent of KEAP1 activity. For example, glycogen synthase kinase-3 (GSK3) is a crucial protein involved in KEAP1-independent NRF2 stabilization and regulation. It phosphorylates NRF2 enhancing the binding β-TrCP that forms the ubiquitin ligase complex with Skp1, Cul1, and Rbx1 proteins, thus promoting the subsequent NRF2 degradation [22,32]. In cell-based ubiquitylation analysis, Hrd1, another ubiquitin ligase, mediates NRF2 ubiquitylation and degradation in the cytosol, independently from KEAP1 and β-TrCP, through specific binding to NRF2 [33]. Ubiquitination and degradation of NRF2 can also be mediated by nuclear-localized WD-repeat protein 23 (WDR23) that interacts with the Cul4-DDB1 ubiquitin ligase complex, proposing that the posttranslational regulation of NRF2 may not be limited to the cytoplasm [34,35].

Furthermore, a noncanonical pathway of NRF2 activation in a p62-dependent manner was carried out. In this pathway, p62 sequesters KEAP1 to autophagic degradation, ultimately leading to the stabilization of NRF2 and the transactivation of NRF2-dependent genes [36–38].

NRF2 signaling in redox homeostasis and inflammation

NRF2 nuclear complex regulates principally the induction of genes encoding phase II detoxifying enzymes that participate in the detoxification of toxic xenobiotics; indeed, these enzymes are down-regulated in NRF2 KO mice [39,40]. Further studies showed that NRF2 controls also the expression of phase I-related genes, such as the family of aldehyde dehydrogenases, NAD(P)H dehydrogenase quinone 1 (NQO1), and cytochrome P450 (CYP), as well as phase III xenobiotic transporters [41,42], such as transporters of the ATP-binding cassette protein superfamily (ABC), thus indicating involvement of NRF2 in the whole process of xenobiotic metabolism.

Moreover, NRF2-dependent transcription is critical not only in maintaining normal redox homeostasis but also in restoring it after an oxidative insult. In this view, NRF2 is a principal transcription factor of two main pathways involved in the restoration of redox homeostasis, the glutathione and thioredoxin antioxidant pathways, since catalytic and modulatory subunits of the glutathione synthesizing enzymes, such as glutamate-cysteine ligase (*GCLC*, *GCLM*) and genes associated with the thioredoxin-based antioxidant system (*TXN1*, *TXNRD1*), are NRF2 target genes [43–45].

During oxidative stress, NRF2 and nuclear factor kappa-light-chain-enhancer of activated B cells (NF-κB) signaling pathways interact to control the transcription and function of downstream target proteins: the crosstalk between NRF2 and NF-κB pathways is even a key point in the regulation of cellular responses to oxidative stress and inflammation [46]. The activation and the nuclear translocation of NF-κB promote the transcription of proinflammatory mediators and drive the inflammatory phenotype, whereas the activation of NRF2 negatively regulates the NF-κB signaling pathway, directly and indirectly [47–50]. Both NRF2 and NF-κB compete for CBP, a cofactor required for transcriptional responses, indicating that, when the activity of one of these transcription factors is increased, the other cannot bind to CBP, and thus transcription of its target genes is reduced [51].

The anti-inflammatory role of NRF2 is linked to the promotion of antioxidant gene expression and the prevention of proinflammatory pathways. Principally, NRF2 promotes the expression of heme oxygenase-1 (HO-1), an inducible 32 kDa enzyme that catalyzes the degradation of heme into three bioactive products: carbon monoxide (CO), free iron, and biliverdin, which is rapidly converted to bilirubin. HO-1 exerts its protective effect through both the enzymatic degradation of proinflammatory free heme and the production of compounds, such as CO and bilirubin, that act as a powerful antioxidant during oxidative stress and cell damage [52,53]. Indeed, the end-products of HO-1 can directly inhibit the nuclear translocation of NF-κB [47]. Furthermore, during inflammation, the regulation of proteolytic activity of matrix metalloproteinases is negatively affected directly by the NRF2 pathway (principally NRF2/HO-1 axis) or indirectly through the NRF2-influenced NF-κB pathway [54–56].

Additionally, when NF-κB is activated by oxidative stress, several proinflammatory cytokines are produced and in turn promote further activation of NF-κB and the overproduction of cytokines. Activation of the NRF2 system plays an important role in disrupting this cycle. For example, NRF2 prevents the LPS-induced transcriptional upregulation of interleukin (IL)-6, IL-1β, and IL-17 [57,58]. Recently, a novel mechanism of suppression of proinflammatory cytokine transcription, through the inhibition of the recruitment of RNA polymerase II, reveals that NRF2 could transactivate specific genes without ARE regulatory sequence [57].

However, the regulatory role of NRF2 on the pyrin domain containing 3 (NLRP3) inflammasome seems more intriguing and complex. NLRP3 is a cytoplasmic multiprotein complex that can be activated by a repertoire of endogenous and exogenous stimuli, leading to enzymatic activation of inflammatory caspases, cysteine-dependent aspartate-directed proteases, which promote the maturation of the cytokines IL-1β and IL-18, and induce a lytic type of cell death, the pyroptosis. Appropriate inflammasome activation is essential for the response to foreign pathogens or tissue damage, while aberrant activation can determine uncontrolled tissue responses that contribute to various diseases, including autoinflammatory disorders, cancer, and neurodegenerative diseases. The role of NRF2 in the regulation of NLRP3 inflammasome activity is paradoxical: on the one hand, NRF2 can negatively modulate NLRP3 transcription, nuclear translocation, and inflammasome assembly [59,60], on the other hand, NRF2 KO mouse macrophages show a defective activation of NLRP3 inflammasome. However, this dual role should not be surprising since NRF2 should not be considered only as an anti-inflammatory factor, but as a fine modulator of aberrant inflammatory pathways to maintain cellular homeostasis [61].

NRF2 and the hallmarks of aging

Aging is associated with a gradual decrease in overall cell signaling pathways, including those related to NRF2. Many factors, such as increased expression of negative regulators, the decline in transcriptional activity and pathway responsiveness, epigenetic silencing, degradation of mRNA and protein, and competition with other transcription factors (e.g., NF-κB), gradually reduce NRF2 signaling with age. The consequent inhibition of expression of its target genes promotes cellular aging phenotype [2].

Given that the NRF2 role is not limited to the expression of detoxifying, antioxidant, and anti-inflammatory enzymes, it should be regarded as a cellular homeostatic factor, regulating several aspects of cellular activity. The loss of NRF2 signaling could potentially drive all key pathological hallmarks associated with mammalian aging, including genomic instability, telomere attrition, epigenetic alterations, loss of proteostasis, deregulated nutrient sensing, mitochondrial dysfunction, cellular senescence, stem cell exhaustion, and altered intercellular communication (Fig. 3.3) [10].

Loss of proteostasis

The dynamic regulation of a balanced and functional proteome is disrupted with age by the intracellular accumulation and aggregation of unfolded and misfolded proteins, impairing the normal function of the cell.

The unfolded protein response (UPR) is activated to combat proteotoxic stress as misfolded proteins accumulate in the endoplasmic reticulum (ER). There are three distinct branches of the UPR: (1) XBP1 mRNA splicing via inositol requiring enzyme 1 (IRE1) that activates transcription of chaperones and endoplasmic reticulum-associated protein degradation (ERAD) proteins; (2) protein kinase RNA-like endoplasmic reticulum kinase (PERK) phosphorylation of eIF2 that activate ATF4-mediated transcription of redox enzymes and cell death proteins while concurrently attenuating translation; and (3) proteolytic cleavage of ATF6 to activate transcription of UPR target genes.

Sodium arsenite and paraquat-induced ROS, if their toxic effects are not opportunely attenuated, inhibit the UPR, increasing ER stress due to the loss of its kinase activity and activating NRF2 in a p38 mitogen-activated protein kinase (MAPK)-dependent manner [62]. On the other hand, UPR activation of PERK induces phosphorylation of NRF2 disrupting the interaction of NRF2-KEAP1 [63]. In both situations, restoration of normal cellular function is obtained by the reduction of ROS in the ER through the induction of redox regulatory proteins. By upregulating target genes including glutathione peroxidase 2 (GPX2), NRF2 activation reduces hydrogen peroxide levels, which may prevent the loss of proteostasis [64]. ATG5, ATG7, and other autophagy-related proteins are regulated by NRF2 to modulate the formation of autophagosomes [65], which means that if NRF2 is reduced, autophagy initiation would be reduced, and misfolded or damaged proteins would accumulate. Considering that NRF2 controls the UPR, proteasome, and autophagy, it follows that a loss of NRF2 signaling may be a major factor causing the proteotoxic phenotype seen in many age-related disorders.

Genomic instability

Lack of DNA damage repair when the NRF2 system is impaired with age causes aging-related genomic instability, resulting in increased frequency of mutations and chromosomal aberrations. Therefore, with aging, the incidence of replication mistakes during DNA duplication increases. Additionally, the base excision repair machinery is less effective, increasing the likelihood of mutations leading to cancer and neurological diseases. Target genes of NRF2 include p53-binding protein (53BP1) and DNA repair protein RAD51 homolog 1 (RAD51), which are important in both repairing pathways, homologous recombination (HR), and nonhomologous end joining (NHEJ).

By binding to the exposed ends of damaged DNA strands and limiting the recruitment of repair complexes, 53BP1, for instance, promotes NHEJ by preventing the resection stage of HR [66]. The DNA strands can subsequently be ligated as a result of the Ku dimeric protein complex being able to attach to the damaged ends of the DNA. On the other hand, RAD51 is a crucial protein in HR because it creates a nucleoprotein filament on DNA that helps with homologous strand pairing [67]. Furthermore, NRF2 is also an activator of ataxia telangiectasia and Rad3-related protein (ATR), whose activation occurs in response to single-strand breaks to ensure genomic integrity [66–68].

These NRF2 target genes aid in DNA repair, preventing aging and illness. Therefore, whether NRF2 is decreased,

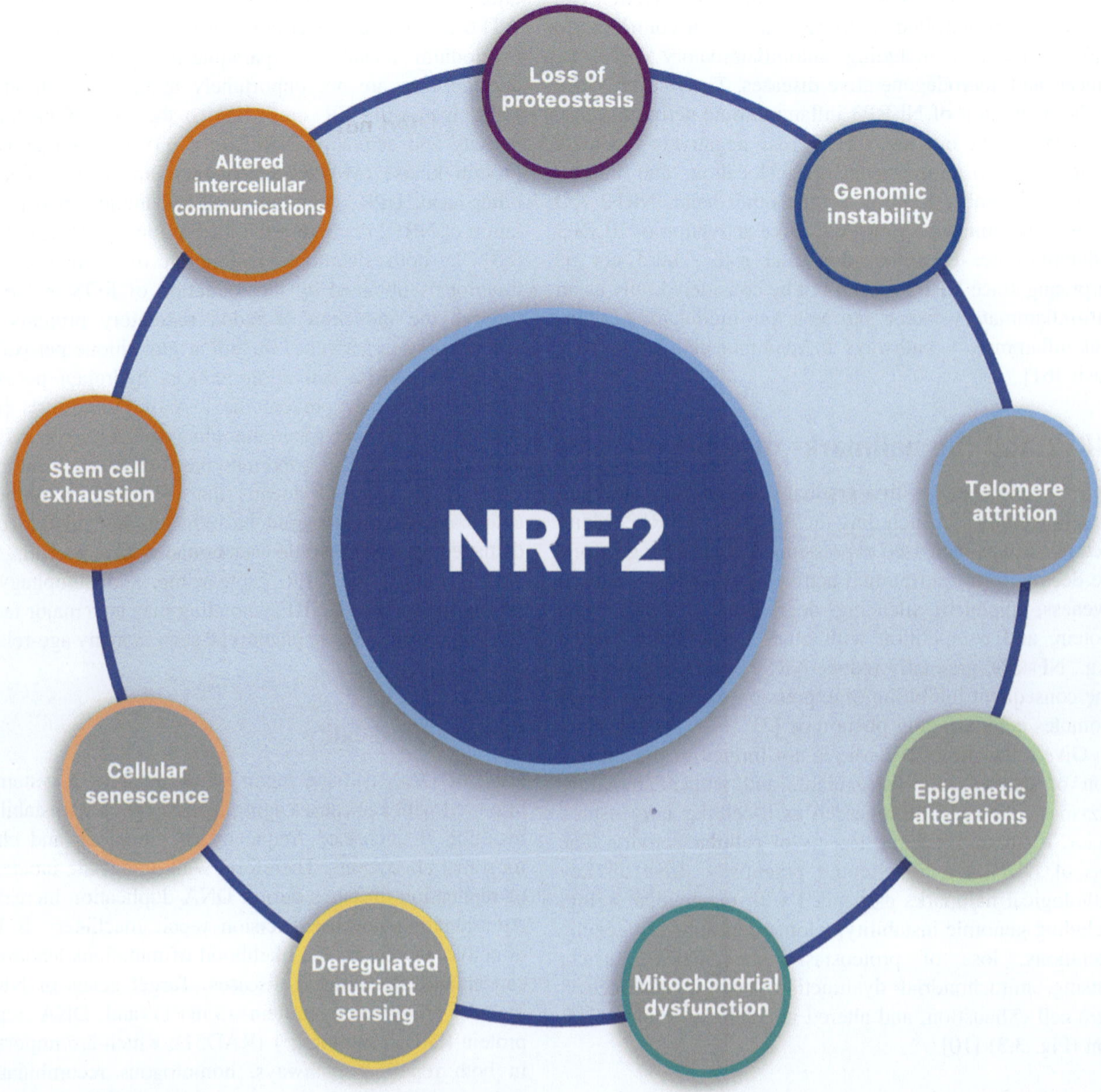

FIGURE 3.3 Age-related reduction of NRF2 contributes to the hallmarks of aging. NRF2 reduction is implicated in loss of proteostasis, genomic instability, telomere attrition, epigenetic alterations, mitochondrial dysfunction, deregulated nutrient sensing, cellular senescence, stem cell exhaustion, and altered intercellular communications.

DNA repair would be prevented, resulting in an overall rise in the number of mutations.

Telomere attrition

Telomere attrition and the resulting reduction of duplication of chromosomes during mitosis are typical hallmarks of aging. Cells that cannot regenerate and divide make them more vulnerable to damage accumulation, which can eventually cause loss of function, senescence, or death. NRF2 and telomerase reverse transcriptase (TERT), an integral component of the telomerase complex, have recently been connected, and it was found that higher NRF2 levels result in higher TERT expression [18]. This complex promotes the lengthening of telomeres, enabling continuous cell division, and preventing chromosomal degradation and apoptosis. It has been demonstrated that the NRF2 and TERT positive loop encourages cell survival. Therefore, a decrease in NRF2-driven TERT expression may be essential in telomeres shortening.

In normal conditions, increased NRF2 levels promote cell survival and division through elevated levels of telomerase reverse transcriptase (TERT), an essential subunit of the telomerase complex that promotes the extension of telomeres at DNA ends: reduced NRF2 expression and activity may contribute to the telomeres shortening in aged cells [69–71].

Epigenetic alterations

Epigenetic alterations, such as DNA methylation and acetylation, are increased during aging. DNA methyltransferases promote the methylation of cytosine residues, particularly those in CpG islands, which prevents transcription from being activated. Increased DNA methylation with age is a result of elevated inflammation and decreased production of metabolic intermediates. Khor et al. demonstrated that the hypermethylation in the NRF2 promoter region inhibits NRF2 transcription and induces cancer [72]. As microRNA (miRNA) regulates the production of essential DNA methyltransferases and histone deacetylases, they have also been demonstrated to play a role in the epigenetic regulation of genes. Accordingly, miRNA-144 could reduce NRF2 expression, which raises hydrogen peroxide levels [73]. Although many of the relationships between epigenetic changes, NRF2, and aging are still unknown, several findings have shown that NRF2 expression is controlled by epigenetic factors, especially in cancer, suggesting that the interaction between NRF2, and these factors may also play a significant role in the aging process.

Mitochondrial dysfunction

The mitochondria, which may create reactive species as a consequence of the electron transport chain, are a significant cause of cellular stress. In aging cells, mitochondrial dysfunction is prominent, and it has been linked to several age-related pathologies [74]. By regulating the cellular redox balance, fatty acid oxidation, membrane potential, and structural integrity of mitochondria, NRF2 is important in preserving the appropriate mitochondrial functions [75]. Therefore, the increasing mitochondrial dysfunction linked to age-related pathologies may be caused by an age-related decrease in NRF2 function. B-cell lymphoma 2 (BCL-2) and B-cell lymphoma-extra-large (BCL-xL) are anti-apoptotic mitochondrial proteins that are expressed in response to cell death [76]. Proapoptotic pathways, including activation of mitochondrial permeability transition pores (MPTP), may start if the expression of these proteins is low. Increased MPTP causes the disruption of the Krebs cycle, reduces ATP production, increases the production of superoxide and hydroxyl radicals, and releases cytochrome C into the cytosol, perpetuating mitochondrial damage and function loss. Accordingly, loss of NRF2 activity could be linked to an increased risk of apoptosis, while induction of NRF2 maintains the mitochondrial function, preventing age-related mitochondrial dysfunction.

Deregulated nutrient sensing

Nutrient sensing pathways play a crucial role in aging and longevity. Among these, the essential nutrient sensor protein AMP-activated protein kinase (AMPK) is activated when ATP levels are decreased. Nevertheless, it has been discovered that AMPK responsiveness declines with aging [77]. Through the nuclear localization of NRF2, induced by serine 550 phosphorylation, AMPK has also been associated with its activation [27]. Therefore, a lack of AMPK activity causes a decrease in NRF2 signaling in aged cells. As a result, the age-related downregulation of NRF2 would substantially affect the flux of metabolites via important metabolic pathways, contributing to the unregulated nutrient metabolism and sensing as seen in age-related pathogenesis. Therefore, target genes of NRF2 are involved in several metabolic processes such as the pentose phosphate pathway and purine biosynthesis [78,79].

Cellular senescence

The senescence of healthy cells promotes the aging phenotype by preventing proliferation. NRF2 was downregulated in older fibroblasts compared to younger cells, demonstrating a relationship between NRF2 and senescence in these cells. Therefore, the effects of general oxidative stress were more prominent in older fibroblasts. Furthermore, proteasome activation prevented the senescence of young cells treated with an NRF2 inducer compared to untreated controls. In detail, NRF2 activation stimulates proteasome production via proteasome maturation protein (POMP) and proteasome subunit alpha type-1 (PSMA1), which extend longevity and avoid senescence. Additionally, treatment of senescent cells with an NRF2 inducer reversed the senescent phenotype and restored proliferation [80]. Senescence and the aging phenotype are exacerbated when NRF2 levels are low because NRF2 generally inhibits cellular senescence.

Stem cell exhaustion

Stem cell renewal and differentiation are essential for sustaining tissue homeostasis and repair. However, the activity of stem cells in all tissues and organs declines with aging. NRF2 seems to have two functions in stem cell renewal. A significant decrease in NRF2 expression is responsible for a dramatic reduction in neural stem progenitor cells (NSPCs) survival and regeneration (proliferation and neuronal differentiation) during middle age. It has been also demonstrated that NRF2 overexpression can enhance NSPC survival and function. Moreover, the overexpression of NRF2 has been linked to enhanced proteasome formation, which aids in the promotion of human embryonic stem cell differentiation [81,82].

Moreover, the pharmacological activation of the NRF2-mediated antioxidative response pathway in mesenchymal stem cells (MSCs) differentiated from induced pluripotent stem cells (iPSCs) [83]. However, persistent NRF2 hyperactivation might cause unchecked regeneration and stem cell depletion [84]. These findings point out the critical role of NRF2 in stem cells and emphasize the need to maintain NRF2 activity during aging to preserve stem cells' viability and functionality as well as to prevent their depletion.

Altered intercellular communications

Inflammation could be considered one of the crucial pathogenic effects that alter intercellular communication between aging cells. The involvement of NRF2 in inflammation is linked to the dualism with NF-κB, a proinflammatory transcription factor that drives the inflammatory phenotype by increasing interleukin levels. This dualism between NRF2 and NF-κB, as described above, is due to competition for the shared cofactor CBP required for both transcriptional responses. This implies that when either of the two factors' activity is upregulated, transcription of the other is downregulated, as during neurodegenerative diseases [51]. Therefore, inflammation is a constant factor during neurodegeneration, and, accordingly, NF-κB is constantly upregulated promoting the inflammation phenotype and reduction of NRF2 transcriptional activity [2].

Intriguingly, α-synuclein, a protein linked to diverse neurodegenerative diseases, promotes NF-κB activation, while NRF2 enhances its clearance preventing the inflammatory phenotype [85,86]. In this case, the decrease of NRF2 activity could be the cause of the altered intercellular communication with the consequent α-synuclein accumulation and inflammatory state during neurodegeneration.

NRF2 modulators

Recently, it has been revealed that NRF2 can be pharmacologically targeted in several age-related diseases, especially those characterized by oxidative stress and inflammation [7,8]. In models of chronic diseases, a reinforcement of homeostasis through NRF2 activators provides a beneficial therapeutic effect. However, many modulators of NRF2 act on its inhibitor KEAP1. Electrophilic molecules that covalently modify the thiol group of cysteine residues (mainly Cys151, Cys273, and Cys288) of KEAP1 protein are the main pharmacological NRF2 modulators [87]. These cysteine modifications generate a nonfunctional closed state with both Neh2 motifs (DLG and ETGE) of NRF2 that interact with KEAP1 dimer, mediating newly synthesized NRF2 escape from KEAP1-mediated ubiquitination and subsequent degradation. An alternative inhibition mechanism of KEAP1 is represented by the disruption of KEAP1 binding with Cul3/RBX1 complex, required for NRF2 ubiquitination, mediated by the adduct formation with Cys151 in the BTB domain [88].

During the last years, the list of electrophilic compounds able to interact with KEAP1 is continuously growing; however, in this chapter, only compounds approved or studied in clinical trials were described.

Pentacyclic triterpenoid 2-cyano-3,12-dioxo-oleana-1,9(11)-dien-28-oate (bardoxolone, CDDO, RTA401) disrupts the interaction of KEAP1 with Cul3, promoting NRF2 escape from ubiquitination [89,90]. A derivative molecule, bardoxolone methyl (CDDO-Me or RTA 402), started clinical trials for advanced chronic kidney disease (CKD) and type 2 diabetes mellitus. Despite demonstrating a long-term increase in glomerular filtration in phase II clinical trials, CDDO-Me was halted in phase III due to its cardiovascular safety. A new phase II clinical trial to better define the safety and efficacy profiles of CDDO-Me has recently begun recruiting patients with rare CKD. CDDO-Me is currently being tested in clinical trials for Alport syndrome and pulmonary hypertension [91,92]. To improve the safety profile, a second-generation difluoromethyl acetamide derivative of bardoxolone methyl called RTA-408 (Omaveloxone) is now being studied in phase II clinical trials for Friedreich's ataxia, ocular inflammation, and pain after ocular surgery [93]. A recent preclinical study evaluated RTA-408 for diabetic wound recovery and found that NRF2 upregulation was responsible for the observed improvement in regenerative capacity [94].

Fumaric acid ester dimethyl fumarate (DMF, BG-12 or Tecfidera, from Biogen) is another successful NRF2 activator approved for relapsing-remitting multiple sclerosis and, previously, for psoriasis. DMF-dependent NRF2 activation improves the clinical course in a multiple sclerosis mouse model, mainly favoring axon preservation and increasing astrocyte activation. Therefore, DMF has been approved in 2013 by FDA for relapsing-remitting multiple sclerosis, and, previously, was authorized for the treatment of psoriasis [95,96]. Moreover, an oral formulation of a monomethyl fumarate (MMF) derivative, diroximel fumarate (2-(2,5-dioxo-1-pyrrolidinyl)ethyl ester; ALKS-8700; Alkermes), which exhibits improved bioavailability and efficacy, is now approved by EMA for treatment in multiple sclerosis. However, some NRF2-independent effects were described, such as anti-inflammatory responses through the activation of the nicotinic receptor hydroxycarboxylic acid receptor 2, mainly expressed in gut epithelial and immune cells [97].

4-Methyl-5(pyrazinyl-2)-1-2-dithiole-3-thione (Oltipraz) is under phase III clinical trial for the treatment of nonalcoholic fatty liver disease. Oltipraz increases GSH biosynthesis and phase II detoxification enzymes, such as NQO1. Ursodeoxycholic acid (Ursodiol) has a not yet explained action mechanism; however, several kinds of research suggest that it exerts its antioxidant and detoxification effects through NRF2 upregulation. For this cytoprotective effect, Ursodiol was approved by FDA for the treatment of primary biliary cirrhosis [98].

Not only synthetic compounds can modulate the NRF2-mediated pathway. Therefore, during the last years, many natural compounds have been described as electrophilic inducers of NRF2, such as curcumin and sulforaphane (SFN). Curcumin, also called diferuloylmethane, is the main natural polyphenol found in the rhizome of *Curcuma longa* (turmeric) and other *Curcuma* spp. Curcumin and its derivatives modulated NFR2-mediated ROS-scavenging through the KEAP1 Cys151 modification, becoming a promising molecule for the treatment of obesity, metabolic syndrome, and prediabetes [99].

SFN, an iso-thiocyanate found in cruciferous vegetables, has been used successfully in the treatment of type II diabetes mellitus [100]. SFN's ability to cross the blood–brain barrier protects against neurodegenerative disorders, as demonstrated in disease models in mice. In terms of acute brain damage, SFN has been shown to protect rats from hypoxic-ischemic injury by lowering the infarct ratio and upregulating NRF2 and HO-1 [101]. SFN improved cognitive impairment in an acute mouse model of Alzheimer's disease (AD) in vivo [102]. SFN protected dopaminergic cells from the cytotoxic effects of 6-hydroxydopamine in PD [103]. SFN prevented astrogliosis and microgliosis in the 1-methyl-4-phenyl-1,2,3,6-tetrahydropyridine PD mouse model [104]. To improve SFN stability, Evgen Pharma developed SFX-01, a cyclodextrin formulation currently in phase II clinical trials for the treatment of subarachnoid hemorrhage. For the treatment of brain ischemia, a hybrid molecule of SFN and melatonin (ITH12674) was developed with a dual "drug-prodrug" mechanism of action [105].

The nitro-fatty acid 9-nitro-octadec-9-enoic acid (OA-NO2), a molecule with anti-inflammatory properties, reacts with a variety of KEAP1 cysteine residues, primarily Cys273 and Cys288, and its activity appears to be independent of Cys151 [106]. CXA-10 (10-nitro-9(E)-octadec-9-enoic acid) is an isomer of OA-NO2 that has demonstrated efficacy in the uninephrectomized deoxycorticosterone acetate-high salt mouse model of chronic kidney disease and is currently being studied in phase I clinical trials for the treatment of this disease, as well as in phase II trials for the treatment of pulmonary arterial hypertension [107].

Conclusions

Many chronic diseases are characterized by the loss of homeostatic responses. NRF2 pathway is critical in the maintenance of redox homeostasis and regulation of inflammation. Loss of NRF2 activity drives aging, allowing reactive species to accumulate in cells shifting them to a pathogenic state. Therefore, a reduction of NRF2 with age increases oxidative stress and contributes to the aging process by influencing numerous processes, such as proteostasis, genomic instability, telomere attrition, epigenetic alterations, mitochondrial dysfunction, deregulated nutrient sensing, cellular senescence, stem cell exhaustion, and intercellular communications. To effectively mitigate the effects of NRF2 loss in aging, the development of effective therapeutics is an important goal. Currently, many biopharmaceutical companies are developing compounds that target NRF2-KEAP1 pathway to restore its activity during aging and induce long-lasting cytoprotective effects. Although there are several concerns about side effects, including an increased cancer risk, over the next few years, the ongoing clinical trials will provide advances to safely restore NRF2 activity during aging.

References

[1] Bruns DR, Drake JC, Biela LM, Peelor FF, Miller BF, Hamilton KL. Nrf2 signaling and the slowed aging phenotype: evidence from long-lived models. Oxid Med Cell Longev 2015;2015. https://doi.org/10.1155/2015/732596.

[2] Schmidlin CJ, Dodson MB, Madhavan L, Zhang DD. Redox regulation by NRF2 in aging and disease. Free Radic Biol Med 2019;134:702–7. https://doi.org/10.1016/j.freeradbiomed.2019.01.016.

[3] Buffenstein R, Edrey YH, Yang T, Mele J. The oxidative stress theory of aging: embattled or invincible? Insights from non-traditional model organisms. Age 2008;30(2–3):99–109. https://doi.org/10.1007/s11357-008-9058-z.

[4] Liguori I, Russo G, Curcio F, Bulli G, Aran L, Della-Morte D, et al. Oxidative stress, aging, and diseases. Clin Interv Aging 2018;13:757–72. https://doi.org/10.2147/CIA.S158513.

[5] Cuadrado A, Rojo AI, Wells G, Hayes JD, Cousin SP, Rumsey WL, et al. Therapeutic targeting of the NRF2 and KEAP1 partnership in chronic diseases. Nat Rev Drug Discov 2019;18(4):295–317. https://doi.org/10.1038/s41573-018-0008-x.

[6] Sykiotis GP, Bohmann D. Stress-activated cap'n'collar transcription factors in aging and human disease. Sci Signal 2010. https://doi.org/10.1126/SCISIGNAL.3112RE3.

[7] Tullet JMA, Green JW, Au C, Benedetto A, Thompson MA, Clark E, et al. The SKN-1/Nrf2 transcription factor can protect against oxidative stress and increase lifespan in *C. elegans* by distinct mechanisms. Aging Cell 2017;16(5):1191–4. https://doi.org/10.1111/acel.12627.

[8] Suh JH, Shenvi SV, Dixon BM, Liu H, Jaiswal AK, Liu RM, et al. Decline in transcriptional activity of Nrf2 causes age-related loss of glutathione synthesis, which is reversible with lipoic acid. Proc Natl Acad Sci USA 2004;101(10):3381−6. https://doi.org/10.1073/pnas.0400282101.

[9] Kensler TW, Wakabayashi N, Biswal S. Cell survival responses to environmental stresses via the Keap1-Nrf2-ARE pathway. Annu Rev Pharmacol Toxicol 2007;47:89−116. https://doi.org/10.1146/annurev.pharmtox.46.120604.141046.

[10] López-Otín C, Blasco MA, Partridge L, Serrano M, Kroemer G. The hallmarks of aging. Cell 2013;153(6):1194. https://doi.org/10.1016/j.cell.2013.05.039.

[11] Robledinos-Antón N, Fernández-Ginés R, Manda G, Cuadrado A. Activators and inhibitors of NRF2: a review of their potential for clinical development. Oxid Med Cell Longev 2019;2019. https://doi.org/10.1155/2019/9372182.

[12] Abrescia P, Treppiccione L, Rossi M, Bergamo P. Modulatory role of dietary polyunsaturated fatty acids in Nrf2-mediated redox homeostasis. Prog Lipid Res 2020;80:101066. https://doi.org/10.1016/j.plipres.2020.101066.

[13] Maher J, Yamamoto M. The rise of antioxidant signaling-the evolution and hormetic actions of Nrf2. Toxicol Appl Pharmacol 2010;244(1):4−15. https://doi.org/10.1016/j.taap.2010.01.011.

[14] Tong KI, Katoh Y, Kusunoki H, Itoh K, Tanaka T, Yamamoto M. Keap1 recruits Neh2 through binding to ETGE and DLG motifs: characterization of the two-site molecular recognition model. Mol Cell Biol 2006;26(8):2887−900. https://doi.org/10.1128/MCB.26.8.2887-2900.2006.

[15] Tong KI, Padmanabhan B, Kobayashi A, Shang C, Hirotsu Y, Yokoyama S, et al. Different electrostatic potentials define ETGE and DLG motifs as hinge and latch in oxidative stress response. Mol Cell Biol 2007;27(21):7511−21. https://doi.org/10.1128/MCB.00753-07.

[16] Sihvola V, Levonen AL. Keap1 as the redox sensor of the antioxidant response. Arch Biochem Biophys 2017;617:94−100. https://doi.org/10.1016/j.abb.2016.10.010.

[17] Saha S, Buttari B, Panieri E, Profumo E, Saso L. An overview of Nrf2 signaling pathway and its role in inflammation. Molecules 2020;25:5474. https://doi.org/10.3390/MOLECULES25225474.

[18] Katoh Y, Itoh K, Yoshida E, Miyagishi M, Fukamizu A, Yamamoto M. Two domains of Nrf2 cooperatively bind CBP, a CREB binding protein, and synergistically activate transcription. Gene Cell 2001;6(10):857−68. https://doi.org/10.1046/j.1365-2443.2001.00469.x.

[19] Nioi P, Nguyen T, Sherratt PJ, Pickett CB. The carboxy-terminal Neh3 domain of Nrf2 is required for transcriptional activation. Mol Cell Biol 2005;25(24):10895−906. https://doi.org/10.1128/MCB.25.24.10895-10906.2005.

[20] Sun Z, Chin YE, Zhang DD. Acetylation of Nrf2 by p300/CBP augments promoter-specific DNA binding of Nrf2 during the antioxidant response. Mol Cell Biol 2009;29(10):2658−72. https://doi.org/10.1128/MCB.01639-08.

[21] Theodore M, Kawai Y, Yang J, Kleshchenko Y, Reddy SP, Villalta F, et al. Multiple nuclear localization signals function in the nuclear import of the transcription factor Nrf2. J Biol Chem 2008;283(14):8984−94. https://doi.org/10.1074/jbc.M709040200.

[22] Rada P, Rojo AI, Chowdhry S, McMahon M, Hayes JD, Cuadrado A. SCF/β-TrCP promotes glycogen synthase kinase 3-dependent degradation of the Nrf2 transcription factor in a Keap1-independent manner. Mol Cell Biol 2011;31(6):1121−33. https://doi.org/10.1128/MCB.01204-10.

[23] Wang H, Liu K, Geng M, Gao P, Wu X, Hai Y, et al. RXRα inhibits the NRF2-ARE signaling pathway through a direct interaction with the Neh7 domain of NRF2. Cancer Res 2013;73(10):3097−108. https://doi.org/10.1158/0008-5472.CAN-12-3386.

[24] Zgorzynska E, Dziedzic B, Walczewska A. An Overview of the Nrf2/ARE pathway and its role in neurodegenerative diseases. Int J Mol Sci 2021;22(17):9592. https://doi.org/10.3390/ijms22179592.

[25] Dinkova-Kostova AT, Holtzclaw WD, Cole RN, Itoh K, Wakabayashi N, Katoh Y, et al. Direct evidence that sulfhydryl groups of Keap1 are the sensors regulating induction of phase 2 enzymes that protect against carcinogens and oxidants. Proc Natl Acad Sci USA 2002;99(18):11908−13. https://doi.org/10.1073/pnas.172398899.

[26] Jaiswal AK. Nrf2 signaling in coordinated activation of antioxidant gene expression. Free Radic Biol Med 2004;36(10):1199−207. https://doi.org/10.1016/j.freeradbiomed.2004.02.074.

[27] Joo MS, Kim WD, Lee KY, Kim JH, Koo JH, Kim SG. AMPK facilitates nuclear accumulation of nrf2 by phosphorylating at serine 550. Mol Cell Biol 2016;36(14):1931−42. https://doi.org/10.1128/MCB.00118-16.

[28] Hirotsu Y, Katsuoka F, Funayama R, Nagashima T, Nishida Y, Nakayama K, et al. Nrf2-MafG heterodimers contribute globally to antioxidant and metabolic networks. Nucleic Acids Res 2012;40(20):10228−39. https://doi.org/10.1093/nar/gks827.

[29] He X, Lai Q, Chen C, Li N, Sun F, Huang W, et al. Both conditional ablation and overexpression of E2 SUMO-conjugating enzyme (UBC9) in mouse pancreatic beta cells result in impaired beta cell function. Diabetologia 2018;61(4):881−95. https://doi.org/10.1007/s00125-017-4523-9.

[30] Sekine H, Okazaki K, Ota N, Shima H, Katoh Y, Suzuki N, et al. The mediator subunit MED16 transduces NRF2-activating signals into antioxidant gene expression. Mol Cell Biol 2016;36(3):407−20. https://doi.org/10.1128/MCB.00785-15.

[31] Kim JH, Yu S, Chen JD, Kong AN. The nuclear cofactor RAC3/AIB1/SRC-3 enhances Nrf2 signaling by interacting with transactivation domains. Oncogene 2013;32(4):514−27. https://doi.org/10.1038/onc.2012.59.

[32] Chowdhry S, Zhang Y, McMahon M, Sutherland C, Cuadrado A, Hayes JD. Nrf2 is controlled by two distinct β-TrCP recognition motifs in its Neh6 domain, one of which can be modulated by GSK-3 activity. Oncogene 2013;32(32):3765−81. https://doi.org/10.1038/onc.2012.388.

[33] Wu T, Zhao F, Gao B, Tan C, Yagishita N, Nakajima T, et al. Hrd1 suppresses Nrf2-mediated cellular protection during liver cirrhosis. Genes Dev 2014;28(7):708−22. https://doi.org/10.1101/gad.238246.114.

[34] Lo JY, Spatola BN, Curran SP. WDR23 regulates NRF2 independently of KEAP1. PLoS Genet 2017;13(4). https://doi.org/10.1371/journal.pgen.1006762.

[35] Spatola BN, Lo JY, Wang B, Curran SP. Nuclear and cytoplasmic WDR-23 isoforms mediate differential effects on GEN-1 and SKN-1 substrates. Sci Rep 2019;9(1). https://doi.org/10.1038/s41598-019-48286-y.

[36] Copple IM, Lister A, Obeng AD, Kitteringham NR, Jenkins RE, Layfield R, et al. Physical and functional interaction of

sequestosome 1 with Keap1 regulates the Keap1-Nrf2 cell defense pathway. J Biol Chem 2010;285(22):16782–8. https://doi.org/10.1074/jbc.M109.096545.

[37] Jain A, Lamark T, Sjøttem E, Larsen KB, Awuh JA, Øvervatn A, et al. p62/SQSTM1 is a target gene for transcription factor NRF2 and creates a positive feedback loop by inducing antioxidant response element-driven gene transcription. J Biol Chem 2010;285(29):22576–91. https://doi.org/10.1074/jbc.M110.118976.

[38] Lau A, Wang XJ, Zhao F, Villeneuve NF, Wu T, Jiang T, et al. A noncanonical mechanism of Nrf2 activation by autophagy deficiency: direct interaction between keap1 and p62. Mol Cell Biol 2010;30(13):3275–85. https://doi.org/10.1128/MCB.00248-10.

[39] Kwak MK, Itoh K, Yamamoto M, Sutter TR, Kensler TW. Role of transcription factor Nrf2 in the induction of hepatic phase 2 and antioxidative enzymes in vivo by the cancer chemoprotective agent, 3H-1, 2-dithiole-3-thione. Mol Med 2001;7(2):135–45. https://doi.org/10.1007/bf03401947.

[40] Ramos-Gomez M, Dolan PM, Itoh K, Yamamoto M, Kensler TW. Interactive effects of nrf2 genotype and oltipraz on benzo[a]pyrene-DNA adducts and tumor yield in mice. Carcinogenesis 2003;24(3):461–7. https://doi.org/10.1093/carcin/24.3.461.

[41] Hayashi A, Suzuki H, Itoh K, Yamamoto M, Sugiyama Y. Transcription factor Nrf2 is required for the constitutive and inducible expression of multidrug resistance-associated protein 1 in mouse embryo fibroblasts. Biochem Biophys Res Commun 2003;310(3):824–9. https://doi.org/10.1016/j.bbrc.2003.09.086.

[42] Vollrath V, Wielandt AM, Iruretagoyena M, Chianale J. Role of Nrf2 in the regulation of the Mrp2 (ABCC2) gene. Biochem J 2006;395(3):599–609. https://doi.org/10.1042/BJ20051518.

[43] Higgins LG, Kelleher MO, Eggleston IM, Itoh K, Yamamoto M, Hayes JD. Transcription factor Nrf2 mediates an adaptive response to sulforaphane that protects fibroblasts in vitro against the cytotoxic effects of electrophiles, peroxides and redox-cycling agents. Toxicol Appl Pharmacol 2009;237(3):267–80. https://doi.org/10.1016/j.taap.2009.03.005.

[44] Reisman SA, Yeager RL, Yamamoto M, Klaassen CD. Increased Nrf2 activation in livers from keap1-knockdown mice increases expression of cytoprotective genes that detoxify electrophiles more than those that detoxify reactive oxygen species. Toxicol Sci 2009;108(1):35–47. https://doi.org/10.1093/toxsci/kfn267.

[45] Wild AC, Moinova HR, Mulcahy RT. Regulation of γ-glutamylcysteine synthetase subunit gene expression by the transcription factor Nrf2. J Biol Chem 1999;274(47):33627–36. https://doi.org/10.1074/jbc.274.47.33627.

[46] Ahmed SMU, Luo L, Namani A, Wang XJ, Tang X. Nrf2 signaling pathway: pivotal roles in inflammation. Biochim Biophys Acta (BBA) Mol Basis Dis 2017;1863(2):585–97. https://doi.org/10.1016/j.bbadis.2016.11.005.

[47] Bellezza I, Tucci A, Galli F, Grottelli S, Mierla AL, Pilolli F, et al. Inhibition of NF-κB nuclear translocation via HO-1 activation underlies α-tocopheryl succinate toxicity. JNB (J Nutr Biochem) 2012;23(12):1583–91. https://doi.org/10.1016/j.jnutbio.2011.10.012.

[48] Hwang YJ, Lee EW, Song J, Kim HR, Jun YC, Hwang KA. MafK positively regulates NF-κB activity by enhancing CBP-mediated p65 acetylation. Sci Rep 2013;3. https://doi.org/10.1038/srep03242.

[49] Lee DF, Kuo HP, Liu M, Chou CK, Xia W, Du Y, et al. KEAP1 E3 ligase-mediated downregulation of NF-κB signaling by targeting IKKβ. Mol Cell 2009;36(1):131–40. https://doi.org/10.1016/j.molcel.2009.07.025.

[50] Thimmulappa RK, Lee H, Rangasamy T, Reddy SP, Yamamoto M, Kensler TW, et al. Nrf2 is a critical regulator of the innate immune response and survival during experimental sepsis. J Clin Invest 2006;116(4):984–95. https://doi.org/10.1172/JCI25790.

[51] Liu GH, Qu J, Shen X. NF-κB/p65 antagonizes Nrf2-ARE pathway by depriving CBP from Nrf2 and facilitating recruitment of HDAC3 to MafK. Biochim Biophys Acta Mol Cell Res 2008;1783(5):713–27. https://doi.org/10.1016/j.bbamcr.2008.01.002.

[52] Campbell NK, Fitzgerald HK, Dunne A. Regulation of inflammation by the antioxidant haem oxygenase 1. Nat Rev Immunol 2021;21(7):411–25. https://doi.org/10.1038/s41577-020-00491-x.

[53] Prestera T, Talalay P, Alam J, Ahn YI, Lee PJ, Choi AM. Parallel induction of heme oxygenase-1 and chemoprotective phase 2 enzymes by electrophiles and antioxidants: regulation by upstream antioxidant-responsive elements (ARE). Mol Med 1995;1(7):827–37. https://doi.org/10.1007/bf03401897.

[54] Gan FF, Ling H, Ang X, Reddy SA, Lee SSH, Yang H, et al. A novel shogaol analog suppresses cancer cell invasion and inflammation, and displays cytoprotective effects through modulation of NF-κB and Nrf2-Keap1 signaling pathways. Toxicol Appl Pharmacol 2013;272(3):852–62. https://doi.org/10.1016/j.taap.2013.07.011.

[55] Kim BC, Jeon WK, Hong HY, Jeon KB, Hahn JH, Kim YM, et al. The anti-inflammatory activity of *Phellinus linteus* (Berk. & M.A. Curt.) is mediated through the PKCδ/Nrf2/ARE signaling to up-regulation of heme oxygenase-1. J Ethnopharmacol 2007;113(2):240–7. https://doi.org/10.1016/j.jep.2007.05.032.

[56] Lee SH, Sohn DH, Jin XY, Kim SW, Choi SC, Seo GS. 2′,4′,6′-Tris(methoxymethoxy) chalcone protects against trinitrobenzene sulfonic acid-induced colitis and blocks tumor necrosis factor-α-induced intestinal epithelial inflammation via heme oxygenase 1-dependent and independent pathways. Biochem Pharmacol 2007;74(6):870–80. https://doi.org/10.1016/j.bcp.2007.06.034.

[57] Kobayashi EH, Suzuki T, Funayama R, Nagashima T, Hayashi M, Sekine H, et al. Nrf2 suppresses macrophage inflammatory response by blocking proinflammatory cytokine transcription. Nat Commun 2016;7. https://doi.org/10.1038/ncomms11624.

[58] Pareek TK, Belkadi A, Kesavapany S, Zaremba A, Loh SL, Bai L, et al. Triterpenoid modulation of IL-17 and Nrf-2 expression ameliorates neuroinflammation and promotes remyelination in autoimmune encephalomyelitis. Sci Rep 2011;1. https://doi.org/10.1038/srep00201.

[59] Liu X, Zhou W, Zhang X, Lu P, Du Q, Tao L, et al. Dimethyl fumarate ameliorates dextran sulfate sodium-induced murine experimental colitis by activating Nrf2 and suppressing NLRP3 inflammasome activation. Biochem Pharmacol 2016;112:37–49. https://doi.org/10.1016/j.bcp.2016.05.002.

[60] Liu X, Zhang X, Ding Y, Zhou W, Tao L, Lu P, et al. Nuclear factor E2-related factor-2 negatively regulates NLRP3 inflammasome activity by inhibiting reactive oxygen species-induced NLRP3 priming. Antioxid Redox Signal 2017;26(1):28–43. https://doi.org/10.1089/ars.2015.6615.

[61] Zhao C, Gillette DD, Li X, Zhang Z, Wen H. Nuclear factor E2-related factor-2 (Nrf2) is required for NLRP3 and AIM2

inflammasome activation. J Biol Chem 2014;289(24):17020–9. https://doi.org/10.1074/jbc.M114.563114.

[62] Hourihan JM, Moronetti Mazzeo LE, Fernández-Cárdenas LP, Blackwell TK. Cysteine sulfenylation directs IRE-1 to activate the SKN-1/Nrf2 antioxidant response. Mol Cell 2016;63(4):553–66. https://doi.org/10.1016/j.molcel.2016.07.019.

[63] Cullinan SB, Zhang D, Hannink M, Arvisais E, Kaufman RJ, Diehl JA. Nrf2 is a direct PERK substrate and effector of PERK-dependent cell survival. Mol Cell Biol 2003;23(20):7198–209. https://doi.org/10.1128/MCB.23.20.7198-7209.2003.

[64] Singh A, Rangasamy T, Thimmulappa RK, Lee H, Osburn WO, Brigelius-Flohé R, et al. Glutathione peroxidase 2, the major cigarette smoke-inducible isoform of GPX in lungs, is regulated by Nrf2. Am J Respir Cell Mol Biol 2006;35(6):639–50. https://doi.org/10.1165/rcmb.2005-0325OC.

[65] Pajares M, Jiménez-Moreno N, García-Yagüe ÁJ, Escoll M, de Ceballos ML, Van Leuven F, et al. Transcription factor NFE2L2/NRF2 is a regulator of macroautophagy genes. Autophagy 2016;12(10):1902–16. https://doi.org/10.1080/15548627.2016.1208889.

[66] Kim SB, Pandita RK, Eskiocak U, Ly P, Kaisani A, Kumar R, et al. Targeting of Nrf2 induces DNA damage signaling and protects colonic epithelial cells from ionizing radiation. Proc Natl Acad Sci USA 2012;109(43):E2949–55. https://doi.org/10.1073/pnas.1207718109.

[67] Jayakumar S, Pal D, Sandur SK. Nrf2 facilitates repair of radiation induced DNA damage through homologous recombination repair pathway in a ROS independent manner in cancer cells. Mutat Res Fundam Mol Mech Mutagen 2015;779:33–45. https://doi.org/10.1016/j.mrfmmm.2015.06.007.

[68] Sun X, Wang Y, Ji K, Liu Y, Kong Y, Nie S, et al. NRF2 preserves genomic integrity by facilitating ATR activation and G2 cell cycle arrest. Nucleic Acids Res 2020;48(16):9109–23. https://doi.org/10.1093/nar/gkaa631.

[69] Ahmad F, Dixit D, Sharma V, Kumar A, Joshi SD, Sarkar C, et al. Nrf2-driven TERT regulates pentose phosphate pathway in glioblastoma. Cell Death Dis 2016;7. https://doi.org/10.1038/cddis.2016.117.

[70] Akino N, Wada-Hiraike O, Isono W, Terao H, Honjo H, Miyamoto Y, et al. Activation of Nrf2/Keap1 pathway by oral Dimethylfumarate administration alleviates oxidative stress and age-associated infertility might be delayed in the mouse ovary. Reprod Biol Endocrinol 2019;17(1). https://doi.org/10.1186/s12958-019-0466-y.

[71] Yilmaz S, Bedir E, Ballar Kirmizibayrak P. The role of cycloastragenol at the intersection of NRF2/ARE, telomerase, and proteasome activity. Free Radic Biol Med 2022;188:105–16. https://doi.org/10.1016/j.freeradbiomed.2022.06.230.

[72] Khor TO, Fuentes F, Shu L, Paredes-Gonzalez X, Yang AY, Liu Y, et al. Epigenetic DNA methylation of antioxidative stress regulator NRF2 in human prostate cancer. Chest 2014;146(6):1186–97. https://doi.org/10.1158/1940-6207.CAPR-14-0127.

[73] Zhou C, Zhao L, Zheng J, Wang K, Deng H, Liu P, et al. MicroRNA-144 modulates oxidative stress tolerance in SH-SY5Y cells by regulating nuclear factor erythroid 2-related factor 2-glutathione axis. Neurosci Lett 2017;655:21–7. https://doi.org/10.1016/j.neulet.2017.06.045.

[74] Streck EL, Czapski GA, Gonçalves Da Silva C. Neurodegeneration, mitochondrial dysfunction, and oxidative stress. Oxid Med Cell Longev 2013. https://doi.org/10.1155/2013/826046.

[75] Dinkova-Kostova AT, Abramov AY. The emerging role of Nrf2 in mitochondrial function. Free Radic Biol Med 2015;88:179–88. https://doi.org/10.1016/j.freeradbiomed.2015.04.036.

[76] Dodson M, De La Vega MR, Cholanians AB, Schmidlin CJ, Chapman E, Zhang DD. Modulating NRF2 in disease: timing is everything. Annu Rev Pharmacol Toxicol 2019;59:555–75. https://doi.org/10.1146/annurev-pharmtox-010818-021856.

[77] Salminen A, Kaarniranta K. AMP-activated protein kinase (AMPK) controls the aging process via an integrated signaling network. Ageing Res Rev 2012;11(2):230–41. https://doi.org/10.1016/j.arr.2011.12.005.

[78] Mitsuishi Y, Taguchi K, Kawatani Y, Shibata T, Nukiwa T, Aburatani H, et al. Nrf2 redirects glucose and glutamine into anabolic pathways in metabolic reprogramming. Cancer Cell 2012;22(1):66–79. https://doi.org/10.1016/j.ccr.2012.05.016.

[79] Singh A, Happel C, Manna SK, Acquaah-Mensah G, Carrerero J, Kumar S, et al. Transcription factor NRF2 regulates miR-1 and miR-206 to drive tumorigenesis. J Clin Invest 2013;123(7):2921–34. https://doi.org/10.1172/JCI66353.

[80] Kapeta S, Chondrogianni N, Gonos ES. Nuclear erythroid factor 2-mediated proteasome activation delays senescence in human fibroblasts. J Biol Chem 2010;285(11):8171–84. https://doi.org/10.1074/jbc.M109.031575.

[81] Corenblum MJ, Ray S, Remley QW, Long M, Harder B, Zhang DD, et al. Reduced Nrf2 expression mediates the decline in neural stem cell function during a critical middle-age period. Aging Cell 2016;15(4):725–36. https://doi.org/10.1111/acel.12482.

[82] Ray S, Corenblum MJ, Anandhan A, Reed A, Ortiz FO, Zhang DD, et al. A role for Nrf2 expression in defining the aging of hippocampal neural stem cells. Cell Transplant 2018;27(4):589–606. https://doi.org/10.1177/0963689718774030.

[83] Kubben N, Zhang W, Wang L, Voss TC, Yang J, Qu J, et al. Repression of the antioxidant NRF2 pathway in premature aging. Cell 2016;165(6):1361–74. https://doi.org/10.1016/j.cell.2016.05.017.

[84] Jang J, Wang Y, Kim HS, Lalli MA, Kosik KS. Nrf2, a regulator of the proteasome, controls self-renewal and pluripotency in human embryonic stem cells. Stem Cell 2014;32(10):2616–25. https://doi.org/10.1002/stem.1764.

[85] Aoki R, Li YR. α-Synuclein promotes neuroprotection through NF-κB-mediated transcriptional regulation of protein kinase Cδ. Sci Signal 2011;4(195). https://doi.org/10.1126/scisignal.2002425.

[86] Skibinski G, Hwang V, Ando DM, Daub A, Lee AK, Ravisankar A, et al. Nrf2 mitigates LRRK2- and α-synuclein-induced neurodegeneration by modulating proteostasis. Proc Natl Acad Sci USA 2017;114(5):1165–70. https://doi.org/10.1073/pnas.1522872114.

[87] Wakabayashi N, Dinkova-Kostova AT, Holtzclaw WD, Kang MI, Kobayashi A, Yamamoto M, et al. Protection against electrophile and oxidant stress by induction of the phase 2 response: fate of cysteines of the Keap1 sensor modified by inducers. Proc Natl Acad Sci USA 2004;101(7):2040–5. https://doi.org/10.1073/pnas.0307301101.

[88] Baird L, Llères D, Swift S, Dinkova-Kostova AT. Regulatory flexibility in the Nrf2-mediated stress response is conferred by conformational cycling of the Keap1-Nrf2 protein complex. Proc

Natl Acad Sci USA 2013;110(38):15259–64. https://doi.org/10.1073/pnas.1305687110.

[89] Cleasby A, Yon J, Day PJ, Richardson C, Tickle IJ, Williams PA, et al. Structure of the BTB domain of Keap1 and its interaction with the triterpenoid antagonist CDDO. PLoS One 2014;9(6). https://doi.org/10.1371/journal.pone.0098896.

[90] Dayalan Naidu S, Muramatsu A, Saito R, Asami S, Honda T, Hosoya T, et al. C151 in KEAP1 is the main cysteine sensor for the cyanoenone class of NRF2 activators, irrespective of molecular size or shape. Sci Rep 2018;8(1). https://doi.org/10.1038/s41598-018-26269-9.

[91] Pergola PE, Raskin P, Toto RD, Meyer CJ, Huff JW, Grossman EB, et al. Bardoxolone methyl and kidney function in CKD with type 2 diabetes. N Engl J Med 2011;365(4):327–36. https://doi.org/10.1056/NEJMoa1105351.

[92] Zhang DD. Bardoxolone brings Nrf2-based therapies to light. Antioxid Redox Signal 2013;19(5):517–8. https://doi.org/10.1089/ars.2012.5118.

[93] Lynch DR, Farmer J, Hauser L, Blair IA, Wang QQ, Mesaros C, et al. Safety, pharmacodynamics, and potential benefit of omaveloxolone in Friedreich ataxia. Ann Clin Transl Neurol 2019;6(1):15–26. https://doi.org/10.1002/acn3.660.

[94] Rabbani PS, Ellison T, Waqas B, Sultan D, Abdou S, David JA, et al. Targeted Nrf2 activation therapy with RTA 408 enhances regenerative capacity of diabetic wounds. Diabetes Res Clin Pract 2018;139:11–23. https://doi.org/10.1016/j.diabres.2018.02.021.

[95] Fox RJ, Miller DH, Phillips JT, Hutchinson M, Havrdova E, Kita M, et al. Placebo-controlled phase 3 study of oral BG-12 or glatiramer in multiple sclerosis. N Engl J Med 2012;367(12):1087–97. https://doi.org/10.1056/NEJMoa1206328.

[96] Höxtermann S, Nüchel C, Altmeyer P. Fumaric acid esters suppress peripheral CD4- and CD8-positive lymphocytes in psoriasis. Dermatology 1998;196(2):223–30. https://doi.org/10.1159/000017903.

[97] von Glehn F, Dias-Carneiro RPC, Moraes AS, Farias AS, Silva VAPG, Oliveira FTM, et al. Dimethyl fumarate downregulates the immune response through the HCA2/GPR109A pathway: implications for the treatment of multiple sclerosis. Mult Scler Relat Disord 2018;23:46–50. https://doi.org/10.1016/j.msard.2018.04.016.

[98] Kawata K, Kobayashi Y, Souda K, Kawamura K, Sumiyoshi S, Takahashi Y, et al. Enhanced hepatic Nrf2 activation after ursodeoxycholic acid treatment in patients with primary biliary cirrhosis. Antioxid Redox Signal 2010;13(3):259–68. https://doi.org/10.1089/ars.2009.2903.

[99] Na LX, Li Y, Pan HZ, Zhou XL, Sun DJ, Meng M, et al. Curcuminoids exert glucose-lowering effect in type 2 diabetes by decreasing serum free fatty acids: a double-blind, placebo-controlled trial. Mol Nutr Food Res 2013;57(9):1569–77. https://doi.org/10.1002/mnfr.201200131.

[100] Axelsson AS, Tubbs E, Mecham B, Chacko S, Nenonen HA, Tang Y, et al. Sulforaphane reduces hepatic glucose production and improves glucose control in patients with type 2 diabetes. Sci Transl Med 2017;9(394). https://doi.org/10.1126/scitranslmed.aah4477.

[101] Ping Z, Liu W, Kang Z, Cai J, Wang Q, Cheng N, et al. Sulforaphane protects brains against hypoxic-ischemic injury through induction of Nrf2-dependent phase 2 enzyme. Brain Res 2010;1343:178–85. https://doi.org/10.1016/j.brainres.2010.04.036.

[102] Kim HV, Kim HY, Ehrlich HY, Choi SY, Kim DJ, Kim YS. Amelioration of Alzheimer's disease by neuroprotective effect of sulforaphane in animal model. Amyloid 2013;20(1):7–12. https://doi.org/10.3109/13506129.2012.751367.

[103] Ji MH, Yong JL, So YL, Eun MK, Moon Y, Ha WK, et al. Protective effect of sulforaphane against dopaminergic cell death. J Pharmacol Exp Therapeut 2007;321(1):249–56. https://doi.org/10.1124/jpet.106.110866.

[104] Jazwa A, Rojo AI, Innamorato NG, Hesse M, Fernández-Ruiz J, Cuadrado A. Pharmacological targeting of the transcription factor NRf2 at the basal ganglia provides disease modifying therapy for experimental parkinsonism. Antioxid Redox Signal 2011;14(12):2347–60. https://doi.org/10.1089/ars.2010.3731.

[105] Egea J, Buendia I, Parada E, Navarro E, Rada P, Cuadrado A, et al. Melatonin-sulforaphane hybrid ITH12674 induces neuroprotection in oxidative stress conditions by a "drug-prodrug" mechanism of action. Br J Pharmacol 2015;172(7):1807–21. https://doi.org/10.1111/bph.13025.

[106] Kansanen E, Bonacci G, Schopfer FJ, Kuosmanen SM, Tong KI, Leinonen H, et al. Electrophilic nitro-fatty acids activate Nrf2 by a Keap1 cysteine 151-independent mechanism. J Biol Chem 2011;286(16):14019–27. https://doi.org/10.1074/jbc.M110.190710.

[107] Arbeeny CM, Ling H, Smith MM, O'Brien S, Wawersik S, Ledbetter SR, et al. CXA-10, a nitrated fatty acid, is renoprotective in deoxycorticosterone acetate-salt nephropathy. J Pharmacol Exp Therapeut 2019;369(3):503–10. https://doi.org/10.1124/jpet.118.254755.

Chapter 4

Fluid redox biomarkers in neurological disease

Carlo Cervellati[1] and Alessandra Pecorelli[2]

[1]*Department of Translational Medicine and for Romagna, University of Ferrara, Ferrara, Italy;* [2]*Department of Environmental Sciences, University of Ferrara, Ferrara, Italy*

Introduction

The term "biomarker" is often improperly used in scientific works, and following a search on PUBMED, it is present in the title of abstract of 1,073,682 (updated on 5th of August 2022) published articles (Fig. 4.1). The reason for this evident abuse is the frequent lack of adherence to the underlying concept of this term. This is an important issue in biomedical research, as the inconsistent use of key terms can hinder the evaluation and interpretation of evidence, which are ultimately used in the development process of drugs and medical devices.

Since 1998 (statement from National Institutes of Health Biomarkers Definitions Working Group), the universally accepted and unequivocal definition of a biomarker is "a characteristic that is objectively measured as an indicator of normal biological processes, pathogenic processes or responses to an exposure or intervention." Sato et al. extended the definition, describing biomarkers as the most objective, quantifiable, and reproducible medical signs.

Biomarkers find applications in several contexts; they play an increasingly important roles in drug discovery and development from target identification and validation to clinical application, stratification and monitoring of enrolled patients, and evaluation of therapeutic response/outcome.

According to the most recent classification proposed by the Food and Drug Administration and the National Institutes of Health as part of their joint Biomarkers, EndpointS, and other Tools (BEST) resource [1], seven categories of biomarkers exist: (1) diagnostic; (2) monitoring; (3) pharmacodynamic/response; (4) predictive; (5) prognostic; (6) safety; and (7) susceptibility/risk.

Oxidative stress (OxS) plays a crucial role in several diseases [2]. These aberrant conditions can be regarded as a

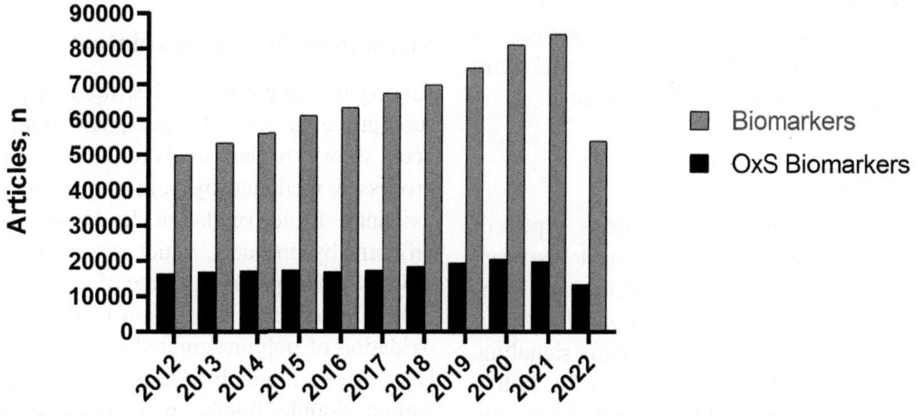

FIGURE 4.1 Number of published papers on biomarkers (*gray*) and the subgroup oxidative stress biomarkers (*black*) from 2012 to 2022 (September 29, 2022). PubMed database was were systematically searched for articles the following terms: "BIOMARKERS" alone or along with "Oxidative stress" OR "Redox."

Modulation of Oxidative Stress. https://doi.org/10.1016/B978-0-443-19247-0.00001-1

rich source of potential disease biomarkers. From the literature, it is clear that OxS or redox biomarkers are mostly used for disease diagnostic and prediction [2,3]. Diagnostic biomarkers are broadly defined as metabolites, genes, proteins, or miRNAs that are capable of identifying the presence of a disease or pathophysiological condition. A biomarker can be considered predictive when it can assess the risk of developing a disease or forecast the treatment effect. Regardless of the biomarker type, it remains imperative that analytical methods allow its detection with sufficient precision and reliability, as measurement objectivity and reproducibility are paramount.

As discussed in the next section, one of the major issues in the discovery and validation of redox biomarkers is the inadequate performance of their measurement procedures. Several methods have been developed and employed in almost all diseases to assess the levels and nature of oxidative stress, ranging from the oxidation of DNA to proteins, lipids, and free amino acids. The lack of standardization, gold standard methods, low analytical and clinical specificity, and poor reproducibility make it challenging to identify the reference range (the value is expected for 95% of the population) and thus the translation of these biomarkers into clinical practice use.

However, there is a growing interest in exploring the potential clinical applications of this family of markers. In particular, over the last 3 decades, researchers have focused on diseases where redox dysregulation and OxS seem to play a proactive role in pathogenesis and pathophysiology. This is the case for neurological diseases, mostly those with an important neurodegenerative component associated with their pathogenesis such as AD, VaD, and PD.

This chapter touches upon the status, analytical issues, and future potential of redox biomarkers as clinical diagnostic and predictive tools for a selection of neurological diseases from the available literature. Notably, the above-mentioned methodological limitations, especially for OxS products, assessed in complex biological milieu such as blood, only a minor part of measurable oxidative damage products can be referred to as biomarkers. Regardless, of this necessary remark, for sake of simplicity the term "biomarker" will be used throughout the chapter.

Redox biomarkers

The generation and accumulation of various types of reactive species (RS), ranging from the most abundant oxygen and nitrogen reactive species (ROS and RNS, respectively), in cells are not adequately copied by antioxidant defense mechanisms, disruption of redox signaling, and oxidative damage [4]. The result of this redox imbalance is commonly referred to as OxS, which is directly responsible for the potentially cytotoxic chemical modifications of biomolecules [4]. The products of these peroxidative and oxidative changes are putative redox biomarkers. Enzymatic and nonenzymatic antioxidants are often included in the category of OxS biomarkers. However, they suffer from very high variability, as their peripheral levels chiefly depend on exogenous (dietary intake, lifestyle habits) and endogenous (blood cell turnover) factors [3,5].

An intuitive question is "Why do we assess the products and not the RS directly?" as direct assessment of RS is the most accurate method to quantify OxS in vivo. This is answered by the fact that the direct assessment of RS is hindered by the technical difficulty of reliably detecting molecular species characterized by a short half-life and high heterogeneity [6]. Several methods have been developed, including the use of fluorescent probes, electron spin resonance, and chemiluminescence, which are able to directly detect RS but are not used in routine clinical practice. For this reason, the most accepted and popular approach is the measurement of stable by-products modified under conditions of OxS that have entered circulation [3,7].

A plethora of markers have been identified for the detection of oxidative damage. RS-induced modification of one biomolecule can produce numerous different measurable products. Unfortunately, detection methods that have been developed for these markers suffer from a number of intrinsic analytical shortcomings related to (1) assay specificity; (2) the product being assessed was not a specific product of lipid peroxidation; (3) inadequate sensitivity to assess levels of the product in nondiseased individuals, thus missing the definition of a normal range; (4) influence of external factors such as diet, subclinical conditions, and lifestyle on the product being measured; and (5) assays that are too expensive and time-consuming to be feasible in clinical practice [3,7–9].

In the next sections, the most commonly used redox biomarkers in studies dealing with neurological diseases (Fig. 4.2) will be briefly described. The main methodological issues were also highlighted.

Markers of lipid peroxidation

Among biological molecules, lipids appear to be the most susceptible to RS influences, and lipid peroxidation has been shown to be involved in neurodegeneration. This process is mediated by both enzymatic and nonenzymatic oxidants. Lipid oxidation leads to a large number of different by-products, which are measurable in biological fluids [8]. The primary source of these potential biomarkers is free radical-mediated chain oxidation, termed lipid peroxidation of polyunsaturated fatty acids (PUFAs) [8]. This is a process in which ROS attack lipids containing carbon-carbon double bonds, particularly PUFAs that involve hydrogen abstraction from a carbon, with oxygen insertion resulting in lipid peroxyl radicals and hydroperoxides [10].

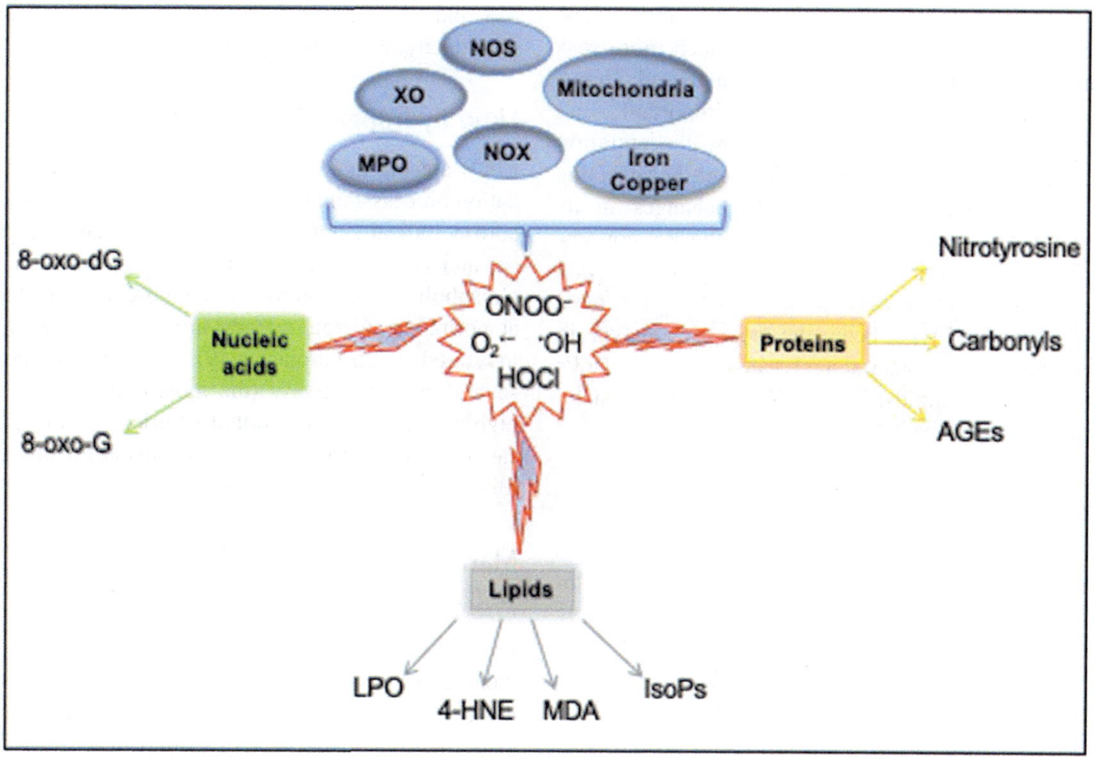

FIGURE 4.2 Main redox biomarkers generated from oxidation of lipids, proteins, and nucleic acids. *8-oxodG*, 8-oxo-7,8-dihydro-2′-deoxyguanosine; *8-oxoG*, 7,8-dihydro-8-oxo-deoxyguanine; *IsoPs*, isoprostanes; *LPO*, lipid hydroperoxides; *MDA*, malondialdehyde; *MPO*, myeloperoxidase; *NOS*, nitric oxide synthetase; *NOX*, NADPH-oxidase; *XO*, xanthine oxidase.

These compounds are also reactive and can propagate peroxidative stress, exacerbating OxS and influencing the shift in lipid signaling, inflammatory pathways, and autoimmune activity [8,11]. Describing the lipid peroxidation process is not within the scope of this chapter; thus, they will not be dealt with in detail.

Glycolipids, phospholipids, and cholesterol are also well-established targets of oxidation, which can be mediated by nonradical oxidants and enzymes such as singlet oxygen, ozone, hypohalous acids, lipoxygenases, cyclooxygenases, and cytochrome P450 [9].

The most studied biomarkers of lipid oxidation are F2-isoprostanes (IsoPs), trans-4-hydroxy-2-nonenal (4-HNE), and malondialdehyde (MDA) and lipid hydroperoxides (LPO). The next paragraphs will focus primarily on these biomarkers with a brief mention of other biomarkers.

Isoprostanes

These stable prostaglandin-like compounds are generated in vivo, mostly via free radical-induced peroxidation of arachidonates (superoxide radical, $O_2^{\cdot-}$, and hydroxyl radical, ·OH) [12,13]. Recent evidence has shown that IsoPs can also be promoted by prostaglandin endoperoxide synthase enzymes, which are induced by inflammation. This alternate pathway is independent of RS concentration [9,13].

There are 64 possible isomers of IsoPs, with 8-iso-PGF2α (also known as iPF2α.-III; 8-epi PGF2α; 8-isoprostane; or 15-F2t-isoprostane) and, in neurological disease, neuroprostanes (Neurop; especially the following steroisomers: (4(RS)-4-F4t-NeuroP, 10-epi-10-F4t-NeuroP, 14(RS)-14-F4t-NeuroP) as the most investigated ones [13,14]. Once IsoPs are released from cell membranes by phospholipases, they circulate in the plasma and are mostly bound to high-density lipoproteins (HDLs) [14]. IsoPs can be reliably detected in almost every biological fluid, including urine, plasma, amniotic fluid, exhaled breath condensate, bile, and cerebrospinal fluid (CSF) [3,14]. These compounds are not mere static biomarkers of OxS, but rather mediators of vasoconstriction and bronchoconstriction that can induce neuronal apoptosis [14].

IsoPs are considered key biomarkers for assessing OxS in vivo and for evaluating human disorder pathogenesis [3,7]. The European Food Safety Authority (EFSA) recommends using IsoPs as biomarkers to assess oxidative damage against lipids [15]. However, as stated in the framework, the reliability of IsoPs depends strictly on the methodology used. Currently, the most accurate detection methods are chromatographic techniques coupled with mass spectrometry (MS) [7,16,17]. These approaches, although labor- and time-consuming, are much more sensitive and specific than the more commonly used immunochemical techniques (ELISA) [7]. An important issue related to the assessment of IsoPs is the low concentration of these compounds in fluids [3,7]. Moreover, because this marker is also produced enzymatically, changes in its concentration may not completely reflect the RS concentration. This scenario is also complicated by the fact that these compounds can be assessed as both free (the most commonly measured type, being the most present type in urine and plasma) and total (an aggregate of free and IsoPs esterified to phospholipids) [7,18]. The latter is normally evaluated upon hydrolysis by phospholipases [7].

Malondialdehyde

MDA is a reactive aldehyde that can form covalent adducts with biomolecules, thereby exerting genotoxic and cytotoxic effects [7]. This compound is the most frequently assessed marker for lipid oxidative damage in vivo [3,7]. Its popularity is mainly due to the ease and low cost of the associated detection method, which allows high-throughput measurement.

Nevertheless, in the most commonly applied method, the spectrophotometric thiobarbituric acid reactive substances (TBARS) assay, up to 98% of the measured MDA can be formed due to the high-temperature conditions during the procedure itself [7,9,19]. Moreover, TBARS assesses not only MDA but also other aldehydes and decomposition products from hydroperoxides present in biological fluids. Therefore, various approaches have been developed to improve assay specificity. The combination of TBARS with chromatographic techniques, HPLC, or gas chromatography (GC), coupled with or without MS detection, has been shown to increase analytical accuracy [7,19]. However, these methods require individual sample processing, and the validity of MDA as a biomarker of in vivo OxS remains uncertain, making it less suitable for routine clinical use.

Trans-4-hydroxy-2-nonenal

As MDA, 4-HNE is a secondary product of the peroxidation cycle [9]. Both bioactive aldehyde species can modify proteins by covalent adduction of the amino acids cysteine, histidine, and lysine [9]. These newly formed adducts can influence protein function and modulate signaling pathways during cell senescence, proliferation, differentiation, apoptosis, and necrosis [9]. The presence of HNE-protein adducts has been demonstrated in a wide range of physiological and pathological conditions. Plasma/serum 4-HNE-protein adducts were accurately assessed using GC/MS and more recently, commercial ELISA have shown good analytical performance [9].

Lipid hydroperoxides

LPOs are the major primary products of the lipid peroxidation process and are formed from the highly reactive lipid peroxy radical (LOO·) [7]. The hydroperoxide group may be attached to various lipid structures, such as FFA, phospholipids, and sterols. In the absence of metal ions and at normal temperature, they are fairly stable and can be measured in serum/plasma [9]. Nevertheless, none of the several available assays (the most popular are simple and highly feasible spectrophotometric methods) provides satisfactory sensitivity/specificity levels for this biomarker [3,9].

Markers of protein oxidation

Protein carbonyls and nitrotyrosine

Protein oxidation leads to irreversible modifications (fragmentation, cross-linkage, etc.) that completely compromise the protein native function or "milder" changes that can cause perturbation of protein biological roles [7]. When the RS levels overwhelm the antioxidant defenses, the formation of amino acid radicals is promoted, which in turn can cross-link or react with O_2 to form peroxyl radicals [7]. This can lead to the generation of other free radicals and protein peroxides, with the consequent exacerbation of oxidative damage [7]. Oxidative modification of proteins can also induce the formation of a series of relatively stable species that can be used as biomarkers for systemic OxS. These include protein carbonyls, alteration of tyrosine residues (including S-glutathionylation, carbonylation, or tyrosine modification to 3-nitro-, 3-chloro-, and 3-bromotyrosine) and as already mentioned, binding of bioactive aldehydes and glycation/glycoxidation [7,20,21].

In this context, protein carbonyls are the most commonly measured markers. Carbonyls are attractive biomarkers due to the easy sampling of plasma proteins and the stability of these oxidative by-products. Protein carbonyls are formed through the oxidative cleavage of protein backbones [3,7]. For instance, the oxidative deamination of lysine and glutamic acid results in protein carbonyl formation. The most frequently used method for assessing carbonyls relies on derivatization with 2,4-dinitrophenylhydrazine (DNPH), which specifically reacts with carbonyls associated with aldehydes and ketones, generating DNPH adducts, which can be easily detected using a spectrophotometric assay [7]. Other methods have been developed for the detection of DNP-derivatized proteins, such as enzyme-linked immunosorbent assay (ELISA) and mass spectroscopy (MS), which, even though more time-consuming, allow for a more accurate quantification of the biomarker [7].

Protein carbonyls and nitrotyrosine

Nitrotyrosine (3-NT) is another reliable biomarker for protein oxidation. It is formed via post-translational modification of proteins due to the highly reactive peroxynitrite (OONO-), which is produced following the reaction between nitric oxide (NO) and $O_2^{\cdot -}$ [21]. Notably, this reaction can also occur with free tyrosine [21]. The main sources of 3-NT are NO metabolism, heme peroxidase, and myeloperoxidase (MPO). The formation of 3-NT is greatly influenced by pH as artifactual nitration can easily occur as a result of acid hydrolysis during sample processing [21]. This, along with the low concentration of the marker in serum/plasma and urine, represents one of the major pitfalls of analytical methods such as ELISA and GC for 3-NT [21].

Advanced glycation end-products

Advanced glycation end-products (AGEs) are proteins or lipids that are glycated following exposure to carbohydrates [22]. AGEs can be generated by a number of chemical pathways, with the Maillard reaction being the most well-known and well described. In addition, there are other well-characterized pathways for AGE formation within cells, tissues, and biological fluids. OxS is one of the main triggers of AGEs production via nonenzymatic glycoxidation reactions [22]. AGE formation causes an impairment in protein structure due to covalent cross-linking, resulting in protein oligomerization and aggregation [7].

The accumulation of AGEs in various tissues (including skin, where the marker is often assessed) progresses with aging and is accelerated in diabetes mellitus patients. Developing a better understating of AGEs' accumulation has confirmed that AGEs interaction with their receptors (RAGE) is implicated not only in the development of diabetic complications but also in neurodegenerative disorders [23].

More than 20 different AGEs have been identified in blood and tissue samples [7]. Several methods have been developed for the measurement of this class of compounds (fluorimetry, HPLC, MS, and commercial ELISA); however, blood measurements of AGEs are indicative of their short-term presence and do not provide information on their accumulation in tissues [24].

Markers of DNA and RNA oxidative damage

8-Oxo-7,8-dihydro-2′-deoxyguanosine and 7,8-dihydro-8-oxo-deoxyguanine

In cells, an important level of DNA damage occurs daily due to exposure to different intracellular and extracellular toxic agents. OxS represents the main endogen factor responsible for these modifications, with the most abundant DNA oxidation by-product being 8-oxo-7,8-dihydro-2′-deoxyguanosine (8-oxodG) [25]. 8-oxodG can be formed by the direct oxidation of guanine through the addition of a hydroxyl radical to C-8 of the imidazole ring of guanine or by reacting with singlet oxygen [25]. This nucleobase is more vulnerable than others to oxidative modification in both RNA and DNA due to its low redox potential compared to those of adenine and pyrimidines [7]. Notably, when repair mechanisms fail, this lesion can result in a G-to-T transversion mutation.

7,8-Dihydro-8-oxo-deoxyguanine (8-OxoG) is formed following the oxidation of RNA nucleotides. This by-product does not prevent nucleic acid synthesis but can induce alternate base pair mismatch [7]. As 8-oxodG, 8-OxoG can be improved by base excision repair, nucleotide excision repair, and mismatch repair. 8-OxoG produced by the repair process can be transported by the cell membrane and excreted into the CSF, plasma, and urine [25,26]. Both 8-oxodG and 8-OxoG have been extensively used as biomarkers of DNA oxidation in several diseases [3]. Although various methods have been used to assess these by-products in a bodily fluid, one of the most frequently used method (ELISA) lacks adequate specificity [7]. Chromatographic methods, including HPLC-electrochemical detection (HPLC-ECD) (liquid chromatography with tandem MS (LC-MS/MS) [25] and GC-MS [26], provide more accurate detection possibilities.

Rationale for measuring fluid redox biomarkers in neurological disease

Neuronal cells are particularly susceptible to oxidative damage due to their various physiological and biochemical features. First, the brain is characterized by an elevated metabolic activity and thus high consumption of oxygen (and consequently more likely leakage of ROS from mitochondria), the used of almost exclusive oxidative phosphorylation (over 25% of circulating glucose to support neuronal function), and no energy reserves [27]. Second, the brain has a comparatively weak endogenous antioxidant defense system and is highly susceptible to disruptions of redox homeostasis [28]. Furthermore, neuronal cells present 50 times lower catalase content than hepatocytes and have constrained glutathione peroxidase 4, along with low glutathione (GSH) content [28]. Third, redox imbalance also occurs easily in the brain because of the abundance of loosely bound redox-active metals (especially copper and iron, which contribute to ferroptosis by catalyzing peroxyl and alkoxyl radical generation) and high concentrations of PUFAs [29]. Forth, neurons preserve their essential physiological functions through neuronal nitric oxide synthase (nNOS) and NADPH oxidase (NOX) [29]. However, overactivation of nNOS (induced by the excitatory neurotransmitter glutamate) is a frequent event, particularly in the aged brain, which leads to an increase in NO· generation, which can be converted to the highly reactive ONOO· when it reacts with $O_2^{\cdot-}/H_2O_2$ generated by NOX and mitochondria [29].

Alzheimer's disease

Role of oxidative stress in the pathogenesis and pathophysiology

Dementia is universally defined as a "group of symptoms affecting memory, thinking, and social abilities severely enough to interfere with individual's daily living" [30]. AD is the primary cause of dementia, with an estimated increase of 9.9 million new cases per year worldwide [31]. AD is characterized by the progressive deterioration of cognitive functions associated with accelerated brain atrophy [31]. The reduction in brain volume results from the degeneration of synapses and the death of neurons, particularly within the hippocampus, a brain region essential for memory [32]. This disorder, as well as other minor forms of dementia such as vascular dementia and frontotemporal dementia, is often preceded by a preclinical phase termed mild cognitive impairment (MCI) [33]. In general, individuals with MCI have a higher rate of progression to dementia over a relatively short period than normal subjects, especially after 60 years of age [34]. As aging is the foremost risk factor for the most common type of AD, the so-called sporadic (also termed late-onset), and life expectancy continues to increase, the number of individuals with this disease is expected to almost triple by 2050 [31].

Several hypotheses have been proposed in an attempt to model the pathogenesis of AD. Among these, the prevailing one is the "amyloid hypothesis" [32] (Fig. 4.3). As the first pathogenic event, β-amyloid (Aβ) is derived from the amyloidogenic pathway. In the predominant and innate nonamyloidogenic pathway, membrane-associated β-amyloid precursor protein (APP) is first hydrolyzed by α-secretase and then by γ-secretase to form nontoxic and putatively protective (sAPPα) fragments [32]. In the amyloidogenic pathway, APP is cleaved by β- and γ-secretases, leading to the formation of full-length Aβ peptides (primarily Aβ1–40/42) [32]. These peptides aggregate to form neurotoxic oligomers and then almost inert senile plaques, which are characteristic to aging brains and constitute a pathological hallmark of AD along with tau neurofibrillary tangles (NTFs) [30,35]. These aberrant peptide aggregates are considered to be responsible for neurodegeneration that leads to memory impairment and dementia [32]. Nevertheless, the exact mechanisms underlying AD remains to be fully elucidated. Thus, further research efforts are needed to shed light on the intricate pathogenesis of AD.

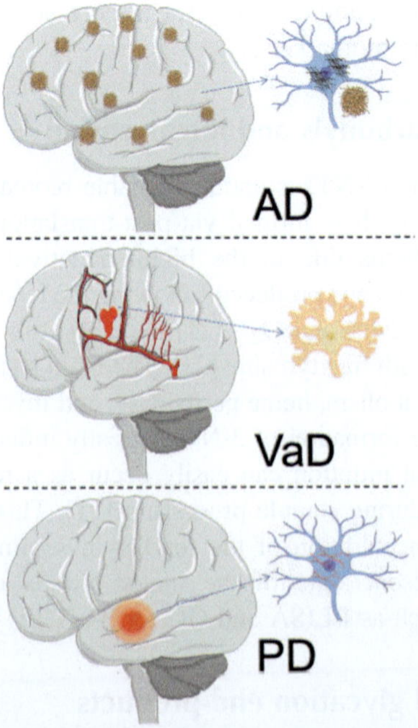

FIGURE 4.3 Main neuropathological hallmarks of Alzheimer's disease (AD), vascular dementia (VaD), and Parkinson's disease (PD). AD: Extracellular **amyloid plaques (brown** fibrillar aggregates) are disseminated in the brain along with intracellular **neurofibrillary tangles (black** fibrillar aggregates); VaD: Hemorrhagic (which is displayed in the Figure) or ischemic micro- and/or macro-infarcts lead to brain **hypoperfusion** and consequent hypoxia and degeneration of neurons; PD: Progressive loss of dopaminergic nigrostriatal neurons in the ***substantia nigra pars compacta*** (highlighted by *red* cycle) with typical formation **of alpha-synuclein aggregates** inside the neurons (*orange* filaments).

One factor that influences AD pathogenesis is the OxS [36]. Accumulating evidence clearly suggests that RS are involved in the onset and progression of AD [29,36,37] (Fig. 4.4). Neuroinflammation, which is now regarded as a typical pathological hallmark of Aβ plaques and NFTs, represents a potent trigger for the redox short circuit occurring in the AD brain [29,38,39].

We recently proposed a novel term, "oxinflammation," to describe the mutual relationship between inflammation and OxS [40]. Biochemical and immune stressors are dynamically connected to each other, and the effect of this vicious cycle is locally (brain) confined but reflects at the systemic level. This concept fits fairly well with AD, since systemic manifestations, including inflammation and OxS, do not merely coexist but drive (and are driven by) neurodegeneration [41].

Several reports have shown that AD is associated with elevated levels of inflammatory markers and risk genes associated with innate immune functions [38]. Moreover, astrocytes and microglial cells, the main types of cells involved in the inflammatory response within the CNS, are highly activated in the AD brain [38]. In particular,

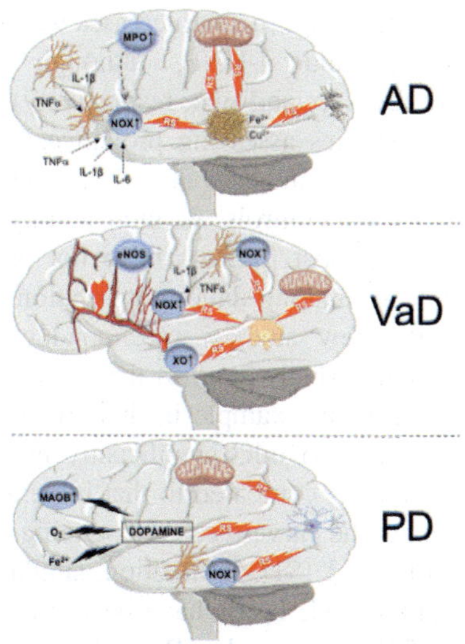

FIGURE 4.4 Principal sources and triggers of reactive species (ROS and RNS) in Alzheimer's disease (AD), vascular dementia (VaD) and Parkinson's disease (PD). AD: RS (e.g., $O_2^{\cdot-}$, ·OH, H_2O_2, HOCl) are generated by: (1) **NOX** of neurons and activated microglia (activation occurs via cytokines coming from other microglia and/or systemic circulation) (2) **MPO** which produces highly toxic HOCl via interaction with NOXs (3) **dysfunctional mitochondria**. RS can contribute to the formation of **Aβ oligomers** that aggregate in **amyloid plaques** (**brown** fibrillar aggregates) which, in turn, are able to generate RS by redox active **iron, copper** and other **free transition metals**. RS from Aβ and other sources may also contribute to the formation of **neurofibrillary tangles** (**black** fibrillar aggregates); VaD: **brain hypoperfusion** leads to decrease in eNOS activity and increase in endothelial and microglial **NOXs**. Further sources of RS are **XO** and dysfunctional **mitochondria**. PD: **dopamine** undergoes auto-oxidation to form dopamine quinones, ROS, and DA-semiquinone radicals. This dopamine breakdown can be catalyzed by **iron**, oxygen, or enzymes such as monoamine oxidase-B (**MAO B**), located in microglia. Other well-documented sources of RS in PD are **mitochondria** and activated microglia (via **NOX**). Excess in RS can contribute to the formation of formation of alpha-synuclein aggregates in the neurons (*orange* filaments) and neurodegeneration. *eNOS*, endothelial nitric oxide synthetase; *MPO*, myeloperoxidase; *NOX*, NADPH-oxidase; *XO*, xanthine oxidase.

microglia, which are brain-resident macrophages that constitute the most significant innate and adaptive immune response, have enhanced sensitivity to inflammatory stimuli [38]. These innate immune cells promptly respond to systemic events, and these responses are exaggerated and uncontrolled in the aging and diseased brain. These extra-brain stimuli can be peripheral inflammatory cytokines (in primis, interleukin (IL)-6, tumor necrosis factor (TNF)-α, and IL-1β) that can easily cross the blood–brain barrier (BBB) [38]. Moreover, elevated brain RS and neurodegenerative processes can contribute to the activation of microglia, which in turn starts to release neurotoxic cytokines, chemokines, and RS36,37.

Specialized enzymes can serve as bridges between OxS and inflammation. NOX, located in microglia, astrocytes, and neurons, is one such enzyme [40]. It generates $O_2^{\cdot-}$ and H_2O_2 upon stimulation by proinflammatory mediators such as TNFα and IL-1β [40]. The NOX-induced elevation in RS levels can activate immune cells as well as redox-sensitive transcription factors in particular AP-1 and NF-kB [40]. Ultimately, this cascade of events leads to the expression of several proinflammatory cytokines that perpetuate NOX activity [42]. In myeloperoxidase (MPO), an important player in host defense against microorganisms, inflammatory signals lead to the release of RS [43]. Furthermore, MPO can convert H_2O_2 into hypochlorous acid (HOCl) in the presence of chloride ions and mounting evidence has shown that increased MPO levels in the frontal cortex are mainly localized in amyloid beta (Aβ)-positive senile plaques and in some activated microglia [44].

The largest contributor of RS in the brain and the rest of the body is the mitochondria. In 2004, Swerdlow and Shaharyar were the first to propose that mitochondrial dysfunction, leading to respiratory chain defects and ultimately excess ROS production, is the earliest event in sporadic AD pathogenesis [45]. According to this hypothesis, the loss of mitochondrial function influences AD chronology by affecting APP expression and processing, Aβ accumulation, tau phosphorylation, and neuroinflammation. The mitochondrial cascade hypothesis has been supported by mounting evidence showing extensive mitochondrial dysfunction in AD-vulnerable regions of the brain [46,47]. Notably, oxidized mitochondrial DNA has been observed in postmortem brain tissue and peripheral nervous system, including cells and isolated mitochondria from individuals with preclinical stages of AD [47].

OxS appears to play an important role in the formation and accumulation of neurotoxic Aβ and NFT. Previous studies have suggested that elevated RS can lead to initiation of the amyloidogenic pathway, which can influence the expression, processing, and intracellular protein trafficking of APP and Aβ peptides [36]. Some of the most solid supporting evidences for this hypothesis were provided by Minosou et al. who showed that OxS cause an increase in the levels of intracellular Aβ in human neuroblastoma cells [37]. Nevertheless, this relationship is not unidirectional as these hallmarks are potential sources of RS. In addition, RS influences the clearance of Aβ from the brain (the main cause of accumulation of these peptides in sporadic AD) through oxidation of low-density lipoprotein receptor-related protein 1 (LRP1), which plays a critical role in this process [48].

The pro-oxidant effects of Aβ, especially in the form of soluble oligomer of the 1–42 subtype (the major component of senile plaques), have mostly been shown in animal models of AD [36,37]. Overexpression of these aberrant peptides has been shown to be associated with an increase in 4-HNE, ROS, and protein carbonyls, as well as decreases in the neuron survival ratio [49]. The increase in ROS caused by Aβ is attributable to the high concentration of pro-oxidant iron and copper as well as the Aβ ability to negatively affect mitochondrial function [49]. Moreover, Aβ localizes to mitochondrial membranes, blocks the transport of nuclear-encoded mitochondrial proteins to mitochondria, interacts with mitochondrial proteins, and disrupts the electron transport chain, thus, inducing mitochondrial damage [49].

As suggested by previous studies [50], Aβ-mediated mitochondrial OxS induces the hyperphosphorylation of tau in AD brains. This is a crucial aspect since tau appears to be the main trigger for neurodegeneration. Several OxS markers have been discovered to be increased in tauopathies (a group of pathologies characterized by the brain deposition of abnormal tau protein), such as MDA or 4-HNE [49,51]. Several in vitro and animal model studies overexpressing tau suggested that inherited tauopathies, besides increasing OxS, enhance the sensitivity of neurons to oxidant molecules such as H_2O_2 or paraquat [52]. OxS may also be a downstream event in tau hyperphosphorylation, and it was observed that 4-HNE and oxidized fatty acids promote the aggregation of phosphorylated tau in vitro and induce tau hyperphosphorylation [52,53]. Similar results were obtained in SOD2-deficient mice, which is a major scavenger of mitochondrial ROS [52,53].

A large body of evidence from postmortem studies has revealed that products of oxidative damage to lipids, proteins, amino acids, RNA, and DNA are significantly more elevated in the brains of patients with AD and MCI than in cognitively healthy controls [49,50,52,53]. The accumulation of these oxidative signatures is mainly detectable in AD-vulnerable regions (e.g., the hippocampus) [47,49,54,55]. In contrast, brain regions with low Aβ levels (e.g., the cerebellum) did not show high concentrations of OxS markers [49,54].

Redox biomarkers in AD

There is a large body of evidence showing alterations in redox biomarkers from blood, urine, and central nervous system (CSF) of AD and MCI patients. One of the most convincing evidence corroborating this claim came from a meta-analysis by Schrag and colleagues. They systematically reviewed case-control studies on OxS markers (protein carbonyls, oxidized LDL, MDA, 4-HNE, 8-OxoG, and 8-oxodG) and the levels of antioxidants, copper, transferrin, and ceruloplasmin in the blood of subjects with AD and MCI [56]. Among the OxS markers, MDA (increase by 25% in AD patients) appeared to be the most robust due to the relatively high number of studies that measured this marker ($n = 27$). However, the reliability of this finding was affected by an important bias, since all studies included in the analysis the MDA assessed using an inaccurate TBARS assay. Other significant increases were detected for 8-OxoG/8-oxodG and 4-HNE, although the studies analyzed were few (six and two, respectively). In contrast, the analysis of studies assessing protein carbonylation in plasma/serum did not indicate any significant differences between patients and controls. As indicated by the authors, for MCI subjects, most findings have not been independently reproduced, making data interpretation challenging.

Subsequently, few studies were conducted on these biomarkers which partially confirm the results of the meta-analysis. An important example in this context is a recent study showing that 8-oxodG significantly increases in the urine of MCI patients compared to that in healthy controls, with an area under the curve-receiver operating characteristic (AUC-ROC) of 0.843 [51]. In addition, similar data evaluating MDA and 4-HNE levels have been presented in previous studies [57]. In particular, Rani et al. discovered that 4-HNE and MDA levels were higher in AD patients than that in SNCs and, most importantly, positively correlated with standard CSF biomarkers (Aβ and Tau) for AD [57].

Although IsoPs are widely considered the gold standard marker for OxS, it was not considered in Schrag's analysis. This gap was filled in a subsequent meta-analysis that included 29 studies, 25 cross-sectional studies, and five longitudinal studies, selectively focusing on the association between 8-iso-PGF2α and AD [58]. This analysis revealed that 8-iso-PGF2α levels were significantly higher in patients with AD than in controls, independently of biological sample types (CSF, plasma, urine, and brain tissue). The difference remained significant in the separated meta-regressions, including studies using the same specimen and detection methods. Among the four longitudinal studies considered in the meta-analysis, two were on CSF and two performed analyses on urine samples. A pooled analysis of the data failed to show significant results. Interestingly, Peña-Bautista et al. showed that some isoprostane isomers assessed in the CSF, although not able to discriminate between AD and non-AD groups, correlate with neuropsychological evaluations and CSF Aβ and tau [59].

Alternatively, the published results on NeuroPs are mixed [60,61]. Lower levels of plasma NeuroPs were observed in patients with AD than in the controls [60]. In contrast, other studies have shown unvaried or increased levels of these compounds in various biological fluids, including CSF, urine, and plasma [61,62]. Recently, plasma NeuroPs have been shown to represent a better AD diagnosis tool when incorporated into a multivariate model that when other isoprostane isomers were incorporated into multivariate models [63]. However, considered alone, it could be more useful for the prognosis than for the diagnosis of AD as suggested by a recent report [64].

Serum LPO have also been investigated by us and other groups [65], with generally consistent results. We discovered that, in a large sample of older individuals ($n = 334$), serum LPO were increased in AD and MCI patients compared to those measured in controls [66]. This difference was independent of potential confounding factors such as age, sex, smoking, and comorbidities. A large longitudinal study investigated the potential association between plasma LPO and cognitive function in community-dwelling older adults ($n = 2882$) [65]. The authors showed that increased levels of this marker were inversely associated with global cognition and verbal fluency in both cross-sectional and prospective analyses.

There have been a number of reports liking type 2 diabetes mellitus (DM) to AD [41,67]. Evidence in support of this relationship comes from preclinical and population-based studies investigating the AGEs blood levels in AD patients. Riviere et al. were among the first to report increased plasma levels of these redox biomarkers in AD patients compared to controls [67]. This result was confirmed by a series of studies on AGEs and RAGEs as assessed in peripheral fluids, including CSF [68].

Vascular dementia

Role of oxidative stress in the pathogenesis and pathophysiology

VaD is the second most common type of dementia (approximately 20% of all cases) [69]. VaD is a disease characterized by cognitive impairment resulting from brain hypoperfusion duc to cerebrovascular diseases and ischemic or hemorrhagic brain damage [69] (Fig. 4.4). Cerebrovascular diseases represent a broad category, including stroke, carotid stenosis, aneurysms, and vascular malformations. There are several subtypes of VaD, with the most common being multi- and single-infarct dementia, small-vessel disease, and AD-VaD mixed dementia (simultaneous presence of cerebrovascular lesions and neuritic plaques) [69]. Notably, cerebrovascular injury is also a pathogenic co-factor and/or a coexisting condition of AD [27,70]. Hypoperfusion is a frequent effect of microangiopathy or macroangiopathy, which, in turn, is caused by common cardiometabolic risk factors (e.g., hypertension, smoking, diabetes) and cerebral amyloid angiopathy (CAA), a major contributor to AD pathogenesis [71]. This form of angiopathy is characterized by amyloid deposition in medium and small cerebral vessels, in addition to the brain parenchyma. CAA leads to changes in the BBB integrity, the release of inflammatory mediators and matrix metalloproteases, and causes (or exacerbates) brain hypoperfusion and consequent hypoxia as well as RS generation [72].

The presence of CAA is not the only common feature of AD and VaD. Although these two diseases are still considered to be different from a nosological point of view, based on current diagnostic criteria, AD and VaD share several clinical presentations, risk factors, and important neuropathological features [27,70]. These commonalities often make differential diagnosis challenging.

OxS in the vasculature appears to be a common feature in diverse cerebrovascular disease and injury models. Overexpression of certain NOXs (in particular isoforms 1 and 4) in the brain vasculature seems to play a prominent role in cerebrovascular disease [73]. Further sources of neurovascular OxS include mitochondria, which are more abundant in the cerebral endothelium than in other cells, xanthine oxidase hypoxia-related activation, and neuroinflammation [74]. Although the release of inflammatory mediators from activated microglia, astrocytes, and neurons occurs rapidly after a stroke, an exaggerated inflammatory response can also occur upstream of RS elevation. Hypoxia-induced elevation of ROS (in particular, $O_2^{\cdot -}$) decreases the nitric oxide (·NO) bioavailability; thus, affecting endothelial relaxation [73]. A decrease in ·NO may also occur via an ROS-induced increase in Rho kinase signaling that interferes with endothelial nitric oxide synthase expression, affecting the production of this potent vasodilator [75]. This phenomenon greatly contributes to endothelial activation, the expression of chemoattractant cytokines, and inflammatory responses. Notably, it is well known that RS can directly cause loss of BBB integrity (most likely due to altered expression of critical tight junction proteins) [40]. This, in turn, allows to the entry of inflammatory cytokines and cells from the systemic circulation into the CNS, thus fueling the neuroinflammatory process [40]. As described for AD, this cytokine cascade inevitably leads to activation of NOXs and an "oxinflammatory" cycle that exacerbates brain damage [40].

Redox biomarkers in VaD

There is a considerable body of literature demonstrating an association between stroke and OxS biomarkers; however, their relationship with VaD has been poorly investigated. Several studies have showed that the MDA levels (as assessed by both spectrophotometric assay and HPLC) are higher in stroke patients than in healthy controls [76]. Moreover, plasma MDA levels were discovered to be related to infarct size, clinical stroke severity, and patient outcomes [77]. Interestingly, Polidori et al. showed that cholesteryl ester hydroperoxides increased in patients that experienced a large ischemic stroke, with their marker being correlated with infarct volume as detected using computed tomography or magnetic resonance imaging scans [78]. The results obtained using blood IsoPs as a marker of OxS were mixed, with increased or unchanged levels in stroke patients compared to those in healthy individuals [77]. One of the last longitudinal studies focusing on this marker suggested that elevated plasma isoP levels independently predicted the occurrence of infarct growth volume in patients with acute ischemic stroke [76]. Plasma oxidized low-density lipoprotein (oxLDL) has also been associated with stroke in several studies [79]. Of note, in one of them, oxLDL levels increased to their maximum 3 days after the ischemic stroke but not hemorrhagic stroke.

Systemic OxS-related diseases, such as diabetes and atherosclerosis, represent important risk factors and comorbidities of VaD, and an association between peripheral redox biomarkers, and these diseases is expected [27,69]. However, as mentioned at the beginning of this section, published data are limited and inconsistent.

One of the few large longitudinal studies investigating IsoPs in VaD was published in 2020 [80]. The authors evaluated the potential associations of urinary IsoPs levels with all-cause, AD and VAD incidence in 5853 older adults and discovered that the levels of this marker were significantly associated with all-cause dementia incidence and AD incidence but not with VaD incidence. A cross-sectional analysis conducted in another study (72 patients with AD, 27 with VaD, 24 with AD-VaD mixed dementia, and 53 controls) suggested that plasma LPO were higher in AD and AD-VaD mixed dementia patients than those in controls [81]. Similarly, we showed that the serum lipid hydroperoxide concentration (assessed with a different spectrophotometric assay) was unchanged in VaD patients when compared to that of controls but significantly lower than that observed in AD patients [82]. Intriguingly, these peripheral markers were able to discriminate between AD and VaD when combined with serum total antioxidant power, uric acid, and homocysteine. This is an interesting finding since the differential diagnosis of these two major forms of dementia is challenging (even in the absence of disease-specific biomarkers).

Another group evaluated serum LPO levels, along with IsoPs and 4-HNE, in 29 possible vascular MCI patients and 89 controls (both patient groups presented stable coronary artery disease) [83]. The authors discovered that the levels of these three markers did not significantly change in patients affected by the prodromal phase of VaD when compared to controls.

In contrast to the aforementioned results, Serra et al. showed that plasma MDA levels (as assessed by spectrophotometric TBARS assay) were increased to a similar extent in both AD and VaD patients when compared to that observed in controls [84]. These findings were corroborated by Casado et al. [85].

Parkinson's disease

Role of oxidative stress in the pathogenesis and pathophysiology

PD is the second most common neurodegenerative disease, after AD [86]. The mechanisms underlying PD-associated neurodegeneration are complex and are yet to be completely elucidated. PD is classified into different types based on its cause and age of onset: idiopathic (the most common form, affecting individuals with an average age of 60 years), early onset (with an onset before the age of 50 years), and familial (inherited form; 10%−15% of total PD cases) [86]. The first familial PD cases were attributed to a point mutation at the gene locus encoding alpha-synuclein, which was identified as the major component of intraneuronal protein aggregates called Lewy bodies. This is a typical neuropathological hallmark of PD disease and Lewy body dementia [86,87]. These abnormal protein aggregates can activate the pathways involved in neuronal dysfunction and cell death. PD is characterized by the progressive loss of dopaminergic nigrostriatal neurons in the substantia nigra pars compacta (SNpc), resulting in an impairment of the dopamine pathways [86,87] (Fig. 4.3). This damage is considered to be responsible for the four classically described motor-related symptoms: resting tremor, rigidity, bradykinesia, and postural instability [86,87]. Nonmotor symptoms include sleep disorders, depression, memory impairment, delayed response, psychosis, and confusion [86,87].

A considerable amount of preclinical evidence indicates that RS might significantly contribute to the PD-specific neuronal loss [88] (Fig. 4.4). The major sources of RS in the PD brain are associated with dopamine metabolism, low GSH, and high levels of iron as well as calcium in the SNpc [88].

After being released from synaptic vesicles into the synaptic cleft, dopamine undergoes auto-oxidation to form dopamine quinones, ROS ($O_2^{\cdot-}$ and $OH^{\cdot-}$), and dopamine semiquinone radicals, which renders dopaminergic neurons highly vulnerable to OxS-induced damage [88,89]. This dopamine breakdown can be catalyzed by iron (which is present in large amount in the striatum of PD brain), oxygen, or enzymes such as monoamine oxidase-B (MAO B), located in microglia [89]. This enzyme plays a pivotal role in the activation of 1-methyl-4-phenyl-1,2,3,6-tetrahydropyridine (MPTP) into 1-methyl-4-phenylpyridinium ions, which is a component of the enzymatic conversion of dopamine into H2O2. ROS are relatively stable and can cross the membrane, entering neighboring dopaminergic neurons, where they can react with reduced iron to form $OH^{\cdot-}$ [88,89].

Dopamine semiquinones can further cyclize into aminochromes, a potent complex I inhibitor, which further produces $O_2^{\cdot-}$ [88,89]. This may be one of the factors accounting for the decreased activity of the complex I within the mitochondrial respiratory chain (accompanied by abnormal morphology of these organelles) in the SNpc, which is often observed in PD patients. It is generally agreed that electron leakage from complex I and complex III represents the main source of mitochondrial $O_2^{\cdot-}$ [88,89]. This type of mitochondrial dysfunction can also occur via dopaminergic neurotoxins, such as MPTP, a contaminant present in synthetic opioids, or environmental herbicides and pesticides [90]. Notably, these toxic compounds can cause nigrostriatal degeneration in animal models [88,90]. An additional source of RS is neuroinflammation (the mechanistic link between this condition and OxS has already been extensively discussed in this chapter), which plays an important role in PD development [38].

Redox biomarkers in PD

Further evidence in favor of the direct involvement of OxS in PD pathogenesis and pathophysiology has emerged from the presence of oxidative damage traces within the brain [36,91,92]. Consistently, 4-HNE-protein adducts were reported to be present in more than half of the dopaminergic neurons from the substantia nigra of PD patients.

The aforementioned convincing preclinical evidence has led to an extensive investigation of the association between blood and CSF OxS biomarkers and PD occurrence. In general, these clinical data appear to corroborate the body of in vitro and in vivo evidence. However, the lack of longitudinal studies limits the capacity to draw definitive conclusions regarding the nature and importance of systemic OxS and PD.

Two meta-analyses and systemic reviews were published on this topic in 2018 and grossly reached the same conclusions [93,94]. The largest study analyzed data on peripheral blood (serum/plasma) and CSF OxS markers gathered from 80 studies encompassing 7212 PD patients and 6037 healthy controls [93]. Of the 22 OxS indicators considered, the random effects meta-analysis showed that blood concentrations of 8-OhdG (as assessed in four studies), TBARS/MDA ($n = 10$), and other less common markers (nitrite and ferritin in addition to various antioxidants) were significantly higher in PD patients than those in controls. The strongest association of a biomarker with PD occurrence was the blood TBARS/MDA levels. The meta-analysis of CSF 8-OhdG (three studies) did not reveal any significant differences between PD patients and controls. As frequently observed by other meta-analyses on this topic, there was a high between-studies heterogeneity; this problem was mostly due to differences in age, sex, sample handling, and detection methods (in particular for MDA/TBARS assessment). A further important point emerging from this study is that there were no associations between the levels of the OxS marker (8-OhdG) in CSF and those in blood.

The other meta-analysis covered almost the same cross-sectional studies (8-OhdG and MDA/TBARS were assessed from three to six studies, respectively), while also including five studies investigating lipid peroxidation markers [94]. The forest plot calculated for these biomarkers indicated a significant association between higher levels on each biomarker and the likelihood of developing PD.

Successive studies on this subject have provided general confirmation of the validity of OxS biomarkers in PD diagnosis and prognosis. However, only few of these studies employed the standard biomarkers of oxidative damage described in this chapter. Two studies reported a positive correlation between plasma MDA levels, clinical presentation, and disease severity [95,96]. Consistently, another study showed that higher CSF levels of lipid peroxidation markers increased in PD patients when they were affected by supranuclear palsy (a condition characterized by problems with balance, movement, vision, speech, and swallowing) compared to those without this clinical complication [97].

Surprisingly, other well-established OxS biomarkers have been poorly investigated. As recently observed by Chang et al. only two studies investigated plasma IsoPs, with one finding that plasma levels of this lipid peroxidation indicator are elevated in PD patients, whereas another study indicating that plasma levels of F2-isoprostanes in PD patients are similar to those in controls and AD patients [92].

Despite the consolidated concept that diabetes is a risk factor for PD and the solid evidence showing that AGEs promote aggregation of alpha-synuclein in the brain, these glycated products were investigated as PD biomarkers only in one study, which indicated that there is a significant difference in AGEs as well as protein carbonyls in PD patients compared to those measured in control women but not in men [98].

Concluding remarks

Redox imbalance is a common early pathophysiological feature of almost every neurological disease. In this chapter, we have focused on AD, VaD, and PD which in our intention may serve as paradigmatic example in this context. In these neurodegenerative diseases, multiple biochemical sources trigger the generation of large amount RS that easily take the lead in the battle with the weak reserve of antioxidants present in the brain. Several lines of evidence clearly show that OxS in these pathologies is not merely confined in the brain but, as inflammation, reflect at systemic level. As effect, peripheral sensors of OxS have the potentials to be early and/or late biomarkers for AD, VaD, and PD. This is a relevant point, since there is still no validated blood-based biomarkers for these diseases. Unfortunately, although some findings are promising, no conclusive evidence of the clinical usefulness of OxS biomarkers has been published yet. The main reasons of this failure stand in the still unsolved methodological issues (in primis, lack of gold-standard biomarker and reference range values) and the scarcity of large longitudinal studies on the topics.

References

[1] Biomarkers Definitions Working Group. Biomarkers and surrogate endpoints: preferred definitions and conceptual framework. Clin Pharmacol Ther 2001;69:89–95. https://doi.org/10.1067/mcp.2001.113989.

[2] Liguori I, Russo G, Curcio F, Bulli G, Aran L, Della-Morte D, et al. Oxidative stress, aging, and diseases. Clin Interv Aging 2018;13:757–72. https://doi.org/10.2147/CIA.S158513.

[3] Dalle-Donne I, Rossi R, Colombo R, Giustarini D, Milzani A. Biomarkers of oxidative damage in human disease. Clin Chem 2006;52:601–23. https://doi.org/10.1373/clinchem.2005.061408.

[4] Sies H. Oxidative stress: a concept in redox biology and medicine. Redox Biol 2015;4:180–3. https://doi.org/10.1016/j.redox.2015.01.002.

[5] Di Renzo L, Di Pierro D, Bigioni M, Sodi V, Galvano F, Cianci R, et al. Is antioxidant plasma status in humans a consequence of the antioxidant food content influence? Eur Rev Med Pharmacol Sci 2007;11:185–92.

[6] Kadiiska MB, Peddada S, Herbert RA, Basu S, Hensley K, Jones DP, et al. Biomarkers of oxidative stress study VI. Endogenous plasma antioxidants fail as useful biomarkers of endotoxin-induced oxidative stress. Free Radic Biol Med 2015;81:100–6. https://doi.org/10.1016/j.freeradbiomed.2015.01.006.

[7] Frijhoff J, Winyard PG, Zarkovic N, Davies SS, Stocker R, Cheng D, et al. Clinical relevance of biomarkers of oxidative stress. Antioxid Redox Signal 2015;23:1144–70. https://doi.org/10.1089/ars.2015.6317.

[8] Ho E, Karimi Galougahi K, Liu C-C, Bhindi R, Figtree GA. Biological markers of oxidative stress: applications to cardiovascular research and practice. Redox Biol 2013;1:483–91. https://doi.org/10.1016/j.redox.2013.07.006.

[9] Niki E. Biomarkers of lipid peroxidation in clinical material. Biochim Biophys Acta Gen Subj 2014;1840:809–17. https://doi.org/10.1016/j.bbagen.2013.03.020.

[10] Forman HJ, Ursini F, Maiorino M. An overview of mechanisms of redox signaling. J Mol Cell Cardiol 2014;73:2–9. https://doi.org/10.1016/j.yjmcc.2014.01.018.

[11] Forman HJ, Davies KJA, Ursini F. How do nutritional antioxidants really work: nucleophilic tone and para-hormesis versus free radical scavenging in vivo. Free Radic Biol Med 2014;66:24–35. https://doi.org/10.1016/j.freeradbiomed.2013.05.045.

[12] De Zwart LL, Meerman JHN, Commandeur JNM, Vermeulen NPE. Biomarkers of free radical damage applications in experimental animals and in humans. Free Radic Biol Med 1999;26:202–26. https://doi.org/10.1016/S0891-5849(98)00196-8.

[13] Leung KS, Galano JM, Durand T, Lee JC-Y. Current development in non-enzymatic lipid peroxidation products, isoprostanoids and isofuranoids, in novel biological samples. Free Radic Res 2015;49:816–26. https://doi.org/10.3109/10715762.2014.960867.

[14] van 't Erve TJ, Kadiiska MB, London SJ, Mason RP. Classifying oxidative stress by F2-isoprostane levels across human diseases: a meta-analysis. Redox Biol 2017;12:582–99. https://doi.org/10.1016/j.redox.2017.03.024.

[15] Turck D, Bresson J, Burlingame B, Dean T, Fairweather-Tait S, Heinonen M, et al. Guidance for the scientific requirements for health claims related to antioxidants, oxidative damage and cardiovascular health. EFSA J 2018;16. https://doi.org/10.2903/j.efsa.2018.5136.

[16] Valacchi G, Pecorelli A, Cervellati C, Hayek J. 4-Hydroxynonenal protein adducts: key mediator in Rett syndrome oxinflammation. Free Radic Biol Med 2017;111:270–80. https://doi.org/10.1016/j.freeradbiomed.2016.12.045.

[17] Brose SA, Thuen BT, Golovko MY. LC/MS/MS method for analysis of E2 series prostaglandins and isoprostanes. J Lipid Res 2011;52:850–9. https://doi.org/10.1194/jlr.D013441.

[18] Klawitter J, Haschke M, Shokati T, Klawitter J, Christians U. Quantification of 15-F2t-isoprostane in human plasma and urine: results from enzyme-linked immunoassay and liquid chromatography/tandem mass spectrometry cannot be compared. Rapid Commun Mass Spectrom 2011;25:463–8. https://doi.org/10.1002/rcm.4871.

[19] Kadiiska MB, Gladen BC, Baird DD, Germolec D, Graham LB, Parker CE, et al. Biomarkers of oxidative stress study II: are oxidation products of lipids, proteins, and DNA markers of CCl4 poisoning? Free Radic Biol Med 2005;38.698–710. https://doi.org/10.1016/j.freeradbiomed.2004.09.017.

[20] Duncan MW. A review of approaches to the analysis of 3-nitrotyrosine. Amino Acids 2003;25:351–61. https://doi.org/10.1007/s00726-003-0022-z.

[21] Bandookwala M, Sengupta P. 3-Nitrotyrosine: a versatile oxidative stress biomarker for major neurodegenerative diseases. Int J Neurosci 2020;130:1047–62. https://doi.org/10.1080/00207454.2020.1713776.

[22] Wei Q, Liu T, Sun D-W. Advanced glycation end-products (AGEs) in foods and their detecting techniques and methods: a review. Trends Food Sci Technol 2018;82:32–45. https://doi.org/10.1016/j.tifs.2018.09.020.

[23] Ahmed N. Advanced glycation endproducts—role in pathology of diabetic complications. Diabetes Res Clin Pract 2005;67:3–21. https://doi.org/10.1016/j.diabres.2004.09.004.

[24] de Vos LC, Lefrandt JD, Dullaart RPF, Zeebregts CJ, Smit AJ. Advanced glycation end products: an emerging biomarker for adverse outcome in patients with peripheral artery disease. Atherosclerosis 2016;254:291–9. https://doi.org/10.1016/j.atherosclerosis.2016.10.012.

[25] Henriksen T, Hillestrøm PR, Poulsen HE, Weimann A. Automated method for the direct analysis of 8-oxo-guanosine and 8-oxo-2′-deoxyguanosine in human urine using ultraperformance liquid chromatography and tandem mass spectrometry. Free Radic Biol Med 2009;47:629–35. https://doi.org/10.1016/j.freeradbiomed.2009.06.002.

[26] Ravanat J-L, Guicherd P, Tuce Z, Cadet J. Simultaneous determination of five oxidative DNA lesions in human urine. Chem Res Toxicol 1999;12:802–8. https://doi.org/10.1021/tx980194k.

[27] De La Torre JC. Pathophysiology of neuronal energy crisis in Alzheimer's disease. Neurodegener Dis 2008;5:126–32. https://doi.org/10.1159/000113681.

[28] Lee KH, Cha M, Lee BH. Neuroprotective effect of antioxidants in the brain. Int J Mol Sci 2020;21:7152. https://doi.org/10.3390/ijms21197152.

[29] Chen Z, Zhong C. Oxidative stress in Alzheimer's disease. Neurosci Bull 2014;30:271–81. https://doi.org/10.1007/s12264-013-1423-y.

[30] Fan L, Mao C, Hu X, Zhang S, Yang Z, Hu Z, et al. New insights into the pathogenesis of Alzheimer's disease. Front Neurol 2019;10:1312. https://doi.org/10.3389/fneur.2019.01312.

[31] Prince M, Ali G-C, Guerchet M, Prina AM, Albanese E, Wu Y-T. Recent global trends in the prevalence and incidence of dementia, and survival with dementia. Alzheimer's Res Ther 2016;8:23. https://doi.org/10.1186/s13195-016-0188-8.

[32] Hampel H, Hardy J, Blennow K, Chen C, Perry G, Kim SH, et al. The amyloid-β pathway in Alzheimer's disease. Mol Psychiatry 2021;26:5481–503. https://doi.org/10.1038/s41380-021-01249-0.

[33] Lopez OL, Jagust WJ, DeKosky ST, Becker JT, Fitzpatrick A, Dulberg C, et al. Prevalence and classification of mild cognitive impairment in the cardiovascular health study cognition study. Arch Neurol 2003;60:1385. https://doi.org/10.1001/archneur.60.10.1385.

[34] Ravaglia G, Forti P, Montesi F, Lucicesare A, Pisacane N, Rietti E, et al. Mild cognitive impairment: epidemiology and dementia risk in an elderly Italian population. J Am Geriatr Soc 2008;56:51–8. https://doi.org/10.1111/j.1532-5415.2007.01503.x.

[35] Hampel H, Caruso G, Nisticò R, Piccioni G, Mercuri NB, Giorgi FS, et al. Biological mechanism-based neurology and psychiatry: a BACE1/2 and downstream pathway model. Curr Neuropharmacol 2021. https://doi.org/10.2174/1570159X19666211201095701.

[36] Barnham KJ, Masters CL, Bush AI. Neurodegenerative diseases and oxidative stress. Nat Rev Drug Discov 2004;3:205–14. https://doi.org/10.1038/nrd1330.

[37] Misonou H, Morishima-Kawashima M, Ihara Y. Oxidative stress induces intracellular accumulation of amyloid β-protein (Aβ) in human neuroblastoma cells. Biochemistry 2000;39:6951–9. https://doi.org/10.1021/bi000169p.

[38] Cervellati C, Trentini A, Pecorelli A, Valacchi G. Inflammation in neurological disorders: the thin boundary between brain and periphery. Antioxid Redox Signal 2020;33:191–210. https://doi.org/10.1089/ars.2020.8076.

[39] Calsolaro V, Edison P. Neuroinflammation in Alzheimer's disease: current evidence and future directions. Alzheimer's Dement 2016;12:719–32. https://doi.org/10.1016/j.jalz.2016.02.010.

[40] Valacchi G, Virgili F, Cervellati C, Pecorelli A. OxInflammation: from subclinical condition to pathological biomarker. Front Physiol 2018;9:858. https://doi.org/10.3389/fphys.2018.00858.

[41] Morris JK, Honea RA, Vidoni ED, Swerdlow RH, Burns JM. Is Alzheimer's disease a systemic disease? Biochim Biophys Acta 2014;1842:1340–9. https://doi.org/10.1016/j.bbadis.2014.04.012.

[42] Forman HJ, Torres M. Reactive oxygen species and cell signaling: respiratory burst in macrophage signaling. Am J Respir Crit Care Med 2002;166. https://doi.org/10.1164/rccm.2206007.

[43] Lefkowitz DL, Mone J, Lefkowitz SS. Myeloperoxidase: the good, the bad, and the ugly. Curr Immunol Rev 2010;6:123–9. https://doi.org/10.2174/157339510791111691.

[44] Üllen A, Singewald E, Konya V, Fauler G, Reicher H, Nusshold C, et al. Myeloperoxidase-derived oxidants induce blood-brain barrier dysfunction in vitro and in vivo. PLoS One 2013;8:e64034. https://doi.org/10.1371/journal.pone.0064034.

[45] Swerdlow RH, Khan SM. A "mitochondrial cascade hypothesis" for sporadic Alzheimer's disease. Med Hypotheses 2004;63:8–20. https://doi.org/10.1016/j.mehy.2003.12.045.

[46] Wang X, Su B, Siedlak SL, Moreira PI, Fujioka H, Wang Y, et al. Amyloid-beta overproduction causes abnormal mitochondrial dynamics via differential modulation of mitochondrial fission/fusion proteins. Proc Natl Acad Sci USA 2008;105:19318–23. https://doi.org/10.1073/pnas.0804871105.

[47] Wang J, Xiong S, Xie C, Markesbery WR, Lovell MA. Increased oxidative damage in nuclear and mitochondrial DNA in Alzheimer's disease. J Neurochem 2005;93:953–62. https://doi.org/10.1111/j.1471-4159.2005.03053.x.

[48] Owen JB, Sultana R, Aluise CD, Erickson MA, Price TO, Bu G, et al. Oxidative modification to LDL receptor-related protein 1 in hippocampus from subjects with Alzheimer disease: implications for Aβ accumulation in AD brain. Free Radic Biol Med 2010;49:1798–803. https://doi.org/10.1016/j.freeradbiomed.2010.09.013.

[49] Tönnies E, Trushina E. Oxidative stress, synaptic dysfunction, and Alzheimer's disease. J Alzheimer's Dis 2017;57:1105–21. https://doi.org/10.3233/JAD-161088.

[50] Liu Z, Li T, Li P, Wei N, Zhao Z, Liang H, et al. The ambiguous relationship of oxidative stress, tau hyperphosphorylation, and autophagy dysfunction in Alzheimer's disease. Oxid Med Cell Longev 2015;2015:1–12. https://doi.org/10.1155/2015/352723.

[51] Cioffi F, Adam RHI, Bansal R, Broersen K. A review of oxidative stress products and related genes in early Alzheimer's disease. J Alzheimer's Dis 2021;83:977–1001. https://doi.org/10.3233/JAD-210497.

[52] Alavi Naini SM, Soussi-Yanicostas N. Tau hyperphosphorylation and oxidative stress, a critical vicious circle in neurodegenerative tauopathies? Oxid Med Cell Longev 2015;2015:1–17. https://doi.org/10.1155/2015/151979.

[53] Melov S, Adlard PA, Morten K, Johnson F, Golden TR, Hinerfeld D, et al. Mitochondrial oxidative stress causes hyperphosphorylation of tau. PLoS One 2007;2:e536. https://doi.org/10.1371/journal.pone.0000536.

[54] Yin J, Liao S-X, He Y, Wang S, Xia G-H, Liu F-T, et al. Dysbiosis of gut microbiota with reduced trimethylamine-N-oxide level in patients with large-artery atherosclerotic stroke or transient ischemic attack. J Am Heart Assoc 2015;4. https://doi.org/10.1161/JAHA.115.002699.

[55] Butterfield DA, Reed T, Perluigi M, De Marco C, Coccia R, Cini C, et al. Elevated protein-bound levels of the lipid peroxidation product, 4-hydroxy-2-nonenal, in brain from persons with mild cognitive impairment. Neurosci Lett 2006;397:170–3. https://doi.org/10.1016/j.neulet.2005.12.017.

[56] Schrag M, Mueller C, Zabel M, Crofton A, Kirsch WM, Ghribi O, et al. Oxidative stress in blood in Alzheimer's disease and mild cognitive impairment: a meta-analysis. Neurobiol Dis 2013;59:100–10. https://doi.org/10.1016/j.nbd.2013.07.005.

[57] Rani P, Krishnan S, Rani Cathrine C. Study on analysis of peripheral biomarkers for Alzheimer's disease diagnosis. Front Neurol 2017;8. https://doi.org/10.3389/fneur.2017.00328.

[58] Trares K, Chen L-J, Schöttker B. Association of F2-isoprostane levels with Alzheimer's disease in observational studies: a systematic review and meta-analysis. Ageing Res Rev 2022;74:101552. https://doi.org/10.1016/j.arr.2021.101552.

[59] Peña-Bautista C, Baquero M, López-Nogueroles M, Vento M, Hervás D, Cháfer-Pericás C. Isoprostanoids levels in cerebrospinal fluid do not reflect Alzheimer's disease. Antioxidants 2020;9:407. https://doi.org/10.3390/antiox9050407.

[60] Ferré-González L, Peña-Bautista C, Baquero M, Cháfer-Pericás C. Assessment of lipid peroxidation in Alzheimer's disease differential

diagnosis and prognosis. Antioxidants 2022;11:551. https://doi.org/10.3390/antiox11030551.

[61] Montine KS, Quinn JF, Zhang J, Fessel JP, Roberts LJ, Morrow JD, et al. Isoprostanes and related products of lipid peroxidation in neurodegenerative diseases. Chem Phys Lipids 2004;128:117–24. https://doi.org/10.1016/j.chemphyslip.2003.10.010.

[62] Montine TJ, Quinn JF, Milatovic D, Silbert LC, Dang T, Sanchez S, et al. Peripheral F2-isoprostanes and F4-neuroprostanes are not increased in Alzheimer's disease. Ann Neurol 2002;52:175–9. https://doi.org/10.1002/ana.10272.

[63] Peña-Bautista C, Vigor C, Galano J-M, Oger C, Durand T, Ferrer I, et al. Plasma lipid peroxidation biomarkers for early and non-invasive Alzheimer disease detection. Free Radic Biol Med 2018;124:388–94. https://doi.org/10.1016/j.freeradbiomed.2018.06.038.

[64] Peña-Bautista C, Álvarez L, Baquero M, Ferrer I, García L, Hervás-Marín D, et al. Plasma isoprostanoids assessment as Alzheimer's disease progression biomarkers. J Neurochem 2021;157:2187–94. https://doi.org/10.1111/jnc.15183.

[65] Horvat P, Kubinova R, Pajak A, Tamosiunas A, Schöttker B, Pikhart H, et al. Blood-based oxidative stress markers and cognitive performance in early old age: the HAPIEE study. Dement Geriatr Cogn Disord 2016;42:297–309. https://doi.org/10.1159/000450702.

[66] Cervellati C, Cremonini E, Bosi C, Magon S, Zurlo A, Bergamini CM, et al. Systemic oxidative stress in older patients with mild cognitive impairment or late onset Alzheimer's disease. Curr Alzheimer Res 2013;10:365–72.

[67] Riviere S, Birlouez-Aragon I, Vellas B. Plasma protein glycation in Alzheimer's disease. Glycoconj J 1998;15:1039–42. https://doi.org/10.1023/a:1006902428776.

[68] Shuvaev VV, Laffont I, Serot J-M, Fujii J, Taniguchi N, Siest G. Increased protein glycation in cerebrospinal fluid of Alzheimer's disease. Neurobiol Aging 2001;22:397–402. https://doi.org/10.1016/S0197-4580(00)00253-0.

[69] Gorelick PB, Scuteri A, Black SE, Decarli C, Greenberg SM, Iadecola C, et al. Vascular contributions to cognitive impairment and dementia: a statement for healthcare professionals from the American Heart Association/American Stroke Association. Stroke 2011;42:2672–713. https://doi.org/10.1161/STR.0b013e3182299496.

[70] de la Torre JC. Is Alzheimer's disease a neurodegenerative or a vascular disorder? Data, dogma, and dialectics. Lancet Neurol 2004;3:184–90. https://doi.org/10.1016/S1474-4422(04)00683-0.

[71] Weller RO, Boche D, Nicoll JAR. Microvasculature changes and cerebral amyloid angiopathy in Alzheimer's disease and their potential impact on therapy. Acta Neuropathol 2009;118:87–102. https://doi.org/10.1007/s00401-009-0498-z.

[72] Ghiso J, Tomidokoro Y, Revesz T, Frangione B, Rostagno A. Cerebral amyloid angiopathy and Alzheimer's disease. Hirosaki Igaku 2010;61:S111–24.

[73] Carvalho C, Moreira PI. Oxidative stress: a major player in cerebrovascular alterations associated to neurodegenerative events. Front Physiol 2018;9. https://doi.org/10.3389/fphys.2018.00806.

[74] Chrissobolis S, Faraci FM. The role of oxidative stress and NADPH oxidase in cerebrovascular disease. Trends Mol Med 2008;14:495–502. https://doi.org/10.1016/j.molmed.2008.09.003.

[75] Ming X-F, Viswambharan H, Barandier C, Ruffieux J, Kaibuchi K, Rusconi S, et al. Rho GTPase/Rho kinase negatively regulates endothelial nitric oxide synthase phosphorylation through the inhibition of protein kinase B/Akt in human endothelial cells. Mol Cell Biol 2002;22:8467–77. https://doi.org/10.1128/MCB.22.24.8467-8477.2002.

[76] Lorenzano S, Rost NS, Khan M, Li H, Lima FO, Maas MB, et al. Oxidative stress biomarkers of brain damage. Stroke 2018;49:630–7. https://doi.org/10.1161/STROKEAHA.117.018440.

[77] Cherubini A, Ruggiero C, Polidori MC, Mecocci P. Potential markers of oxidative stress in stroke. Free Radic Biol Med 2005;39:841–52. https://doi.org/10.1016/j.freeradbiomed.2005.06.025.

[78] Polidori MC, Frei B, Rordorf G, Ogilvy CS, Koroshetz WJ, Beal MF. Increased levels of plasma cholesteryl ester hydroperoxides in patients with subarachnoid hemorrhage. Free Radic Biol Med 1997;23:762–7. https://doi.org/10.1016/s0891-5849(97)00053-1.

[79] Husseini NE, Laskowitz DT. Clinical application of blood biomarkers in cerebrovascular disease. Expert Rev Neurother 2010;10:189–203. https://doi.org/10.1586/ern.09.151.

[80] Trares K, Gào X, Perna L, Rujescu D, Stocker H, Möllers T, et al. Associations of urinary 8-iso-prostaglandin $F_{2\alpha}$ levels with all-cause dementia, Alzheimer's disease, and vascular dementia incidence: results from a prospective cohort study. Alzheimer's Dement 2020;16:804–13. https://doi.org/10.1002/alz.12081.

[81] Hatanaka H, Hanyu H, Fukasawa R, Hirao K, Shimizu S, Kanetaka H, et al. Differences in peripheral oxidative stress markers in Alzheimer's disease, vascular dementia and mixed dementia patients. Geriatr Gerontol Int 2015;15:53–8. https://doi.org/10.1111/ggi.12659.

[82] Cervellati C, Romani A, Seripa D, Cremonini E, Bosi C, Magon S, et al. Oxidative balance, homocysteine, and uric acid levels in older patients with Late Onset Alzheimer's Disease or Vascular Dementia. J Neurol Sci 2014;337:156–61. https://doi.org/10.1016/j.jns.2013.11.041.

[83] Suridjan I, Herrmann N, Adibfar A, Saleem M, Andreazza A, Oh PI, et al. Lipid peroxidation markers in coronary artery disease patients with possible vascular mild cognitive impairment. J Alzheimer's Dis 2017;58:885–96. https://doi.org/10.3233/JAD-161248.

[84] Serra JA, Domínguez RO, Marschoff ER, Guareschi EM, Famulari AL, Boveris A. Systemic oxidative stress associated with the neurological diseases of aging. Neurochem Res 2009;34:2122–32. https://doi.org/10.1007/s11064-009-9997-5.

[85] Casado Á, Encarnación López-Fernández M, Concepción Casado M, De La Torre R. Lipid peroxidation and antioxidant enzyme activities in vascular and Alzheimer dementias. Neurochem Res 2008. https://doi.org/10.1007/s11064-007-9453-3.

[86] Ascherio A, Schwarzschild MA. The epidemiology of Parkinson's disease: risk factors and prevention. Lancet Neurol 2016;15:1257–72. https://doi.org/10.1016/S1474-4422(16)30230-7.

[87] Kalia LV, Lang AE. Parkinson's disease. Lancet 2015;386:896–912. https://doi.org/10.1016/S0140-6736(14)61393-3.

[88] Dias V, Junn E, Mouradian MM. The role of oxidative stress in Parkinson's disease. J Parkinsons Dis 2013;3:461–91. https://doi.org/10.3233/JPD-130230.

[89] Ma L, Gholam Azad M, Dharmasivam M, Richardson V, Quinn RJ, Feng Y, et al. Parkinson's disease: alterations in iron and redox biology as a key to unlock therapeutic strategies. Redox Biol 2021;41:101896. https://doi.org/10.1016/j.redox.2021.101896.

[90] Dionísio PA, Amaral JD, Rodrigues CMP. Oxidative stress and regulated cell death in Parkinson's disease. Ageing Res Rev 2021;67:101263. https://doi.org/10.1016/j.arr.2021.101263.

[91] Yoritaka A, Hattori N, Uchida K, Tanaka M, Stadtman ER, Mizuno Y. Immunohistochemical detection of 4-hydroxynonenal protein adducts in Parkinson disease. Proc Natl Acad Sci 1996;93:2696–701. https://doi.org/10.1073/pnas.93.7.2696.

[92] Chang K-H, Chen C-M. The role of oxidative stress in Parkinson's disease. Antioxidants 2020;9:597. https://doi.org/10.3390/antiox9070597.

[93] Wei Z, Li X, Li X, Liu Q, Cheng Y. Oxidative stress in Parkinson's disease: a systematic review and meta-analysis. Front Mol Neurosci 2018;11. https://doi.org/10.3389/fnmol.2018.00236.

[94] Khan Z, Ali SA. Oxidative stress-related biomarkers in Parkinson's disease: a systematic review and meta-analysis. Iran J Neurol 2018;17:137–44.

[95] Sanyal J, Bandyopadhyay SK, Banerjee TK, Mukherjee SC, Chakraborty DP, Ray BC, et al. Plasma levels of lipid peroxides in patients with Parkinson's disease. Eur Rev Med Pharmacol Sci 2009;13:129–32.

[96] Shukla R, Rajani M, Srivastava N, Barthwal MK, Dikshit M. Nitrite and malondialdehyde content in cerebrospinal fluid of patients with Parkinson's disease. Int J Neurosci 2006;116:1391–402. https://doi.org/10.1080/00207450500513989.

[97] Takahashi K, Iwaoka K, Takahashi K, Suzuki Y, Taguchi K, Yamahara K, et al. Cerebrospinal fluid levels of oxidative stress measured using diacron-reactive oxygen metabolites and biological antioxidant potential in patients with Parkinson's disease and progressive supranuclear palsy. Neurosci Lett 2021;757:135975. https://doi.org/10.1016/j.neulet.2021.135975.

[98] Sharma A, Weber D, Raupbach J, Dakal TC, Fließbach K, Ramirez A, et al. Advanced glycation end products and protein carbonyl levels in plasma reveal sex-specific differences in Parkinson's and Alzheimer's disease. Redox Biol 2020;34:101546. https://doi.org/10.1016/j.redox.2020.101546.

Chapter 5

CCM proteins are key players in redox signaling and oxidative stress regulation in Cerebral Cavernous Malformations

Federica Finetti, Lucrezia Paradisi and Lorenza Trabalzini
Department of Biotechnology, Chemistry and Pharmacy, University of Siena, Siena, Italy

Introduction

Cerebral cavernous malformations (CCMs) are vascular lesions predominantly affecting neurovasculature. CCMs consist of mulberry-like, thin-walled sinusoidal capillaries lacking mature vessel structural components [1,2]. Clustered capillaries are characterized by an inhomogeneous vessel wall due to the presence of defective cell−cell junctions. This condition results in the impairment of the blood−brain barrier that predisposes it to episodes of thrombosis and bleeding. CCM lesions are typically found in the brain and spinal cord with a prevalence of 0.3%−0.5%, but they are also seen in the retina, liver, kidney, and on skin as hyperkeratotic cutaneous capillary venous malformations [3].

CCMs can occur as single or multiple lesions with sizes ranging from a few millimeters to a few centimeters. Despite the high prevalence of CCM lesions, only 30% of affected people develop clinical symptoms, including recurrent headaches, neurological deficits, seizures, stroke, and intracerebral hemorrhage, while up to 70% of mutation carriers remain clinically asymptomatic during their entire life [4,5].

CCMs can arise sporadically (80%) or may be inherited as an autosomal dominant condition with incomplete penetrance and variable clinical expressivity (20%). Sporadic cases, which occur in individuals with no family history of CCM, are mostly associated with the presence of a single lesion, while multiple lesions are frequently detected in familial CCM [6]. Both familial and sporadic CCM have been attributed to mutations in three different genes known as *CCM1/KRIT1*, *CCM2/MGC4607*, and *CCM3/PDCD10*, which account for about 50%, 20%, and 10% of the cases, respectively. The remaining 20% of cases have been attributed either to not yet detected genetic alterations of the three known CCM genes or to an additional and not yet identified gene correlated to the disease [7,8].

More than 350 distinct *CCM1/CCM2/CCM3* mutations have been detected to date [9], most of which typical of a single family.

It has been suggested that CCM lesion genesis requires homozygous loss-of-function (LOF) mutations in a CCM gene by a Knudsonian two-hit mechanism, whereby an inactivating germline mutation in one allele (first hit) is accompanied by a somatic mutation in the other (second hit) [10−14]. However, the somatic second-hit loss-of-heterozygosity mutation was detected only in a subset of the endothelial cells lining cavernous vessels with germline CCM gene mutations [11], which appears antithetical to the Knudson's two-hit model of CCM pathogenesis. On the other hand, as a plausible refutation of this apparent discrepancy, it has been recently reported that CCM lesions may develop through clonal expansion of mutant endothelial cells accompanied by incorporation in the growing malformation of normal nonmutated endothelial cells [15−17]. Furthermore, more recent evidence has unequivocally demonstrated that homozygous loss of CCM genes is indeed not fully sufficient to cause CCM lesion formation and disease progression in the absence of additional critical stimulants [18]. The major limitation of this model is that lesions only form during early development, in contrast to human CCM disease onset where lesions may form at any moment of life [19,20]. Recently, the discovery that many human CCMs harbor gain of function (GOF) mutations in the oncogene PIK3CA in addition to the previously noted LOF somatic mutations in the CCM genes suggest that the etiology of CCM may be more complex and consistent with a three-hit model. In fact, somatic GOF mutations in

Modulation of Oxidative Stress. https://doi.org/10.1016/B978-0-443-19247-0.00018-7

PIK3CA are present in both sporadic and familial CCMs of all three genotypes [21–23]. Consistently, several previous studies have noted a link between CCM pathogenesis and PI3K signaling activation [14,24]. However, even if PIK3CA activation seems to be a common feature of human CCM lesions, further studies are necessary to better understand this mechanism [25].

Overall, the different clinical penetrance between the three CCM genes and large variability of clinical features of CCM disease, including lesion number and size, rate of recurrent bleeding, age-of-onset, and severity of symptoms, even between family members carrying the same causative gene mutation, strongly suggest that CCM disease onset and progression is determined by a combination of multiple factors, including disease-associated mutations, environmental risk factors, and interindividual genetic modifiers of vascular sensitivity to stressful conditions [26–29].

Currently, there are no direct therapeutic approaches for CCM disease, besides the neurosurgical removal of accessible CCM lesions in patients with recurrent hemorrhage or intractable seizures [1,30,31]. However, based on the great multidisciplinary research advances in the identification of pathobiological mechanisms of CCM disease made in the last decade, some imaging and plasma biomarkers of prognostic value and distinct promising pharmacological strategies for preventing or limiting symptomatic disease onset and severity in susceptible individuals have been recently proposed and tested in animal models and pilot small clinical trials [1,32,33].

CCM1, *CCM2*, and *CCM3* genes encode for KRIT1, CCM2/Malcavernin, and PDCD10 proteins, respectively. These three proteins are structurally unrelated and do not share sequence homology, in addition, lack defined catalytic domains, and contain well-characterized protein-protein interaction motifs and domains. The presence of distinct binding motifs and domains suggests that CCM proteins can interact with multiple binding partners to regulate complex signaling pathways. Indeed, many of the roles of the distinct domains of the three CCM proteins have been revealed by structure–function relationship and functional proteomic studies, which showed that the CCM proteins can directly interact with one another to form an either dimeric (KRIT1/CCM2) or trimeric (KRIT1/CCM2/CCM3) scaffold complex that functions in distinct signal transduction pathways by interacting with a range of other binding partners, including ICAP1, RAP1, and MEKK3 [34–37]. Moreover, such studies showed also that CCM3 can independently heterodimerize with proteins of the GCKIII (germinal center kinase III) family of Sterile 20 (Ste20)-like serine/threonine kinases, including MST3/STK24, SOK1/STK25, and MST4/STK26, forming a stable complex that may function in a separate pathway from the KRIT1/CCM2 complex, suggesting additional independent roles for CCM3 [38–42]. Accordingly, CCM3 has been described as residing in the STRiatin-interacting phosphatase and kinase (STRIPAK) complex, which contains STK25 and MST4, but not CCM1 or CCM2 [43,44].

A schematic representation of CCM1, CCM2, and CCM3 architecture and interaction partners is shown in Fig. 5.1.

Thanks to their ability to establish multiple interactions CCM proteins play critical roles in many cellular events, including cell polarity, cytoskeletal reorganization, cell proliferation, cellular adhesion and migration, angiogenesis, cell–cell junction integrity, vascular permeability, and apoptosis, whether as part of the ternary complex or not, suggesting that CCM proteins act as pleiotropic regulators of cellular homeostasis. Based on their ability to regulate several signaling pathways and their ubiquitous expression, CCM proteins are likely to be involved in other pathological conditions than CCM. Growing evidence indicates the implication of CCM proteins in different pathologies including cardiovascular diseases [45], diabetes [46], intestinal epithelial barrier dysregulation [47], and cancer [48–55].

Furthermore, accumulated evidence in cellular and animal models indicates that the emerged pleiotropic functions of CCM proteins are mainly due to their ability to modulate redox-sensitive pathways and mechanisms involved in adaptive responses to oxidative stress and inflammation, thus contributing to the preservation of cellular homeostasis and stress defenses.

CCM proteins regulate redox signaling and oxidative stress in CCM

A pathological hallmark of the CCM disease is the structural and functional alteration of vascular endothelium. In the central nervous system, the endothelium is part of the neurovascular unit (NVU) where it is in close contact with pericytes, astrocytes, neurons, and the extracellular matrix. All components of this unit constitute the structural basis of the blood–brain barrier and interact with each other in a multidimensional process in which mediators released from multiple cells engage distinct signaling pathways and effector systems in a highly orchestrated manner and safeguard the integrity of the structure itself by regulating immune response, angiogenesis, vasculogenesis, oligodendrogenesis, neuroprotection, and neuroplasticity [48,56–58]. Several studies have demonstrated that endothelial expression of the CCM proteins contributes to proper angiogenesis and blood vessel integrity, supporting the hypothesis that CCM lesion onset is consequent to primary defects intrinsic to the endothelium. However, the effect of CCM protein loss on the NVU function is not completely known to date.

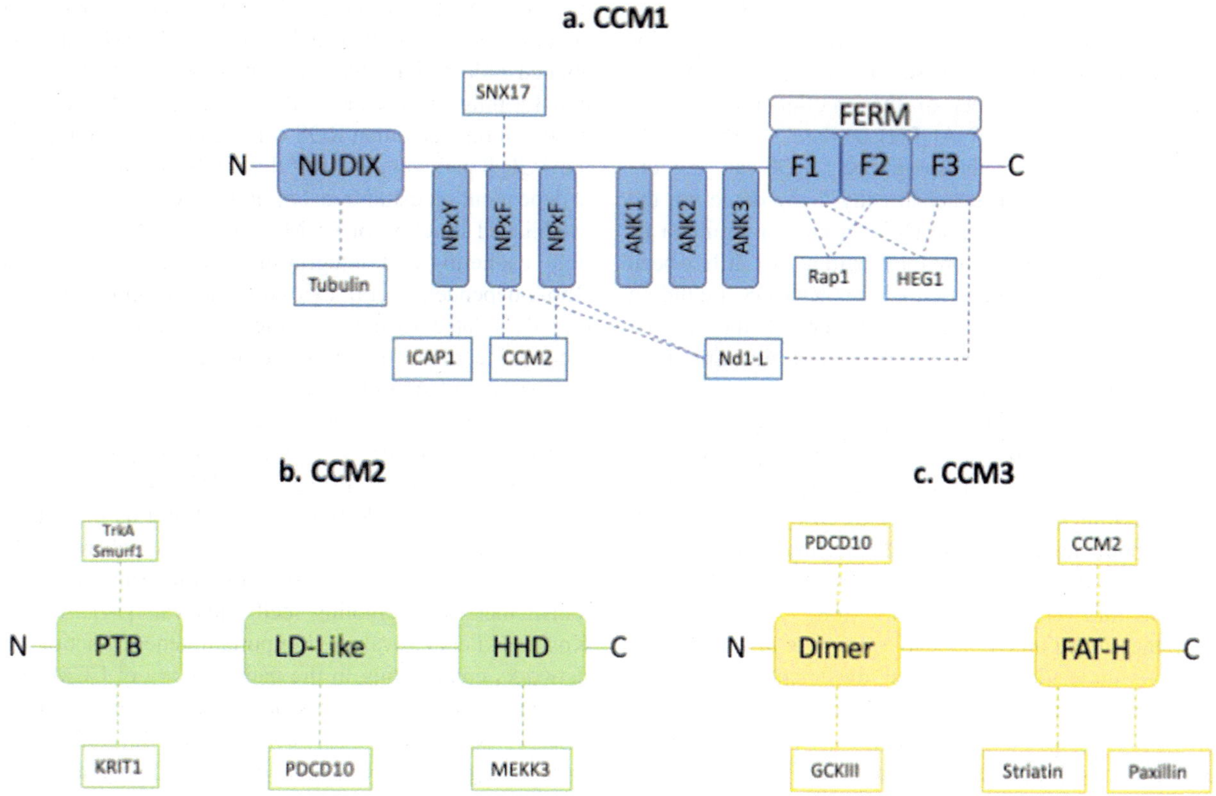

FIGURE 5.1 **Schematic representation of CCM1, CCM2, CCM3 architecture and interaction partners.** (A). CCM1/KRIT1 consists of a Nudix domain, three NPxF motifs, three ankyrin repeats (ANK), and a FERM domain, which comprises three subdomains (F1, F2 and F3). Tubulin binds the Nudix domain, ICAP1 binds the first NPxY motif, SNX17 binds the second NPxF motif, CCM2 binds the second or the third NPxF motif, Nd1-L binds through the second and the third NPxF motif and the F3 subdomain, Rap1 binds through the F1 and F3 subdomains, and HEG1 binds through the F1 and F3 subdomains. (B). CCM2 consists of an N-terminal phosphotyrosine binding domain (PTB), an LD-like motif, and a C- terminal harmonin homology domain (HHD). The PTB domain binds KRIT1, TrkA, and Smurf1, the LD-like motif binds PDCD10, and the HHD domain binds MEKK3. (C). CCM3/ PDCD10 consists of an N-terminal dimerization domain and a C-terminal focal adhesion targeting-homology (FAT-H) domain. The dimerization domain binds another PDCD10 protein and GCKIII, through the FAT-H domain binds CCM2, striatin and paxillin.

Recent evidence outlines the importance of the microenvironment in the development of vascular lesions observed in familial CCM. It has been demonstrated in an animal model that neural deletion of *CCM3* has cell autonomous effects resulting in the formation of multiple vascular lesions closely resembling cavernomas. In addition, it has been shown that vascular lesions originate from clonal expansion of few *CCM3* KO endothelial cells that attract surrounding wild-type endothelial cells thus contributing to the growth of the cavernoma [17,59].

These and other evidence suggest that CCM lesions may develop because of altered and functional interactions within the NVU due to the combination of genetic predisposition with local stressful events [32]. Oxidative stress has been widely shown to promote endothelial dysfunction and cerebrovascular disease by affecting multiple redox-sensitive molecular mechanisms [60,61].

It is well known that oxidative stress is generated by an imbalance of the physiological equilibrium between the generation of reactive oxygen species (ROS) and the capacity of the cellular antioxidant system to quickly detoxify the reactive intermediates or repair the resulting damage.

ROS are highly reactive oxygen-containing molecules generated as common by-products of oxidative metabolism or in response to the activation of several oxidative enzyme complexes.

At physiological concentrations ROS act as signaling molecules implicated in cellular processes and signaling pathways, including regulation of cell metabolism, adhesion, migration, proliferation, and differentiation. Conversely, unphysiologically high levels of ROS cause the oxidative stress status that induces damage to proteins, membrane lipids, and nucleic acids with consequent cellular dysfunctions and pathological states [62].

ROS can be produced by all vascular cell types, including endothelial and periendothelial cells and migrating inflammatory cells [63–65]. In the cell, ROS are generated by multiple systems, including the mitochondrial electron-transport chain (mECT), cytochrome P450 monooxygenases (CYP), nitric oxide synthases (NOS), cyclooxygenase (COX), lipoxygenases (LOX), xanthine oxidase (XOD), and the members of the nicotinamide adenine dinucleotide phosphate (NADPH) oxidase (NOX) family [62]. Above determined threshold levels, ROS can promote endothelial dysfunction either directly or by depleting the bioavailability of nitric oxide (NO), a known regulator of vascular integrity and vasomotor function [66]. It has been shown that the overproduction of distinct ROS, including O_2^-, HO^-, and H_2O_2 can elicit endothelial barrier dysfunction by affecting the cytoskeletal architecture of the endothelial monolayer [67].

On the other hand, ROS production is counteracted by several constitutive or inducible antioxidant defense systems whose function is that of preventing oxidative stress and maintaining cellular homeostasis. In mitochondria are present both nonenzymatic and enzymatic antioxidant systems, including the superoxide dismutase 2 (SOD2), and the glutathione (GSH) redox system [68].

As mentioned above, oxidative stress is involved in all the major molecular and cellular dysfunctions related to CCM disease, including destabilization of endothelial cell-cell junctions, increased β1 integrin activation, increased vascular permeability, and angiogenic activity, suggesting that it may represent a significant triggering factor involved in the onset and progression of CCM [32]. Several studies show that CCM proteins are involved in protecting cells against oxidative stress. In 2010, Goitre et al. demonstrated that KRIT1 protein plays an antioxidant and cytoprotective role by maintaining mitochondrial homeostasis and modulating important regulators of cell responses to oxidative stress such as the transcription factor FoxO1 and its downstream target SOD2 and Sirt1 [69]. These findings have been then corroborated by the identification of a novel molecular interactor of KRIT1, Nd1-L, known to be implicated in the regulation of both Rho GTPase and cellular responses to oxidative stress [70]. In addition, it has been shown that KRIT1 loss-of-function induces the up-regulation of c-Jun, a basic component of the redox-sensitive transcription factor AP-1 and that this up-regulation can be reversed by either KRIT1 re-expression or ROS scavenging with antioxidant compounds. Thus, KRIT1 may play a protective role against oxidative stress by limiting prooxidant and proinflammatory pathways [71]. Interestingly, the up-regulation of c-Jun induced by KRIT1 loss is associated with the induction of cycloxygenase 2 (COX-2), a major oxidative stress biomarker and inflammatory mediator involved in vascular dysfunctions, indicating the implication of KRIT1 in synergistic oxidative stress and inflammatory responses [71].

These observations might be connected to the ones of Maddaluno et al. showing that endothelial-specific disruption of the *CCM1* gene in mice induces endothelial-to-mesenchymal transition (EndMT), which contributes to the development of vascular malformations. EndMT in *CCM1*-ablated endothelial cells is mediated by the activation of the transforming growth factor-β (TGF-β) [72]. Indeed, it has been demonstrated that ROS can stimulate the activation of the TGF-β pathway, and that this ROS-mediated regulation is dependent on c-Jun transcription activity. In addition, the established function of CCM proteins in the regulation of both cadherin- and integrin-mediated cell adhesion and RhoA-dependent actin cytoskeleton dynamics might be directly related to the key role of ROS signaling in the modulation of the functional crosstalk between integrins, cadherins, and small GTPases [32,68,73].

To further substantiate these data, it has been demonstrated that also PDCD10 plays a role in protecting cells from oxidative stress. In fact, PDCD10 is required for the activation of the GCKIII kinase Mst4 and its relocation to the cell periphery after oxidative stress, where it phosphorylates and activates ezrin/radixin/moesin (ERM) proteins, thereby promoting cell survival [74]. Recently Koskimäki et al., evaluated important genes, functions, and networks contributing to the pathobiology of CCM by using transcriptomic analyses across three species and two disease genotypes. Cross-comparisons of differentially expressed genes (DEGs) between species and genotypes, as well as network and gene ontology (GO) enrichment analyses, highlighted that in Ccm3/Pdcd10 KO models, the dysregulated genes are associated with apoptosis, ROS metabolism, and intracellular vesicle trafficking [75].

In addition, CCM2 loss-of-function in endothelial cells induces increased levels of ROS and down-regulates FoxO1 expression, reflecting a physiopathological mechanism common to KRIT1 and suggesting that oxidative stress may be a driving force in CCM at the level of individual cells [76].

Based on these observations, new promising preventive and therapeutic options were suggested involving two available repurposed drugs: Tempol, an SOD-mimetic ROS scavenger, and cholecalciferol (Vitamin D3), endowed with autophagy-inducing and antioxidant properties that have been shown to exert protective effects against oxidative damage in different cell types, including vascular endothelial cells, neurons, and glial cells [32].

To further support the pleiotropic effect of KRIT1 loss-of-function on multiple redox-sensitive mechanisms, other cellular pathways and enzymatic systems involved in cytoprotective mechanisms of adaptive responses to oxidative stress have been investigated, including the Nrf2 antioxidant defense pathway and its downstream target glyoxalase 1 (Glo1), a stress-responsive defense enzyme involved in cellular protection against glycative and oxidative stress through the metabolism of methylglyoxal (MG) [46]. KRIT1 loss induces a redox-sensitive up-regulation of Nrf2 and Glo, leading to chronic adaptative redox homeostasis that counteracts intrinsic oxidative stress but increases susceptibility to oxidative DNA damage and apoptosis, sensitizing cells to further oxidative challenges [46].

Furthermore, it has been found that KRIT1 loss-of-function affects the GSH redox system, causing a significant decrease in total GSH levels and an increase in oxidized glutathione disulfide (GSSG), with a consequent deficit in the GSH/GSSG redox ratio and GSH-mediated antioxidant capacity [77]. These effects are associated with increased S-glutathionylation of distinct proteins involved in adaptative responses to oxidative stress, including redox-sensitive chaperonins, metabolic enzymes, and cytoskeletal proteins, suggesting novel molecular targets of KRIT1 loss-of-function [77].

An important advance in the understanding of the mechanisms by which KRIT1 regulates the function of the vascular barrier was given by the study by Goitre et al. where it has been shown that endothelial ROS production directly contributes to the loss of barrier function in KRIT1 deficient animal and cellular models [78]. In vitro, KRIT1 depletion increased endothelial ROS production via NOX signaling, up-regulated NOX4 expression, and promoted NF-kB-dependent promoter activity. The treatment with an antioxidant and inhibitor of NF-kB signaling rescued barrier function in KRIT1 deficient cells, indicating that ROS signaling is critical for the loss of barrier function following the genetic deletion of KRIT1 and supporting the potentiality of antioxidant therapy in the treatment for CCM [78].

A subsequent study demonstrated that KRIT1 loss-of-function in stromal cells (fibroblasts) causes the up-regulation of NOX1 and the activation of inflammatory pathways, which in turn promote an enhanced production of proangiogenic factors, including vascular endothelial growth factor (VEGF) and prostaglandin E2 (PGE2). Furthermore, conditioned media from KRIT1 null fibroblasts induce proliferation, migration, matrix metalloproteinase 2 (MMP2) activation, and VE-cadherin redistribution in wild-type human endothelial cells [79]. These findings suggest a novel role for endothelial cell-non autonomous effects of KRIT1 mutation in CCM pathogenesis and point to NOX1 as a major regulator of these effects, thus opening interesting therapeutical perspectives.

A summary of the imbalance in redox homeostasis induced by KRIT1 loss-of-function on redox homeostasis is shown in Fig. 5.2.

In accordance with the proposed pleiotropic functions of *CCM* genes, defective autophagy has been linked to enhanced endothelial cell sensitivity to oxidative stress [32]. About this, it has been shown that KRIT1 loss-of-function causes defective autophagy and consequent molecular and cellular dysfunctions, including accumulation of the autophagy adapter p62, and abnormal persistence of

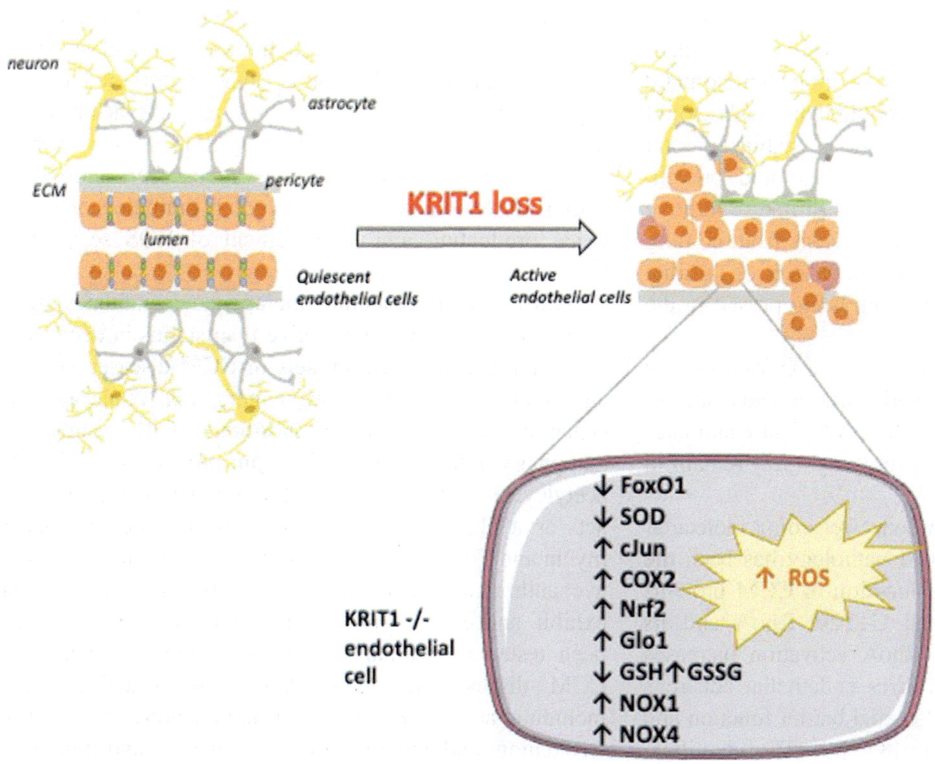

FIGURE 5.2 KRIT1 loss-of-function induces oxidative stress. The oxidative stress consequent to KRIT1 loss-of-function is linked to the modification of expression and activity of enzymes and transcription factors involved in redox homeostasis.

dysfunctional mitochondria, leading to a strong increase of ROS intracellular levels [80–82].

Finally, it is important to point out that several genes encoding proteins involved in ROS metabolism and vascular responses to oxidative stress are characterized by single nucleotide polymorphisms (SNPs) that confer substantial interindividual variability in susceptibility to various oxidative stress-related pathologies, including vascular diseases [32]. Oxidative stress-related genetic modifiers with a significant impact on interindividual variability in onset and severity of familial CCM have been identified and include highly polymorphic genes such as cytochrome P450 mono-oxygenase (CYP) and extracellular matrix metalloproteinase (MMP) genes [27]. These genes have a potential prognostic value and open new perspectives for risk stratification and personalized medicine strategies.

Therapeutic perspectives

At present, pharmacological treatment of CCM is limited to antiepileptic drugs for CCM patients exhibiting seizures, with many of these patients ultimately becoming resistant to the therapy, while the most effective treatment that is used to treat CCM disease remains the neurosurgical removal of accessible CCM lesions in patients with recurrent hemorrhage or intractable seizures. However, the surgical approach is risky since remnants may rupture if the lesion is not completely removed, is limited by lesion accessibility, and can be associated with significant rates of morbidity and mortality [83]. Thus, effective pharmacological strategies aimed to prevent or limit symptomatic disease onset and severity in susceptible individuals would be necessary to treat inaccessible lesions, stabilize blood vessels to reduce the risk of hemorrhage and prevent rehemorrhage after an acute hemorrhage, shrink, or remove lesions without surgery or to prevent lesions from coming back after surgery; to prevent systemic effects of familial CCM; and to stop familial CCM from being passed to the next generation.

Insight from multidisciplinary research carried out by different groups around the world has already led to rationally designed preclinical pharmacological candidates and prognostic biomarkers; however, only a few remain in clinical trials [84].

One of the first pieces of evidence regarding molecular mechanisms underlying the CCM pathology has been the correlation between the loss-of-function of CCM proteins and the activation of the small GTPase RhoA and its effector Rho kinase (ROCK). RhoA activation increases cellular contractility and destabilizes endothelial adherens junctions, thereby reducing endothelial barrier function and increasing vascular permeability [85–89]. The identification of this mechanism has initially suggested a potential therapy for CCM disease based on inhibitors of the RhoA-ROCK signaling, including statins (simvastatin, fluvastatin, and atorvastatin) [62,68,85,90], fasudil [88,90,91], and BA-1049, a ROCK2-selective kinase inhibitor [92]. Notably, atorvastatin is part of an enrolling phase I/II clinical trial [93]. In addition, other putative therapeutic compounds and strategies have been also proposed with the potentiality to be effective at least in limiting CCM disease severity, including inhibitors of β-catenin and TGF-β pathways (sulindac sulfide and its analogs) [94]; distinct angiogenesis inhibitors (sorafenib [94], semaxanib [95], anti-angiogenic thrombospondin1 (TSP1) fragment [96]); ANGPT2-neutralizing antibodies [97]; ponatinib, an inhibitor of MEKK3-KLF signaling with antiangiogenic effects [98]; blocking antibodies against the anticoagulant endothelial receptors thrombomodulin (TM) and endothelial protein C receptor (EPCR) [99]; and propranolol, a nonselective β-adrenergic blocker and antiangiogenic agent used as first-line treatment for infantile hemangiomas [100–103]. The anti-VEGF-A antibody bevacizumab and propranolol are among the few clinical trials candidate [104,105].

It has to be noted that, whereas accumulated evidence points to oxidative stress and inflammation as driving forces in CCM pathogenesis, and support the tight correlation between autophagy and oxidative stress, there is also clear evidence that all of the different therapeutic candidates for CCM disease proposed so far are endowed with either antioxidant or autophagy-inducing properties or both, suggesting that their reported effectiveness may be directly or indirectly related to the modulation of the tight crosstalk between autophagy and redox homeostasis and signaling [32,82]. Indeed, both statins and fasudil reduce the expression and activity of c-Jun, and the RhoGTPase pathway can be directly activated by ROS. Moreover, both statins, fasudil, and sulindac derivatives exert antioxidant activity in endothelial cells, including inhibition of superoxide production and improvement of ROS scavenging [32].

Other major potential therapeutic candidates were shown to be even more effective than statins in decreasing lesion burden in mouse models of CCM disease: Tempol, an SOD-mimetic ROS scavenger, and cholecalciferol (vitamin D3), a steroid hormone with established autophagy-inducing and antioxidant properties [32,76]. N-acetylcysteine (NAC), a potent antioxidant compound that acts as a glutathione precursor, mTOR inhibitors (Rapamycin and Torin1) which act as inducers of autophagy, and avenanthramides, phenolic compounds present in oats that exhibit antioxidant and anti-inflammatory activity, have been tested in cellular models and shown to counteract CCM disease phenotypes linked to oxidative stress, including actin stress fiber formation, adherens junction weakening, endothelial barrier dysfunction, and inflammatory responses [32,45,106,107].

TABLE 5.1 Pharmacological approaches for Cerebral Cavernous Malformations.

Mechanism	Drug	Pre-clinical	Phase I	Phase II	Phase III	References
RHO kinase inhibitor	Atorvastatin			✓		[84]
Superoxide dismutase mimetic	Rec-994 (Tempol)		✓			[32,76]
Nutritional supplement	Vitamin D3	✓				[32,76]
Beta blocker	Propranolol			✓		[104]
RHO kinase inhibitor	Simvastatin	✓				[85,89]
ROCK2-kinase inhibitor	Fasudil	✓				[88,98]
	BA-1049	✓				[99]
Inflammatory inhibitor	Sulindac	✓				[94]
Angiogenesis inhibitor	Thrombospondin1	✓				[96]
MEKK3-KLF inhibitor	Ponatinib	✓				[101]

In addition, a screen of 5268 compounds applied to animal and cellular models of CCM identified dozens of new and already identified candidates involved in processes including angiogenesis and the oxidative stress/redox system [108]. In Table 5.1 are reported the currently proposed pharmacological approaches for the treatment of CCM disease.

Taken together with the emerging evidence that the interplay between defective autophagy and redox imbalance may be integral to the development and progression of CCM lesions by sensitizing endothelial cells to local oxidative stress and inflammatory events [32,82], these findings suggest that a novel and promising option for the pharmacological treatment of CCM would be the development of a combinatorial treatment that targets both oxidative and inflammation state and autophagic dysfunction [109].

Concluding remarks

CCM1/KRIT1, CCM2/Malcavernin, and CCM3/PDCD10 are three structurally unrelated scaffolding proteins that lack catalytic activity and contain well characterized protein–protein interaction motifs and domains. Their loss of function has been associated with the pathogenesis of CCM; however, growing evidence indicates the implication of CCM proteins in different pathologies including cardiovascular diseases, diabetes, intestinal epithelial barrier dysregulation, and cancer.

The presence of distinct binding motifs and domains suggests that CCM proteins can interact with multiple binding partners to regulate complex signaling pathways and play critical roles in many cellular events, including cell polarity, cytoskeletal reorganization, cell proliferation, cellular adhesion and migration, angiogenesis, cell-cell junction integrity, vascular permeability, and apoptosis, suggesting that CCM proteins act as pleiotropic regulators of cellular homeostasis.

Accumulated evidence in cellular and animal models indicates that the emerged pleiotropic functions of CCM proteins are mainly due to their ability to modulate redox-sensitive pathways and mechanisms involved in adaptive responses to oxidative stress and inflammation, thus contributing to the preservation of cellular homeostasis and stress defenses.

Indeed, oxidative stress is involved in all the major molecular and cellular dysfunctions related to CCM disease, including destabilization of endothelial cell-cell junctions, increased β1 integrin activation, increased vascular permeability and angiogenic activity, suggesting that it may represent a significant triggering factor involved in the onset and progression of CCM.

Furthermore, it is known that oxidative stress and inflammatory events have a focal nature and can occur locally in the brain vasculature, triggering focal endothelial dysfunction in genetically predisposed blood vessels. In this regards many studies suggest that CCM disease pathogenesis involves an intricate interplay between multiple factors, including genetic and environmental risk factors associated with enhanced susceptibility to oxidative stress and inflammation.

Recent findings have also linked defective autophagy to enhanced endothelial cell sensitivity to oxidative stress and suggest that the interplay between defective autophagy and redox imbalance may play a decisive role in the development and progression of CCM lesions by sensitizing endothelial cells to local oxidative stress events.

In the complicated interplay between these processes, CCM proteins play a key role in the regulation of the stability of endothelial barriers by regulating the complex machinery governing cellular redox homeostasis and responses to oxidative stress and inflammation, and it is clear that redox signaling is the common link between the various pathogenic mechanisms associated with CCM onset and progression.

A further and comprehensive characterization of the multifaceted role of CCM proteins is fundamental to design novel options for the pharmacological treatment of CCM, including combinatorial treatments targeting both oxidative and inflammation states and autophagic dysfunction.

Acknowledgments

This work was supported by MIUR (Ministero dell'Istruzione dell'Università e della Ricerca, Italy) grant "Dipartimento di Eccellenza 2018 -2022".

References

[1] Awad IA, Polster SP. Cavernous angiomas: deconstructing a neurosurgical disease: JNSPG 75th anniversary invited review article. J Neurosurg 2019;131:1−13. https://doi.org/10.3171/2019.3.JNS181724.

[2] Padarti A, Zhang J. Recent advances in cerebral cavernous malformation research. Vessel Plus 2018;2:21. https://doi.org/10.20517/2574-1209.2018.34.

[3] Riolo G, Ricci C, Battistini S. Molecular genetic features of cerebral cavernous malformations (CCM) patients: an overall view from genes to endothelial cells. Cells 2021;10:1−19.

[4] Faurobert E, Albiges-Rizo C. Recent insights into cerebral cavernous malformations: a complex jigsaw puzzle under construction. FEBS J 2010;277:1084−96. https://doi.org/10.1111/j.1742-4658.2009.07537.x.

[5] Revencu N, Vikkula M. Cerebral cavernous malformation: new molecular and clinical insights. J Med Genet 2006;43:716−21.

[6] Fischer A, Zalvide J, Faurobert E, Albiges-Rizo C, Tournier-Lasserve E. Cerebral cavernous malformations: from CCM genes to endothelial cell homeostasis. Trends Mol Med 2013;19:302−8.

[7] Bergametti F, Denier C, Labauge P, Arnoult M, Boetto S, Clanet M, et al. Mutations within the programmed cell death 10 gene cause cerebral cavernous malformations. Am J Hum Genet 2005;76:42−51. https://doi.org/10.1086/426952.

[8] Denier C, Labauge P, Bergametti F, Marchelli F, Riant F, Arnoult M, et al. Genotype-phenotype correlations in cerebral cavernous malformations patients. Ann Neurol 2006;60:550−6. https://doi.org/10.1002/ana.20947.

[9] Stenson PD, Mort M, Ball EV, Chapman M, Evans K, Azevedo L, et al. The human gene mutation database (HGMD®): optimizing its use in a clinical diagnostic or research setting. Hum Genet 2020;139:1197−207.

[10] Gault J, Shenkar R, Recksiek P, Awad IA. Biallelic somatic and germ line *CCM1* truncating mutations in a cerebral cavernous malformation lesion. Stroke 2005;36:872−4. https://doi.org/10.1161/01.STR.0000157586.20479.fd.

[11] Akers AL, Johnson E, Steinberg GK, Zabramski JM, Marchuk DA. Biallelic somatic and germline mutations in cerebral cavernous malformations (CCMs): evidence for a two-hit mechanism of CCM pathogenesis. Hum Mol Genet 2009;18:919−30. https://doi.org/10.1093/hmg/ddn430.

[12] Pagenstecher A, Stahl S, Sure U, Felbor U. A two-hit mechanism causes cerebral cavernous malformations: complete inactivation of CCM1, CCM2 or CCM3 in affected endothelial cells. Hum Mol Genet 2009;18:911−8. https://doi.org/10.1093/hmg/ddn420.

[13] McDonald DA, Shenkar R, Shi C, Stockton RA, Akers AL, Kucherlapati MH, et al. A novel mouse model of cerebral cavernous malformations based on the two-hit mutation hypothesis recapitulates the human disease. Hum Mol Genet 2011;20:211−22. https://doi.org/10.1093/hmg/ddq433.

[14] McDonald DA, Shi C, Shenkar R, Gallione CJ, Akers AL, Li S, et al. Lesions from patients with sporadic cerebral cavernous malformations harbor somatic mutations in the CCM genes: evidence for a common biochemical pathway for CCM pathogenesis. Hum Mol Genet 2014;23:4357−70. https://doi.org/10.1093/hmg/ddu153.

[15] Detter MR, Snellings DA, Marchuk DA. Cerebral cavernous malformations develop through clonal expansion of mutant endothelial cells. Circ Res 2018;123:1143−51. https://doi.org/10.1161/CIRCRESAHA.118.313970.

[16] Rath M, Pagenstecher A, Hoischen A, Felbor U. Postzygotic mosaicism in cerebral cavernous malformation. J Med Genet 2020;57:212−6. https://doi.org/10.1136/jmedgenet-2019-106182.

[17] Malinverno M, Maderna C, Abu Taha A, Corada M, Orsenigo F, Valentino M, et al. Endothelial cell clonal expansion in the development of cerebral cavernous malformations. Nat Commun 2019;10:2761. https://doi.org/10.1038/s41467-019-10707-x.

[18] Tang AT, Choi JP, Kotzin JJ, Yang Y, Hong CC, Hobson N, et al. Endothelial TLR4 and the microbiome drive cerebral cavernous malformations. Nature 2017;545:305−10. https://doi.org/10.1038/nature22075.

[19] Detwiler PW, Porter RW, Zabramski JM, Spetzler RF. De novo formation of a central nervous system cavernous malformation: implications for predicting risk of hemorrhage. Case report and review of the literature. J Neurosurg 1997;87. https://doi.org/10.3171/jns.1997.87.4.0629.

[20] Brunereau L, Levy C, Laberge S, Houtteville JP, Labauge P. De novo lesions in familial form of cerebral cavernous malformations: clinical and MR features in 29 non-hispanic families. Surg Neurol 2000;53. https://doi.org/10.1016/S0090-3019(00)00218-4.

[21] Hong T, Xiao X, Ren J, Cui B, Zong Y, Zou J, et al. Somatic MAP3K3 and PIK3CA mutations in sporadic cerebral and spinal cord cavernous malformations. Brain 2021;144. https://doi.org/10.1093/brain/awab117.

[22] Ren AA, Snellings DA, Su YS, Hong CC, Castro M, Tang AT, et al. PIK3CA and CCM mutations fuel cavernomas through a cancer-like mechanism. Nature 2021;594. https://doi.org/10.1038/s41586-021-03562-8.

[23] Weng J, Yang Y, Song D, Huo R, Li H, Chen Y, et al. Somatic MAP3K3 mutation defines a subclass of cerebral cavernous malformation. Am J Hum Genet 2021;108. https://doi.org/10.1016/j.ajhg.2021.04.005.

[24] Zhu Y, Peters C, Hallier-Neelsen M, Miller D, Pagenstecher A, Bertalanffy H, et al. Phosphatase and tensin homolog in cerebral cavernous malformation: a potential role in pathological angiogenesis - laboratory investigation. J Neurosurg 2009;110:530−9. https://doi.org/10.3171/2008.7.17626.

[25] Snellings DA, Hong CC, Ren AA, Lopez-Ramirez MA, Girard R, Srinath A, et al. Cerebral cavernous malformation: from mechanism to therapy. Circ Res 2021;129:195–215.

[26] Trapani E, Retta SF. Cerebral cavernous malformation (CCM) disease: from monogenic forms to genetic susceptibility factors. J Neurosurg Sci 2015;59:201–9.

[27] Choquet H, Trapani E, Goitre L, Trabalzini L, Akers A, Fontanella M, et al. Cytochrome P450 and matrix metalloproteinase genetic modifiers of disease severity in cerebral cavernous malformation type 1. Free Radic Biol Med 2016;92:100–9. https://doi.org/10.1016/j.freeradbiomed.2016.01.008.

[28] Perrelli A, de Luca E, Swamy H, Nitti M, Passalacqua M, Furfaro AL, et al. Protein kinase cα regulates the nucleocytoplasmic shuttling of KRIT1. Free Radic Biol Med 2021;177. https://doi.org/10.1016/j.freeradbiomed.2021.08.050.

[29] Fontes-Dantas FL, da Fontoura Galvão G, Veloso da Silva E, Alves-Leon S, Cecília da Silva Rêgo C, Garcia DG, et al. Novel CCM1 (KRIT1) mutation detection in Brazilian familial cerebral cavernous malformation: different genetic variants in inflammation, oxidative stress, and drug metabolism genes affect disease aggressiveness. World Neurosurg 2020;138:535–540.e8. https://doi.org/10.1016/j.wneu.2020.02.119.

[30] Fontanella MM, Panciani PP, Spena G, Roca E, Migliorati K, Ambrosi C, et al. Professional athletes and cerebral cavernomas: an obstacle to overcome. J Sports Med Phys Fit 2015;55:1046–7.

[31] Fontanella M, Bacigaluppi S. Treatment of cerebral cavernous malformations: where do we stand? J Neurosurg Sci 2015;59:199–200.

[32] Retta SF, Glading AJ. Oxidative stress and inflammation in cerebral cavernous malformation disease pathogenesis: two sides of the same coin. Int J Biochem Cell Biol 2016. https://doi.org/10.1016/j.biocel.2016.09.011.

[33] Mabray MC, Caprihan A, Nelson J, McCulloch CE, Zafar A, Kim H, et al. Effect of simvastatin on permeability in cerebral cavernous malformation type 1 patients: results from a pilot small randomized controlled clinical trial. Transl Stroke Res 2019. https://doi.org/10.1007/s12975-019-00737-4.

[34] Draheim KM, Fisher OS, Boggon TJ, Calderwood DA. Cerebral cavernous malformation proteins at a glance. J Cell Sci 2014;127:701–7. https://doi.org/10.1242/jcs.138388.

[35] Fisher OS, Boggon TJ. Signaling pathways and the cerebral cavernous malformations proteins: lessons from structural biology. Cell Mol Life Sci 2014;71:1881–92.

[36] Draheim KM, Li X, Zhang R, Fisher OS, Villari G, Boggon TJ, et al. CCM2-CCM3 interaction stabilizes their protein expression and permits endothelial network formation. J Cell Biol 2015;208:987–1001. https://doi.org/10.1083/jcb.201407129.

[37] Fisher OS, Deng H, Liu D, Zhang Y, Wei R, Deng Y, et al. Structure and vascular function of MEKK3-cerebral cavernous malformations 2 complex. Nat Commun 2015;6. https://doi.org/10.1038/ncomms8937.

[38] Fidalgo M, Fraile M, Pires A, Force T, Pombo C, Zalvide J. CCM3/PDCD10 stabilizes GCKIII proteins to promote Golgi assembly and cell orientation. J Cell Sci 2010;123:1274–84. https://doi.org/10.1242/jcs.061341.

[39] Yoruk B, Gillers BS, Chi NC, Scott IC. Ccm3 functions in a manner distinct from Ccm1 and Ccm2 in a zebrafish model of CCM vascular disease. Dev Biol 2012;362:121–31. https://doi.org/10.1016/j.ydbio.2011.12.006.

[40] Zalvide J, Fidalgo M, Fraile M, Guerrero A, Iglesias C, Floridia E, et al. The CCM3-GCKIII partnership. Histol Histopathol 2013;28:1265–72.

[41] Zhang M, Dong L, Shi Z, Jiao S, Zhang Z, Zhang W, et al. Structural mechanism of CCM3 heterodimerization with GCKIII kinases. Structure 2013;21:680–8. https://doi.org/10.1016/j.str.2013.02.015.

[42] Voss K, Stahl S, Schleider E, Ullrich S, Nickel J, Mueller TD, et al. CCM3 interacts with CCM2 indicating common pathogenesis for cerebral cavernous malformations. Neurogenetics 2007;8:249–56. https://doi.org/10.1007/s10048-007-0098-9.

[43] Lant B, Yu B, Goudreault M, Holmyard D, Knight JDR, Xu P, et al. CCM-3/STRIPAK promotes seamless tube extension through endocytic recycling. Nat Commun 2015;6:6449. https://doi.org/10.1038/ncomms7449.

[44] Pal S, Lant B, Yu B, Tian R, Tong J, Krieger JR, et al. CCM-3 promotes C. Elegans germline development by regulating vesicle trafficking cytokinesis and polarity. Curr Biol 2017;27:868–76. https://doi.org/10.1016/j.cub.2017.02.028.

[45] Vieceli Dalla Sega F, Mastrocola R, Aquila G, Fortini F, Fornelli C, Zotta A, et al. KRIT1 deficiency promotes aortic endothelial dysfunction. Int J Mol Sci 2019;20. https://doi.org/10.3390/ijms20194930.

[46] Antognelli C, Trapani E, Delle Monache S, Perrelli A, Daga M, Pizzimenti S, et al. KRIT1 loss-of-function induces a chronic nrf2-mediated adaptive homeostasis that sensitizes cells to oxidative stress: implication for cerebral cavernous malformation disease. Free Radic Biol Med 2018. https://doi.org/10.1016/j.freeradbiomed.2017.11.014.

[47] Wang Y, Li Y, Zou J, Polster SP, Lightle R, Moore T, et al. The cerebral cavernous malformation disease causing gene KRIT1 participates in intestinal epithelial barrier maintenance and regulation. FASEB J 2019. https://doi.org/10.1096/fj.201800343R.

[48] Ercoli J, Finetti F, Woodby B, Belmonte G, Miracco C, Valacchi G, et al. KRIT1 as a possible new player in melanoma aggressiveness. Arch Biochem Biophys 2020;691. https://doi.org/10.1016/j.abb.2020.108483.

[49] Abou-Fadel J, Qu Y, Gonzalez EM, Smith M, Zhang J. Emerging roles of CCM genes during tumorigenesis with potential application as novel biomarkers across major types of cancers. Oncol Rep 2020;43:1945–63. https://doi.org/10.3892/or.2020.7550.

[50] Glading AJ, Ginsberg MH. Rap1 and its effector KRIT1/CCM1 regulate β-catenin signaling. DMM Dis Models Mechanisms 2010;3:73–83. https://doi.org/10.1242/dmm.003293.

[51] Orso F, Balzac F, Marino M, Lembo A, Retta SF, Taverna D. MiR-21 coordinates tumor growth and modulates KRIT1 levels. Biochem Biophys Res Commun 2013;438:90–6. https://doi.org/10.1016/j.bbrc.2013.07.031.

[52] Park S, Lee HY, Kim J, Park H, Ju YS, Kim EG, et al. Cerebral cavernous malformation 1 determines YAP/TAZ signaling-dependent metastatic hallmarks of prostate cancer cells. Cancers 2021;13. https://doi.org/10.3390/cancers13051125.

[53] He Q, Ye A, Ye W, Liao X, Qin G, Xu Y, et al. Cancer-secreted exosomal MiR-21-5p induces angiogenesis and vascular permeability by targeting KRIT1. Cell Death Dis 2021;12. https://doi.org/10.1038/s41419-021-03803-8.

[54] Zhu Y, Zhao K, Prinz A, Keyvani K, Lambertz N, Kreitschmann-Andermahr I, et al. Loss of endothelial programmed cell death 10 activates glioblastoma cells and promotes tumor growth. Neuro Oncol 2016;18. https://doi.org/10.1093/neuonc/nov155.

[55] Nickel AC, Wan XY, Saban DV, Weng YL, Zhang S, Keyvani K, et al. Loss of programmed cell death 10 activates tumor cells and leads to temozolomide-resistance in glioblastoma. J Neuro Oncol 2019;141. https://doi.org/10.1007/s11060-018-03017-7.

[56] Huang L, Nakamura Y, Lo EH, Hayakawa K. Astrocyte signaling in the neurovascular unit after central nervous system injury. Int J Mol Sci 2019;20:282. https://doi.org/10.3390/ijms20020282.

[57] Iadecola C. The neurovascular unit coming of age: a journey through neurovascular coupling in health and disease. Neuron 2017;96:17–42. https://doi.org/10.1016/j.neuron.2017.07.030.

[58] Winkler EA, Lu AY, Raygor KP, Linzey JR, Jonzzon S, Lien Bv, et al. Defective vascular signaling & prospective therapeutic targets in brain arteriovenous malformations. Neurochem Int 2019;126:126–38. https://doi.org/10.1016/j.neuint.2019.03.002.

[59] Louvi A, Chen L, Two AM, Zhang H, Min W, Günel M. Loss of cerebral cavernous malformation 3 (Ccm3) in neuroglia leads to CCM and vascular pathology. Proc Natl Acad Sci U S A 2011;108:3737–42. https://doi.org/10.1073/pnas.1012617108.

[60] Carvalho C, Moreira PI. Oxidative stress: a major player in cerebrovascular alterations associated to neurodegenerative events. Front Physiol 2018;9:1–14. https://doi.org/10.3389/fphys.2018.00806.

[61] Chrissobolis S, Miller AA, Drummond GR, Kemp-Harper BK, Sobey CG. Oxidative stress and endothelial dysfunction in cerebrovascular disease. Front Biosci 2011;16. https://doi.org/10.2741/3816.

[62] Ferro E, Goitre L, Baldini E, Retta SF, Trabalzini L. Ras GTPases are both regulators and effectors of redox agents. Methods Mol Biol 2014;1120.

[63] Taniyama Y, Griendling KK. Reactive oxygen species in the vasculature: molecular and cellular mechanisms. Hypertension 2003;42:1075–81.

[64] Kim YW, Byzova TV. Oxidative stress in angiogenesis and vascular disease. Blood 2014;123:625–31.

[65] Forrester SJ, Kikuchi DS, Hernandes MS, Xu Q, Griendling KK. Reactive oxygen species in metabolic and inflammatory signaling. Circ Res 2018;122:877–902.

[66] Sumpio BE, Timothy Riley J, Dardik A. Cells in focus: endothelial cell. Int J Biochem Cell Biol 2002;34:1508–12.

[67] Antognelli C, Perrelli A, Armeni T, Talesa VN, Retta SF. Dicarbonyl stress and S-glutathionylation in cerebrovascular diseases: a focus on cerebral cavernous malformations. Antioxidants 2020;9:124.

[68] Goitre L, Pergolizzi B, Ferro E, Trabalzini L, Retta SF. Molecular crosstalk between integrins and cadherins: do reactive oxygen species set the talk? J Signal Transduct 2012;2012:1–12. https://doi.org/10.1155/2012/807682.

[69] Goitre L, Balzac F, Degani S, Degan P, Marchi S, Pinton P, et al. KRIT1 regulates the homeostasis of intracellular reactive oxygen species. PLoS One 2010. https://doi.org/10.1371/journal.pone.0011786.

[70] Guazzi P, Goitre L, Ferro E, Cutano V, Martino C, Trabalzini L, et al. Identification of the kelch family protein Nd1-L as a novel molecular interactor of KRIT1. PLoS One 2012;7:e44705. https://doi.org/10.1371/journal.pone.0044705.

[71] Goitre L, de Luca E, Braggion S, Trapani E, Guglielmotto M, Biasi F, et al. KRIT1 loss of function causes a ROS-dependent upregulation of c-Jun. Free Radic Biol Med 2014. https://doi.org/10.1016/j.freeradbiomed.2013.11.020.

[72] Maddaluno L, Rudini N, Cuttano R, Bravi L, Giampietro C, Corada M, et al. EndMT contributes to the onset and progression of cerebral cavernous malformations. Nature 2013;498:492–6. https://doi.org/10.1038/nature12207.

[73] Ferro E, Goitre L, Retta SF, Trabalzini L. The interplay between ROS and ras GTPases: physiological and pathological implications. J Signal Transduct 2011;2012:1–9. https://doi.org/10.1155/2012/365769.

[74] Fidalgo M, Guerrero A, Fraile M, Iglesias C, Pombo CM, Zalvide J. Adaptor protein cerebral cavernous malformation 3 (CCM3) mediates phosphorylation of the cytoskeletal proteins ezrin/radixin/moesin by mammalian ste20-4 to protect cells from oxidative stress. J Biol Chem 2012;287. https://doi.org/10.1074/jbc.M111.320259.

[75] Koskimäki J, Girard R, Li Y, Saadat L, Zeineddine HA, Lightle R, et al. Comprehensive transcriptome analysis of cerebral cavernous malformation across multiple species and genotypes. JCI Insight 2019;4. https://doi.org/10.1172/jci.insight.126167.

[76] Gibson CC, Zhu W, Davis CT, Bowman-Kirigin JA, Chan AC, Ling J, et al. Strategy for identifying repurposed drugs for the treatment of cerebral cavernous malformation. Circulation 2015;131:289–99. https://doi.org/10.1161/CIRCULATIONAHA.114.010403.

[77] Cianfruglia L, Perrelli A, Fornelli C, Magini A, Gorbi S, Salzano A, et al. KRIT1 loss-of-function associated with cerebral cavernous malformation disease leads to enhanced S-glutathionylation of distinct structural and regulatory proteins. Antioxidants 2019;8:27. https://doi.org/10.3390/antiox8010027.

[78] Goitre L, DiStefano PV, Moglia A, Nobiletti N, Baldini E, Trabalzini L, et al. Up-regulation of NADPH oxidase-mediated redox signaling contributes to the loss of barrier function in KRIT1 deficient endothelium. Sci Rep 2017;7:8296. https://doi.org/10.1038/s41598-017-08373-4.

[79] Finetti F, Schiavo I, Ercoli J, Zotta A, Boda E, Retta SF, et al. KRIT1 loss-mediated upregulation of NOX1 in stromal cells promotes paracrine pro-angiogenic responses. Cell Signal 2020;68. https://doi.org/10.1016/j.cellsig.2020.109527.

[80] Marchi S, Corricelli M, Trapani E, Bravi L, Pittaro A, Delle Monache S, et al. Defective autophagy is a key feature of cerebral cavernous malformations. EMBO Mol Med 2015;7:1403–17. https://doi.org/10.15252/emmm.201505316.

[81] Marchi S, Retta SF, Pinton P. Cellular processes underlying cerebral cavernous malformations: autophagy as another point of view. Autophagy 2016;12:424–5. https://doi.org/10.1080/15548627.2015.1125073.

[82] Marchi S, Trapani E, Corricelli M, Goitre L, Pinton P, Retta SF. Beyond multiple mechanisms and a unique drug: defective autophagy as pivotal player in cerebral cavernous malformation pathogenesis and implications for targeted therapies. Rare Dis 2016;4:e1142640. https://doi.org/10.1080/21675511.2016.1142640.

[83] Su VL, Calderwood DA. Signalling through cerebral cavernous malformation protein networks: CCM protein signaling. Open Biol 2020;10. https://doi.org/10.1098/rsob.200263.

[84] Chohan MO, Marchiò S, Morrison LA, Sidman RL, Cavenee WK, Dejana E, et al. Emerging pharmacologic targets in cerebral cavernous malformation and potential strategies to alter the natural history of a difficult disease: a review. JAMA Neurol 2019;76:492–500. https://doi.org/10.1001/jamaneurol.2018.3634.

[85] Whitehead KJ, Chan AC, Navankasattusas S, Koh W, London NR, Ling J, et al. The cerebral cavernous malformation signaling pathway promotes vascular integrity via Rho GTPases. Nat Med 2009;15:177–84. https://doi.org/10.1038/nm.1911.

[86] Crose LES, Hilder TL, Sciaky N, Johnson GL. Cerebral cavernous malformation 2 protein promotes smad ubiquitin regulatory factor 1-mediated RhoA degradation in endothelial cells. J Biol Chem 2009;284:13301–5. https://doi.org/10.1074/jbc.C900009200.

[87] Borikova AL, Dibble CF, Sciaky N, Welch CM, Abell AN, Bencharit S, et al. Rho kinase inhibition rescues the endothelial cell cerebral cavernous malformation phenotype. J Biol Chem 2010;285:11760–4. https://doi.org/10.1074/jbc.C109.097220.

[88] Stockton RA, Shenkar R, Awad IA, Ginsberg MH. Cerebral cavernous malformations proteins inhibit Rho kinase to stabilize vascular integrity. J Exp Med 2010;207:881–96. https://doi.org/10.1084/jem.20091258.

[89] Richardson BT, Dibble CF, Borikova AL, Johnson GL. Cerebral cavernous malformation is a vascular disease associated with activated RhoA signaling. Biol Chem 2013;394:35–42. https://doi.org/10.1515/hsz-2012-0243.

[90] Castro M, Laviña B, Ando K, Álvarez-Aznar A, Abu Taha A, Brakebusch C, et al. CDC42 deletion elicits cerebral vascular malformations via increased MEKK3-dependent KLF4 expression. Circ Res 2019;124:1240–52. https://doi.org/10.1161/CIRCRESAHA.118.314300.

[91] Li DY, Whitehead KJ. Evaluating strategies for the treatment of cerebral cavernous malformations. Stroke 2010;41:S92–4. https://doi.org/10.1161/STROKEAHA.110.594929.

[92] Nishimura S, Mishra-Gorur K, Park J, Surovtseva Yv, Sebti SM, Levchenko A, et al. Combined HMG-COA reductase and prenylation inhibition in treatment of CCM. Proc Natl Acad Sci USA 2017;114:5503–8. https://doi.org/10.1073/pnas.1702942114.

[93] Polster SP, Stadnik A, Akers AL, Cao Y, Christoforidis GA, Fam MD, et al. Atorvastatin treatment of cavernous angiomas with symptomatic hemorrhage exploratory proof of concept (AT CASH EPOC) trial. Neurosurgery 2018. https://doi.org/10.1093/neuros/nyy539.

[94] Shenkar R, Peiper A, Pardo H, Moore T, Lightle R, Girard R, et al. Rho kinase inhibition blunts lesion development and hemorrhage in murine models of aggressive *pdcd10/ccm3* disease. Stroke 2019;50:738–44. https://doi.org/10.1161/STROKEAHA.118.024058.

[95] DiStefano PV, Kuebel JM, Sarelius IH, Glading AJ. KRIT1 protein depletion modifies endothelial cell behavior via increased vascular endothelial growth factor (VEGF) signaling. J Biol Chem 2014;289:33054–65. https://doi.org/10.1074/jbc.M114.582304.

[96] Lopez-Ramirez MA, Fonseca G, Zeineddine HA, Girard R, Moore T, Pham A, et al. Thrombospondin1 (TSP1) replacement prevents cerebral cavernous malformations. J Exp Med 2017;214:3331–46. https://doi.org/10.1084/jem.20171178.

[97] Zhou HJ, Qin L, Zhang H, Tang W, Ji W, He Y, et al. Endothelial exocytosis of angiopoietin-2 resulting from CCM3 deficiency contributes to cerebral cavernous malformation. Nat Med 2016;22:1033–42. https://doi.org/10.1038/nm.4169.

[98] McDonald DA, Shi C, Shenkar R, Stockton RA, Liu F, Ginsberg MH, et al. Fasudil decreases lesion burden in a murine model of cerebral cavernous malformation disease. Stroke 2012;43:571–4. https://doi.org/10.1161/STROKEAHA.111.625467.

[99] McKerracher L, Shenkar R, Abbinanti M, Cao Y, Peiper A, Liao JK, et al. A brain-targeted orally available ROCK2 inhibitor benefits mild and aggressive cavernous angioma disease. Transl Stroke Res 2019. https://doi.org/10.1007/s12975-019-00725-8.

[100] Bravi L, Rudini N, Cuttano R, Giampietro C, Maddaluno L, Ferrarini L, et al. Sulindac metabolites decrease cerebrovascular malformations in *CCM3* -knockout mice. Proc Natl Acad Sci USA 2015;112:8421–6. https://doi.org/10.1073/pnas.1501352112.

[101] Choi JP, Wang R, Yang X, Wang X, Wang L, Ting KK, et al. Ponatinib (AP24534) inhibits MEKK3-KLF signaling and prevents formation and progression of cerebral cavernous malformations. Sci Adv 2018;4:eaau0731. https://doi.org/10.1126/sciadv.aau0731.

[102] Shi C, Shenkar R, Zeineddine HA, Girard R, Fam MD, Austin C, et al. B-cell depletion reduces the maturation of cerebral cavernous malformations in murine models. J Neuroimmune Pharmacol 2016;11:369–77. https://doi.org/10.1007/s11481-016-9670-0.

[103] Lopez-Ramirez MA, Pham A, Girard R, Wyseure T, Hale P, Yamashita A, et al. Cerebral cavernous malformations form an anticoagulant vascular domain in humans and mice. Blood 2019;133:193–204. https://doi.org/10.1182/blood-2018-06-856062.

[104] Zabramski JM, Kalani MYS, Filippidis AS, Spetzler RF. Propranolol treatment of cavernous malformations with symptomatic hemorrhage. World Neurosurg 2016;88:631–9. https://doi.org/10.1016/j.wneu.2015.11.003.

[105] Zhu L, Xie J, Liu Z, Huang Z, Huang M, Yin H, et al. Pigment epithelium-derived factor/vascular endothelial growth factor ratio plays a crucial role in the spontaneous regression of infant hemangioma and in the therapeutic effect of propranolol. Cancer Sci 2018;109. https://doi.org/10.1111/cas.13611.

[106] de Luca E, Pedone D, Moglianetti M, Pulcini D, Perrelli A, Retta SF, et al. Multifunctional Platinum@BSA–rapamycin nanocarriers for the combinatorial therapy of cerebral cavernous malformation. ACS Omega 2018;3:15389–98. https://doi.org/10.1021/acsomega.8b01653.

[107] Apra C, Dumot C, Bourdillon P, Pelissou-Guyotat I. Could propranolol be beneficial in adult cerebral cavernous malformations? Neurosurg Rev 2019;42:403–8. https://doi.org/10.1007/s10143-018-01074-0.

[108] Otten C, Knox J, Boulday G, Eymery M, Haniszewski M, Neuenschwander M, et al. Systematic pharmacological screens uncover novel pathways involved in cerebral cavernous malformations. EMBO Mol Med 2018;10:e9155. https://doi.org/10.15252/emmm.201809155.

[109] Retta SF, Perrelli A, Trabalzini L, Finetti F. From genes and mechanisms to molecular-targeted therapies: the long climb to the cure of cerebral cavernous malformation (CCM) disease. In: Methods in molecular biology, vol 2152. Humana Press Inc.; 2020. p. 3–25.

Chapter 6

The effect of maternal and early-life nutrition on redox homeostasis

Ufuk Ersoy[1], Moussira Alameddine[1], Ioannis Kanakis[1,2], Caroline Amy Staunton[1], Mandy Jayne Peffers[1], Malcolm J. Jackson[1], Katarzyna Goljanek-Whysall[1,3] and Aphrodite Vasilaki[1]

[1]Institute of Life Course and Medical Sciences, The MRC - Versus Arthritis Centre for Integrated Research into Musculoskeletal Ageing (CIMA), University of Liverpool, Liverpool, United Kingdom; [2]Chester Medical School, Faculty of Medicine and Life Sciences, University of Chester, Chester, United Kingdom; [3]Department of Physiology, School of Medicine and REMEDI, CMNHS, NUI Galway, Galway, Ireland

Key takeaways

1. There is a strong association between early-life suboptimal growth and enhanced risk of developing chronic disorders in later life.
2. Maternal undernutrition-induced early life growth restriction followed by accelerated growth increases the probability of age-related diseases in later life.
3. Maternal overnutrition is associated with long-term effects on offspring health and an increased risk of the development of age-related diseases such as cardiovascular diseases, type 2 diabetes, and metabolic syndrome.
4. Redox dysregulation and mitochondrial dysfunction play a pivotal role in the development of maternal nutrition-induced age-related diseases later in life in the offspring.
5. It is now emerging that modification in the epigenome is also a possible underlying mechanism that governs the effects of maternal nutrition on the development of age-related diseases.
6. Both maternal iron deficiency or maternal iron excess can cause free radical damage, and leading to functional alterations.

Introduction

Reactive oxygen species (ROS) have a pivotal role in maintenance and regulation of cellular homeostasis. During its development, the embryo is exposed to various levels of ROS. This fluctuation in ROS levels affects cellular function, proliferation, differentiation, and apoptosis. Over the course of embryonic development, the delicate balance of redox homeostasis can be disturbed by exogenous factors. Early life environment has been shown as a factor that affects redox homeostasis during development. Epidemiological studies and studies in animal models have suggested that there is an association between early environment, especially maternal nutrition, and subsequent risk of age-related diseases in later life, including cardiovascular diseases (CVD), type 2 diabetes, and sarcopenia. Maternal nutrition has been shown to be an important factor for embryo development and in maintaining embryonic redox homeostasis during embryonic growth. Therefore, in this chapter, we will discuss the effects of maternal nutrition on redox homeostasis of the offspring at different stages of their life and oxidative stress as a potential underlying mechanism in mediating the effects of early life nutrition on the development of diseases in later life.

Oxidative stress signaling and embryonic development

ROS (e.g., superoxide ($O_2^{\cdot -}$), hydrogen peroxide (H_2O_2), and hydroxyl radical ($OH^{\cdot}$)) are radical or nonradical reactive derivative forms of atmospheric oxygen (Fig. 6.1) [2]. ROS are often considered as molecules that induce pathology by damaging lipids, DNA, and proteins. However, recently, it has become clear that they also serve as signaling molecules in regulation of biological and physiological processes [3]. It has been reported that ROS work as signal transducers to enable organisms to adapt to changes in an oxidative environment as well as in the presence of environmental nutrients [4]. There are well-defined mechanisms whereby ROS directly up-regulate transcription factors for stress adaptation in prokaryotes [1,5]. In order to maintain redox homeostasis and keep ROS in physiological levels, organisms have adapted antioxidant defense systems that include both enzymatic and nonenzymatic antioxidants [2]. Superoxide dismutase, peroxiredoxins, glutathione peroxidase, and catalase are the principal antioxidant enzymes, whereas nonenzymatic antioxidants include glutathione, uric acid, and bilirubin [6].

Normal embryonic development of mammals is a complex process that starts with fusion of sperm to oocyte and

Modulation of Oxidative Stress. https://doi.org/10.1016/B978-0-443-19247-0.00002-3

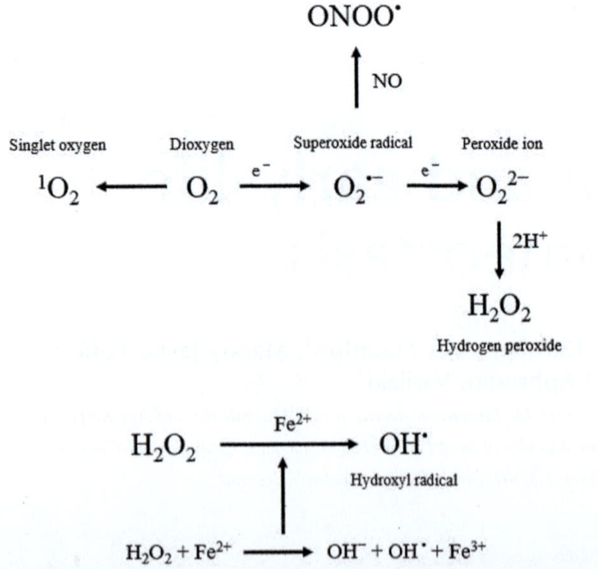

FIGURE 6.1 Formation of reactive oxygen species from atmospheric oxygen. Dioxygen is reduced or excited to create superoxide radical ($O_2^{\bullet-}$) or singlet oxygen ($^1O_2$), respectively. Superoxide radical are converted to hydrogen peroxide (H_2O_2) or peroxynitrite ($ONOO^\bullet$). H_2O_2 generates hydroxyl radicals ($OH^\bullet$) via the Fenton reaction as shown [1].

ends with birth. Ovulation, fertilization, organogenesis, organ maturation, and birth compose the normal developmental process. After the sperm-oocyte fusion, the fertilized egg divides into two cells. The morula is an early embryonic stage consisting of 16 blastomeres formed by numerous divisions of a zygote, or fertilized egg. Next, blastulation process occurs to form a thin-walled hollow structure called blastocyst. This attaches to the uterus. Next, implantation of blastocyst and formation of egg cylinder takes place. Gastrulation refers to embryonic transformation from a one-dimensional layer of blastula into a multilayered and multidimensional form called the gastrula. The primary germ layers; endoderm, mesoderm, and ectoderm are formed during gastrulation. The nervous system is the first system that develops during embryogenic development. Neural plate forms a neural tube which marks the beginning of the formation of the central nervous system. Next, embryonic folding occurs, and the cardiovascular system starts developing. Lastly, organogenesis takes place. The timing of these processes differs in different mammalian organisms [7].

The embryo is exposed to varying levels of ROS during its development; the source of these by-products is not only the developing embryo itself but also maternal processes [7]. Physiological levels of ROS play a crucial role in regulation of embryogenesis, embryonic implantation, and fetoplacental development. In contrast, dysregulation of redox equilibrium is considered to be responsible for the development or initiation of pathological processes [8]. It has been proposed that a firmly monitored redox homeostasis is required for normal embryonic and placental growth, and imbalance of this homeostasis significantly hinders growth [7,9]. Oxygen requirement and energy metabolism change throughout embryogenesis, and the levels of ROS production appear to follow oxygen consumption [10]. Early in development, the single cell embryo relies on the tricarboxylic acid (TCA) cycle, whereas the blastocyst primarily relies on anaerobic metabolism and glycolysis to meet energy demands (Fig. 6.2) [11].

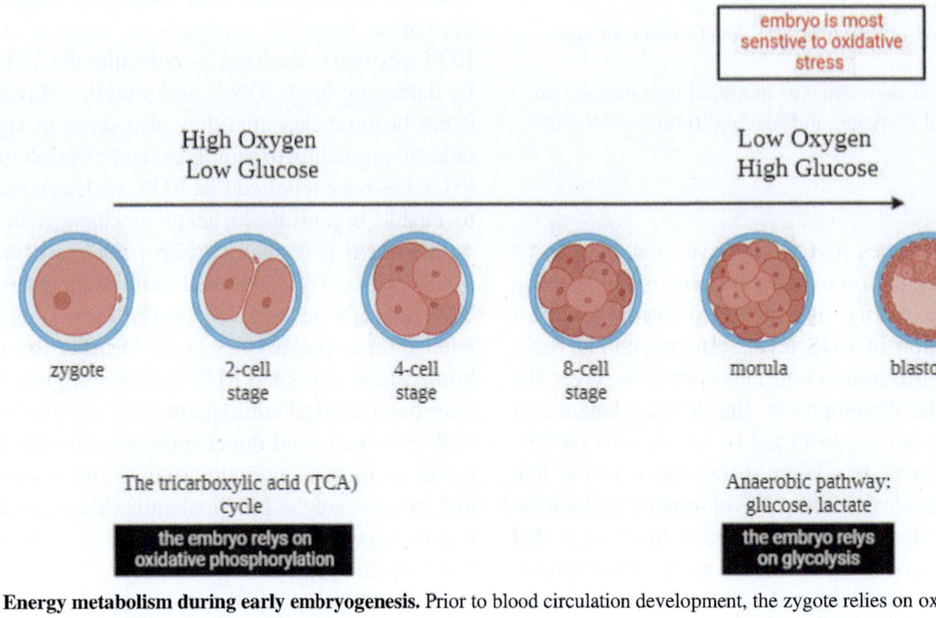

FIGURE 6.2 Energy metabolism during early embryogenesis. Prior to blood circulation development, the zygote relies on oxidative phosphorylation to meet energy demands. However, the blastocyst uses anaerobic pathways; glucose, lactate to produce energy. Embryo is most sensitive to oxidative stress during formation of morula and blastocyst [7].

During this time, the environment is relatively hypoxic and the embryo is most sensitive to oxidative stress [7]. This is important for early organogenesis, as hypoxia leads embryonic and placental development [7]. It has been shown that hypoxic environment regulates peri-implantation angiogenesis (the formation of new blood vessels) in humans, sheep, and mice during early organogenesis [12–14]. Once the circulation between the uterus and the placenta is established, there is a higher reliance on aerobic metabolism and relatively more ROS are produced from mitochondria. Moreover, antioxidant defense systems are improved, and the embryo becomes more resistant to oxidative stress [10].

The cellular redox fluctuations in embryo have a great impact on a number of cellular functions, energy metabolism, and the gene expression cascade during embryogenesis [7]. These fluctuations in oxidative tone modify the fate of the embryonic cells toward proliferation, differentiation, apoptosis, or necrosis [10]. Even though proliferating cell response to oxidative stress is dependent on the cell type, metabolic state and on stress intensity and duration, it has been reported that a reduced oxidative state stimulates cell proliferation [15]. On the other hand, higher concentrations of hydrogen peroxide (H_2O_2) actuate a temporary cell growth arrest which in turn may result in an adaptive response upregulating the expression of the genes for DNA repair and antioxidant enzymes [16]. However, further oxidation may lead the cell into a permanently growth-arrested state and even apoptosis [16]. Cell differentiation and maturation are lethal for embryogenesis. During the exit from the pluripotent state, embryonic stem cells undergo a programmed differentiation process that has been optimized during evolution [7].

Apart from having a direct impact on cells, ROS function as second messengers by regulating pivotal transcriptional factors in the embryo. It is now emerging that ROS can also control changes in the epigenetic landscape (discussed below) resulting in alterations in transcriptional activities and interfere with embryonic development [17]. The regulation of hypoxia inducible factor (HIF-1) by intracellular redox state is well-defined. HIF-1 has two subunits; the oxygen-sensitive HIF-1α and continuously produced HIF-1β. HIF-1α is degraded under normal conditions, whereas it is stabilized under hypoxic conditions, which allow the formation of heterodimeric HIF-1 protein. This transcription factor can translocate into the nucleus to enable transcription of the genes that regulate activation of erythropoietin, vascular endothelial growth factor, glucose transporter 1, and glycolytic enzymes [18]. Nuclear factor kappa B (NF-κB) constitute a family of transcription factors composed of five members—p50 (NF-κB1), p52 (NF-κB2), p65 (RelA), c-Rel and RelB [19]. Inflammatory cytokines and ROS can regulate the activation of NF-κB which play a key role in immune response and inflammation through regulation of gene expression. The possible role of NF-κB in regulating the response of an embryo to embryonic stress has been reported because of its ability to activate cell proliferation and its anti-apoptotic effect [20]. Activator protein-1 (AP-1) is another transcription factor activated during oxidative stress. This transcription factor has four subunits—c-fos, c-jun, junB, and junD whose activation is increased during mid-organogenesis. Oxidative stress-induced dysregulation of AP-1 may alter the profile of gene transcription leading to abnormal development and apoptosis [10]. Nuclear factor (NF)-E2 related factor 1 (Nrf-1), nuclear factor (NF)-E2 related factor 2 (Nrf-2), and redox effector factor-1 (Ref-1) are among the redox-sensitive transcription factors that can also have an impact on the embryo during the its development and knocking out these gene could result in embryonic mortality in mice [7].

Maternal nutrition and the chronic disorders in later life

There is a strong association between early life suboptimal growth and enhanced risk of development of chronic disorders in later life. Hales and Barker reported that low birth weight and a lower weight at 1 year are strongly linked with impaired glucose metabolism and type 2 diabetes in 468 male subjects [21]. Moreover, they demonstrated that CVD, hypertension, and type 2 diabetes have a fetal suboptimal development origin [22,23]. Low birth weight has been associated with grip strength in later life, suggesting the factors associated with sarcopenia development may be affected already in early life [24,25]. A number of similar studies reported this association between early life growth and chronic disorders in later life. One of these studies with 70,297 women participants observed that stroke and coronary heart disease were associated with birth weight [26]. However, it has become clear that high weight at birth is also an apparent indicator of enhanced risk of chronic disorders in later life [27]. Developing a metabolic syndrome risk was shown to be increased in children who had higher birth weight and were exposed to intrauterine maternal obesity or diabetes [28]. A more recent human study from Sweden has reported that high birth weight raises type 2 diabetes risk in young males and enhances the risk of obesity in both genders [29]. There are also other studies showing the relation between high birth weight and an increased risk of developing chronic disorders such as insulin resistance, CVD, and heart hypertrophy in later life [30–32]. Maternal nutrition has been shown to be one of the most important factors on development and growth in early life. Animal studies have shown that maternal undernutrition or maternal overnutrition increase the risk of developing chronic disorders [33]. The Thrifty Phenotype Hypothesis has been proposed to explain this relationship between maternal nutrition and chronic disorders; the fetus adapts to current metabolic conditions by permanently modifying its organ structure in the suboptimal in-utero environment to ensure the survival of the organism [34]. It is now emerging that modification in the epigenome is also a possible underlying mechanism that governs the effects of maternal nutrition on the development of age-related diseases. Oxidative stress can modify DNA methylations or histone modifications, affecting gene expression. It is feasible to think that oxidative stress is another underlying mechanism for this concept [27].

Maternal undernutrition, intrauterine growth restriction, and redox homeostasis

Newborns experiencing in utero growth restriction (IUGR) demonstrated impaired organ growth with long-lasting effects into old age [35]. IUGR occurs as a consequence of suboptimal prenatal environment, whereby the placenta does not meet metabolic requirements of the growing organism. Placental suboptimal environment is often secondary to insults of maternal origin, including maternal malnutrition, drug use, maternal infection, and maternal hypoxia [27]. There are many studies focused on the role of the maternal factors on the growth of the embryo and metabolic outcomes of IUGR on the offspring at different stages of life [22,23,35]. While the clinical evidence supporting the adverse effects of IUGR on the offspring is plentiful, the underlying mechanisms of IUGR and the mechanisms that govern the relation between IUGR and adverse outcomes are still relatively unknown. Oxidative stress and mitochondrial dysfunction have been reported to play a major role in adverse outcomes in various models of IUGR [27,35]. Mitochondria generate ROS in aerobic respiration via "leaking" of single electrons from the electron transport chain (ETC) to oxygen and converting them into superoxide anion. Mitochondrial ETC is both a source and target of ROS. During cellular respiration, superoxide anions are predominantly converted H_2O_2 by manganese superoxide dismutase (MnSOD) in mitochondria. If ROS production is in excess, the antioxidant defense system cannot eliminate excessive ROS production, which causes harmful effects on mitochondria. Mitochondrial dysfunction is often considered to coexist with dysregulated redox equilibrium [36]. It has been reported that a placental suboptimal environment can cause mitochondrial dysfunction in IUGR offspring [37–39]. We outline the latest findings on oxidative stress and mitochondrial dysfunction that are prevalent in maternal malnutrition-induced IUGR offspring during postnatal life.

IUGR offspring demonstrate mitochondrial dysfunction and oxidative stress in different organs at different stages of life. Rat offspring from dams fed a protein-restricted diet during gestation have demonstrated IUGR. These were significantly smaller than the control group on postnatal day (PND) 3. However, they underwent accelerated catch-up growth and were similar to the control offspring at PND 14 and at 12 months of age. These adult offspring were reported to have had increased protein contents of NADPH oxidase 2 (NOX2), NF-κB, xanthine oxidase (XO), and antioxidant enzymes; MnSOD, copper-zinc superoxide dismutase (CuZnSOD), catalase, and heme oxygenase-1 (HO1) at 12 months of age in their skeletal muscle, suggesting an increased response to oxidative stress [40]. Offspring from gestational calorie-restricted dams had a reduced body weight and demonstrated reduced mitochondrial number and content in mixed skeletal muscle fibers at 10 weeks of age [41]. 50% maternal calorie restriction from gestational day 11 to PND 21 (i.e., weaning point) caused an enhanced hepatic oxidative stress in pups, as they had an elevated level of oxidized 4-hydroxynonenal (4HNE) and decreased glutathione levels at PND 21 [42]. It has been reported that both pre- and postnatal maternal nutrition have a great impact in liver redox state in rats. Offspring fed by gestational and lactational protein-restricted mothers displayed an increase in oxidative stress markers (i.e., increased 4HNE, SOD1, SOD2) in the liver [35]. Antioxidant enzyme activities were also affected in pancreatic islet of IUGR offspring suggesting that modification in antioxidant defences could serve as a possible underlying mechanism responsible for pancreatic islet dysfunction later in life [43]. Tarry-Adkins et al. have reported that poor maternal nutrition-induced IUGR followed by accelerated growth in rats resulted in increased expression of peroxiredoxin 1 (PRDX1), peroxiredoxin 3 (PRDX3), HO1, and MnSOD, which are up-regulated under stress conditions [44].

It is debated whether catch-up growth may be the greater detriment to offspring redox homeostasis and mitochondrial function rather than IUGR in the offspring. Poor maternal nutrition may be detrimental in postnatal conditions of adequate nutrition or overnutrition. A human study has demonstrated that children who were born small, but who underwent accelerated postnatal growth had poor glucose tolerance, higher average body mass, increased cardiovascular risk factors, and were insulin resistant in childhood [27]. Ozanne et al. have reported IUGR mice nursed by normally fed dams during lactation experienced an accelerated catch-up growth and had shorter lifespan than the control group. However, mice that had normal in utero growth but were fed by low-protein fed mothers during lactation demonstrated enhanced longevity [45]. In a developmental rat model, dams were fed by low protein diet during pregnancy, thereby inducing IUGR. Offspring that were maintained on a protein-restricted diet postnatally did not demonstrate a rapid catch-up growth and remained relatively smaller. Hepatic ROS production was decreased in these offspring that were metabolically healthy in adulthood. Other offspring that were exposed to a normal protein diet either at birth or at weaning underwent postnatal rapid growth and had increased lipid peroxidation and increased SOD1 and SOD2 levels in their liver [38].

The effects of maternal undernutrition on the offspring might be gender-dependent. Maternal low-protein diet during gestation led to mitochondrial dysfunction in pancreatic islets of 3-month-old rats. Interestingly, the alteration of mitochondrial function was shown in sex-dependent manner as ROS production and mitochondrial dysfunction were more evident in males [46]. Male rat offspring were more susceptible to oxidative stress induced by a maternal low protein diet than females. The detrimental effects of maternal poor nutrition on oxidative balance in heart were showed to be mitigated by increased levels of oestradiol in female rats. The authors suggested that estrogen may act as an antioxidant in protection against oxidative stress levels elevated by maternal nutritional manipulation [47]. In another study, ovariectomy was conducted to evaluate the effects of estrogen in the aging process in rats with a maternal low-protein diet. It has been reported that the absence of female hormones accelerates kidney damage and increase levels of inflammatory markers and oxidative markers in the maternal low-protein rat model. Female rats exposed to maternal protein restriction had no alteration in plasma antioxidant status and no adverse outcome in the medulla oblongata, whereas male rats demonstrated medullary oxidative dysfunction at mRNA level and impaired antioxidant capacity [48]. Moreover, maternal nutritional suboptimal environment has led to reduced mitochondrial content and respiration particularly in the male kidney [49].

In contrast, the effects of maternal undernutrition on redox homeostasis and development in the brain are not well-understood [50,51]. Contrary to other organs, gestational calorie restriction has been shown to improve redox homeostasis in the brain of Wistar rats. Pups from 20% calorie restricted mice were monitored at PND0, PND7, PND21, and PND60. A decrease was observed in carbonyl levels in the hippocampus at PND60 and in malondialdehyde (MDA) levels in prefrontal cortex of pups suggesting reduced oxidative damage to lipids and proteins [51]. This evidence suggests that different organs can be affected in different ways. This can be explained by the Thrifty Phenotype Hypothesis; under suboptimal conditions, the organism permanently modifies its organ structure to provide sufficient nutrients to vital organs such as the brain [52]. This occurs through the "sparing" of vital organs, particularly brain, at the cost of other organs, including skeletal muscle, liver, pancreas, and heart. There is evidence that a lactational low protein diet resulted in a reduction in body weight, vastus lateralis muscle weight, pancreas weight, liver weight, and heart weight of mouse offspring but the brain and thymus weight were similar to the control group suggesting the brain might be protected from the adverse effect of a suboptimal nutritional early life environment [53]. Further studies are needed clarify the effects of maternal undernutrition on the brain.

It is becoming obvious that maternal nutrition has a great impact on the metabolic outcome of offspring. Animal studies have established the inverse relationship between IUGR and oxidative stress and mitochondrial dysfunction. Even though IUGR is an important factor in development of these adverse metabolic effects, accelerated catch-up growth, and the timing of the nutritional manipulation appear to be crucial in mediating oxidative stress driven poor health outcome. Moreover, the effects of poor maternal diet on different organs and gender are not well-established (Fig. 6.3).

Maternal overnutrition and redox homeostasis

The deleterious effects of IUGR on long-term metabolic health are well-established; however, it has become clear that high birth weight is also an apparent indicator of an increased risk of age-related diseases. Many epidemiological studies have shown a relation between maternal obesity, gestational diabetes, and elevated risk of diseases in later life [30,32]. Hyperglycemia and hyperinsulinemia are common outcomes in offspring of mothers with gestational diabetes and maternal obesity, as insulin regulation mechanism is impaired [54]. Studies have revealed that offspring exposed to maternal obesity and gestational diabetes in utero had higher incidence of insulin resistance, metabolic syndrome, type 2 diabetes, heart hypertrophy, and CVD in later life [28,31,32,55]. Numerous processes appear to be compromised which may lead to early signs of age-related diseases in response to maternal obesity and gestational diabetes including altered regulation of food intake, altered glucose homeostasis, altered adipose physiology, oxidative stress, mitochondrial function, and epigenetic modifications. Association of oxidative stress markers with insulin resistance, obesity, and diabetes has been shown through insulin signaling [54]. It is reported that oxidative stress may have a pivotal role in developing insulin resistance and obesity in response to maternal obesity and gestational diabetes by modifying gene expression and insulin metabolism [54]. Mitochondrial dysfunction and mutations in mitochondrial DNA are also implicated in development of a range of disorders including insulin resistance and type 2 diabetes [56].

Increased oxidative stress and mitochondrial dysfunction have been reported in offspring from mothers with obesity, gestational diabetes, and overnourished mothers. A human study which recruited 242 pregnant women measured

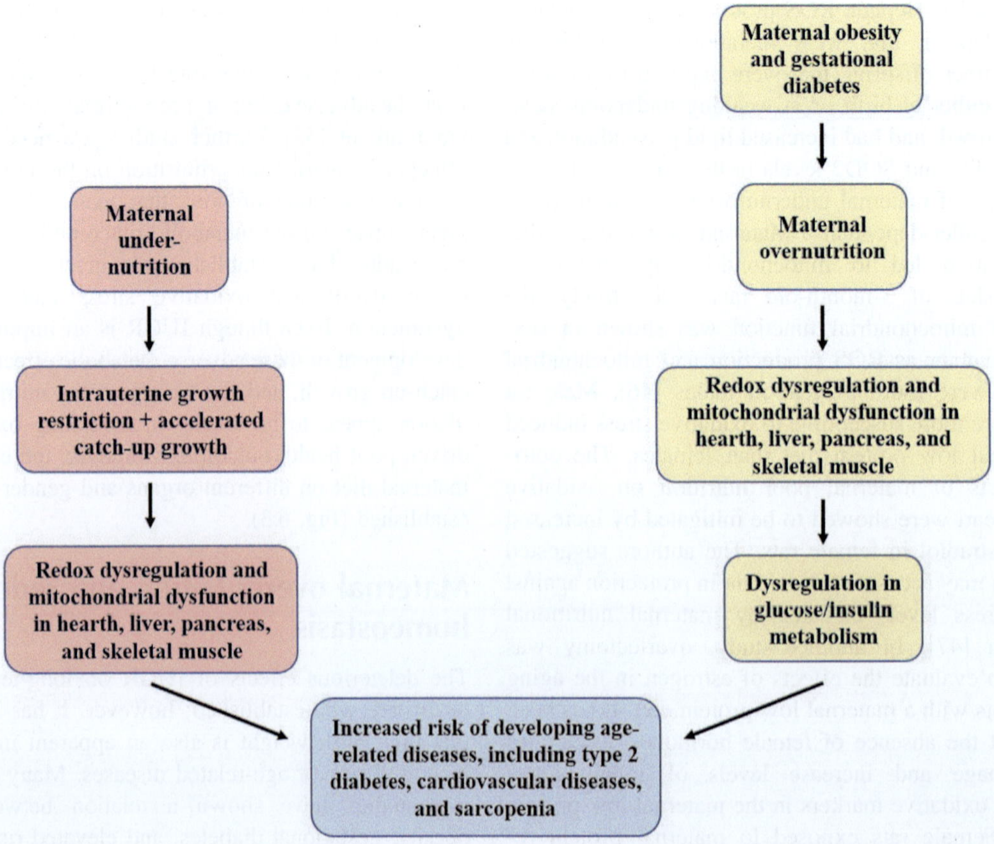

FIGURE 6.3 Effects of maternal under-nutrition and maternal overnutrition on development of age-related diseases.

plasma levels of nitric oxide (NO) and malondialdehyde (MDA) as markers of oxidative stress. Offspring from mothers with pregestational obesity and overweight had higher levels of oxidative stress markers [57]. As gestation is an important period for redox homeostasis, it has been suggested that elevated oxidative stress may be responsible for epigenetic modifications and in turn altered regulation of gene expression during development [57]. The placenta plays a crucial role in fetal growth and development during gestation. A study using MALDI-TOF Mass spectrometry technique has shown that pre-existing maternal obesity enhanced the expression of proteins that are involved in ROS production and proteins with antioxidant properties. Ferritin is involved in the formation of the hydroxyl radical ($OH^{\cdot}$). Ferritin light chain and ferritin heavy chain expressions were increased in the placenta of mothers with obesity. Moreover, the adenosine triphosphate (ATP) synthase subunit beta (ATBP) expression decreased in the placenta. It was suggested that this may lead to mitochondrial dysfunction [58]. Effects of gestational diabetes on the proteome, redox status, and antioxidant defences in human fetal endothelial cells have been investigated. Proteins involved in mitochondrial superoxide generation, protein oxidation, and DNA damage were significantly increased while glutathione (GSH) synthesis was diminished [59]. The detrimental effects of overnutrition on redox homeostasis during fetal and early life have also been shown in animal models. Oocytes and zygotes of obese female mice had altered mitochondrial distribution, noticeable hyperpolarization of the mitochondrial membrane, oxidized redox state, and increased oxidative stress. As embryos are extremely susceptible to fluctuations in redox state during early embryogenesis, these alterations may underlie poor reproductive outcomes often reported in obese mothers [60]. Lactational maternal high-fat diet to increased lipid peroxidation and resulted in a persistent synaptic instability in mouse offspring. Synaptic impairments were ameliorated by treatment with ascorbic acid suggesting that oxidative stress play a pivotal role [61]. Ventricular hypertrophy, increased fibrosis, and cardiac dysfunction were reported in overfed rat offspring. It was proposed that these changes are driven by oxidative stress as these animals demonstrated enhanced SOD1 and Ras-related protein (Rab-1B) [62]. Another study has found that maternal high-fat feeding increased the mRNA expression of enzymes involved in oxidative stress and mitochondrial dysfunction in 15-week-old mice offspring [63]. Increased oxidative stress and induced DNA damage were also shown in the liver of rabbit offspring from mothers on high-fat and high carbohydrates diet before and during gestation [64]. Moreover, a recent meta-analysis looking at oxidative stress profile after maternal high-fat diet consumption during early life in rodents (77 studies in total) found elevated MDA levels and ROS levels and decreased levels of antioxidant enzymes such as SOD and CAT [65].

Maternal nutrition, epigenetics, and oxidative stress

Epigenetics can be defined as heritable changes in phenotype or gene expression regulated by DNA methylation or histone modifications (methylation, acetylation, phosphorylation, and ubiquitination) which is independent of changes in DNA sequence. DNA methylation is the most mechanistically understood epigenetic modification; DNA methyltransferases (DNMTs) are enzymes that methylate the DNA by transferring a methyl group from S-adenyl methionine (SAM) to the C5 position of a cytosine residue in order to form 5-methylcytosine (5 mC). Chromatin consists of DNA and proteins known as histones that package DNA. Histone modifications establish different chromatin transcriptional states. All these modifications put together compose "the epigenetic landscape." Early life environment can have an impact on epigenetic landscape that can be "remembered" during the lifespan. There is evidence supporting that epigenetic changes are associated with aging [17]. Oxidative stress can influence the epigenetic landscape by having an impact on DNA, histone, and histone modifiers. Oxidant-caused DNA breaks can open up access sites to DNMTs, which enhance DNA methylation. It has been reported that ROS can directly modify histone proteins, causing disturbance of normal mRNA expression [27]. ROS can also indirectly regulate the epigenetic activity as intracellular levels of ROS regulated-metabolites such as Acetyl-CoA, Fe, and NAD^+ control the activity of histone-modifying enzymes [66]. It is suggested that a molecular mechanism for the changes in the epigenetic landscape in several early-life programming models may be oxidative stress. Epigenetic alterations in peroxisomal proliferator-activated receptor (PPAR)-α have been shown in rat offspring from mothers fed a low-protein diet [67]. Maternal high-fat diet is associated with impaired antioxidant defense mechanisms and DNA methylation in adult mouse offspring suggesting maternal diet has long-lasting effects [68]. Even though the role of oxidative stress on maternal nutrition-induced epigenetic modifications is not well-established, it is feasible to think that oxidative stress is one of the possible underlying mechanisms.

Maternal iron and oxidative stress

Iron is an essential element for cellular functions including oxygen delivery, electron transport, and enzymatic activity. There is a dramatic increase in iron requirement during pregnancy. Hence, iron deficiency is very common during fetus growth and development and results in many abnormalities including long-term neurocognitive and mental health impairments [69]. An association between maternal iron deficiency and enhanced incidence of IUGR has been reported by epidemiological studies [70]. Moreover, low maternal iron intake during gestation is associated with hypertension, abnormal brain structure, and autism in the offspring [69].

Iron and iron derivatives have a crucial role in the formation and destruction of ROS including superoxide ($O_2^{\cdot -}$), peroxides (H_2O_2 and ROOH), and free radicals ($HO^{\cdot}$ and $RO^{\cdot}$) by controlling the function of ROS-producing enzymes such as xanthine oxidase and nicotinamide adenine dinucleotide phosphate hydride (NADPH) oxidases (NOXs). The free radical formation can also be directly catalyzed by intracellular redox-active iron pools via the Fenton reaction [71]. Therefore, oxidative stress could have a potential role in the development of abnormalities in the offspring of maternal iron deficient-mothers. A rat study has shown that offspring from mothers who had an iron-restricted diet during pregnancy were smaller than the control group at PD1. It has also been reported that male offspring had dysregulation in renal mitochondrial function and an increase in mitochondrial and cytosolic superoxide levels at 6 months of age [72]. An increase in oxidative stress biomarkers including lipid peroxidation products and protein carbonyl content in brain, blood, and liver of iron-deficient offspring also been indicated in another animal study [73]. Even though there are human studies indicating the adverse effects of maternal iron-deficiency in the offspring, a recent study which recruited 57 pregnant women showed a positive correlation between the oxidative stress levels in the offspring and the iron concentration in maternal serum [74]. According to Casanueva and Viteri, both iron deficiency and iron excess can cause free radical damage, and leading to functional alterations [75]. Finally, although it is not well-established, there is evidence of a U-shaped curve between iron concentrations during pregnancy and birth outcomes. It has been reported that oxidative stress is a possible underlying mechanism through which gestational iron statues may have adverse effects on birth outcomes [76]. However, further studies are needed to establish the potential role of oxidative stress in iron deficiency or iron excess lead impairments.

Concluding remarks

Maternal nutrition has a great impact on the metabolic outcome of offspring. Animal studies have established the inverse relationship between IUGR and oxidative stress and mitochondrial dysfunction. Even though IUGR is an important factor in the development of these adverse metabolic effects, accelerated catch-up growth and the timing of the nutritional manipulation appear to be crucial in mediating oxidative stress-driven poor health outcome. Moreover, the effects of poor maternal diet on different organs and sex are not well-established. Maternal over-nutrition is also associated with long-term effects on offspring health and increased risk of development of age-related diseases such as CVD, type 2 diabetes, and metabolic syndrome. Human and animal studies have demonstrated an association between increased oxidative stress levels with maternal overnutrition in the placenta and offspring. These findings suggest that maternal overnutrition-driven redox dysregulation may play a pivotal role in the development of age-related diseases later in life in the offspring. Maternal iron intake has impact on the growth and development of the fetus. As iron is an important element in the formation of ROS, it is proposed that oxidative stress plays a pivotal role in emerging of gestational iron statutes-induced adverse effects on birth outcomes.

References

[1] Powers SK, Ji LL, Kavazis AN, Jackson MJ. Reactive oxygen species: impact on skeletal muscle. Compr Physiol 2011;1(2):941.

[2] Schieber M, Chandel NS. ROS function in redox signaling and oxidative stress. Curr Biol 2014;24(10):R453–62.

[3] Finkel T. Signal transduction by reactive oxygen species. J Cell Biol 2011;194(1):7–15.

[4] Wood ZA, Poole LB, Karplus PA. Peroxiredoxin evolution and the regulation of hydrogen peroxide signaling. Science 2003;300(5619):650–3.

[5] Kiley PJ, Storz G. Exploiting thiol modifications. PLoS Biol 2004;2(11):e400.

[6] Powers SK, Jackson MJ. Exercise-induced oxidative stress: cellular mechanisms and impact on muscle force production. Physiol Rev 2008;88(4):1243–76.

[7] Ufer C, Wang CC, Borchert A, Heydeck D, Kuhn H. Redox control in mammalian embryo development. Antioxid Redox Signal 2010;13(6):833–75.

[8] Agarwal A, Gupta S, Sekhon L, Shah R. Redox considerations in female reproductive function and assisted reproduction: from molecular mechanisms to health implications. Antioxid Redox Signal 2008;10(8):1375–404.

[9] Al-Gubory KH, Fowler PA, Garrel C. The roles of cellular reactive oxygen species, oxidative stress and antioxidants in pregnancy outcomes. Int J Biochem Cell Biol 2010;42(10):1634–50.

[10] Dennery PA. Effects of oxidative stress on embryonic development. Birth Defects Res C Embryo Today Rev 2007;81(3):155–62.

[11] Hansen JM. Oxidative stress as a mechanism of teratogenesis. Birth Defects Res C Embryo Today Rev 2006;78(4):293–307.

[12] De Marco CS, Caniggia I. Mechanisms of oxygen sensing in human trophoblast cells. Placenta 2002;23:S58–68.

[13] Nau PN, Van Natta T, Ralphe JC, Teneyck CJ, Bedell KA, Caldarone CA, et al. Metabolic adaptation of the fetal and postnatal ovine heart: regulatory role of hypoxia-inducible factors and nuclear respiratory factor-1. Pediatr Res 2002;52(2):269–78.

[14] Daikoku T, Matsumoto H, Gupta RA, Das SK, Gassmann M, DuBois RN, et al. Expression of hypoxia-inducible factors in the peri-implantation mouse uterus is regulated in a cell-specific and ovarian steroid hormone-dependent manner: evidence for differential function of HIFs during early pregnancy. J Biol Chem 2003;278(9):7683–91.

[15] Ruiz-Gines J, Lopez-Ongil S, Gonzalez-Rubio M, Gonzalez-Santiago L, Rodriguez-Puyol M, Rodriguez-Puyol D. Reactive oxygen species induce proliferation of bovine aortic endothelial cells. J Cardiovasc Pharmacol 2000;35(1):109–13.

[16] Davies KJ. The broad spectrum of responses to oxidants in proliferating cells: a new paradigm for oxidative stress. IUBMB Life 1999;48(1):41–7.

[17] Guillaumet-Adkins A, Yañez Y, Peris-Diaz MD, Calabria I, Palanca-Ballester C, Sandoval J. Epigenetics and oxidative stress in aging. Oxid Med Cell Longev 2017;2017.

[18] Semenza GL. Regulation of mammalian O_2 homeostasis by hypoxia-inducible factor 1. Annu Rev Cell Dev Biol 1999;15:551.

[19] Liu T, Zhang L, Joo D, Sun S-C. Therapy T. NF-κB signaling in inflammation. Signal Transduct Target Ther 2017;2(1):1–9.

[20] Torchinsky A, Toder V. To die or not to die: the function of the transcription factor NF-κB in embryos exposed to stress. Am J Reprod Immunol 2004;51(2):138–43.

[21] Hales CN, Barker DJ, Clark PM, Cox LJ, Fall C, Osmond C, et al. Fetal and infant growth and impaired glucose tolerance at age 64. Br Med J 1991;303(6809):1019–22.

[22] Barker DJ, Hales CN, Fall C, Osmond C, Phipps K, Clark P. Type 2 (non-insulin-dependent) diabetes mellitus, hypertension and hyperlipidaemia (syndrome X): relation to reduced fetal growth. Diabetologia 1993;36(1):62–7.

[23] Osmond C, Barker D, Winter P, Fall C, Simmonds SJ. Early growth and death from cardiovascular disease in women. Br Med J 1993;307(6918):1519–24.

[24] Sayer A, Stewart C, Patel H, Cooper C. The developmental origins of sarcopenia: from epidemiological evidence to underlying mechanisms. J Dev Orig Health Dis 2010;1(3):150–7.

[25] Sayer AA, Syddall HE, Gilbody HJ, Dennison EM, Cooper C. Does sarcopenia originate in early life? Findings from the Hertfordshire cohort study. J Gerontol A Biol Sci Med Sci 2004;59(9):M930–4.

[26] Curhan GC, Chertow GM, Willett WC, Spiegelman D, Colditz GA, Manson JE, et al. Birth weight and adult hypertension and obesity in women. Circulation 1996;94(6):1310–5.

[27] Tarry-Adkins JL, Ozanne SE. The impact of early nutrition on the ageing trajectory. Proc Nutr Soc 2014;73(2):289–301.

[28] Boney CM, Verma A, Tucker R, Vohr BR. Metabolic syndrome in childhood: association with birth weight, maternal obesity, and gestational diabetes mellitus. Pediatrics 2005;115(3):e290–6.

[29] Johnsson IW, Haglund B, Ahlsson F, Gustafsson J. A high birth weight is associated with increased risk of type 2 diabetes and obesity. Pediatr Obes 2015;10(2):77–83.

[30] Boerschmann H, Pflüger M, Henneberger L, Ziegler A-G, Hummel S. Prevalence and predictors of overweight and insulin resistance in offspring of mothers with gestational diabetes mellitus. Diabetes Care 2010;33(8):1845–9.

[31] Zielinsky P, Piccoli Jr AL. Myocardial hypertrophy and dysfunction in maternal diabetes. Early Hum Dev 2012;88(5):273–8.

[32] Krishnaveni GV, Veena SR, Hill JC, Kehoe S, Karat SC, Fall CH. Intrauterine exposure to maternal diabetes is associated with higher adiposity and insulin resistance and clustering of cardiovascular risk markers in Indian children. Diabetes Care 2010;33(2):402–4.

[33] Langley-Evans S. Nutrition in early life and the programming of adult disease: a review. J Hum Nutr Diet 2015;28:1–14.

[34] Hales CN, Barker DJ. Type 2 (non-insulin-dependent) diabetes mellitus: the thrifty phenotype hypothesis. Diabetologia 1992;35(7):595–601.

[35] Oke SL, Hardy DB. The role of cellular stress in intrauterine growth restriction and postnatal dysmetabolism. Int J Mol Sci 2021;22(13):6986.

[36] Cui H, Kong Y, Zhang H. Oxidative stress, mitochondrial dysfunction, and aging. J Signal Transduct 2012;2012.

[37] Park KS, Kim SK, Kim MS, Cho EY, Lee JH, Lee K-U, et al. Fetal and early postnatal protein malnutrition cause long-term changes in rat liver and muscle mitochondria. J Nutr 2003;133(10):3085–90.

[38] Oke SL, Sohi G, Hardy DBJR. Perinatal protein restriction with postnatal catch-up growth leads to elevated p66Shc and mitochondrial dysfunction in the adult rat liver 2020;159(1):27–39.

[39] Pendleton AL, Wesolowski SR, Regnault TR, Lynch RM, Limesand SW. Dimming the powerhouse: mitochondrial dysfunction in the liver and skeletal muscle of intrauterine growth restricted fetuses. Front Endocrinol 2021;12:612888.

[40] Tarry-Adkins JL, Fernandez-Twinn DS, Chen JH, Hargreaves IP, Neergheen V, Aiken CE, et al. Poor maternal nutrition and accelerated postnatal growth induces an accelerated aging phenotype and oxidative stress in skeletal muscle of male rats. Dis Model Mech 2016;9(10):1221–9.

[41] Beauchamp B, Ghosh S, Dysart M, Kanaan GN, Chu A, Blais A, et al. Low birth weight is associated with adiposity, impaired skeletal muscle energetics and weight loss resistance in mice. Int J Obes 2015;39(4):702–11.

[42] Devarajan A, Rajasekaran NS, Valburg C, Ganapathy E, Bindra S, Freije WA, et al. Maternal perinatal calorie restriction temporally regulates the hepatic autophagy and redox status in male rat. Free Radic Biol Med 2019;130:592–600.

[43] Theys N, Clippe A, Bouckenooghe T, Reusens B, Remacle C. Early low protein diet aggravates unbalance between antioxidant enzymes leading to islet dysfunction. PLoS One 2009;4(7):e6110.

[44] Tarry-Adkins J, Chen J, Smith N, Jones R, Cherif H, Ozanne S. Poor maternal nutrition followed by accelerated postnatal growth leads to telomere shortening and increased markers of cell senescence in rat islets. FASEB J 2009;23(5):1521–8.

[45] Ozanne SE, Hales CN. Catch-up growth and obesity in male mice. Nature 2004;427(6973):411–2.

[46] Theys N, Bouckenooghe T, Ahn M-T, Remacle C, Reusens B. Maternal low-protein diet alters pancreatic islet mitochondrial function in a sex-specific manner in the adult rat. Am J Physiol Regul Integr Comp Physiol 2009;297(5):R1516–25.

[47] Braz G, Emiliano A, Sousa S, Pedroza A, Santana D, Fernandes M, et al. Maternal low-protein diet in female rat heart: possible protective effect of estradiol. J Dev Orig Health Dis 2017;8(3):322–30.

[48] de Brito Alves JL, de Oliveira JM, Ferreira DJ, Barros MADV, Nogueira VO, Alves DS, et al. Maternal protein restriction induced-hypertension is associated to oxidative disruption at transcriptional and functional levels in the medulla oblongata. Clin Exp Pharmacol Physiol 2016;43(12):1177–84.

[49] Woodman AG, Mah R, Keddie D, Noble RM, Panahi S, Gragasin FS, et al. Prenatal iron deficiency causes sex-dependent mitochondrial dysfunction and oxidative stress in fetal rat kidneys and liver. FASEB J 2018;32(6):3254–63.

[50] Tarry-Adkins JL, Martin-Gronert MS, Fernandez-Twinn DS, Hargreaves I, Alfaradhi MZ, Land JM, et al. Poor maternal nutrition followed by accelerated postnatal growth leads to alterations in DNA damage and repair, oxidative and nitrosative stress, and oxidative defense capacity in rat heart. FASEB J 2013;27(1):379–90.

[51] Stone V, Crestani MS, Saccomori AB, Dal Magro BM, Maurmann RM, August PM, et al. Gestational caloric restriction improves redox homeostasis parameters in the brain of Wistar rats: a screening from birth to adulthood. J. Nutr. Biochem. 2019;67:138–48.

[52] Hales CN, Barker DJ. The thrifty phenotype hypothesis: type 2 diabetes. Br Med Bull 2001;60(1):5–20.

[53] Chen J-H, Martin-Gronert MS, Tarry-Adkins J, Ozanne SE. Maternal protein restriction affects postnatal growth and the expression of key proteins involved in lifespan regulation in mice. PLoS One 2009;4(3):e4950.

[54] Alfaradhi MZ, Ozanne SE. Developmental programming in response to maternal overnutrition. Front Genet 2011;2:27.

[55] Pettitt DJ, Moll PP, Knowler WC, Mott DM, Nelson RG, Saad MF, et al. Insulinemia in children at low and high risk of NIDDM. Diabetes Care 1993;16(4):608–15.

[56] Wang CH, Wang CC, Wei YH. Mitochondrial dysfunction in insulin insensitivity: implication of mitochondrial role in type 2 diabetes. Ann N Y Acad Sci 2010;1201(1):157–65.

[57] Lopez-Yañez Blanco A, Díaz-López KM, Vilchis-Gil J, Diaz-Garcia H, Gomez-Lopez J, Medina-Bravo P, et al. Diet and maternal obesity are associated with increased oxidative stress in newborns: a cross-sectional study. Nutrients 2022;14(4):746.

[58] Oliva K, Barker G, Riley C, Bailey MJ, Permezel M, Rice GE, et al. The effect of pre-existing maternal obesity on the placental proteome: two-dimensional difference gel electrophoresis coupled with mass spectrometry. J Mol Endocrinol 2012;48(2):139–49.

[59] Cheng X, Chapple SJ, Patel B, Puszyk W, Sugden D, Yin X, et al. Gestational diabetes mellitus impairs Nrf2-mediated adaptive antioxidant defenses and redox signaling in fetal endothelial cells in utero. Diabetes 2013;62(12):4088–97.

[60] Igosheva N, Abramov AY, Poston L, Eckert JJ, Fleming TP, Duchen MR, et al. Maternal diet-induced obesity alters mitochondrial activity and redox status in mouse oocytes and zygotes. PLoS One 2010;5(4):e10074.

[61] Hatanaka Y, Wada K, Kabuta T. Maternal high-fat diet leads to persistent synaptic instability in mouse offspring via oxidative stress during lactation. Neurochem Int 2016;97:99–108.

[62] Junior MDF, Cavalcante KVN, Ferreira LA, Lopes PR, Pontes CNR, de Bessa ADSM, et al. Postnatal early overfeeding induces cardiovascular dysfunction by oxidative stress in adult male Wistar rats. Life Sci 2019;226:173–84.

[63] Bruce KD, Cagampang FR, Argenton M, Zhang J, Ethirajan PL, Burdge GC, et al. Maternal high-fat feeding primes steatohepatitis in

adult mice offspring, involving mitochondrial dysfunction and altered lipogenesis gene expression. Hepatology 2009;50(6):1796–808.

[64] Salazar AM, Sordo M, Navarrete-Monroy E, Pánico P, Díaz-Villaseñor A, Montúfar-Chaveznava R, et al. Maternal over-nutrition before and during pregnancy induces DNA damage in male offspring: a rabbit model. Mutat Res/Genet Toxicol Environ Mutagen 2021;865:503324.

[65] Moraes-Souza R, Vesentini G, Paula VG, Sinzato YK, Soares T, Gelaleti RB, et al. Oxidative stress profile of mothers and their offspring after maternal consumption of high-fat diet in rodents: a systematic review and meta-analysis. Oxid Med Cell Longev 2021;2021.

[66] Simpson NE, Tryndyak VP, Pogribna M, Beland FA, Pogribny IP. Modifying metabolically sensitive histone marks by inhibiting glutamine metabolism affects gene expression and alters cancer cell phenotype. Epigenetics 2012;7(12):1413–20.

[67] Lillycrop KA, Phillips ES, Jackson AA, Hanson MA, Burdge GC. Dietary protein restriction of pregnant rats induces and folic acid supplementation prevents epigenetic modification of hepatic gene expression in the offspring. J Nutr 2005;135(6):1382–6.

[68] Keleher MR, Zaidi R, Shah S, Oakley ME, Pavlatos C, El Idrissi S, et al. Maternal high-fat diet associated with altered gene expression, DNA methylation, and obesity risk in mouse offspring. PLoS One 2018;13(2):e0192606.

[69] Georgieff MK. Iron deficiency in pregnancy. Am J Obstet Gynecol 2020;223(4):516–24.

[70] Lee H, Kim M, Kim M, Kim Y, Kim W. Iron status and its association with pregnancy outcome in Korean pregnant women. Eur J Clin Nutr 2006;60(9):1130–5.

[71] Dixon SJ, Stockwell BR. The role of iron and reactive oxygen species in cell death. Nat Chem Biol 2014;10(1):9–17.

[72] Woodman AG, Mah R, Keddie DL, Noble RM, Holody CD, Panahi S, et al. Perinatal iron deficiency and a high salt diet cause long-term kidney mitochondrial dysfunction and oxidative stress. Cardiovasc Res 2020;116(1):183–92.

[73] Vieyra-Reyes P, Millán-Aldaco D, Palomero-Rivero M, Jiménez-Garcés C, Hernández-González M, Caballero-Villarraso J. An iron-deficient diet during development induces oxidative stress in relation to age and gender in Wistar rats. J Physiol Biochem 2017;73(1):99–110.

[74] Rak K, Łoźna K, Styczyńska M, Bobak Ł, Bronkowska M. Oxidative stress at birth is associated with the concentration of iron and copper in maternal serum. Nutrients 2021;13(5):1491.

[75] Casanueva E, Viteri FE. Iron and oxidative stress in pregnancy. J Nutr 2003;133(5):1700S–8S.

[76] Dewey KG, Oaks BM. U-shaped curve for risk associated with maternal hemoglobin, iron status, or iron supplementation. Am J Clin Nutr 2017;106(Suppl. 1_6):1694S–702S.

Chapter 7

Mitochondria-associated membranes (MAMs) as modulators of oxidative stress in Alzheimer disease

Tânia Fernandes[1,2,3,4], M. Rosário Domingues[5], Cláudia F. Pereira[1,3,4] and Paula I. Moreira[1,3,4]

[1]*CNC - Center for Neuroscience and Cell Biology, CIBB - Center for Innovative Biomedicine and Biotechnology, University of Coimbra, Coimbra, Portugal;* [2]*IIIUC - Institute for Interdisciplinary Research, University of Coimbra, Coimbra, Portugal;* [3]*CACC - Clinical Academic Center of Coimbra, Coimbra, Portugal;* [4]*Faculty of Medicine, University of Coimbra, Coimbra, Portugal;* [5]*Mass Spectrometry Centre, LAQV REQUIMTE, Department of Chemistry, Centre for Environmental and Marine Studies (CESAM), University of Aveiro, Santiago University Campus, Aveiro, Portugal*

Introduction

Mitochondria and the endoplasmic reticulum (ER) communicate by establishing physical and biochemical contacts with an intermembrane distance [1]. These structures, called mitochondria-associated membranes (MAMs) or mitochondria-endoplasmic reticulum contacts (MERCs), are enriched in proteins and lipids and modulate several cellular processes, including Ca^{2+} signaling, lipid synthesis and trafficking, mitochondria and ER dynamics, ER stress response, autophagy, redox status, inflammation, and apoptosis [2]. Alterations at MAMs can increase the Ca^{2+} transfer between the ER and mitochondria, which trigger mitochondrial Ca^{2+} overload and increased reactive oxygen species (ROS) production. Subsequently, high ROS levels can impair lipid biosynthesis and promote oxidative lipid damage, referred as lipid peroxidation, exacerbating mitochondrial dysfunction [3].

Structural and functional alterations of MAMs have been described in neurodegenerative diseases, including Alzheimer disease (AD), which are characterized by aberrant Ca^{2+} homeostasis, ER stress, mitochondrial dysfunction, and increased ROS production. The impairment of MAM-related features occurs years before the appearance of AD pathological hallmarks [4]. Therefore, strategies or therapies to prevent or slowdown AD progression may include the use of drugs able to modulate MAMs, which will in turn regulate ER to mitochondria Ca^{2+} flux, lipid biosynthesis, and/or interorganelle transport, as well as production of ROS, among other processes [3].

In this chapter, we provide an overview of MAMs structure and functions and discuss their involvement in ROS production and oxidative stress/damage in AD, with an emphasis on lipid peroxidation. Finally, the therapeutic potential of MAMs modulation in AD will be also discussed.

Structure and function of mitochondria-associated membranes

The physical interplay between the ER membrane and the outer mitochondrial membrane (OMM) was observed for the first time in mammalian ovary tissue using transmission electron microscopy, by Ruby and co-workers [5]. However, the knowledge about this structure started only in 1990 when Jean Vance isolated the contact sites between the ER and mitochondria from rat liver tissue through cell fractionation [6].

It is currently established that the ER and mitochondria communicate through physical and biochemical juxtaposition of their membranes, with a distance ranging from 10 to 80 nm between both organelles [1]. These close contact sites, called MAMs or MERCs, are dynamic structures that are sensitive to the physiological conditions of the cell, which results in a transient and highly variable MAMs composition [7]. Several protein complexes are responsible for the ER−mitochondria tethering, namely the complex formed by the ER 1,4,5-triphosphate receptor (IP3R), the chaperone 75-kDa glucose-regulated protein (Grp75), and

Modulation of Oxidative Stress. https://doi.org/10.1016/B978-0-443-19247-0.00012-6

the voltage-dependent anion-selective channel (VDAC) in the OMM [1,2,8]. Other tethering complexes result from the interaction between the ER-localized vesicle-associated membrane protein-associated protein B (VAPB) or the B-cell receptor-associated protein 31 (BAP31) with the mitochondrial protein tyrosine phosphatase interacting protein 51 (PTPIP51) and the mitochondrial fission 1 protein (FIS1), respectively. The mitofusin 2 (MFN2) protein present in the ER membrane can also form homodimers or heterodimers with MFN2 or with mitofusin 1 (MFN1), respectively, present in the OMM [1,2]. The ER–mitochondria contact sites regulate the function of both organelles and, consequently, modulate multiple cellular activities such as energy metabolism, Ca^{2+} signaling, lipid synthesis and trafficking, mitochondrial and ER dynamics, ER stress response, autophagy, inflammation, and apoptosis [2,7,8]. Several proteins located at MAMs are implicated in the regulation of Ca^{2+} homeostasis, including the protein complex IP3R-GRP75-VDAC that mediates Ca^{2+} fluxes between the ER and the mitochondria [8], as well as the ryanodine receptor (RyR) and sarco/endoplasmic reticulum Ca^{2+}-ATPase (SERCA), which are responsible for ER Ca^{2+} release and uptake, respectively [1,2]. Another ER protein involved in Ca^{2+} signaling is the chaperone Sigma-1 receptor (Sigma1R) that upon ER Ca^{2+} release dissociates from the chaperone binding immunoglobulin protein (BiP) to stabilize the IP3R, which leads to sustained Ca^{2+} transfer into mitochondria [9]. On MAMs, the ER chaperones calnexin and calreticulin also regulate Ca^{2+} flux through the IP3R [8]. Another protein present in the MAMs is BiP, which is involved in the ER stress–induced unfolded protein response (UPR) to reestablish proteostasis upon accumulation of misfolded proteins. The proteins inositol-requiring enzyme 1 alpha (IRE1α) and protein kinase RNA-like ER kinase (PERK) that act as sensors of ER stress and upregulate UPR mediators upon activation are also components of MAMs [10]. Other proteins involved in quality control pathways are present at MAMs, such as the phosphoinositide 3-kinase (PI3K) that is implicated in autophagosome formation [11]. In addition, the antiapoptotic factors B-cell CLL/lymphoma 2 (BCL-2), Bcl-2 associated X protein (BAX), and Bcl-2 antagonist/killer (BAK), as well as components of the inflammasome, namely the activated NOD-like receptor protein 3 (NLRP3) and its adaptor protein caspase-recruitment domain (ASC), are located at MAMs to regulate apoptosis and inflammation [2]. The proteins MFN1, MFN2, dynamin-related protein 1 (DRP1), BAP31, and FIS1 are also present in MAMs and regulate mitochondrial dynamics [2]. ER redox status is regulated by disulfide isomerase (PDI) and ER oxidoreduction 1 α (ERO1α) found at MAMs [12].

Since the ER is the major site of biosynthesis of membranes phospholipids, MAMs represent an important platform for nonvesicular phospholipids and cholesterol transport between the ER and mitochondria [2,3]. Due to this, MAMs are highly enriched in proteins involved in lipid metabolism, such as: (1) acyl-CoA cholesterol acyltransferase/sterol O-acyltransferase 1 (ACAT1/SOAT1) that catalyzes the esterification of cholesterol into cholesteryl ester [13]; (2) steroidogenic acute regulatory lipid transfer domain (STARD1) and translocator protein (TSPO) involved in cholesterol transport from the ER to the inner mitochondrial membrane (IMM) [14,15]; (3) diacylglycerol O-acyltransferase 2 (DGAT2) that catalyzes the synthesis of triacylglycerols (TG) and formation of lipid droplets [16]; (4) phosphatidylserine synthases 1 and 2 (PSS1 and PSS2) and phosphatidylethanolamine methyltransferase (PEMT) involved in phospholipid synthesis [17,18]; and (5) fatty acid CoA ligase 4 (FACL4/ACSL4) involved in long-chain free fatty acids (FA) metabolism [19]. So, MAMs represent a critical metabolic and trafficking hub in lipid metabolism.

Phosphatidylcholine (PC), that is the most abundant phospholipid present in the outer layer of cellular membranes, can be converted into phosphatidylserine (PS) by PSS1 at the ER. Then, PS is imported to mitochondria where it can be transformed to phosphatidylethanolamine (PE) through the action of phosphatidylserine decarboxylase (PSD). PE synthesized in the mitochondria can be translocated to the ER where it is converted to PC by PEMT or, in a lower extent, to PS by PSS2 [2,20,21]. PC formed in ER can be translocated to the mitochondrial membrane [21]. The increase of ER–mitochondria contacts and the enrichment of biosynthetic enzymes in these structures affect lipid transfer between both organelles and their function. For instance, PSS1/2 enriched at MAMs enhances the transfer of PS to the mitochondria [20], and it has been shown that PE deficiency affects mitochondrial morphology and oxidative phosphorylation (OXPHOS) [22]. In yeast, the loss of components of ER-mitochondria contacts was found to impair PS transport between these organelles [23], further demonstrating the importance of MAMs in lipid trafficking.

Cardiolipin (CL), which is synthesized from phosphatidic acid (PA), is essential for mitochondrial protein import, dynamics, OXPHOS, and apoptosis [3]. PA is translocated from the ER to IMM via MAMs and converted into cytidinediphosphate-diacylglycerol (CDP-DAG) by the CDP-DAG synthase TAMM41. Then, phosphatidylglycerol phosphate synthase (PGS1) catalyzes the conversion of CDP-DAG to phosphatidylglycerol phosphate (PGP). Phosphatidylglycerol (PG) is produced by the phosphatase protein-tyrosine phosphatase mitochondrial 1 (PTPMT1) and the enzyme CL synthase (CLS) catalyzes the bound of one molecule of CDP-DAG to PG to produce one molecule of CL [24]. Depletion of CL and remodeling of its FA composition have been associated to aging, since an increase in unsaturated FAs, predominantly arachidonic and docosahexaenoic acids (ARA and DHA, respectively), was observed in the heart of aged mice [25].

Besides lipid trafficking between the ER and mitochondria, MAMs contain lipid raft microdomains enriched in cholesterol, ceramides, and glycosphingolipids that interact with proteins present in this region [20,26]. For example, ceramides are physically associated with the Sigma1R contributing to IP3R stabilization [26] and cholesterol or ceramide depletion causes the relocation of these proteins to the bulk of the ER membrane, suggesting that lipids play an important role in the formation of specialized protein assemblies at MAMs [27]. Treatment of isolated rat liver mitochondria with methyl-β-cyclodextrin (an agent that depletes membrane cholesterol) was shown to disrupt MAMs structure and subsequently impair mitochondrial bioenergetics [28].

Alterations in proteins involved in lipid metabolism at MAMs affect other protein complexes and, therefore, biological processes regulated in this region, which in turn disturb the interaction between the ER and the mitochondria further disturbing lipid trafficking between both organelles [2]. During aging, the failure of the ER stress response (e.g., UPR activation) dysregulates lipid metabolism and homeostasis [29]. These alterations impact mitochondria function contributing to energy deficits, increased oxidative stress and damage of lipids (peroxidation), proteins and nucleic acids that, in turn, exacerbate mitochondrial dysfunction [3] (Fig. 7.1).

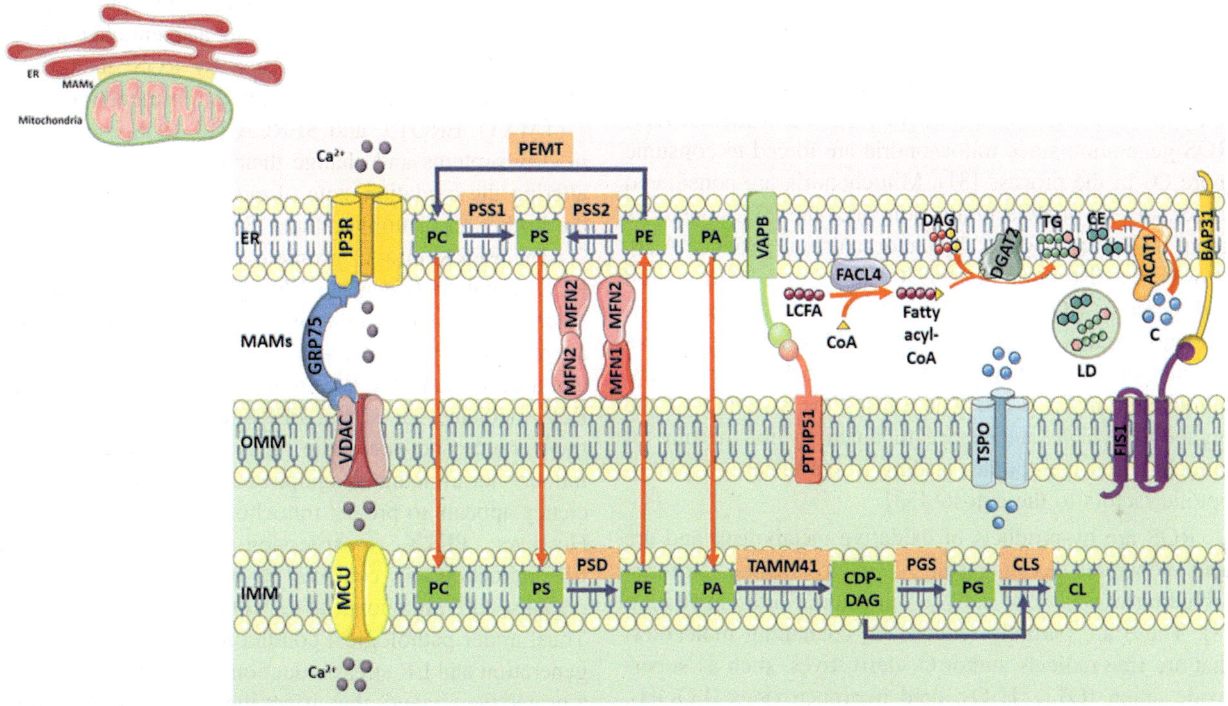

FIGURE 7.1 ER–mitochondria tethering and lipid metabolism. The platform responsible for the physical connection between the ER and the mitochondria, known as MAMs, is formed by several protein complexes such as IP3R-GRP75-VDAC, VAPB-PTPI51, BAP31-FIS1, and MFN2-MFN1/2. This region regulates Ca^{2+} signaling and lipid synthesis and trafficking. The Ca^{2+} transfer between the ER and mitochondria is mediated by the ER protein IP3R and by the mitochondrial proteins VDAC in the OMM, and MCU in the IMM. GRP75 acts as a linker between IP3R and VDAC. MAMs are enriched in proteins involved in lipid metabolism, including FACL4 that plays a key role in fatty acid metabolism, DGAT2 that catalyzes the synthesis of TG from DAG and LD formation, ACAT1 that is involved in the esterification of cholesterol into CE that can be store in LD, and TSPO that is responsible for cholesterol transport from the ER to IMM. Phospholipid PC can be directly transferred from the ER to mitochondria or converted into PS by PSS1 at the ER, then PS is imported to the mitochondria and converted to PE by PSD. PE synthesized in mitochondria can be translocated to the ER and converted to PC or PS by PEMT or PSS2, respectively. PA transferred from the ER to the mitochondria is transformed into CDP-DAG through the action of TAMM41 and converted to PG by PGS. To produce CL, the enzyme CLS catalyzes the binding of CDP-DAG to PG. *ACAT1*, acyl-CoA cholesterol acyltransferase; *BAP31*, B-cell receptor-associated protein 31; *C*, cholesterol; *CDP-DAG*, cytidine diphosphate-diacylglycerol; *CE*, cholesteryl esters; *CL*, cardiolipin; *CLS*, cardiolipin synthase; *CoA*, coenzyme A; *DAG*, diacylglycerol; *DGAT2*, diacylglycerol O-acyltransferase; *ER*, endoplasmic reticulum; *FACL4*, fatty acid CoA ligase 4; *FIS1*, mitochondrial fission 1; *GRP75*, glucose regulated protein 75; *IMM*, inner mitochondrial membranes; *IP3R*, inositol 1,4,5 trisphosphate receptor; *LCFA*, long chain fatty acid; *LD*, lipid droplets; *MAMs*, mitochondria-associated membranes; *MCU*, mitochondrial calcium uniporter protein; *MFN1/2*, mitofusin 1/2; *OMM*, outer mitochondrial membranes; *PA*, phosphatidic acid; *PC*, phosphatidylcholine; *PE*, phosphatidylethanolamine; *PEMT*, PE N-methyltransferase; *PG*, phosphatidylglycerol; *PGS*, phosphatidylglycerol phosphate synthase; *PSD*, PS decarboxylase; *PSS1/2*, PS synthases 1/2; *PTPIP51*, protein tyrosine phosphatase interacting protein 51; *TAMM41*, phosphatidate cytidylyl transferase mitochondrial; *TG*, triacylglycerol; *TSPO*, translocator protein; *VAPB*, vesicle-associated membrane protein-associated protein B; *VDAC*, voltage-dependent anion channel.

MAMs and ROS production

As previously referred, MAMs are responsible for Ca^{2+} transport from the ER, the major intracellular Ca^{2+} store, to mitochondria. Therefore, these structures play an essential role in the regulation of mitochondrial Ca^{2+} homeostasis and modulate many aspects of mitochondrial function, such as OXPHOS and ATP production, ROS generation and signaling, and activation of the mitochondrial apoptotic cell death pathway [8]. Ca^{2+} released from the ER through the IP3R is transported to the mitochondrial intermembrane space by the VDAC1 channel, then entering into mitochondrial matrix through the mitochondrial Ca^{2+} uniporter (MCU) [2,21]. Ca^{2+} flux to the mitochondrial matrix can be potentiated by ROS generated in the mitochondria via MCU oxidation that enhances its oligomerization and activity. MCU oxidation causes persistent mitochondrial Ca^{2+} uptake and disrupts mitochondrial bioenergetics, culminating in loss of function and viability [30]. Indeed, increased levels of mitochondrial Ca^{2+} stimulate the activity of the electron transport chain (ETC), which elevates ROS generation since mitochondria are forced to consume more O_2 in the process [31]. Mitochondria are considered major sources of ROS production since the ETC consumes about 85% of all O_2 used by the organism to produce ATP. However, a disruption in the ETC decreases ATP formation and increases ROS production, which affect the reduction-oxidation (redox) potential of the cell [32]. When excessive transfer of Ca^{2+} from the ER to mitochondria occurs, mitochondrial Ca^{2+} overload causes the swelling of the organelle, which can be accompanied by the rupture of mitochondrial membranes leading to the release of proapoptotic factors to the cytosol [33].

ROS are by-products of oxidative metabolism and are also generated as a result of environmental stresses, including exposure of cells to oxidants or ultraviolet light [8]. These are partially reduced O_2-containing molecules, that are free radicals and/or O_2 derivatives, such as superoxide anion ($O_2^{\bullet-}$), H_2O_2, lipid hydroperoxides (LOOH), hydroxyl ($OH^{\bullet}$), and peroxyl (ROO^{-}) radicals [34]. Moreover, ROS are involved in many redox-dependent processes, such as cell signaling, oxidative homeostasis, immune responses, energy metabolism, and tissue remodeling [35]. The deleterious effects of high levels of ROS include disruption of mitochondrial structure and function [36], which is involved in the progression of neurodegenerative diseases [34–36]. In fact, neurons are highly susceptible to oxidative stress due to their high dependence on OXPHOS to obtain energy, high Ca^{2+} trafficking, enrichment of neuronal membranes in PUFAs, presence of redox active transition metals, exposure to auto-oxidation of neurotransmitters, and modest antioxidant defenses [35].

High levels of ROS are able to induce ER stress and, under these conditions, ER–mitochondria contacts are increased and their protein composition change, which include an upregulation of stress response mediators (e.g., PERK) [8]. In unstressed cells, antiapoptotic proteins (e.g., BCL-2) bind and inhibit the IP3R, maintaining Ca^{2+} signaling between the ER and mitochondria at basal levels [37]. During prolonged ER stress, ER chaperones bind and stimulate IP3R increasing Ca^{2+} transfer between the ER and the mitochondria, which triggers Ca^{2+} overload and ROS production leading to apoptosis [8]. The mitochondrial respiration promotes the accumulation of H_2O_2 at IMM/mitochondrial cristae space and Ca^{2+} uptake induces compression of dilated cristae and stimulates the translocation of H_2O_2 to MAMs, contributing to the existence of redox nanodomains at the ER-mitochondria contacts. The MAMs' nanodomains of H_2O_2 regulate IP3R via the oxidation of specific thiol groups, which results in a positive redox feedback on IP3R activation that promotes Ca^{2+} efflux from the ER [38]. MAMs are also enriched in redox-active proteins that are regulated by ROS, including the oxidoreductases thioredoxin-related transmembrane protein 1 (TMX1), ERO1α, and SERCA [8]. ROS can reversibly modify proteins and change their function, particularly by altering the oxidation state of cysteine residues or causing the formation of thiol adducts [8,38].

The PERK protein promotes the transfer of Ca^{2+} and ROS signals between the ER and mitochondria, and it is essential for MAMs integrity. Thus, $PERK^{-/-}$ cells show alterations in the ER morphology and Ca^{2+} homeostasis and a decrease in the ER–mitochondria interaction. Under ROS-mediated ER stress, PERK deficiency reduces ROS transference between the ER and mitochondria and mitochondria-mediated apoptosis. Moreover, PERK deficiency appears to protect mitochondria from ROS damage. However, PERK re-expression in these cells restores ER–mitochondria contacts as well as the deleterious response of mitochondria to ROS originated in the ER. Thus, under pathological conditions characterized by ROS generation and ER stress induction, loss of PERK can act as a protective strategy that affect the transfer of ROS signals between the ER and mitochondria and consequently can induce apoptosis [10]. The ERO1α protein, located at MAMs, together with PDI, is responsible for disulfide bonds formation during protein folding, resulting in H_2O_2 production [7]. ERO1α oxidizes PDI, and, subsequently, PDI catalyzes the formation of disulfide bonds in newly synthesized proteins. In this process, ERO1α uses O_2, which is reduced to H_2O_2, as the electron acceptor during PDI oxidation [7]. The MAMs proteins ERO1α, PDI, and NADPH oxidase complexes (especially Nox4) are the major ROS producers during UPR induction [31].

The proapoptotic p66Shc is a ROS-generating protein present in MAMs, that under physiological conditions is involved in Ras-mediated signal transduction pathways [7,39]. However, under oxidative stress conditions, p66Shc can be phosphorylated at Ser36 residue by serine-threonine kinases, such as the protein kinase C β (PKCβ), c-Jun N-terminal kinase (JNK), or extracellular signal-regulated kinase (ERK), and induces apoptosis [7]. Phosphorylation of p66Shc initiates a cascade of events, namely: (1) isomerization of phosphorylated p66Sch (p-p66Sch) at Ser36 residue by the prolyl isomerase Pin1; (2) dephosphorylation of p-p66Sch at Ser36 residue by phosphatase A2 (PP2A); and (3) translocation of p66Sch to mitochondria, where it interacts with cytochrome *c* and, as a redox enzyme, transfers electrons from cytochrome *c* to O_2 generating H_2O_2 [7]. The reduction of O_2 by electrons derived from the respiratory chain can lead to the opening of the mitochondrial permeability transition pore (mPTP), which promotes caspases activation and apoptosis [40]. Moreover, p66Shc present at MAMs can interact with OMM proteins stimulating ROS production through the activation of membrane-bound NADPH-oxidases and down-regulation of antioxidant enzymes [39]. So, the MAMs-resident p66Sch can trigger apoptosis through the generation of mitochondrial H_2O_2 and the opening of the mPTP [41]. Levels of p66Sch at MAMs, as well as H_2O_2 production, increase in an age-dependent manner indicating that this protein contributes to mitochondrial oxidative stress during the aging process [42]. In mice, *p66shc* knockout decreases the levels of intracellular ROS and the oxidative damage of DNA and proteins [39,43], and upregulates antioxidant enzymes [44]. However, mouse embryonic fibroblasts (MEFs) that express p66Shc have increased mitochondrial OXPHOS and ROS production [45]. Moreover, p66Shc can interact directly with mitochondria, since cells with *p66shc* deletion are resistant to several inducers of mitochondria-mediated apoptosis [39].

Under physiological conditions, ROS accumulation and oxidative damage are prevented by the endogenous antioxidant system, which include enzymes [e.g., superoxide dismutase (SOD), catalase (CAT), glutathione peroxidase, and thioredoxin reductase] and nonenzymatic components, such as vitamins (e.g., vitamins A, C, and E, coenzyme Q10, and flavonoids), minerals (e.g., selenium and zinc), and metabolites (e.g., bilirubin and melatonin) [31]. However, under stressful conditions, ROS overproduction, and/or the imbalance between antioxidants and oxidants induce damage of cellular components [46]. Lipid membranes provide a physical barrier against ROS diffusion; however, they are the primary targets for oxidative damage [47]. ROS generation is very high in cellular and organelles membranes due to the low solubility of molecular O_2 and, consequently, the components of the membranes, particularly the lipid components, are especially susceptible to ROS attack, which is called "lipid peroxidation" [34]. This process consists in ROS-mediated oxidation of lipids that contain carbon-carbon double bound(s), such as polyunsaturated FA (PUFAs), glycolipids, phospholipids, and cholesterol [3,36,48]. Membrane phospholipids contain unsaturated FA residues being many of them PUFAs. The presence of a methylene group between two double bonds makes FAs sensitive to ROS oxidation, and the high concentration of PUFAs in phospholipids makes them targets for oxidizing agents [49].

Lipid peroxidation is initiated by $OH^{\cdot}$, $O_2^{\bullet -}$, ROO^-, nitric oxide (NO), peroxynitrite ($ONOO^-$), or nitrogen dioxide (NO_2) radicals and precedes via hydrogen abstraction (removal of an atom or group from a molecule by a radical) at the methylene group adjacent to the carbon–carbon double bond of PUFAs [3,34,48]. The generated lipid radicals initiate a self-perpetuating chain reaction that amplifies the initial oxidative event through the oxidation of other PUFAs in the proximity [3,48]. Moreover, PUFAs can themselves convert into reactive free radicals after reacting with free radicals and propagate the lipid peroxidation chain reaction [50]. Lipid peroxidation will continue until the (1) substrate is consumed, (2) radical-radical neutralization occurs, or (3) the interaction of the radical with chain-breaking antioxidants happens [34,48]. This biological process results in intermediate unstable oxidized lipid species and stable end products that act as bioactive lipid mediators [3]. Since lipid peroxides are more polar and highly unstable, they can react with neighboring FAs and trigger a chain reaction that propagates through the membrane unless stopped by free radical scavengers, such as antioxidants [51].

Lipid oxidation is responsible for the loss of the membrane permeability barrier function, phospholipid phase transitions and phase separation, cross-linking of phospholipid head groups, and augmented phospholipid flip-flop [52]. For example, ROS can lead to CL peroxidation activating intrinsic apoptosis [34]. The nonenzymatic oxidation of esterified PUFAs of PS, initiated by free radicals or nonradical ROS under pathological conditions, can lead to PS externalization in plasma membrane, which is essential for the engulfment of apoptotic cells and serves as an "eat-me" signal for phagocytes [46,53]. So, the oxidation of anionic phospholipid molecules is important for efficient apoptosis execution and removal of the apoptotic cells by phagocytes. However, under pathological conditions, elevated ROS levels oxidize high amounts of PS and the innate mechanisms cannot efficiently metabolize the oxidized PS preventing apoptosis of the affected cells [46]. For example, it is known that null mutations of ABHD12, a lipase capable of hydrolyzing oxidized PS, is associated with the neurodegenerative disease PHARC (polyneuropathy, hearing loss, ataxia, retinitis pigmentosa, and cataract) [46].

Phospholipids peroxidation and their products decrease the membrane fluidity, inactivate membrane-bound proteins and, subsequently, lead to membrane disruption. They also affect the interactions lipid–lipid and lipid–protein, which in turn affect cells function [3,46,54]. In fact, it was reported that lipid peroxidation disrupts the biophysical properties of membranes changing the lipid structure and organization [51]. Furthermore, the same authors observed that lipid peroxidation induces the formation of cholesterol domains and reduces the lipid bilayer width [51].

The disruption of the lipid composition, structure, and function of biological membranes caused by lipid peroxidation is intimately associated to aging and disease, namely, age-related neurodegenerative disorders [51]. Indeed, lipid peroxidation is a key marker of oxidative stress in the central nervous system (CNS) due to its high content of PUFAs and the high rate of O_2 utilization; these features making the CNS sensitive to ROS attack [54,55]. PUFAs like ARA and DHA are vulnerable to hydrogen removal and addition of O_2 producing the ROO^- radicals isoprostane and neuroprostane isomers, respectively [48]. These ROO^- radicals undergo numerous secondary reactions causing the production of lipid aldehydes, including malondialdehyde (MDA), 4-hydroxy-nonenal (HNE), 4-hydroxy-hexenal (HHE), 4-oxo-nonenal (ONE), methylglyoxal (MGO), and isolevuglandins (IsoLGs) [56]. The HNE is produced during lipid peroxidation of *n*-6 PUFAs, such as linoleic acid and ARA, while lipid peroxidation of *n*-3 PUFAs, including α-linolenic acid (ALA) and DHA, generates HHE [54]. Furthermore, lipid peroxidation of ARA and DHA is considered an early alteration in AD [48] (Fig. 7.2).

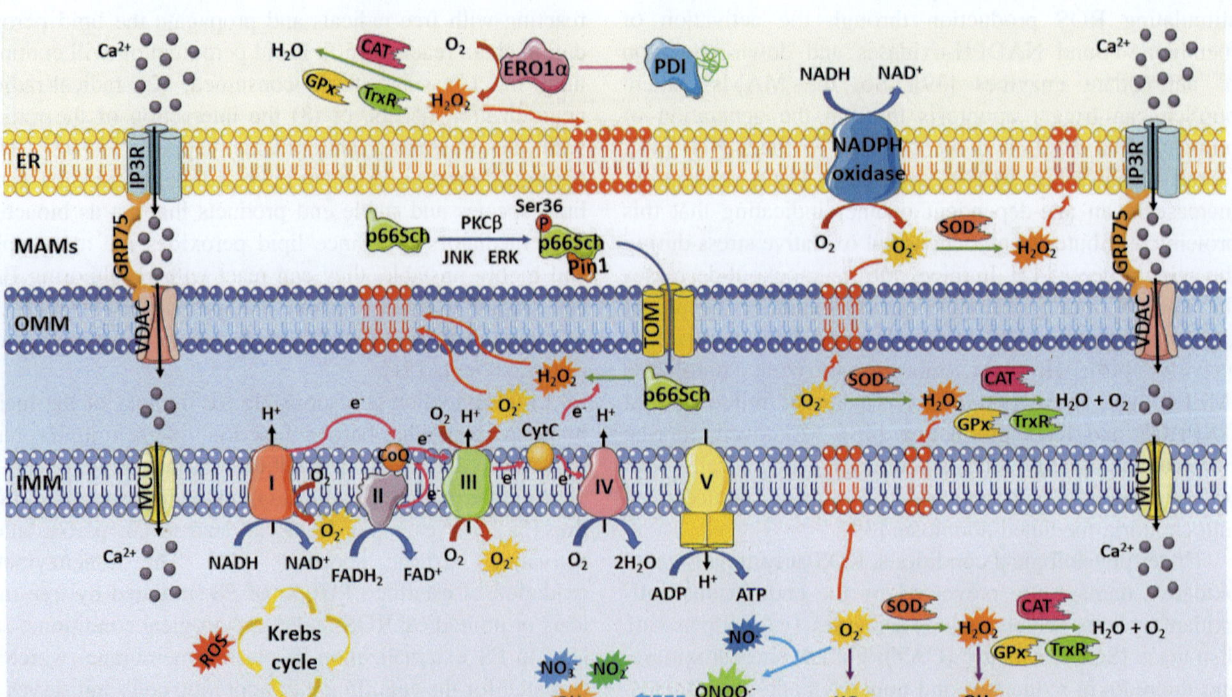

FIGURE 7.2 MAMs' involvement in ROS production. During protein folding, ERO1α reduces O_2 to H_2O_2 and oxidizes PDI that in turn catalyzes the formation of disulfide bonds in de novo synthesized proteins. The NADPH oxidase complexes are also ROS producers, since they catalyze the transfer of electrons from NADPH to O_2 through the Nox catalytic subunit. MAMs protein p66Shc can be phosphorylated at Ser36 by PKCβ, JNK or ERK, isomerated by Pin1, and translocated to the mitochondria through the TOM complex. In mitochondria, p66Sch interacts with cytC allowing the transfer of electrons from cytC to O_2 generating H_2O_2. The Ca^{2+} released from the ER through the IP3R is transported to the mitochondria by VDAC and MCU present in the OMM and IMM, respectively. The increase of mitochondrial Ca^{2+} levels stimulates the activity of the ETC and, consequently, increases ROS generation, specially $O_2^{\cdot-}$ production at the level of complexes I and III. Other free radicals, such as $OH^{\cdot}$, $HO_2^{\cdot}$, $NO^{\cdot}$, $ONOO^{\cdot-}$, $NO_2^{\cdot}$, and NO_3^- can be generated by $O_2^{\cdot-}$ and H_2O_2 reduction. The ROS produced through these cellular processes can attack lipids present in membranes and disrupt their biophysical properties. Under physiological conditions, antioxidant enzymes, including SOD, CAT, GPx, and TrxR, prevent ROS overproduction and subsequent damage. *CAT*, catalase; *CoQ*, coenzyme Q10; *CytC*, cytochrome C; *ER*, endoplasmic reticulum; *ERK*, extracellular signal-regulated kinase; *ERO1α*, endoplasmic reticulum oxidoreductase 1 alpha; *ETC*, electron transport chain; *GPx*, glutathione peroxidase; *GRP75*, glucose regulated protein 75; *H_2O_2*, hydrogen peroxide; *HO_2*, hydroperoxyl; *IMM*, inner mitochondrial membranes; *IP3R*, inositol 1,4,5 trisphosphate receptor; *JNK*, c-Jun N-terminal kinase; *MAMs*, mitochondria-associated membranes; *MCU*, mitochondrial calcium uniporter protein; *$NO^{\cdot}$*, nitric oxide; *$NO_2^{\cdot}$*, nitrogen dioxide; *NO_3^-*, nitrate; *O_2*, oxygen; *$O_2^{\cdot-}$*, superoxide; *$OH^{\cdot}$*, hydroxyl; *OMM*, outer mitochondrial membranes; *$ONOO^{\cdot-}$*, peroxynitrite; *PDI*, protein disulfide isomerase; *Pin1*, peptidyl-prolyl cis-trans isomerase NIMA-interacting 1; *PKCβ*, protein kinase C β; *ROS*, reactive oxygen species; *Ser36*, serine 36; *SOD*, superoxide dismutase; *TOM*, translocase of the outer membrane; *TrxR*, thioredoxin reductase; *VDAC*, voltage-dependent anion channel.

Alzheimer disease, oxidative stress, and MAMs

AD is the most common cause of dementia over the age of 65 years, affecting more than 44 million people worldwide, and it is characterized by progressive memory loss, cognitive dysfunction, and behavioral changes [36,55]. The incidence and prevalence of this neurodegenerative disease increase with age from 3% to 50% among individuals aged 65−74 and ≥85, respectively. It is expected that the number of people suffering from AD quadruple by 2050, once the worldwide population gets older and older [36]. There are two forms of AD, the sporadic AD (SAD) and the familial AD (FAD). SAD is usually diagnosed in people aged ≥65 and represents >95% of all AD cases. The main risk factor for SAD is aging, but there are other risk factors such as metabolic and cardiovascular diseases [57]. The main genetic risk factor for SAD is the presence of the allele ε4 of the apolipoprotein E (ApoE4) [58]. ApoE is a protein responsible for phospholipid and cholesterol transport [35]. FAD affects individuals aged <65 and represents <5% of all AD cases, and it is associated with mutations in the genes that encode the amyloid-β (Aβ) precursor protein (APP) or presenilins 1 or 2 (PS1 and PS2) [57,58]. APP is cleaved by α-secretase or β-secretase (also known as BACE; β-site amyloid precursor protein cleaving enzyme) to produce C-terminal fragments of 83 aa (C83) or 99 aa (C99) long, respectively. Then, C83 and C99 are cleaved by the catalytic subunits of the γ-secretase complex (PS1 and PS2) to produce p3 or Aβ, respectively, along with the APP intracellular domain (AICD) [59]. Neuropathologically, AD is characterized by the accumulation of Aβ peptide in senile plaques due to its overproduction or impaired clearance and by the deposition of neurofibrillary tangles, mainly formed by hyperphosphorylated tau protein, which are associated to synaptic loss and neuronal degeneration and death [55]. The APP, β-secretase, and γ-secretase are present in lipid rafts (membrane regions enriched in cholesterol and sphingolipids), including MAMs, and these regions serve as platforms for the interaction between Aβ and ApoE and promote the aggregation of Aβ oligomers and hyperphosphorylated tau [55,60]. MAMs lipid composition and their oxidation status modulate APP processing, since lipid rafts play an essential role in APP trafficking [61]. During aging, a gradual reduction in cholesterol and PUFAs in lipid rafts occurs, which is exacerbated in neurodegenerative diseases. In AD, the alteration in the composition of lipid rafts potentiates APP processing and Aβ generation and aggregation [35].

In the last years, the ER−mitochondria axis has emerged as a fundamental component of the physiopathology of several diseases [4]. Alterations in MAMs-associated functions have been implicated in AD, contributing to impaired lipid and glucose metabolism, aberrant Ca^{2+} homeostasis, ER stress, mitochondrial dysfunction, and oxidative stress, and have been reported to occur years before the appearance of the pathological hallmarks [62,63]. In 2012, Area-Gomez and colleagues showed that mutations in PS1/2 in MEFs cells affect MAMs function, and these alterations are also observed in fibroblasts from FAD patients with mutations in PS1, PS2, or APP, as well as in SAD patients with unknown genetic etiology [64]. Hedskog and colleagues observed by proximity ligation assay (PLA) a decrease in the distance between the ER-resident proteins IP3R and the mitochondrial VDAC and an increase in Ca^{2+} transfer from the ER to mitochondria in mouse primary cortical neurons and SH-SY5Y cells, respectively, incubated with conditioned medium derived from CHO cells overexpressing APP with the Indiana mutation (AAPPV717F) [65]. The increase in ER-mitochondria connectivity was also observed in SH-SY5Y cells overexpressing APP with the Swedish mutation (APPswe) [60]. A recent study from our laboratory showed that neuro-2a cells overexpressing APPswe present several changes in MAMs composition that are associated with mitochondrial dysfunction and energy deficits [66]. Furthermore, other authors reported an increase in ROS production in the same cell line [67], supporting the link between MAMs alterations and ROS accumulation in AD. Other studies support a link between impaired MAMs and generation of ROS in in vitro models of AD. Calvo-Rodrigues and colleagues observed an increase in ER-mitochondria contacts, Ca^{2+} transfer between these organelles, ROS production, and apoptosis in rat primary hippocampal neurons incubated with $A\beta_{42}$ [68]. It was also demonstrated in SH-SY5Y cells that Aβ induces mitochondrial Ca^{2+} uptake, causing an increase in ROS production, inhibition of ATP synthesis, mPTP opening, release of cytochrome *c*, activation of caspases, and apoptosis [69]. A mitochondrial Ca^{2+} overload after Aβ deposition was also observed in the APP/PS1 transgenic (Tg) mouse model of AD and the blockage of MCU with the inhibitor Ru360 prevented Ca^{2+} overload and, consequently, avoided mitochondrial dysfunction [69]. In immortalized hippocampal astrocytes from 3xTg-AD mice, it was observed an increase in mitochondria−ER interaction and ROS production, simultaneously with Ca^{2+} homeostasis deregulation [70]. A recent study in a *Drosophila* model of AD shows that an increased physical coupling between the ER and mitochondria enhances mitochondrial Ca^{2+} levels and ROS production [71]. So, Ca^{2+} transfer and ROS accumulation at MAMs could maintain a vicious cycle contributing to neurodegeneration by amplifying oxidative stress [72].

During the aging process, mitochondrial dysfunction causes a redox imbalance due to an increased production of ROS and loss of cellular antioxidant defenses predisposing to cell death [41]. Markers of oxidative stress and damage and of mitochondrial dysfunction have also been observed in *postmortem* brain and blood, urine, and cerebrospinal fluid samples from AD patients [36].

The brain is a lipid-rich organ and cerebral lipids account for, at least, 50% of brain dry weight and represent the basic structural component of neuronal cells membranes [55]. The brain contains sphingolipids, glycerophospholipids, cholesterol, and FAs. The most prominent long-chain PUFAs in the brain are the DHA and eicosapentaenoic acid (EPA) derived from ALA, an *n*-3 FA, and ARA and docosatetraenoic acid (DPA) derived from linolenic acid (LNA), an *n*-6 FA [35,55]. During the aging process, a decrease in *n*-3 FAs, which have antioxidant properties, and an increase in lipid peroxidation were observed [35]. Along with the formation of Aβ plaques and neurofibrillary tangles, an increase in lipid peroxidation markers has been also observed in the AD brain [56]. In hippocampal samples from AD human *postmortem* brain, increased levels of the lipid peroxidation product IsoLG-Lys were observed in correlation with the severity of the disease [73]. Transgenic mice overexpressing the APPswe mutation or presenting the deletion of exon 9 of the PS1 (APP-PS1) show an increase of the reactive lipid aldehyde IsoLG-Lys in the posterior cortex at 4 months of age that correlates with Aβ deposition and memory impairment [74]. An increase in IsoLG-Lys adducts was also observed in transgenic mice expressing the human ApoE4, which is associated with the loss of spatial working memory in mice older than 12 months. In these mice, long-term treatment with 2-hydroxybenzylamine (2-HOBA), that block the formation of IsoLG protein adducts, avoided the loss of working memory [75].

Altered mechanisms of cell death control, metabolism, and redox homeostasis have been associated to mitochondrial dysfunction during the physiological process of aging [32]. The DNA damage caused by lipid peroxidation products can increase the number of mitochondrial mutations altering the function of these organelles, which exacerbate ROS production and oxidative damage in a vicious cycle. This situation has been described in several neurodegenerative disorders [76]. Mitochondrial dysfunction underlies brain energy deficits and failure to adapt to stress in AD. The decrease in glucose metabolism associated to inhibition of mitochondrial ETC and oxidative stress appear decades before the pathological hallmarks and symptoms of the disease [77].

Due to their important role in brain aging and neurodegenerative diseases, dysfunctional mitochondria and lipid dysmetabolism are emerging therapeutic targets to alleviate their negative impact in the brain [3]. So, strategies or therapies aimed to stop or delay aging and age-related diseases may include the use of drugs that prevent mitochondrial uncoupling, inhibit inflammatory lipid synthesis, modulate lipid transport or storage, and decrease mitochondrial oxidative stress [3], which are features related with the activity of MAMs (Fig. 7.3).

MAMs as therapeutic target in AD

Mitochondrial dysfunction contributes to oxidative damage, including lipid peroxidation and impaired lipid biosynthesis, among others, which accelerate aging and the development of age-related diseases. Numerous studies suggest that alterations in MAMs occur upstream of mitochondrial dysfunction, ROS generation, and oxidative damage [78]. Therefore, therapies capable of stabilizing and restoring mitochondrial function can be beneficial for reducing the age-related decline [78]. Accordingly, agents that improve mitochondrial bioenergetics and glucose metabolism and decrease oxidative stress/damage are potential therapeutic approaches [3]. More importantly, therapies focusing the composition and function of MAMs could be very relevant to fight brain aging and neurodegeneration.

AD patients present a decrease of carotenoids concentrations, including lutein, lycopene, and zeaxanthin, in blood serum with a consequent increase of lipid peroxidation products. The enzymes responsible for carotenoids metabolization are present in the mitochondrial membranes and chronic lycopene administration reestablishes the activity of mitochondrial ETC in $A\beta_{1-42}$-treated rats [79]. $A\beta_{1-42}$-treated animals show poor memory retention and increased oxidative stress, mitochondrial damage, and an increase in interleukin (IL)-6, tumor necrosis factor (TNF)-α, and caspase-3 activity. However, lycopene improves memory retention, decreases mitochondrial oxidative damage and neuro-inflammation, and restores brain-derived neurotrophic factor (BDNF) levels [80].

Enzymatic antioxidants have a protective effect against oxidative attack by decomposing ROS. For example, SOD catalyzes the conversion of $O_2^{\bullet-}$ into O_2 and H_2O_2 and CAT decomposes H_2O_2 into molecular O_2 and H_2O [81]. Vitamin A, that results from the breakdown of β-carotene, can interact with ROO^- radicals forming free carbon-centered radical adducts and scavenge ROO^- radicals by electron transfer before they interact with lipids [34]. Coenzyme Q10, essential for electron transport in the mitochondrial respiratory chain, prevents oxidative damage by lipid ROO^- radicals and improves mitochondrial biogenesis [82]. Furthermore, vitamin C (ascorbic acid) can scavenge O_2 free radicals and vitamin E (α-tocopherol) protects membrane PUFAs from oxidation [34]. It was previously shown that neurons treated with α-tocopherol before the exposure to Aβ show decreased HNE adducts and ceramides levels when compared with untreated neurons [83]. Flavonoids present in beverages, vegetables, and fruits also have antioxidant activity by inhibiting enzymes, such as NADPH oxidases, involved in $O_2^{\bullet-}$ production [84]. Selenium and zinc also have

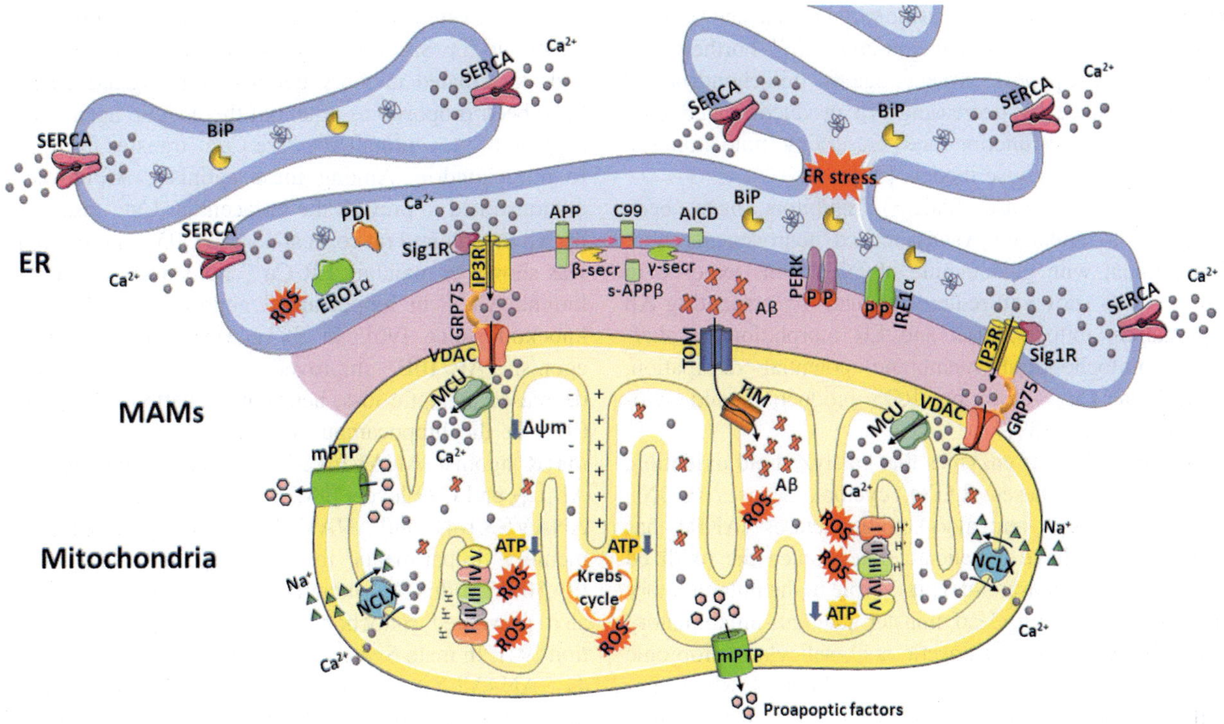

FIGURE 7.3 MAMs and Alzheimer disease. MAMs serve as platforms for APP processing and Aβ formation. In Alzheimer disease, APP is cleaved by β-secretase to produce C99 and s-APPβ, then C99 is cleaved by γ-secretase to produce Aβ and AICD. The Aβ accumulated at MAMs can be transported to mitochondria through the TOM/TIM complex. Alterations at MAMs and Aβ accumulation induce mitochondrial Ca^{2+} uptake via IP3R-GRP75-VDAC-MCU causing an increase in ROS production, a decrease of ATP synthesis through the ETC, mitochondrial membrane depolarization, mPTP opening, and release of proapoptotic factors. The accumulation of misfolded proteins in the lumen of ER results in ER stress, which induces BiP dissociation from the PERK and IRE1α proteins located at MAMs to bind unfolded proteins. This leads to spontaneous dimerization of PERK and IRE1α and activation of UPR. The accumulation of unfolded proteins also activates ERO1α and PDI and increases ROS generation. *Δψm*, mitochondrial membrane potential; *β-secr*, β-secretase; *γ-secr*, γ-secretase; *Aβ*, amyloid-β; *AICD*, APP intracellular domain; *APP*, Aβ protein precursor; *BiP*, binding immunoglobulin protein; *C99*, C-terminal fragments of 99 aa long; *ER*, endoplasmic reticulum; *ERO1α*, endoplasmic reticulum oxidoreductase 1 alpha; *ETC*, electron transport chain; *GRP75*, glucose regulated protein 75; *IP3R*, inositol 1,4,5 trisphosphate receptor; *IRE1α*, inositol-requiring enzyme 1 alpha; *MAMs*, mitochondria-associated membranes; *MCU*, mitochondrial calcium uniporter protein; *mPTP*, mitochondrial permeability transition pore; *NCLX*, mitochondrial sodium/calcium exchanger protein; *PDI*, protein disulphide isomerase; *PERK*, PKR-like endoplasmic reticulum kinase; *ROS*, reactive oxygen species; *s-APPβ*, soluble APPβ; *SERCA*, sarco/endoplasmic reticulum Ca^{2+} ATPase; *Sig1R*, sigma 1 receptor; *TIM*, translocase of the inner membrane; *TOM*, translocase of the outer membrane; *UPR*, unfolded protein response; *VDAC*, voltage-dependent anion channel.

antioxidant activity due their role in the maintenance of many antioxidant enzymes [85]. Besides, antioxidants like vitamins E and C and β-carotene decrease free radicals-mediated damage caused by toxic chain reactions in neuronal cells and can help prevent AD in humans and mouse models [31]. In cultured rat cortical neurons, lycopene provides protection against $Aβ_{25-35}$ neurotoxicity by inhibiting mitochondrial membrane depolarization and ROS overproduction and by decreasing apoptosis [86]. Although the natural antioxidants show some therapeutic potential in in vitro and animal models, very few antioxidants present effective results in clinical trials, and some therapeutic approaches involving natural antioxidants have been disappointing about their neuroprotective efficacy [36,41]. There are several reasons for this failure such as the stage of the disease when the therapy is initiated, since therapies should begin as early as possible, and the concentration of the compounds that reach the target tissue/cells/organelles, which may be insufficient to exert beneficial effects.

Suppressing lipid peroxidation using robust antioxidants is one potential strategy to stop the formation of lipid oxidant products, such as IsoLGs. However, chemical antioxidants do not only suppress lipid peroxidation but also affect the levels of ROS like H_2O_2 that are essential secondary messengers that control key cellular processes, creating adverse effects that counterbalance the beneficial ones [56]. The use of small molecules to scavenge and sequester IsoLGs could protect proteins and PE from oxidative modifications without inhibiting critical cell signaling events; however, these molecules need to have a good bioavailability [56]. The synthetic antioxidant peptide SS31 can bind and protect CL from oxidation, which improves mitochondrial function in aged muscle and maintains the structure of mitochondrial cristae and protects neurons from hypoxia reperfusion injury [87]. Furthermore, this antioxidant peptide protects against mitochondria and synaptic damage by decreasing Aβ production, reducing mitochondrial dysfunction and preserving mitochondrial dynamics in AD mouse models [88].

Acetylcholinesterase (AChE) inhibitors have been suggested to attenuate AD-associated neurodegeneration. Pretreatment with galantamine of PC12 cells exposed to $A\beta_{25-35}$ was shown to reduce apoptosis by preventing Aβ aggregation, mitochondrial and ER morphological alterations, mitochondrial membrane potential dissipation, intracellular Ca^{2+} elevation, ROS production, and cytochrome *c* release [89].

The inhibition of enzymes that catalyze lipid oxidation, such as lipoxygenases (LOX), cyclooxygenases (COX), cytochrome P450, and aldo-keto reductases (AKR), has been found to have beneficial effects since the oxidized ARA products (eicosanoids) play a role in the inflammatory process during aging. Also, nonsteroidal anti-inflammatory drugs (NSAIDs), such as acetic acid, salicylate, propionic acid, fenamate, oxicam, and COX-2 inhibitors, which present analgesic, antipyretic, and anti-inflammatory properties, were shown to promote benefits in neurodegenerative disorders [90]. These findings suggest that inhibition of the lipid peroxidation-inflammation axis is a potential therapeutic strategy.

The increase in ER–mitochondria contacts after Aβ exposure augments Ca^{2+} transfer between both organelles [65]. So, the regulation of Ca^{2+} flux from ER to mitochondria is considered a promising strategy to avoid the accumulation of mitochondrial ROS in AD. Lee et al. showed that urolithin A (produced by the gut microbiome) alleviates high glucose-induced mitochondrial ROS accumulation through the reduction of mitochondrial Ca^{2+} influx and decreases the expression of enzymes involved in Aβ production in neuronal cells. Urolithin A was also found to modulate MAMs formation due to downregulation of transglutaminase type 2 (TGM2) in diabetes-associated AD pathogenesis. Furthermore, *TGM2* silencing inhibits the interaction between the IP3R and the VDAC and, consequently, prevents Ca^{2+} influx and accumulation of ROS by mitochondria triggered by high glucose [91]. Thus, urolithin A, which targets MAMs, has been considered a novel promising antioxidant and neuroprotective compound [92].

Another therapeutic target that should be considered in AD is Sigma1R that regulates Ca^{2+} flux between the ER and mitochondria by the interaction with the IP3R [9]. Sigma1R activation has been related with several cellular processes, such as Ca^{2+} homeostasis, ER stress, excitotoxity, mitochondrial dysfunction, ROS scavenging, and structural and functional stability of MAMs [93]. In *post-mortem* brain tissue from AD patients low levels of Sigma1R were found [65], and a mouse model of AD knockout for Sigma1R shows increased oxidative stress and exacerbated memory deficits [94]. Sigma1R agonists have been proposed as potential therapeutic agents for AD capable of preventing excessive Ca^{2+} transfer from the ER to mitochondria. Among these agonists, Afobazole was demonstrated to prevent the intracellular Ca^{2+} rise induced by Aβ on cultured rat cortical neurons [95], and pridopidine was shown to maintain ER Ca^{2+} homeostasis by reducing luminal Ca^{2+} in hippocampal neurons from PS double-knockout mice [96]. In 3xTg-AD mice, the Sigma1R agonist AF710B improved cognitive function and decreased synaptic loss, neuroinflammation and Aβ levels [97]. In the hippocampus of Aβ-injected mice, the Sigma1R agonist ANAVEX2-73 prevented the increase of $A\beta_{1-42}$ and C99 levels [98]. Similarly, PRE-084, SA4503, ANAVEX1-41, and ANAVEX2-73 prevented learning and memory impairments in mice injected with $A\beta_{25-35}$ [99,100]. In this AD model, PRE-084 and ANAVEX2-73 also prevented mitochondrial respiratory chain dysfunction [94]. In male Swiss OF-1 mice PRE-084, ANAVEX1-41, ANAVEX3-71, and DHEA promoted a moderate increase in mitochondrial ROS levels under physiological conditions, which could represent an increase in ROS-mediated signaling; however, under AD mimicking conditions ($A\beta_{1-42}$ exposure), the compounds reduced mitochondrial ROS levels [101].

In the last years, the MAMs protein p66Sch has also been appointed as a possible therapeutic target for AD treatment due to its role in ROS generation. Lone et al. showed that neuronal cells (HT-22 and B12 immortalized cell lines and primary cortical neurons from C57/BL6 mice embryos) expressing activated p66Sch are more sensitive to Aβ-induced toxicity (98). However, the silencing of p66Shc in HT-22 and B12 cells changes their metabolic state from OXPHOS toward aerobic glycolysis decreasing ROS levels and promoting stress resistance against Aβ [102]. In SK-N-SH neuroblastoma cells treated during 30 min with acrolein, the most reactive aldehyde product resulting from lipid peroxidation, an activation of p66Shc and increased oxidative stress were observed [103]. Another study performed in SH-SY5Y cells under oxidative stress caused by the exposure to anisomycin showed an increase in $A\beta_{1-42}$ secretion and upregulation of p66Sch expression levels [104]. However, the treatment with the antioxidant gallic acid decreased p66Shc expression, and subsequently reduced the deposition of Aβ, enhanced SOD activity, and increased the release of acetylcholine [104]. Another in vitro study showed that p66Sch induces ROS production and that vitamin C is capable to downregulate p66Sch through the increase of its ubiquitination, which reduces ROS levels [105]. In vivo studies demonstrated that the ablation of p66Sch in APP-PS1 Tg mice improved brain mitochondrial respiration, restored mitochondrial complex I activity and ATP production, and reduced ROS levels [106]. MEFs cells derived from p66Shc$^{-/-}$ embryos presented low levels of intracellular ROS and a decrease of oxidative stress markers (8-oxo-guanosine, isoprostane, and nitrotyrosine) [40]. Furthermore, in an in vivo model of intestinal ischemia/reperfusion injury, an up-regulation of p66Sch was observed resulting in mitochondrial ROS accumulation and, consequently, enhanced epithelial apoptosis. However, the inhibition of Pin1, which is responsible for p66Sch translocation to mitochondria, with the juglone compound, caused a reduced translocation of p66Sch to mitochondria and a decrease in ROS production and apoptosis [107]. These results show that p66Sch or Pin1 represent possible therapeutic targets to fight oxidative stress and damage in aging or pathological conditions (Fig. 7.4).

Concluding remarks

MAMs, or MERCS, provide an important platform for several signaling pathways to carry out many cellular processes that are important for neuronal function, such as regulation of Ca^{2+} homeostasis, phospholipid synthesis and exchange, mitochondrial biogenesis and dynamics, stress response, autophagy, and apoptosis. Due to key role of MAMs in mitochondria–ER interaction, alterations in this region have been implicated in the physiopathology of AD. During AD asymptomatic stages, changes at MAMs may represent a compensatory response, while chronic MAMs alterations occurring during the progression of AD, contribute to deregulate Ca^{2+} and redox homeostasis, as well as to impair proteostasis triggering apoptotic cell death pathways. Moreover, mitochondrial dysfunction caused by

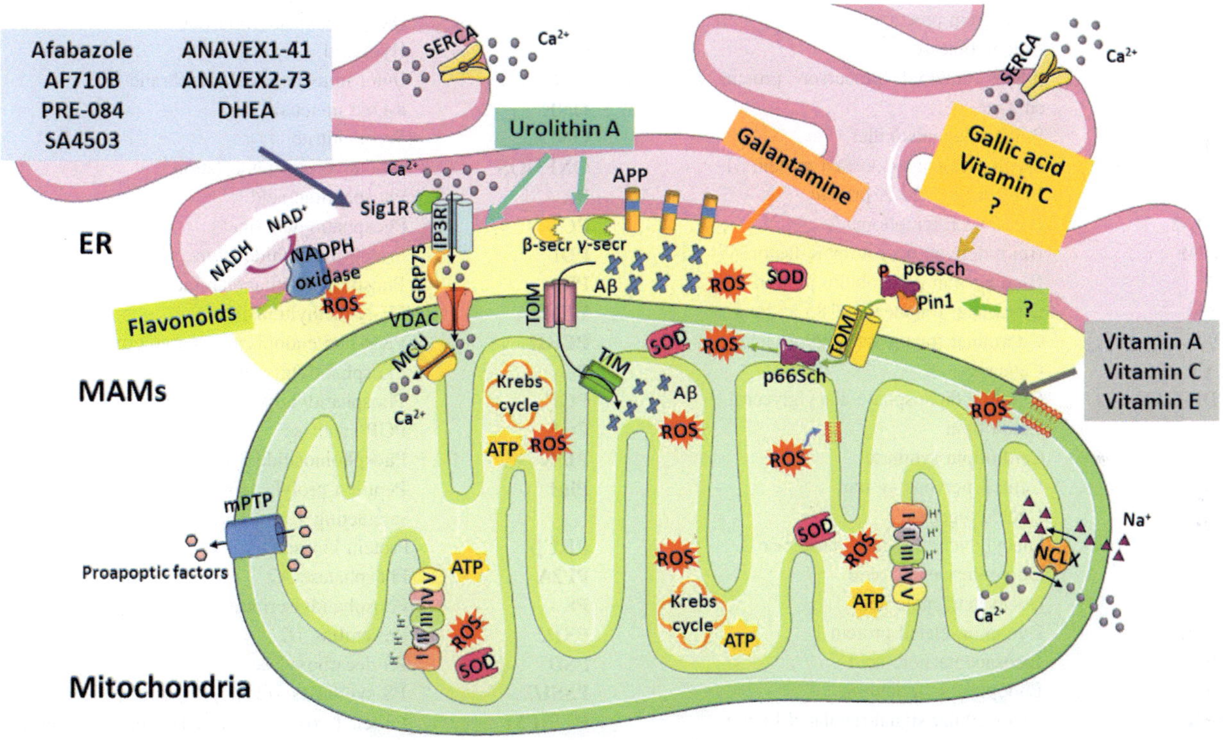

FIGURE 7.4 Targets at MAMs to decrease ROS production in Alzheimer disease. Alterations in MAMs occur before oxidative damage and mitochondrial dysfunction, so strategies focusing on the composition and function of MAMs and capable of decreasing oxidative damage are potential therapeutic agents in Alzheimer disease. Galantamine prevents Aβ aggregation and urolithin A modulates MAMs formation, reduces the mitochondrial Ca^{2+} influx, decreases the expression of enzymes involved in Aβ production, and consequently reduces ROS generation. The MAMs protein Sig1R interacts with the IP3R and regulates Ca^{2+} flux between the ER and the mitochondria. Sig1R agonists, such as afobazole, AF710B, PRE-084, SA4503, ANAVEX1-41, ANAVEX2-73, and DHEA, avoid excessive Ca^{2+} transfer from the ER to the mitochondria and decrease Aβ-induced mitochondrial ROS production. Another possible therapeutic target for AD treatment is the MAMs' protein p66Shc due its role in ROS generation. Inhibition or down-regulation of p66Shc expression levels with gallic acid or vitamin C reduce the deposition of Aβ, increase SOD activity, and reduce ROS levels. Pin1 can be another target to fight oxidative stress, since it is responsible for p66Sch translocation to mitochondria. Enzymatic antioxidants, such as SOD, also have a protective effect against oxidative damage by decomposing ROS. Nonenzymatic antioxidants, including vitamin A, C, and E can neutralize ROS and protect membranes from lipid peroxidation, and flavonoids can inhibit enzymes that are responsible for ROS production, such as the NADPH oxidases. *β-secr*, β-secretase; *γ-secr*, γ-secretase; *Aβ*, amyloid-β; *APP*, Aβ protein precursor; *ER*, endoplasmic reticulum; *GRP75*, glucose regulated protein 75; *IP3R*, inositol 1,4,5 trisphosphate receptor; *MAMs*, mitochondria-associated membranes; *MCU*, mitochondrial calcium uniporter protein; *mPTP*, mitochondrial permeability transition pore; *NCLX*, mitochondrial sodium/calcium exchanger protein; *Pin1*, peptidyl-prolyl cis-trans isomerase NIMA-interacting 1; *ROS*, reactive oxygen species; *SERCA*, sarco/end plasmatic reticulum Ca^{2+} ATPase; *Sig1R*, sigma 1 receptor; *SOD*, superoxide dismutase; *TIM*, translocase of the inner membrane; *TOM*, translocase of the outer membrane; *VDAC*, voltage-dependent anion channel.

changes in MAMs functions contributes to oxidative damage, including lipid peroxidation and impaired lipid biosynthesis. In this line, drugs capable of modulating MAMs components and, consequently, of controlling Ca^{2+} and lipids flux from ER to mitochondria, oxidative and ER stress responses, and ROS generation can provide preventive and therapeutic benefits.

Abbreviations

Aβ	Amyloid-β
ACAT1/SOAT1	Acyl-CoA, cholesterol acyltransferase/sterol O-acyltransferase 1
ACS	Caspase-recruitment domain
AD	Alzheimer disease
AICD	APP intracellular domain
AKR	Aldo-keto reductases
ALA	α-Linolenic acid
ApoE	Apolipoprotein E
APP	Aβ protein precursor
ARA	Arachidonic acid
BACE	β-Site amyloid precursor protein cleaving enzyme
BAK	Bcl-2 antagonist/killer
BAP31	B-cell receptor-associated protein 31
BAX	Bcl-2 associated X protein
BCL-2	B-cell CLL/lymphoma 2
BDNF	Brain-derived neurotrophic factor
BiP	Binding immunoglobulin protein
C83	C-terminal fragments of 83 aa long
C99	C-terminal fragments of 99 aa long
CAT	Catalase
CDP-DAG	Cytidine diphosphate-diacylglycerol
CL	Cardiolipin
CLS	Cardiolipin synthase
CNS	Central nervous system
COX	Cyclooxygenase
DGAT2	Diacylglycerol O-acyltransferase 2
DHA	Docosahexaenoic acid
DPA	Docosatetraenoic acid
DRP1	Dynamin-related protein 1
EPA	Eicosapentaenoic acid
ER	Endoplasmic reticulum
ERK	Extracellular signal-regulated kinase
ERO1α	Endoplasmic reticulum oxidoreductase 1 alpha
ETC	Electron transport chain
FA	Fatty acid
FACL4/ACSL4	Fatty acid CoA ligase 4
FAD	Familial AD
FIS1	Mitochondrial fission 1
GRP75	Glucose regulated protein 75
H_2O_2	Hydrogen peroxide
HHE	4-Hydroxy-hexenal
HNE	4-Hydroxy-nonenal
IL-6	Interleukin 6
IMM	Inner mitochondrial membrane
IP3R	Inositol 1,4,5 trisphosphate receptor
IRE1α	Inositol-requiring enzyme 1 alpha
IsoLGs	Isolevuglandins
JNK	c-Jun N-terminal kinase
LNA	Linolenic acid
LOOH	Lipid hydroperoxides
LOX	Lipoxygenases
MAMs	Mitochondria-associated membranes
MCU	Mitochondrial calcium uniporter protein
MDA	Malondialdehyde
MEFs	Mouse embryonic fibroblasts
MERCs	Mitochondria-ER contacts
MFN1/2	Mitofusin 1/2
MGO	Methylglyoxal
mPTP	Mitochondrial permeability transition pore
NLRP3	NOD-like receptor protein 3
NO	Nitric oxide
NO_2	Nitrogen dioxide
NSAIDs	Nonsteroidal anti-inflammatory drugs
O_2	Oxygen
O_2	Superoxide
OCR	Oxygen consumption rate
OH	Hydroxyl
OMM	Outer mitochondrial membrane
ONE	4-Oxo-nonenal
ONOO	Peroxynitrite
OXPHOS	Oxidative phosphorylation
PA	Phosphatidic acid
PC	Phosphatidylcholine
PDI	Protein disulphide isomerase
PE	Phosphatidylethanolamine
PEMT	PE N-methyltransferase
PERK	PKR-like endoplasmic reticulum kinase
PG	Phosphatidylglycerol
PGP	Phosphatidylglycerol phosphate
PGS	PGP synthase
PI3K	Phosphoinositide 3-kinase
Pin1	Peptidyl-prolyl cis-trans isomerase NIMA-interacting 1
PKCβ	Protein kinase C β
PP2A	Phosphatase A2
PS	Phosphatidylserine
PS1/2	Presenilins 1/2
PSD	PS decarboxylase
PSS1/2	PS synthases 1/2
PTPIP51	Protein tyrosine phosphatase interacting protein 51
PTPMT1	Protein tyrosine phosphatase mitochondrial 1
PUFAs	Polyunsaturated FA
ROO	Peroxyl
ROS	Reactive oxygen species
RyR	Ryanodine receptor
SAD	Sporadic AD
SERCA	Sarco/endoplasmic reticulum Ca^{2+} ATPase
Sigma1R	Sigma 1 receptor
SOD	Superoxide dismutase
STARD1	Steroidogenic acute regulatory lipid transfer domain
TAMM41	Phosphatidate cytidylyl transferase mitochondrial

TG	Triacylglycerol
Tg	Transgenic
TGM2	Transglutaminase type 2
TMX1	Thioredoxin-related transmembrane protein 1
TNFα	Tumor necrosis factor-α
TSPO	Translocator protein
UPR	Unfolded protein response
VAPB	Vesicle-associated membrane protein-associated protein B
VDAC	Voltage-dependent anion channel

Acknowledgments

We apologize to researchers in the field whose work could not be cited to space constraints. This work was funded by the European Regional Development Fund (ERDF), through the Centro 2020 Regional Operational Program: project CENTRO-01-0145-FEDER-000012-HealthyAging2020, the COMPETE 2020—Operational Program for Competitiveness and Internationalization, and the Portuguese national funds via FCT—Fundação para a Ciência e a Tecnologia, I.P.: projects POCI-01-0145-FEDER-028214/PTDC/MED-NEU/28214/2017 and POCI-01-0145-FEDER-029369/PTDC/MED-FAR/29369/2017 and UIDB/04539/2020 and UIDP/04539/2020 and EXPL/MED-FSL/0033/2021. Tânia Fernandes is recipient of Ph.D. fellow from the FCT (SFRH/BD/148801/2019).

References

[1] Simmen T, Herrera-Cruz MS. Plastic mitochondria-endoplasmic reticulum (ER) contacts use chaperones and tethers to mould their structure and signaling. Curr Opin Cell Biol 2018;53:61–9. https://doi.org/10.1016/j.ceb.2018.04.014.

[2] Gordaliza-Alaguero I, Cantó C, Zorzano A. Metabolic implications of organelle–mitochondria communication. EMBO Rep 2019;20:1–27. https://doi.org/10.15252/embr.201947928.

[3] Ademowo OS, Dias HKI, Burton DGA, Griffiths HR. Lipid (per) oxidation in mitochondria: an emerging target in the ageing process? Biogerontology 2017;18:859–79. https://doi.org/10.1007/s10522-017-9710-z.

[4] Area-Gomez E, Schon EA. On the pathogenesis of Alzheimer's disease: the MAM hypothesis. FASEB J 2017;31:864–7. https://doi.org/10.1096/fj.201601309.

[5] Ruby JR, Dyer RF, Skalko RG. Continuities between mitochondria and endoplasmic reticulum in the mammalian ovary. Z Zellforsch Mikrosk Anat 1969;97:30–7. https://doi.org/10.1007/BF00331868.

[6] Vance JE. Phospholipid synthesis in a membrane fraction associated with mitochondria. J Biol Chem 1990;265:7248–56. https://doi.org/10.1016/S0021-9258(19)39106-9.

[7] Giorgi C, Missiroli S, Patergnani S, Duszynski J, Wieckowski MR, Pinton P. Mitochondria-associated membranes: composition, molecular mechanisms, and physiopathological implications. Antioxid Redox Signal 2015;22:995–1019. https://doi.org/10.1089/ars.2014.6223.

[8] Prinz WA, Toulmay A, Balla T. The functional universe of membrane contact sites. Nat Rev Mol Cell Biol 2020;21:7–24. https://doi.org/10.1038/s41580-019-0180-9.

[9] Hayashi T, Su TP. Sigma-1 receptor chaperones at the ER-mitochondrion interface regulate Ca^{2+} signaling and cell survival. Cell 2007;131:596–610. https://doi.org/10.1016/j.cell.2007.08.036.

[10] Verfaillie T, Rubio N, Garg AD, Bultynck G, Rizzuto R, Decuypere J-P, et al. PERK is required at the ER-mitochondrial contact sites to convey apoptosis after ROS-based ER stress. Cell Death Differ 2012;19:1880–91. https://doi.org/10.1038/cdd.2012.74.

[11] Hamasaki M, Furuta N, Matsuda A, Nezu A, Yamamoto A, Fujita N, et al. Autophagosomes form at ER–mitochondria contact sites. Nature 2013;495:389–93. https://doi.org/10.1038/nature11910.

[12] Sevier CS, Kaiser CA. Ero1 and redox homeostasis in the endoplasmic reticulum. Biochim Biophys Acta Mol Cell Res 2008;1783:549–56. https://doi.org/10.1016/j.bbamcr.2007.12.011.

[13] Xu L, Wang X, Tong C. Endoplasmic reticulum–mitochondria contact sites and neurodegeneration. Front Cell Dev Biol 2020;8. https://doi.org/10.3389/fcell.2020.00428.

[14] Prasad M, Kaur J, Pawlak KJ, Bose M, Whittal RM, Bose HS. Mitochondria-associated endoplasmic reticulum membrane (MAM) regulates steroidogenic sctivity via steroidogenic acute regulatory protein (StAR)-voltage-dependent anion channel 2 (VDAC2) interaction. J Biol Chem 2015;290:2604–16. https://doi.org/10.1074/jbc.M114.605808.

[15] Rone MB, Midzak AS, Issop L, Rammouz G, Jagannathan S, Fan J, et al. Identification of a dynamic mitochondrial protein complex driving cholesterol import, trafficking, and metabolism to steroid hormones. Mol Endocrinol 2012;26:1868–82. https://doi.org/10.1210/me.2012-1159.

[16] Harris CA, Haas JT, Streeper RS, Stone SJ, Kumari M, Yang K, et al. DGAT enzymes are required for triacylglycerol synthesis and lipid droplets in adipocytes. J Lipid Res 2011;52:657–67. https://doi.org/10.1194/jlr.M013003.

[17] Cui Z, Vance JE, Chen MH, Voelker DR, Vance DE. Cloning and expression of a novel phosphatidylethanolamine N-methyltransferase. A specific biochemical and cytological marker for a unique membrane fraction in rat liver. J Biol Chem 1993;268:16655–63. https://doi.org/10.1016/S0021-9258(19)85468-6.

[18] Stone SJ, Vance JE. Phosphatidylserine synthase-1 and -2 are localized to mitochondria-associated membranes. J Biol Chem 2000;275:34534–40. https://doi.org/10.1074/jbc.M002865200.

[19] Kuwata H, Hara S. Role of acyl-CoA synthetase ACSL4 in arachidonic acid metabolism. Prostaglandins Other Lipid Mediat 2019;144:106363. https://doi.org/10.1016/j.prostaglandins.2019.106363.

[20] Xu J, Huang X. Lipid metabolism at membrane contacts: dynamics and functions beyond lipid homeostasis. Front Cell Dev Biol 2020;8:1–14. https://doi.org/10.3389/fcell.2020.615856.

[21] Muallem S, Chung WY, Jha A, Ahuja M. Lipids at membrane contact sites: cell signaling and ion transport. EMBO Rep 2017;18:1893–904. https://doi.org/10.15252/embr.201744331.

[22] Tasseva G, Bai HD, Davidescu M, Haromy A, Michelakis E, Vance JE. Phosphatidylethanolamine deficiency in mammalian mitochondria impairs oxidative phosphorylation and alters mitochondrial morphology. J Biol Chem 2013;288:4158–73. https://doi.org/10.1074/jbc.M112.434183.

[23] Kojima R, Endo T, Tamura Y. A phospholipid transfer function of ER-mitochondria encounter structure revealed in vitro. Sci Rep 2016;6:30777. https://doi.org/10.1038/srep30777.

[24] Blunsom NJ, Cockcroft S. CDP-diacylglycerol synthases (CDS): gateway to phosphatidylinositol and cardiolipin synthesis. Front Cell Dev Biol 2020;8:63. https://doi.org/10.3389/fcell.2020.00063.

[25] Lee H-J, Mayette J, Rapoport SI, Bazinet RP. Selective remodeling of cardiolipin fatty acids in the aged rat heart. Lipids Health Dis 2006;5:2. https://doi.org/10.1186/1476-511X-5-2.

[26] Hayashi T, Fujimoto M. Detergent-resistant microdomains determine the localization of σ-1 receptors to the endoplasmic reticulum-mitochondria junction. Mol Pharmacol 2010;77:517–28. https://doi.org/10.1124/mol.109.062539.

[27] Fujimoto M, Hayashi T, Su T-P. The role of cholesterol in the association of endoplasmic reticulum membranes with mitochondria. Biochem Biophys Res Commun 2012;417:635–9. https://doi.org/10.1016/j.bbrc.2011.12.022.

[28] Ziolkowski W, Szkatula M, Nurczyk A, Wakabayashi T, Kaczor JJ, Olek RA, et al. Methyl-beta-cyclodextrin induces mitochondrial cholesterol depletion and alters the mitochondrial structure and bioenergetics. FEBS Lett 2010;584:4606–10. https://doi.org/10.1016/j.febslet.2010.10.023.

[29] Bhattarai KR, Chaudhary M, Kim H-R, Chae H-J. Endoplasmic reticulum (ER) stress response failure in diseases. Trends Cell Biol 2020;30:672–5. https://doi.org/10.1016/j.tcb.2020.05.004.

[30] Dong Z, Shanmughapriya S, Tomar D, Siddiqui N, Lynch S, Nemani N, et al. Mitochondrial Ca^{2+} uniporter is a mitochondrial luminal redox sensor that augments MCU channel activity. Mol Cell 2017;65:1014–1028.e7. https://doi.org/10.1016/j.molcel.2017.01.032.

[31] Bhandary B, Marahatta A, Kim HR, Chae HJ. An involvement of oxidative stress in endoplasmic reticulum stress and its associated diseases. Int J Mol Sci 2013;14:434–56. https://doi.org/10.3390/ijms14010434.

[32] Yin F, Sancheti H, Liu Z, Cadenas E. Mitochondrial function in ageing: coordination with signalling and transcriptional pathways. J Physiol 2016;594:2025–42. https://doi.org/10.1113/JP270541.

[33] Giorgi C, Baldassari F, Bononi A, Bonora M, De Marchi E, Marchi S, et al. Mitochondrial Ca^{2+} and apoptosis. Cell Calcium 2012;52:36–43. https://doi.org/10.1016/j.ceca.2012.02.008.

[34] Su L-J, Zhang J-H, Gomez H, Murugan R, Hong X, Xu D, et al. Reactive oxygen species-induced lipid peroxidation in apoptosis, autophagy, and ferroptosis. Oxid Med Cell Longev 2019;2019:1–13. https://doi.org/10.1155/2019/5080843.

[35] Chew H, Solomon VA, Fonteh AN. Involvement of lipids in Alzheimer's disease pathology and potential therapies. Front Physiol 2020;11:1–28. https://doi.org/10.3389/fphys.2020.00598.

[36] Fernández-Moriano C, González-Burgos E, Gómez-Serranillos MP. Lipid peroxidation and mitochondrial dysfunction in Alzheimer's and Parkinson's diseases: role of natural products as cytoprotective agents. In: Neuroprotective Natural Products. Weinheim, Germany: Wiley-VCH Verlag GmbH & Co. KGaA; 2017. p. 107–51.

[37] Eckenrode EF, Yang J, Velmurugan GV, Foskett JK, White C. Apoptosis protection by Mcl-1 and Bcl-2 modulation of inositol 1,4,5-trisphosphate receptor-dependent Ca^{2+} signaling. J Biol Chem 2010;285:13678–84. https://doi.org/10.1074/jbc.M109.096040.

[38] Booth DM, Enyedi B, Geiszt M, Várnai P, Hajnóczky G. Redox nanodomains are induced by and control calcium signaling at the ER-mitochondrial interface. Mol Cell 2016;63:240–8. https://doi.org/10.1016/j.molcel.2016.05.040.

[39] Galimov ER. The role of p66shc in oxidative stress and apoptosis. Acta Naturae 2010;2:44–51. https://doi.org/10.32607/20758251-2010-2-4-44-51.

[40] Giorgio M, Migliaccio E, Orsini F, Paolucci D, Moroni M, Contursi C, et al. Electron transfer between cytochrome c and p66Shc generates reactive oxygen species that trigger mitochondrial apoptosis. Cell 2005;122:221–33. https://doi.org/10.1016/j.cell.2005.05.011.

[41] Lee YM, He W, Liou Y-C. The redox language in neurodegenerative diseases: oxidative post-translational modifications by hydrogen peroxide. Cell Death Dis 2021;12:58. https://doi.org/10.1038/s41419-020-03355-3.

[42] Lebiedzinska M, Duszynski J, Rizzuto R, Pinton P, Wieckowski MR. Age-related changes in levels of p66Shc and serine 36-phosphorylated p66Shc in organs and mouse tissues. Arch Biochem Biophys 2009;486:73–80. https://doi.org/10.1016/j.abb.2009.03.007.

[43] Camici GG, Schiavoni M, Francia P, Bachschmid M, Martin-Padura I, Hersberger M, et al. Genetic deletion of p66Shc adaptor protein prevents hyperglycemia-induced endothelial dysfunction and oxidative stress. Proc Natl Acad Sci 2007;104:5217–22. https://doi.org/10.1073/pnas.0609656104.

[44] Galimov ER, Chernyak BV, Sidorenko AS, Tereshkova AV, Chumakov PM. Prooxidant properties of p66Shc are mediated by mitochondria in human cells. PLoS One 2014;9:e86521. https://doi.org/10.1371/journal.pone.0086521.

[45] Nemoto S, Combs CA, French S, Ahn B-H, Fergusson MM, Balaban RS, et al. The mammalian longevity-associated gene product p66 regulates mitochondrial metabolism. J Biol Chem 2006;281:10555–60. https://doi.org/10.1074/jbc.M511626200.

[46] Kelkar DS, Ravikumar G, Mehendale N, Singh S, Joshi A, Sharma AK, et al. A chemical–genetic screen identifies ABHD12 as an oxidized-phosphatidylserine lipase. Nat Chem Biol 2019;15:169–78. https://doi.org/10.1038/s41589-018-0195-0.

[47] Imlay JA. The molecular mechanisms and physiological consequences of oxidative stress: lessons from a model bacterium. Nat Rev Microbiol 2013;11:443–54. https://doi.org/10.1038/nrmicro3032.

[48] Bradley-Whitman MA, Lovell MA. Biomarkers of lipid peroxidation in Alzheimer disease (AD): an update. Arch Toxicol 2015;89:1035–44. https://doi.org/10.1007/s00204-015-1517-6.

[49] Pamplona R. Membrane phospholipids, lipoxidative damage and molecular integrity: a causal role in aging and longevity. Biochim Biophys Acta Bioenerg 2008;1777:1249–62. https://doi.org/10.1016/j.bbabio.2008.07.003.

[50] Spiteller G, Afzal M. The action of peroxyl radicals, powerful deleterious reagents, explains why neither cholesterol nor saturated fatty acids cause atherogenesis and age-related diseases. Chem A Eur J 2014;20:14928–45. https://doi.org/10.1002/chem.201404383.

[51] Jacob RF, Mason RP. Lipid peroxidation induces cholesterol domain formation in model membranes. J Biol Chem 2005;280:39380–7. https://doi.org/10.1074/jbc.M507587200.

[52] Volinsky R, Kinnunen PKJ. Oxidized phosphatidylcholines in membrane-level cellular signaling: from biophysics to physiology and molecular pathology. FEBS J 2013;280:2806–16. https://doi.org/10.1111/febs.12247.

[53] Matsura T. Oxidized phosphatidylserine: production and bioactivities. Yonago Acta Med 2014;57:119–27.

[54] Catalá A. Lipid peroxidation of membrane phospholipids generates hydroxy-alkenals and oxidized phospholipids active in physiological and/or pathological conditions. Chem Phys Lipids 2009;157:1–11. https://doi.org/10.1016/j.chemphyslip.2008.09.004.

[55] Kao Y, Ho P, Tu Y, Jou I, Tsai K. Lipids and Alzheimer's disease. Int J Mol Sci 2020;21:1505. https://doi.org/10.3390/ijms21041505.

[56] Davies SS, May-Zhang LS, Boutaud O, Amarnath V, Kirabo A, Harrison DG. Isolevuglandins as mediators of disease and the

development of dicarbonyl scavengers as pharmaceutical interventions. Pharmacol Ther 2020;205:107418. https://doi.org/10.1016/j.pharmthera.2019.107418.

[57] Cardoso S, Carvalho C, Correia SC, Seiça RM, Moreira PI. Alzheimer's disease: from mitochondrial perturbations to mitochondrial medicine. Brain Pathol 2016;26:632–47. https://doi.org/10.1111/bpa.12402.

[58] Dorszewska J, Prendecki M, Oczkowska A, Dezor M, Kozubski W. Molecular basis of familial and sporadic Alzheimer's disease. Curr Alzheimer Res 2016;13:952–63. https://doi.org/10.2174/1567205013666160314150501.

[59] Pera M, Larrea D, Guardia-Laguarta C, Montesinos J, Velasco KR, Agrawal RR, et al. Increased localization of APP-C99 in mitochondria-associated ER membranes causes mitochondrial dysfunction in Alzheimer disease. EMBO J 2017;36:3356–71. https://doi.org/10.15252/embj.201796797.

[60] Del Prete D, Suski JM, Oulès B, Debayle D, Gay AS, Lacas-Gervais S, et al. Localization and processing of the amyloid-β protein precursor in mitochondria-associated membranes. J Alzheimers Dis 2017;55:1549–70. https://doi.org/10.3233/JAD-160953.

[61] Ehehalt R, Keller P, Haass C, Thiele C, Simons K. Amyloidogenic processing of the Alzheimer β-amyloid precursor protein depends on lipid rafts. J Cell Biol 2003;160:113–23. https://doi.org/10.1083/jcb.200207113.

[62] Area-Gomez E, de Groof A, Bonilla E, Montesinos J, Tanji K, Boldogh I, et al. A key role for MAM in mediating mitochondrial dysfunction in Alzheimer disease. Cell Death Dis 2018;9:335. https://doi.org/10.1038/s41419-017-0215-0.

[63] Schon EA, Area-Gomez E. Mitochondria-associated ER membranes in Alzheimer disease. Mol Cell Neurosci 2013;55:26–36. https://doi.org/10.1016/j.mcn.2012.07.011.

[64] Area-Gomez E, del Carmen Lara Castillo M, Tambini MD, Guardia-Laguarta C, de Groof AJC, Madra M, et al. Upregulated function of mitochondria-associated ER membranes in Alzheimer disease. EMBO J 2012;31:4106–23. https://doi.org/10.1038/emboj.2012.202.

[65] Hedskog L, Pinho CM, Filadi R, Ronnback A, Hertwig L, Wiehager B, et al. Modulation of the endoplasmic reticulum-mitochondria interface in Alzheimer's disease and related models. Proc Natl Acad Sci 2013;110:7916–21. https://doi.org/10.1073/pnas.1300677110.

[66] Fernandes T, Resende R, Silva DF, Marques AP, Santos AE, Cardoso SM, et al. Structural and functional alterations in mitochondria-associated membranes (MAMs) and in mitochondria activate stress response mechanisms in an in vitro model of Alzheimer's disease. Biomedicines 2021;9:881. https://doi.org/10.3390/biomedicines9080881.

[67] Park J, Choi H, Min JS, Kim B, Lee SR, Yun JW, et al. Loss of mitofusin 2 links beta-amyloid-mediated mitochondrial fragmentation and Cdk5-induced oxidative stress in neuron cells. J Neurochem 2015;132:687–702. https://doi.org/10.1111/jnc.12984.

[68] Calvo-Rodriguez M, Hernando-Perez E, Nuñez L, Villalobos C. Amyloid β oligomers increase ER-Mitochondria Ca^{2+} cross talk in young hippocampal neurons and exacerbate aging-induced intracellular Ca^{2+} remodeling. Front Cell Neurosci 2019;13. https://doi.org/10.3389/fncel.2019.00022.

[69] Calvo-Rodriguez M, Hou SS, Snyder AC, Kharitonova EK, Russ AN, Das S, et al. Increased mitochondrial calcium levels associated with neuronal death in a mouse model of Alzheimer's disease. Nat Commun 2020;11:2146. https://doi.org/10.1038/s41467-020-16074-2.

[70] Dematteis G, Vydmantaitė G, Ruffinatti FA, Chahin M, Farruggio S, Barberis E, et al. Proteomic analysis links alterations of bioenergetics, mitochondria-ER interactions and proteostasis in hippocampal astrocytes from 3xTg-AD mice. Cell Death Dis 2020;11:645. https://doi.org/10.1038/s41419-020-02911-1.

[71] Garrido-Maraver J, Loh SHY, Martins LM. Forcing contacts between mitochondria and the endoplasmic reticulum extends lifespan in a Drosophila model of Alzheimer's disease. Biol Open 2019;9. https://doi.org/10.1242/bio.047530.

[72] De Mario A, Quintana-Cabrera R, Martinvalet D, Giacomello M. (Neuro)degenerated mitochondria-ER contacts. Biochem Biophys Res Commun 2017;483:1096–109. https://doi.org/10.1016/j.bbrc.2016.07.056.

[73] Zagol-Ikapitte I, Masterson TS, Amarnath V, Montine TJ, Andreasson KI, Boutaud O, et al. Prostaglandin H2-derived adducts of proteins correlate with Alzheimer's disease severity. J Neurochem 2005;94:1140–5. https://doi.org/10.1111/j.1471-4159.2005.03264.x.

[74] Woodling NS, Wang Q, Priyam PG, Larkin P, Shi J, Johansson JU, et al. Suppression of Alzheimer-associated inflammation by microglial prostaglandin-E2 EP4 receptor signaling. J Neurosci 2014;34:5882–94. https://doi.org/10.1523/JNEUROSCI.0410-14.2014.

[75] Davies SS, Bodine C, Matafonova E, Pantazides BG, Bernoud-Hubac N, Harrison FE, et al. Treatment with a γ-ketoaldehyde scavenger prevents working memory deficits in hApoE4 mice. J Alzheimer's Dis 2011;27:49–59. https://doi.org/10.3233/JAD-2011-102118.

[76] Nissanka N, Moraes CT. Mitochondrial DNA damage and reactive oxygen species in neurodegenerative disease. FEBS Lett 2018;592:728–42. https://doi.org/10.1002/1873-3468.12956.

[77] Selfridge JE, Lezi E, Lu J, Swerdlow RH. Role of mitochondrial homeostasis and dynamics in Alzheimer's disease. Neurobiol Dis 2013;51:3–12. https://doi.org/10.1016/j.nbd.2011.12.057.

[78] Zhang Z-W, Xu X-C, Liu T, Yuan S. Mitochondrion-permeable antioxidants to treat ROS-burst-mediated acute diseases. Oxid Med Cell Longev 2016;2016:1–10. https://doi.org/10.1155/2016/6859523.

[79] Horvath SE, Daum G. Lipids of mitochondria. Prog Lipid Res 2013;52:590–614. https://doi.org/10.1016/j.plipres.2013.07.002.

[80] Prakash A, Kumar A. Implicating the role of lycopene in restoration of mitochondrial enzymes and BDNF levels in β-amyloid induced Alzheimer's disease. Eur J Pharmacol 2014;741:104–11. https://doi.org/10.1016/j.ejphar.2014.07.036.

[81] Wang Y, Branicky R, Noë A, Hekimi S. Superoxide dismutases: dual roles in controlling ROS damage and regulating ROS signaling. J Cell Biol 2018;217:1915–28. https://doi.org/10.1083/jcb.201708007.

[82] Grenier-Larouche T, Galinier A, Casteilla L, Carpentier AC, Tchernof A. Omental adipocyte hypertrophy relates to coenzyme Q10 redox state and lipid peroxidation in obese women. J Lipid Res 2015;56:1985–92. https://doi.org/10.1194/jlr.P058578.

[83] Jembrek MJ, Hof PR, Šimić G. Ceramides in Alzheimer's disease: key mediators of neuronal apoptosis induced by oxidative stress and Aβ accumulation. Oxid Med Cell Longev 2015;2015:1–17. https://doi.org/10.1155/2015/346783.

[84] Maraldi T. Natural compounds as modulators of NADPH oxidases. Oxid Med Cell Longev 2013;2013:1–10. https://doi.org/10.1155/2013/271602.

[85] Marreiro D, Cruz K, Morais J, Beserra J, Severo J, de Oliveira A. Zinc and oxidative stress: current mechanisms. Antioxidants 2017;6:24. https://doi.org/10.3390/antiox6020024.

[86] Qu M, Li L, Chen C, Li M, Pei L, Chu F, et al. Protective effects of lycopene against amyloid β-induced neurotoxicity in cultured rat cortical neurons. Neurosci Lett 2011;505:286–90. https://doi.org/10.1016/J.NEULET.2011.10.048.

[87] Birk AV, Chao WM, Bracken C, Warren JD, Szeto HH. Targeting mitochondrial cardiolipin and the cytochrome c/cardiolipin complex to promote electron transport and optimize mitochondrial ATP synthesis. Br J Pharmacol 2014;171:2017–28. https://doi.org/10.1111/bph.12468.

[88] Reddy PH, Manczak M, Kandimalla R. Mitochondria-targeted small molecule SS31: a potential candidate for the treatment of Alzheimer's disease. Hum Mol Genet 2017;26:1483–96. https://doi.org/10.1093/hmg/ddx052.

[89] Liu X, Xu K, Yan M, Wang Y, Zheng X. Protective effects of galantamine against Aβ-induced PC12 cell apoptosis by preventing mitochondrial dysfunction and endoplasmic reticulum stress. Neurochem Int 2010;57:588–99. https://doi.org/10.1016/j.neuint.2010.07.007.

[90] Hajeyah AA, Griffiths WJ, Wang Y, Finch AJ, O'Donnell VB. The biosynthesis of enzymatically oxidized lipids. Front Endocrinol (Lausanne) 2020;11:910. https://doi.org/10.3389/fendo.2020.591819.

[91] Lee HJ, Jung YH, Choi GE, Kim JS, Chae CW, Lim JR, et al. Urolithin A suppresses high glucose-induced neuronal amyloidogenesis by modulating TGM2-dependent ER-mitochondria contacts and calcium homeostasis. Cell Death Differ 2021;28:184–202. https://doi.org/10.1038/s41418-020-0593-1.

[92] González-Sarrías A, Núñez-Sánchez MÁ, Tomás-Barberán FA, Espín JC. Neuroprotective effects of bioavailable polyphenol-derived metabolites against oxidative stress-induced cytotoxicity in Human neuroblastoma SH-SY5Y cells. J Agric Food Chem 2017;65:752–8. https://doi.org/10.1021/acs.jafc.6b04538.

[93] Shi M, Chen F, Chen Z, Yang W, Yue S, Zhang J, et al. Sigma-1 receptor: a potential therapeutic target for traumatic brain injury. Front Cell Neurosci 2021;15:402. https://doi.org/10.3389/fncel.2021.685201.

[94] Lahmy V, Long R, Morin D, Villard V, Maurice T. Mitochondrial protection by the mixed muscarinic/σ1 ligand ANAVEX2-73, a tetrahydrofuran derivative, in Aβ25-35 peptide-injected mice, a nontransgenic Alzheimer's disease model. Front Cell Neurosci 2014;8:463. https://doi.org/10.3389/fncel.2014.00463.

[95] Behensky AA, Yasny IE, Shuster AM, Seredenin SB, Petrov AV, Cuevas J. Afobazole activation of σ-1 receptors modulates neuronal responses to amyloid-β 25–35. J Pharmacol Exp Ther 2013;347:468–77. https://doi.org/10.1124/jpet.113.208330.

[96] Ryskamp D, Wu L, Wu J, Kim D, Rammes G, Geva M, et al. Pridopidine stabilizes mushroom spines in mouse models of Alzheimer's disease by acting on the sigma-1 receptor. Neurobiol Dis 2019;124:489–504. https://doi.org/10.1016/j.nbd.2018.12.022.

[97] Fisher A, Bezprozvanny I, Wu L, Ryskamp DA, Bar-Ner N, Natan N, et al. AF710B, a novel M1/σ1 agonist with therapeutic efficacy in animal models of Alzheimer's disease. Neurodegener Dis 2016;16:95–110. https://doi.org/10.1159/000440864.

[98] Lahmy V, Meunier J, Malmström S, Naert G, Givalois L, Kim SH, et al. Blockade of Tau hyperphosphorylation and Aβ1–42 generation by the aminotetrahydrofuran derivative ANAVEX2-73, a mixed muscarinic and σ1 receptor agonist, in a nontransgenic mouse model of Alzheimer's disease. Neuropsychopharmacology 2013;38:1706–23. https://doi.org/10.1038/npp.2013.70.

[99] Maurice T. Protection by sigma-1 receptor agonists is synergic with donepezil, but not with memantine, in a mouse model of amyloid-induced memory impairments. Behav Brain Res 2016;296:270–8. https://doi.org/10.1016/j.bbr.2015.09.020.

[100] Maurice T, Su T-P, Privat A. Sigma1 (σ1) receptor agonists and neurosteroids attenuate β25–35-amyloid peptide-induced amnesia in mice through a common mechanism. Neuroscience 1998;83:413–28. https://doi.org/10.1016/S0306-4522(97)00405-3.

[101] Goguadze N, Zhuravliova E, Morin D, Mikeladze D, Maurice T. Sigma-1 receptor agonists induce oxidative stress in mitochondria and enhance complex I activity in physiological condition but protect against pathological oxidative stress. Neurotox Res 2019;35:1–18. https://doi.org/10.1007/s12640-017-9838-2.

[102] Lone A, Harris RA, Singh O, Betts DH, Cumming RC. p66Shc activation promotes increased oxidative phosphorylation and renders CNS cells more vulnerable to amyloid beta toxicity. Sci Rep 2018;8:17081. https://doi.org/10.1038/s41598-018-35114-y.

[103] Thanh Nam D, Arseneault M, Zarkovic N, Waeg G, Ramassamy C. Molecular regulations induced by acrolein in neuroblastoma SK-N-SH cells: relevance to Alzheimer's disease. J Alzheimer's Dis 2010;21:1197–216. https://doi.org/10.3233/JAD-2010-100417.

[104] Wang Y, Liu T, Pan W, Chi H, Chen J, Yu Z, et al. Small molecule compounds alleviate anisomycin-induced oxidative stress injury in SH-SY5Y cells via downregulation of p66shc and Aβ1–42 expression. Exp Ther Med 2016;11:593–600. https://doi.org/10.3892/etm.2015.2921.

[105] Kirmani D, Bhat HF, Bashir M, Zargar MA, Khanday FA. P66Shc-rac1 pathway-mediated ROS production and cell migration is downregulated by ascorbic acid. J Recept Signal Transduct 2013;33:107–13. https://doi.org/10.3109/10799893.2013.770527.

[106] Derungs R, Camici GG, Spescha RD, Welt T, Tackenberg C, Späni C, et al. Genetic ablation of the p66Shc adaptor protein reverses cognitive deficits and improves mitochondrial function in an APP transgenic mouse model of Alzheimer's disease. Mol Psychiatry 2017;22:605–14. https://doi.org/10.1038/mp.2016.112.

[107] Feng D, Yao J, Wang G, Li Z, Zu G, Li Y, et al. Inhibition of p66Shc-mediated mitochondrial apoptosis via targeting prolyl-isomerase Pin1 attenuates intestinal ischemia/reperfusion injury in rats. Clin Sci 2017;131:759–73. https://doi.org/10.1042/CS20160799.

Chapter 8

Oxidative stress biomarkers in human health and disease

Catalina Rojas-Solé, José Lillo-Moya and Ramón Rodrigo
Molecular and Clinical Pharmacology Program, Institute of Biomedical Sciences, Faculty of Medicine, University of Chile, Santiago, Chile

Introduction

Redox processes are present in a myriad of reactions occurring in every cell. Physiologically, it is essential to maintain this balance to carry out different biological functions. The development of oxidative stress occurs when the rate of production of reactive species overwhelms the capacity of the antioxidant defense system. This redox alteration can produce derangements in cell signaling and molecular damage [1]. The pro-oxidant components contain reactive oxygen species (ROS) and reactive nitrogen species (RNS), which are formed by enzymatic and nonenzymatic pathways. Oxidative stress has been described as one of the pathophysiological mechanisms of various diseases, such as cardiovascular diseases, cancer, metabolic, and neurodegenerative diseases, among others. Because of this, during the last decades, extensive research has been carried out on the description and validation of different biomarkers of oxidative stress and thus allow to know the follow up during the treatment of diseases in which oxidative stress is involved. The World Health Organization definition establishes that "A biomarker is any substance, structure, or process that can be measured in the body or its products and influence or predict the incidence of outcome or disease" [2]. However, it is worth noting that biomarkers also allow the evaluation of treatments and interventions [3], as well as the generation of new pharmacological strategies by demonstrating the relationship between the processes of the generation of specific molecules and the pathophysiology of diseases.

Regarding oxidative stress, to date, there is a high level of accumulated evidence on biomarkers, which have shown a certain degree of association. Nevertheless, it has also been reported that their clinical relevance remains inconclusive, as well as their specificity [4]. The aim of this chapter is to present an overview of available data influencing biomarkers related to the involvement of reactive oxygen and nitrogen species in cellular processes of health and disease. In addition, the role of biomarkers as therapeutic targets of diseases is analyzed.

Reactive oxygen species and oxidative stress

Reactive oxygen species are molecules produced in cellular physiological states by different redox processes. It has been described that mammals metabolize 95% of oxygen into H_2O, and 5% of oxygen undergoes univalent reductions, successively generating superoxide radical anion ($O2^{\cdot -}$), hydrogen peroxide (H_2O_2), hydroxyl radical ($\cdot OH$), and finally H_2O [5]. Under normal conditions, the production of ROS is in balance with respect to the antioxidant system to avoid the subsequent generation of damage. On the other hand, in pathological states, there may be an unbalance between these two components in favor of the pro-oxidant, ranging from the eustress linked to the healthy physiological state, to distress, defined as a state of damaging oxidative stress, linked to the pathophysiology of the disease, where redox signaling is disrupted. Within the pro-oxidant component, in addition to ROS, there are also reactive nitrogen, sulfur, electrophilic, and halogen species [6], being ROS and RNS the most described and associated with the pathophysiological mechanisms of certain diseases. Enzymatic pathways can mediate ROS generation from NADPH oxidase (NOX), xanthine oxidase (XO), mitochondrial enzymes, uncoupled nitric oxide synthase (unc-eNOS), myeloperoxidase (MPO), lipoxygenases/cyclo-oxygenases, among others, as well as nonenzymatic pathways, such as Fenton and Haber-Weiss reactions.

Increased reactive species concentration in the steady state can produce an elevation of the probability that they

Modulation of Oxidative Stress. https://doi.org/10.1016/B978-0-443-19247-0.00003-5

attack and damage cellular biomolecules, such as lipids, proteins, and nucleic acids. The process subsequently leads to the alteration of the redox signaling of the cell and its entire functioning, which can lead to pathological effects, even reaching cell death. Thus, ROS have been involved in cell death by apoptosis, necrosis, pyroptosis, and ferroptosis [7], processes crucial in developing diseases by causing damage at the cellular level, what is accompanied by structural and functional alterations at the tissue and organ level.

Enzymatic ROS sources

NADPH oxidase is an enzyme that catalyzes the transfer of electrons through biological membranes, generating radical superoxide anion from oxygen, oxidizing NADPH during this process. Due to this function, the role of NADPH oxidase has been involved in multiple physiological functions, such as host defense and inflammation, cellular signaling, ROS-mediated gene expression, cell death and senescence, among many others [8]. This enzyme has multiple isoforms (NOX 1, NOX2, NOX3, NOX4, NOX 5, DUOX1, and DUOX 2) that are differentially expressed in the different tissues of our body. The general structure of NOX is composed of the membrane subunits gp61, Nox, and p22phox and the cytosolic subunits p47phox, p67phox, p40phox, and Rac2. In addition to its physiological functions, NOX has been described as part of the pathophysiology of different disease models where oxidative stress plays a key role, such as hypertension, ischemia-reperfusion, or stroke.

Xanthine oxidase (XO). This enzyme catalyzes the reactions of the last two steps of purine metabolism, converting hypoxanthine to xanthine and the latter to uric acid. The enzyme is considered as a xanthine oxidoreductase system, as it exerts either the function of dehydrogenase or oxidase due to the occurrence of these two isoforms. Xanthine dehydrogenase, which preferentially uses NAD^+, is an electron acceptor, and XO, which usually uses O_2 as substrate, is an acceptor, being the form involved in the production of superoxide and hydrogen peroxide. Xanthine dehydrogenase is converted to XO by oxidation of the sulfhydryl residues or proteolysis [9]. Physiologically, XO is expressed in different tissues of the human body; however, it has higher levels in the intestine and liver [10].

Nitric oxide synthase has three recognized isoforms: neuronal NOS (nNOS), endothelial NOS (eNOS), and inducible NOS (iNOS). The structure of NOS consists of an oxygenase, which contains heme and tetrahydrobiopterin (BH4) and binds substrates L-arginine and oxygen, and a reductase domain, which binds NADPH [5]. NO synthesized by eNOS avidly reacts with superoxide formed via NOX to produce $ONOO^-$. The latter is capable of uncoupling eNOS by oxidizing and decreasing the synthesis of BH4, being a cofactor for the regulation of eNOS activity that is easily oxidized under conditions of a prevailing pro-oxidant state. In turn, unc-eNOS forms superoxide in a higher proportion than NO, simultaneously diminishing the availability of NO and promoting the formation of ROS, due to the oxidation of BH4 and thus the uncoupling of eNOS [11,12].

Nonenzymatic ROS production

Fenton and Haber-Weiss reactions

Physiologically, the concentrations of free metal ions in our bodies are finely regulated so that they can fulfill their functions, as well as the place where they are stored. However, under certain stimuli, this regulation can be altered, generating variations that can be deleterious for our cells. An example of the consequences of this type of situation corresponds to the **Fenton reaction**, where hydrogen peroxide and iron are involved. The increase in Fe^{2+} triggers this metal ion to react with hydrogen peroxide, giving a hydroxyl radical as reaction product, which has been described as the most dangerous free radical due to its high reactivity. In recent years, this reaction has become relevant after the description of a new cell death pathway, called Ferroptosis, which has generated new lines of research to be able to explain pathophysiologically the mechanisms of certain damage processes, including cell death, derived from processes such as myocardial ischemia/reperfusion and acute kidney injury.

$$Fe^{2+} + H_2O_2 \rightarrow Fe^{3+} + {}^{\cdot}OH + -OH$$

Fenton reaction.

In the **Haber–Weiss** reaction, iron catalyzes the reaction to increase the production of hydroxyl radical:

$$Fe^{3+} + {}^{-\cdot}O_2 \rightarrow Fe^{2+} + O_2$$

$$Fe^{2+} + H_2O_2 \rightarrow Fe^{3+} + OH^- + {}^{\cdot}OH$$

Net reaction:

$${}^{-\cdot}O_2 + H_2O_2 \rightarrow O_2 + {}^{\cdot}OH + {}^{-}OH$$

Haber-Weiss reaction.

Oxidative stress biomarkers

One of the attractions of oxidative stress is its medical application, which has given way to a new perspective on the consequences of free radicals and the use of antioxidants. Exposure of tissues to low levels of ROS and RNS confers protection for cells, generating an adaptive and survival response [13]. On the other hand, chronic oxidative stress is harmful to the cell, since it causes oxidation of macromolecules and generates changes in cell signaling pathways due to modifications in the redox balance, altering cell function and even causing death through various mechanisms [14]. Because of this, certain diseases have been categorized as "redox diseases" [15] and several biomarkers have been investigated to assess the progression or status of oxidative damage and are common between the diseases. So far, there are methods such as electron spin resonance, fluorescence, magnetic resonance, and mass spectrometry techniques to approximate a measurement of ROS levels. However, these are methods that are used in research, and their clinical use in humans is limited [16,17]. Table 8.1 summarizes the main biomarkers of oxidative stress.

Biomarkers based in ROS modification

Lipid peroxidation

As previously, it should be noted that ROS attack to different components of the cell, such as plasma membrane lipids, where the end products of lipid peroxidation have been widely used as biomarkers. Polyunsaturated fatty acids (PUFAs) correspond to the lipids most susceptible of undergoing lipid peroxidation, being linoleic acid the main exponent, which is present in an amount 5 times greater than arachidonic acid [5]. Lipid peroxidation consists of three main stages: initiation, propagation, and termination [18]. First, ROS attack a double bond located in the PUFA aliphatic chain, abstracting hydrogen and forming a lipid radical (L·). Then, this radical will react with the oxygen surrounding it, forming peroxyl radical (LOO·), which is capable of reacting with other lipids by abstracting a hydrogen from them and spreading the generation of new lipid radicals that will also react with the oxygen that surrounds them. Finally, the propagation stage continues until peroxyl reacts with another free radical or a free radical scavenger antioxidant agent that reduces it, ending the propagation chain (Fig. 8.1). LOO· and LO· are then cyclized and/or degraded to form more stable products such

TABLE 8.1 Prooxidant biomarkers.

Prooxidant biomarkers	Characteristic	Location	Reference
3-Nitrotyrosine	Relatively specific marker of oxidative damage mediated by peroxynitrite	Extracellular	[125]
4-Hydroxynonenal	One of the most specific and sensitive measures of lipid autoxidation	Extracellular	[126]
Carbonyls	Protein carbonylation is produced by direct damage to proteins during oxidative stress	Extracellular	[127]
Uncoupled eNOS	Production of $O_2\cdot^-$instead of NO	Intracellular	[128]
F2 isoprostane	Result of nonenzymatic peroxidation of arachidonic acid. It is a reliable biomarker of lipid peroxidation in clinical settings for studies in vivo	Extracellular	[129]
Malondialdehyde	Result of peroxides decomposition Assessment of lipid peroxidation	Extracellular	[130]
NADPH oxidase	Catalyzes the one electron reduction of O_2 to generate $O_2\cdot^-$, using NADPH as the source of electrons It is the main ROS source in the vasculature	Intracellular	[131]
Xanthine oxidase	Plays a major role in cell oxidative stress. Catalyzes the oxidation of hypoxanthine to xanthine as well as the catalysis of xanthine to uric acid	Intracellular	[132]

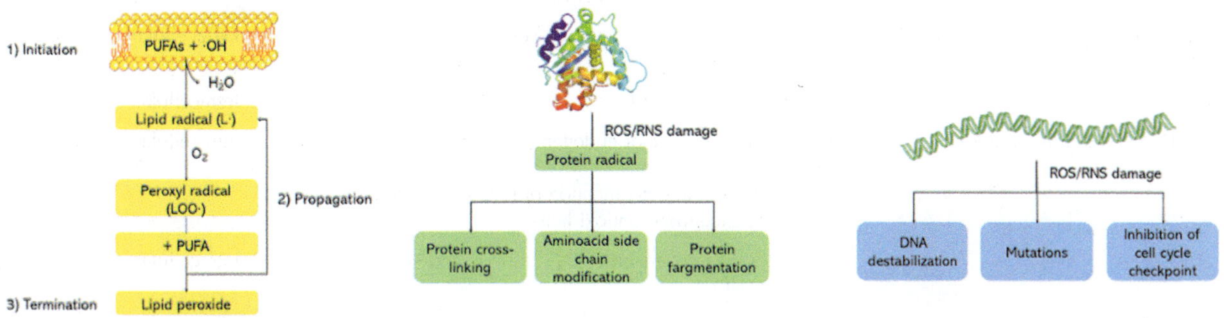

FIGURE 8.1 General mechanism of lipid, protein and DNA damage induced by oxidative stress. L·, lipid radical; ·OH, hydroxyl radical; LOO·, peroxyl radical; PUFAs, polyunsaturated fatty acids; ROS, reactive oxygen species; RNS, reactive nitrogen species.

as different aldehydes including trans-4-hydroxy-2-nonenal (4-HNE), trans-4-oxo-2-nonenal, acrolein, and malondialdehyde (MDA) [18,19]. MDA and HNE represent the most investigated end products of lipid peroxidation [16,20].

Protein oxidation

Proteins are another example of molecules susceptible to ROS attack, especially in the side chains of the amino acids that compose it (Fig. 8.1). The functional damages caused to proteins by oxidative stress corresponds to loss of enzymatic activity, altered cellular functions such as energy production, interference with the creation of membrane potentials, and changes in the type and level of cellular proteins [18]. The chemical and structural changes due to protein oxidation will result in the formation of carbonyl groups, which can be measured and have been described as a promising biomarker of oxidative stress [21]. The early formation of carbonylated proteins and their high stability provide an advantage over other biomarkers of oxidative stress. Protein carbonylation is suitable to be measured in different types of samples, such as blood or urine, although those extracted from the specific tissue or cell will be much more representative and accurate [16]. However, other authors report that its relevance as a biomarker is lower because these are produced by various mechanisms, so they can often be quite high [19,22], and the clinical and biological relevance of oxidations of proteins as a biomarker depends on the availability of the methodologies able to identify and quantify specific protein oxidative modifications, so now this biomarker is still limited. Also, 3-nitro-tyrosine is another oxidation protein product generated by reaction with RNS. ELISA assay can measure this molecule, but its utility as a clinical biomarker is still questioned [16].

DNA oxidation

DNA damage caused by ROS is considered one of the most serious modifications, where the hydroxyl radical reacts with all components of the DNA molecule, including the purine and pyrimidine bases and the deoxyribose backbone. However, nitrosative stress also plays a key role through peroxynitrite and nitric oxide. In addition, other RNS can cause damage either indirectly or directly (Fig. 8.1). Thus, the endogenous formation of carcinogenic N-nitrosamine molecules can occur by bases oxidation [5]. DNA damage is severe because it is not synthesized de novo, and the modifications are perpetuated as the DNA strand is copied. These modifications induce mutations that destabilize DNA, causing alterations in the functioning of the cell and can ultimately lead to the development of cancer [4,5]. It has been reported an association between 7,8-dihydroxy-8-oxo-2′-deoxyguanosine excretion, the most common DNA oxidation product, with the risk of suffering from lung cancer as well as breast cancer [23–26]. The DNA oxidation products can be measured using commercial assays on urine samples by ELISA [4].

Antioxidant system status biomarkers

The maintenance of the reducing environment within our cells is in charge of the antioxidant system, which is the defense system against oxidative stress made up of different components, either enzymatic or nonenzymatic ones. These, before the unbalance of the redox state of our cells, are capable of acting to avoid the oxidative damage that this disturbance could imply and with the trend to return to the physiological balance. Table 8.2 summarizes the main antioxidant biomarkers.

TABLE 8.2 Antioxidant system status biomarkers.

Biomarkers of antioxidant system status	Characteristic	Location	Reference
CAT	Metabolizes H_2O_2 into H_2O and O_2 Also, it can act in the decomposition of small substrates CAT exhibits low oxidase activity	Intracellular	[31]
Ferric reducing ability of plasma (FRAP)	Measure of "total antioxidant power"	Extracellular	[44]
GPx	Reduces H_2O_2 to H_2O	Intracellular	[133]
GSH/GSSG ratio (thiol index)	GSH: GSH is the major endogenous antioxidant produced by the cells Participates in the detoxification of H_2O_2 and free radicals Maintains exogenous antioxidants	Intracellular	[42]
SOD	Catalyzes the conversion of $O_2^{-}\cdot$ into O_2 and H_2O_2 Preserves NO	Intracellular	[134]
Vitamin C	Acts as an ROS scavenger and regenerates vitamin E	Extracellular	[92]

Enzymatic antioxidant biomarkers

The induction of many cytoprotective and antioxidant enzymes in response to reactive stress is regulated at the transcriptional level. A very relevant transcription factor of antioxidant response is the nuclear factor erythroid 2-related factor 2 (Nrf2), which modulates the expression of antioxidant proteins that protect cells and tissues against oxidative, electrophilic, and xenobiotic stress.

Nrf2 is regulated by Kelch-like ECH-associated protein 1 (Keap1), which facilitates the ubiquitination and subsequent proteolysis of Nrf2. The dissociation of Keap1 and Nrf2 in the cytoplasm is followed by the translocation of Nrf2 to the nucleus. Finally, Nrf2 binds to an enhancer termed antioxidant response element (ARE), which promotes detoxification, antioxidant, and expression of anti-inflammatory genes. In conclusion, the interaction between Keap1-Nrf2-ARE is in a redox-sensitive manner [27,28] (Fig. 8.2).

As previously mentioned in this chapter, the oxygen in its reduction pathway to water forms ROS, which are in turn reduced by antioxidant enzymes, being the main responsible enzymes: Superoxide dismutase (SOD), catalase (CAT) and glutathione peroxidase (GPx).

Superoxide dismutase. This enzyme corresponds to a family of enzymes (Mn-SOD and Cu−Zn SOD), which differ in structure and cofactor [13]. In humans, there are three isoforms of SOD. SOD1 (Cu−Zn SOD) is found in the cytoplasm, SOD2 (Mn SOD) in the mitochondria, and SOD3 (EcSOD, extracellular isoform) in the extracellular space [29]. These enzymes reduce the radical anion superoxide to hydrogen peroxide and can be measured using the Misra and Fridovich technique [30] (Fig. 8.3).

Catalase. It is a human enzyme formed by four identical subunits that are located within cells, mainly in peroxisomes. This enzyme can catalyze the dismutation of H_2O_2, converting it into water and oxygen and thus avoiding the oxidative damage that H_2O_2 can generate by forming hydroxyl radical through the Fenton reaction, as well as the damage pathways that H_2O_2 can activate by acting as a second messenger [31,32] (Fig. 8.3). The activity of this enzyme can be measured by the Aebi technique using the nonspontaneous decomposition of hydrogen peroxide [33].

Glutathione peroxidase. It is a family of antioxidant enzymes consisting of GPx1, GPx2, GPx3 and GPx4. GPx is capable of reducing both hydrogen peroxide and those organic molecules that ROS attacks, such as lipid peroxides, to water or corresponding alcohols using GSH [34] (Fig. 8.3). The activity of this enzyme can be measured by the method described by Flohé and Günzler [35].

Nonenzymatic antioxidant biomarkers

The main biomarkers or nonenzymatic parameters correspond to the different antioxidant vitamins and other antioxidant compounds, the levels of reduced glutathione, and the total antioxidant capacity of the plasma.

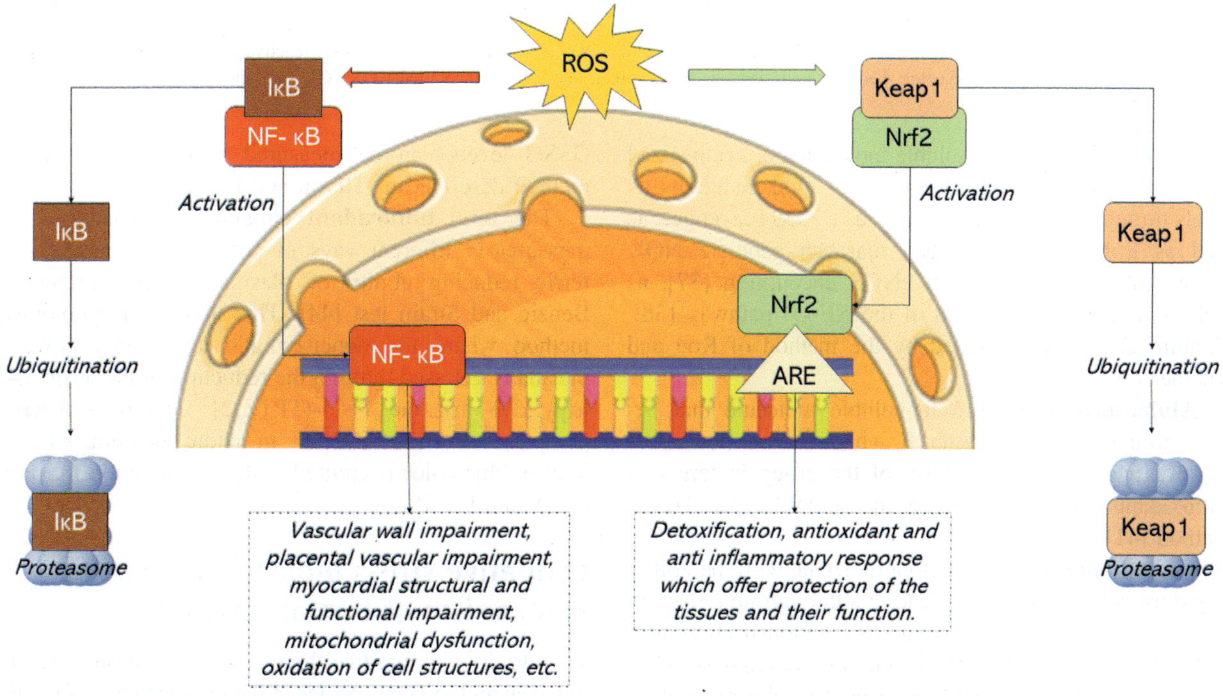

FIGURE 8.2 Genetic and molecular mechanisms of the response to oxidative stress by tissues. ARE, antioxidant response element; IκB, IkappaB kinase; Keap1, kelch-like ECH-associated protein one; NF-κB, nuclear factor kappa-light-chain-enhancer; Nrf2, nuclear factor erythroid 2-related factor 2; ROS, reactive oxygen species.

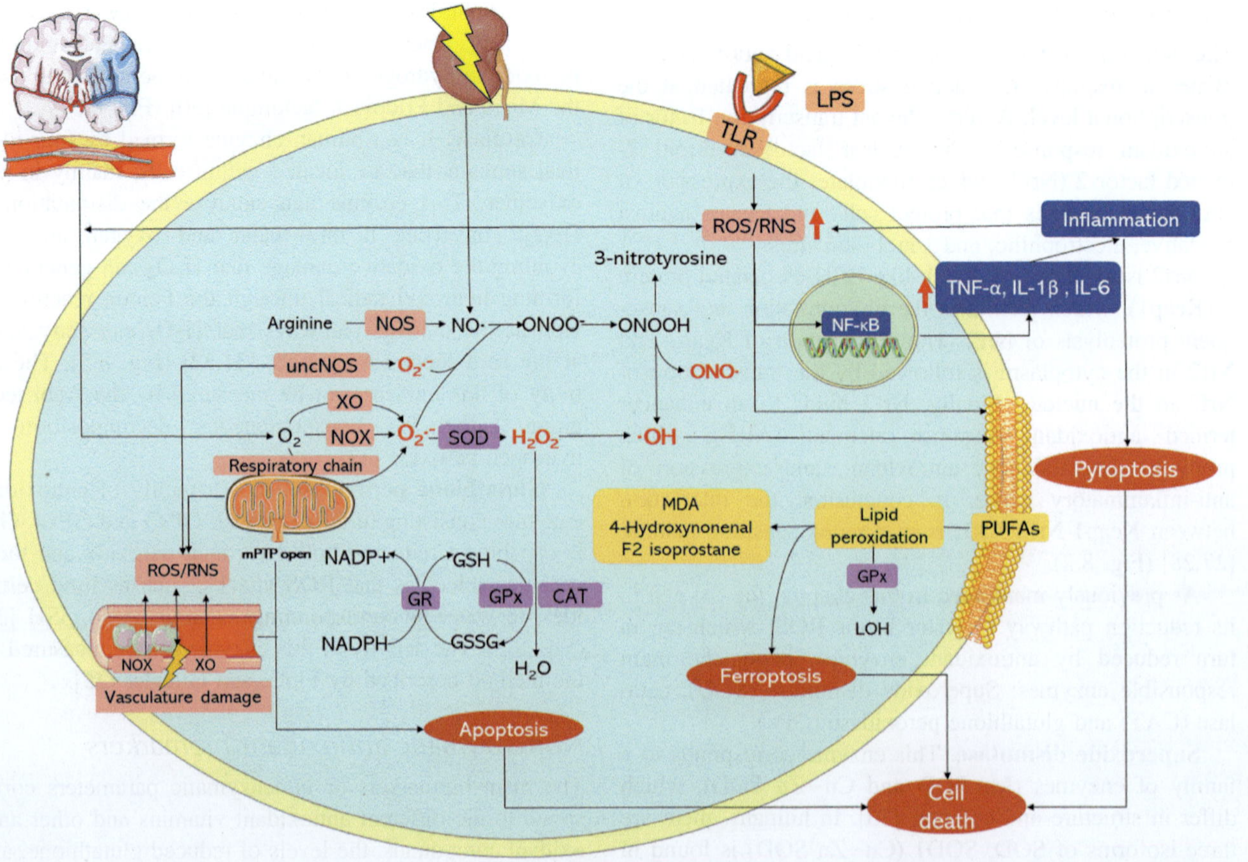

FIGURE 8.3 Molecular mechanisms of the deleterious effects of oxidative stress at cellular level in various diseases. CAT, catalase; GR, glutathione reductase; GPx, glutathione peroxidase; GSH, reduced glutathione; GSSG, oxidized glutathione; IL-1β, interleukin one beta; IL.-6, interleukin six; LPS, lipopolysaccharide; LOH, lipid alcohol; mPTP, mitochondrial permeability transition pore; MDA, malondialdehyde; NF-κB, nuclear factor kappa-light-chain-enhancer of the activated B cells; NO·, nitric oxide; NOS, nitric oxide synthase; NOX, NADPH oxidase; ·OH, hydroxyl radical; H_2O, water; H_2O_2, hydrogen peroxide; ONOO-, peroxynitrite; ONOOH, peroxynitrous acid; SOD, superoxide dismutase; ROS, reactive oxygen species; RNS, reactive nitrogen species; TLR, toll like receptor; TNF-α, tumor necrosis factor alpha; unc-eNOS, uncoupled NOS; XO, xanthine oxidase.

Vitamin C is a water-soluble molecule not synthesized by human cells, so the contribution of food maintains its levels through the daily diet. It acts as a ROS scavenger, as well as it has been described that can generate NOX downregulation [36], prevent eNOS uncoupling [37], as well as inhibit the activation of the NF-κB pathway [38]. Vitamin C can be estimated by the method of Roe and Kuether [39].

Alpha-tocopherol is a fat-soluble molecule that belongs to the family of vitamin E, which is described as the most active and effective form of the group in terms of antioxidants [40] and can be measured by the HPLC method [41].

Glutathione corresponds to a molecule with the ability to reduce compounds by presenting a thiol group (−SH) of the cysteine, and while the vitamins mentioned previously had to be ingested through the diet, GSH is synthesized by the cell [42]. This is usually measured by the ratio of its reduced to the oxidized form (GSH/GSSH ratio), giving us information on the intracellular redox state. GSH and GSSG levels can be measured in erythrocytes by the method described by Hissin and Hilf [43].

The **total antioxidant capacity of plasma** can be measured in different ways, one of the main ones being the ferric reducing ability of plasma (FRAP) through the Benzie and Strain test [44]. This is a spectrophotometric method where the nonenzymatic antioxidant power of plasma is assessed through the reduction of the ferric 2,4,6-tripyridyl-s-triazine [Fe^{3+}-(TPTZ)2] $^{3+}$complex to ferrous complex [Fe^{2+}-(TPTZ)2] $^{2+}$ in acidic medium, where an intense blue color is emitted with an absorption maximum at 593 nm [13,45].

Oxidative stress biomarkers and the mechanism of human diseases

To date, it is known that there is a contribution of reactive nitrogen and oxygen species in the pathogenesis of multiple acute and chronic diseases. However, it is necessary to take into account that the redox balance is a change that is constantly dynamic and can be modified according to the protective or risk factors or the drugs that each patient consumes. Oxidative stress can even contribute to disease development if people are exposed to toxic compounds found daily in air pollution and cigarette smoke [46]. The different biomarkers are classically measured in blood or urine.

Next in the chapter, some classic pathologies in the clinical field and their relationship with oxidative stress and biomarkers will be presented.

Hypertension

Among the human pathologies closely related to oxidative stress, it can be mentioned that arterial hypertension (Fig. 8.3) is a very common one that is a risk factor for cardiovascular diseases and the most important contributor to the global burden of disease and mortality. So far, the number of people living with hypertension has doubled to 1.28 billion since 1990 [47,48]. Hypertension is associated with the accumulation of cellular senescence markers in the vascular wall; these conditions are often associated with vascular dysfunction, inflammation, hypertrophy, apoptosis, cell migration, fibrosis, and angiogenesis [49]. ROS and RNS play a key role in the pathophysiology of hypertension, especially as mediators of endothelial injury and in the modulation of the vasomotor system. In general, hypertensive patients show higher values of lipid peroxidation and lower values of antioxidant status (FRAP and GSH/GSSG ratio) [50].

Indeed, in the vascular wall, there is a high activity of NOX, which produces most of the ROS, such as $O_2^{-}\cdot$. Although ROS are produced principally by NOX and XO, other enzymatic sources such as mitochondrial electron transport chain and unc-eNOS also contribute in the vasculature damage involving decreased vasodilation, increased vasoconstriction, adhesion of proinflammatory monocytes with coagulation, production of thiobarbituric acid–reactive substances (TBARS), H_2O_2, and loss of integrity of the endothelial monolayer [51,52]. Furthermore, it has been shown that there is a decrease in antioxidant activity, reduced levels of ROS scavengers, and decrease in NO availability [53–55].

An essential component of the renin-angiotensin system in the regulation of blood pressure is **Ang II**, which stimulates adrenal cortical cells to produce aldosterone, which binds to renal mineralocorticoid receptors (MR) in order to maintain hydroelectrolytic homeostasis Aldosterone can produce its effects via the MR through genomic and nongenomic signals [56].

In addition, it interacts with extrarenal MRs that influence vascular tone, adipose tissue function, cardiac contraction, and cardiovascular fibrosis. Elevated aldosterone levels are associated with hypertension, obesity and increased risk of cardiovascular and cardiometabolic diseases. In aldosterone-dependent hypertension (primary hyperaldosteronism), there is an increase in oxidative stress through overexpression of NOX, especially NOX4 in endothelial cells and NOX1 in vascular smooth muscle cells, leading to increased vascular ROS production and elevated levels of TBARS, effects that improve with treatment with MR antagonists such as spironolactone [56–58].

Aldosterone also produces fibrinolytic effects and influences the activity of immune cells and adipocytes, which is related to cardiac and vascular fibrosis and the remodeling of hypertension through increased production of H_2O_2, an up-regulation of SOD genes and an increase in 3-nitrotyrosine production in lymphocytes. Also, it occurs a proinflammatory process which involves CD4+ cells that invade intramural coronary arteries and MR activation in macrophages and adipocytes [59,60].

In addition, we know that people can suffer hypertensive emergencies either in patients with or without known preexisting hypertension, and these, despite being episodic, cause organ dysfunction and also cause oxidative damage as well as elevated markers of inflammation, coagulation, platelet activation, and enhanced fibrinolytic activity. On the other hand, patients with hypertensive urgencies, defined as an elevation of blood pressure without organ damage, show levels of biomarkers similar to normotensive patients [61].

Due to the extensive studies on hypertension and its treatments, different drugs (angiotensin-converting enzyme inhibitors or angiotensin receptor blockers) have been proposed for its management, as well as diuretics and antioxidants such as ROS scavengers, and NOX inhibitors, antioxidant vitamins (vitamins C and E), SOD mimetics, and free radical scavengers (NAC) [55].

In addition, beta-blocking drugs such as carvedilol or nebivolol have been shown to exert pleiotropic effects beyond beta-receptor blockade and the treatment of hypertension and involve different mechanisms. First, both increase the response to endothelium-dependent vasodilatation. On the one hand, nebivolol induces vasodilation through a pathway dependent on the increase in nitric oxide, through activation of the L-arginine/NO pathway, which in turn decreases changes in arterial thickness and stiffness [62]. On the other hand, carvedilol has been shown to have antioxidant and anti-inflammatory properties [63], and patients under this treatment showed lower levels of MDA and erythrocyte F2-isoprostane, and higher levels of FRAP and GSH/GSSG ratio, which can provide vascular protection by improving endothelial function and decreasing the production of reactive endothelial species [50].

However, the clinical method to follow depends on the patient, and it is aimed to reduce their risk factors, reduce oxidative stress, and prevent the development of hypertension.

Preeclampsia

During pregnancy, oxidative stress increases physiologically due to a normal systemic inflammatory response and the primary source of ROS is the placenta; however, a local balance is achieved with antioxidant species [64,65]. In contrast to physiology, preeclampsia is a pregnancy-specific clinical syndrome with multisystem disorder that progresses over time, characterized by new-onset hypertension and proteinuria or new-onset hypertension and significant end-stage organ dysfunction with or without proteinuria after the 20th week of pregnancy or postpartum in a previously patient without hypertension [66,67].

Regarding oxidative stress, preeclampsia is associated with poorly placental perfusion due to placental vascular impairment [68]. It is caused by maternal and placental vascular dysfunction and usually resolves after birth. However, the mother and child are still at increased risk of serious morbidity or mortality. Furthermore, patients with preeclampsia are at increased risk of developing cardiovascular and renal diseases in the future [69,70].

Patients may also present with thrombocytopenia, hemolysis, hemoconcentration, hyperuricemia, and impaired liver function [71–73].

In preeclampsia, there are also genetic risk factors that are associated with oxidative stress that involve ROS and RNS, renin-angiotensin system, endothelin system, and inflammatory factors [74]. Moreover, iron homeostasis is disturbed, and ferroptosis pathways may play an important role in the development and progress of the disease [75].

Oxidative stress biomarkers depend on the stage of pregnancy. In the first trimester, placentas have significantly higher MDA and 4-HNE levels and an increase in fibronectin and ET-1 levels. Nevertheless, the use of antioxidants such as MitoQ, an orally mitochondrial-targeted antioxidant, reduces the blood vessel density and angiogenesis pathway. MitoQ selectively concentrates in this organelle and prevents mitochondrial oxidative stress damage and also may play a role in prolongation the half-life of SOD in the context of SOD deficiency [68,76,77]. It should be taken into account that a huge amount of ROS is generated by ETC, which produces $O_2^{-}\cdot$ through oxygen reduction.

On the other hand, the angiogenesis process is mediated by moderate ROS due to the up-regulation pathway of vascular endothelial growth factor that promotes the activation of metalloproteinases. ROS also could activate mitogen-activated protein kinases (MAPK). MAPK signal is necessary for the correct development, differentiation, and morphogenesis [78,79].

However, in pregnant women with preeclampsia, there is an increase in the placental production of soluble Fms-like tyrosine kinase (sFlt-1), which is a biomolecule with antiangiogenic properties and functions as a receptor for vascular endothelial growth factor and placental growth factor [80]. Overexpression of serum sFlt-1 levels is related to poor placental angiogenesis [68]. Moreover, antioxidant capacity is reduced which traduces that GPx activity, CAT activity, glutathione S-transferase, as well as EcSOD activity are not present in patients with preeclampsia [81,82] (Fig. 8.4).

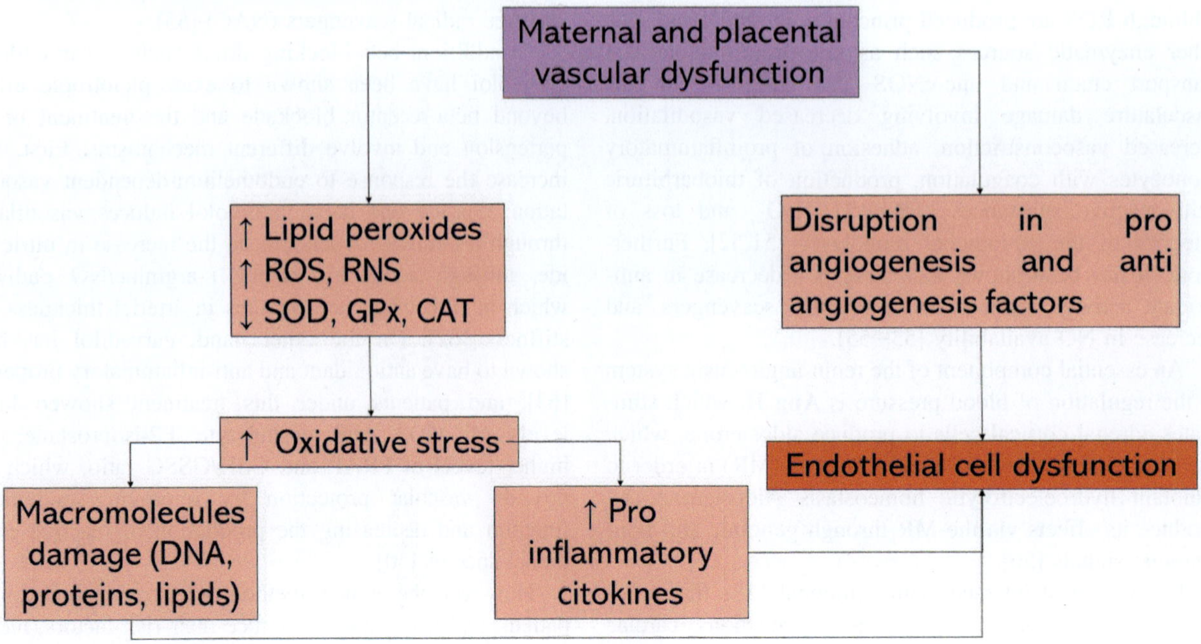

FIGURE 8.4 Pathophysiology of preeclampsia. CAT, catalase; GPx, glutathione peroxidase; SOD, superoxide dismutase; ROS, reactive oxygen species; RNS, reactive nitrogen species.

Ischemia/reperfusion

An adequate blood supply to the tissues is necessary for the proper functioning of the body. Otherwise, ischemia occurs, and blood flow must be restored as soon as possible to avoid tissue necrosis. However, the reperfusion can cause more negative collateral damage than ischemia itself because it produces a phenomenon called ischemia-reperfusion injury (IRI) [83] (Fig. 8.3). This injury is associated with several clinical settings, such as acute heart failure, especially with the development of atherosclerotic plaque; organ transplantation; cerebral dysfunction; gastrointestinal dysfunction; systemic inflammatory response syndrome; and multiple organ dysfunction syndromes [84].

Ischemia causes hypoxia and hypoperfusion of the tissues, which generates a decrease in antioxidative agents and ATP production due to the anaerobic environment and a dysfunction of the mitochondrial electron transport chain. One of the consequences is pump failure (Na^+/K^+ ATPase, Ca^{2+} ATPase), causing retention of sodium in cells, retention of potassium out of cells, and limiting calcium uptake. A higher level of sodium within the cells decreases the activity of Na^+/H^+ exchangers, retaining hydrogen, which reduces intracellular pH, affecting enzyme activity and protein synthesis. Inside the cells, ion accumulation causes hyperosmolarity, leading to water influx and cell swelling [84].

On the other hand, reperfusion induces an oxygen burst that is essential for ROS production, giving rise to the activation of different pathways of cellular damage such as endothelial dysfunction, DNA damage, local inflammatory responses, and even a cytokine storm resulting in cell death through apoptosis, autophagy, necrosis, necroptosis, and ferroptosis [7,84].

Three major enzymatic systems are involved in IRI: NOX, nitric oxide synthase, and XO.

NADPH oxidases are involved in ROS production in IRI by their overexpression and increased activity which immediately produce $O_2^-\cdot$ that is transferred to H_2O_2 via enzymes. In turn, increased $O_2^-\cdot$ leads to NO degradation and ONOO− production. During reperfusion, cells release several chemical mediators that activate NOX, and some of them promote local inflammation, leading to IRI in organs [85,86].

During xanthine formation, $O_2^-\cdot$ and H_2O_2 are released, and they aggravate oxidative stress as well as inflammation process by triggering cytokine cascade and pathological changes by expression of adhesion proteins [87,88].

Although there are different NOS isoforms, all of them produce NO by converting L-arginine to L-citrulline. Their role characterizes nitric oxide as an antioxidant and anti-inflammatory agent [89]. In a hypoxic state, NOS is converted to uncoupled NOS that produces ROS instead of NO, thereby inducing IRI. Moreover, oxidative stress oxidizes BH4 and reduces its level in the tissue, causing uncoupling of NOS, further O_2—· production and cell death [90].

Particular forms of IRI are myocardial ischemia-reperfusion injury (MIRI) and stroke (which is addressed in a separate point below). Both account for up to four out of five deaths [91]. MIRI occurs after a percutaneous coronary intervention (PCI), the gold standard therapy to recover blood flow after an acute myocardial infarction. However, paradoxically, this action induces additional injury in which ROS and RNS play a deleterious role in tissue, producing cellular death, changes in hemodynamic parameters and myocardial enzymes, a decrease in the left ventricular ejection fraction, and left fractional ventricular shortening [92–94].

The treatments in MIRI, such as PCI in the heart or thrombolytic and anticoagulant therapy, generally aim to recover flow after an ischemic phase. Although there are studies with different antioxidant drugs to reduce MIRI, there is still no effective therapy. This may indicate that there are numerous mechanisms of action where both ischemia and reperfusion cause activation of signaling cascades and tissue damage. In addition to antioxidant therapy, other drugs such as empagliflozin have been reported to protect endothelial cell function in patients with or without diabetes who suffer from ischemia-reperfusion events since it improves mitochondrial homeostasis by preventing the fission mechanism. It also improves endothelial function and reduces the formation of microthrombi [95].

SOD isoforms are also related to certain cardiovascular diseases and might serve as biomarkers, especially the plasma activities of SOD1 and SOD2 [96].

In recent years, ischemia-modified albumin (IMA) has been investigated as a novel marker in ischemic heart disease. It is an indirect indicator of hypoxic conditions and increased oxidative stress. This biomarker can also be used as a short- and long-term prognosis and can also be used in other pathologies that will be discussed later, such as stroke, sepsis, or other thromboembolic complications [97].

On the other hand, in kidney IRI, mitochondrial oxidative damage is a key point and antioxidants such as MitoQ are potential therapies for renal dysfunction due to IRI [98]. However, this molecule might also have adverse effects, such as mitochondrial swelling and depolarization in kidney tissue [99].

Ischemia-reperfusion events also occur in patients undergoing cardiac surgery with extracorporeal circulation, which is associated with increases in biomarkers of oxidative stress and inflammation such as MDA, protein carbonylation, lower GSH/GSSG ratio, increase in C reactive protein and leukocyte count, and higher activation of NF-κB under proinflammatory conditions [100].

Stroke

A stroke occurs when the blood supply to part of brain tissue is interrupted or reduced. It is classified into two types: ischemic and hemorrhagic, and it is kind of pathology with high morbidity and mortality. Annually, 15 million people worldwide suffer a stroke, and there are several risk factors such as race, age, ethnicity, tobacco, and high blood pressure. In the United States, more than 795,000 people have a stroke, and approximately 87% have an ischemic cause, in which blood flow to the brain is blocked. Among the main pathological processes are oxidative stress and excitotoxicity. Indeed, the phenomenon of IRI also occurs, causing ROS, RNS production, and inflammation [101–103].

The brain is one of the organs with the highest oxygen consumption and the lowest antioxidant capacity. Therefore, it is very susceptible to ROS damage (Fig. 8.3). Neuronal cells have a heterogeneous distribution in the brain and also vary in their morphology and biochemical function. Due to this, each cell population can have its own vulnerability to oxidative stress, which can modulate tissue damage [104]. Overactivation of glutamate receptors in neurons leads to massive calcium uptake that generates ROS and also produces energy depletion mainly by the alteration of the mitochondrial respiratory function. Moreover, ROS production is increased in the central nervous system (CNS) compared with other tissues. One of the most important ROS in CNS is $O_2^{-}\cdot$, generated by NOX, XO or as a product of the respiratory chain. As for other markers of oxidative damage in stroke, F2-isoprostanes, which are considered the best biomarkers of oxidative stress and lipid peroxidation in vivo, are found increased with the damage generated by stroke. In the case of vitamin E and vitamin C, both show a significant decrease [105].

Upon ischemia, NOX4 is induced in the human and mouse brain. Indeed, brain damage in mice with stroke has been found dramatically reduced by NOX4 blockade, protecting against oxidative stress, neuronal apoptosis, and blood–brain barrier leakage [106].

The two pathophysiological processes mentioned above, oxidative stress and excitotoxicity, activate cytoprotective and cell death–inducing pathways, particularly those involved in programmed cell death or apoptosis. AMPK plays important roles in excitotoxicity and ischemic brain injury, with zinc neurotoxicity representing at least one mechanism of ischemic neuronal death. The protein kinase AMPK is activated by energy depletion and exerts essential prosurvival functions during excitotoxicity. However, when a chronic activation occurs, AMPK can cause detrimental effects and can stimulate apoptosis by inducing the expression of the proapoptotic protein Bim [107,108]. On the other hand, heat shock proteins (Hsp) are cytoprotective during oxidative stress, and high levels of Hsp27 prevent neuronal apoptosis by up-regulating the proapoptotic protein Bim [109]. So, various cellular mechanisms are involved either in neuronal protection or in neuronal death during oxidative stress or excitotoxic lesions, making treatment and prevention very complex.

Despite numerous clinical trials performed in patients with stroke and the research work of the pharmaceutical industries, only a thrombolytic therapy with intravenous administration of recombinant tissue plasminogen activator (rt-PA) is approved for the recovery of the blood flow in the ischemic stroke [110], causing the ROS/RNS cascade activation [101,106,111]. Moreover, rt-PA therapy has contraindications that exclude 90% of the patients, and the efficacy is suboptimal [106]. On the other hand, despite the body of evidence supporting oxidative stress as a pathogenic factor in neurological diseases, the use of antioxidants for neuroprotection has generally been negative, mainly with classic antioxidants such as vitamin C and E [112].

Sepsis

Sepsis is an uncontrolled and exacerbated systemic inflammation in response to infection and can progress to multiple organ dysfunction syndromes, related to organ dysfunction or tissue hypoperfusion. It remains a major cause of morbidity and mortality in hospitalized patients, especially in the pediatric intensive care unit [113]. Oxidative stress is known to participate in the progression and ROS/RNS play a key role in the pathogenesis of sepsis by inducing endothelial cell injuries such as vascular permeability impairment, mitochondrial dysfunction, and oxidation of cell structures (Fig. 8.3). In this context, the information provided by the biomarkers is essential for diagnosis and prognosis for being a critical condition [114].

In general, ROS sepsis pathogenesis include $O_2^{-}\cdot$, H_2O_2, and $\cdot OH$, whereas RNS include the free radical NO and the ONOO– [115] and both are associated with an amplification of the proinflammatory state of sepsis in nearby tissues, causing a vicious circle that increases their production in these cells [116]. Hydrogen peroxide enhances the migration and activation of immune cells through increasing the endothelium permeability and expressing adhesion molecules [114]. In sepsis, neutrophils are the most crucial part of the treatment. However, a different type of cell death called pyroptosis exists and depends on the neutrophil activity. Indeed, neutrophils play a dual role in the pathogenesis and progression of the condition. Pyroptosis is a programmed cell death associated with inflammation, which starts by inflammasomes or cytosolic LPS in innate immunity [117] and can be a target against the development of the sepsis.

The biomarkers depend on the stage of the time-course of sepsis, and further it could be investigated that these are associated with a severity scale according to the positive biomarker. Elevated markers of lipid, especially TBARS and protein oxidative damage, have been observed in septic patients. Patients with nonsevere and severe sepsis have high levels of plasma antioxidant capacity, GPx activity, and plasma F2-isoprostanes concentration, as well as decreased erythrocyte thiol index, GSH, vitamins E and C,

SOD, and CAT activity. On the other hand, patients with severe sepsis have more NF-κB activation [113,118].

So far, therapies have been proposed such as the use of selenium, ascorbic acid, N-acetylcysteine, mitochondria-targeted antioxidants, NOS inhibitors, and melatonin, but the outcomes are not still sufficient for the implementation into a clinical setting.

Acute renal failure

Acute renal failure is characterized by a rapid decrease (hours to days) in global kidney function, especially defined by a reduction in renal function or glomerular filtration rate, generally reversible, accompanied by retention of nitrogenous products, electrolyte, acid-base, and extracellular volume alterations. General or regional decreases in renal blood flow cause acute hypoxia and ischemia, encompassing most causes of acute renal failure [119,120]. Aging and the widespread use of nephrotoxic therapies make this pathology more prevalent, especially in hospitalized patients. In this group, hospitalization time increases and is associated with higher long- and short-term mortality, as well as a higher risk of developing chronic kidney disease (CKD) [121]. Both the acute and chronic phases of kidney disease have detrimental effects mainly in the cardiovascular area. IMA biomarker could be used to measure the cardiovascular and CKD disease [122].

Oxidative stress has been identified as an important pathological mediator, causing oxidative damage to tubular cells and renal tissue. Hypoxia and ischemia perturb microcirculation, cellular enzymes, metabolic and mitochondrial function, supporting production of ROS such as $O_2^{-}\cdot$, $\cdot OH$ and H_2O_2, causing signal disruption, organelle dysfunction, mitochondrial damage, depletion of ATP, and activation of cell death pathways. Moreover, hypochlorous acid and ONOO− may be relevant oxidants in AKI. Results showed increased circulating biomarkers of protein and lipid oxidation that correlate with markers of proinflammatory, pro-oxidative mediators, and cytokines [123]. Lipid peroxidation and DNA damage in ischemia are associated with the formation of 3-nitrotyrosine, a biomarker for ROS/RNS, suggesting that NO·, $O_2^{-}\cdot$, and ONOO-, contribute to renal oxidative damage.

The treatment to stop the progression is discussed; however, the elimination of noxa, maintaining normal blood volume, and taking care of the plasma electrolyte levels are the main management [124].

Conclusion and perspectives

The relevance of the clinical analyses of oxidative stress biomarkers arises from the fact that there exists considerable evidence supporting the view that oxidative stress is involved in the pathophysiology of several diseases. In this chapter, some of the best known pathologies that have a mechanism with component of oxidative stress as substantial damage were briefly addressed. However, it is important to mention that there are more diseases (not discussed in this chapter) in which oxidative stress also plays an important role in their pathogenesis.

On the other hand, the use of biomarkers to detect or measure the evolution of human diseases is being more currently used in clinical settings. However, it is important to consider the profile of the patients and their physiology as well as their previous illnesses. Although numerous applications of different methodologies for the determination of oxidative stress are described, many of these methods have been shown to be ineffective, insensitive, or require complex protocols and specific and expensive equipment that is not routinely available in clinical or research settings.

There are pro-oxidant or antioxidant oxidative stress-related biomarkers, and these can be extracellular and intracellular. Extracellular oxidative stress-related biomarkers include FRAP, carbonyls, plasma antioxidants, vitamin levels, and lipid peroxidation product levels, among others. Intracellular oxidative stress—related biomarkers principally include the activity of antioxidant enzymes, prooxidant enzymes, GSH levels, and lipid peroxidation biomarkers.

Although it is still a subject under study, cardiovascular pathologies, for example, such as hypertension or MIRI have a well-known component of ROS-mediated progression damage. In hypertension, there is an endothelial dysfunction that is a source of ROS and produces an increase in vasoconstriction. Consequently, the use of cellular biomarkers of endothelial dysfunction has the potential to produce a powerful mechanistic understanding of disease progression. In MIRI, the contribution of ROS to the oxidative damage of the myocardium caused by infarction is due to the direct and cell-mediated effects of ROS. It deserves special mention the effect derived from reperfusion and its oxygen boom that produce damage to the endothelial wall and the attraction and adhesion of leukocytes, foam cell formation, proliferation of various cell types, and induction of an inflammatory response.

In summary, the applicability of oxidative stress-related biomarkers to study the pathogenesis and clinical outcome can be applied to a wide variety of clinical settings. It is important to consider oxidative stress and chronic inflammation in patients with multiple comorbidities. The challenge is to improve the techniques for measuring current biomarkers and to study novel biomarkers for additional pathological processes, considering oxidative stress and inflammation as central processes.

Acknowledgments

This study was supported by the Agencia Nacional de Investigación y Desarrollo (ANID) to a project of the Fondo Nacional de Desarrollo Científico y Tecnológico (FONDECYT, grant number 1211850).

References

[1] Sies H. Oxidative stress: a concept in redox biology and medicine. Redox Biol 2015;4:180–3. https://doi.org/10.1016/j.redox.2015.01.002.

[2] WHO. Biomarkers in risk assessment: validity and validation. 2001. https://inchem.org/documents/ehc/ehc/ehc222.htm.

[3] Strimbu K, Tavel JA. What are biomarkers? Curr Opin HIV AIDS 2010;5:463–6. https://doi.org/10.1097/COH.0b013e32833ed177.

[4] Frijhoff J, Winyard PG, Zarkovic N, Davies SS, Stocker R, Cheng D, et al. Clinical relevance of biomarkers of oxidative stress. Antioxidants Redox Signal 2015;23:1144–70. https://doi.org/10.1089/ars.2015.6317.

[5] Rodrigo R. Oxidative stress and antioxidants: their role in human disease. Hauppauge, New York, USA: Nova Science Publishers; 2009.

[6] Sies H. Oxidative stress: concept and some practical aspects. Antioxidants 2020;9:1–6. https://doi.org/10.3390/antiox9090852.

[7] Lillo-Moya J, Rojas-Solé C, Muñoz-Salamanca D, Panieri E, Saso L, Rodrigo R. Targeting ferroptosis against ischemia/reperfusion cardiac injury. Antioxidants 2021;10:1–25. https://doi.org/10.3390/antiox10050667.

[8] Bedard K, Krause KH. The NOX family of ROS-generating NADPH oxidases: physiology and pathophysiology. Physiol Rev 2007;87:245–313. https://doi.org/10.1152/PHYSREV.00044.2005.

[9] Nishino T, Okamoto K, Kawaguchi Y, Hori H, Matsumura T, Eger BT, et al. Mechanism of the conversion of xanthine dehydrogenase to xanthine oxidase identification of the two cysteine disulfide bonds and crystal structure of a non-convertible rat liver xanthine dehydrogenase MUTANT*□ S. J Biol Chem 2005;280:24888–94. https://doi.org/10.1074/jbc.M501830200.

[10] Parks DA, Granger DN. Xanthine oxidase: biochemistry, distribution and physiology. Acta Physiol Scand Suppl 1986;548:87–99.

[11] Vásquez-Vivar J, Kalyanaraman B, Martásek P, Hogg N, Masters BSS, Karoui H, et al. Superoxide generation by endothelial nitric oxide synthase: the influence of cofactors. Proc Natl Acad Sci USA 1998;95:9220–5. https://doi.org/10.1073/PNAS.95.16.9220.

[12] Xia Y, Zweier JL. Superoxide and peroxynitrite generation from inducible nitric oxide synthase in macrophages. Proc Natl Acad Sci USA 1997;94:6954–8. https://doi.org/10.1073/PNAS.94.13.6954.

[13] Rodrigo R, Libuy M, Feliú F, Hasson D. Oxidative stress-related biomarkers in essential hypertension and ischemia-reperfusion myocardial damage. Dis Markers 2013;35:773–90. https://doi.org/10.1155/2013/974358.

[14] Poblete-Aro C, Russell-Guzmán J, Parra P, Soto-Muñoz M, Villegas-González B, Cofré-Bola-Dos C, et al. Exercise and oxidative stress in type 2 diabetes mellitus. Rev Med Chile 2018;146:362–72. https://doi.org/10.4067/S0034-98872018000300362.

[15] Watson JD. Type 2 diabetes as a redox disease. Lancet 2014;383:841–3. https://doi.org/10.1016/S0140-6736(13)62365-X.

[16] Marrocco I, Altieri F, Peluso I. Measurement and clinical significance of biomarkers of oxidative stress in humans. Oxid Med Cell Longev 2017;2017. https://doi.org/10.1155/2017/6501046.

[17] Winterbourn C. The challenges of using fluorescent probes to detect and quantify specific reactive oxygen species in living cells. Biochim Biophys Acta 2014;1840:730–8. https://doi.org/10.1016/J.BBAGEN.2013.05.004.

[18] Kohen R, Nyska A. Oxidation of biological systems: oxidative stress phenomena, antioxidants, redox reactions, and methods for their quantification. Toxicol Pathol 2002;30:620–50. https://doi.org/10.1080/01926230290166724.

[19] Gasparovic AC, Milkovic L, Sunjic SB, Zarkovic N. Cancer growth regulation by 4-hydroxynonenal. Free Radic Biol Med 2017;111:226–34. https://doi.org/10.1016/J.FREERADBIOMED.2017.01.030.

[20] Sousa BC, Pitt AR, Spickett CM. Chemistry and analysis of HNE and other prominent carbonyl-containing lipid oxidation compounds. Free Radic Biol Med 2017;111:294–308. https://doi.org/10.1016/J.FREERADBIOMED.2017.02.003.

[21] Stadtman ER. Importance of individuality in oxidative stress and aging. Free Radic Biol Med 2002;33:597–604. https://doi.org/10.1016/S0891-5849(02)00904-8.

[22] Dean RT, Fu S, Stocker R, Davies MJ. Biochemistry and pathology of radical-mediated protein oxidation. Biochem J 1997;324(Pt 1):1–18. https://doi.org/10.1042/BJ3240001.

[23] Loft S, Svoboda P, Kasai H, Tjønneland A, Vogel U, Møller P, et al. Prospective study of 8-oxo-7,8-dihydro-2'-deoxyguanosine excretion and the risk of lung cancer. Carcinogenesis 2006;27:1245–50. https://doi.org/10.1093/CARCIN/BGI313.

[24] Loft S, Svoboda P, Kawai K, Kasai H, Sørensen M, Tjønneland A, et al. Association between 8-oxo-7,8-dihydroguanine excretion and risk of lung cancer in a prospective study. Free Radic Biol Med 2012;52:167–72. https://doi.org/10.1016/j.freeradbiomed.2011.10.439.

[25] Sova H, Jukkola-Vuorinen A, Puistola U, Kauppila S, Karihtala P. 8-Hydroxydeoxyguanosine: a new potential independent prognostic factor in breast cancer. Br J Cancer 2010;102:1018–23. https://doi.org/10.1038/sj.bjc.6605565.

[26] Loft S, Olsen A, Møller P, Poulsen HE, Tjønneland A. Association between 8-oxo-7,8-dihydro-2'-deoxyguanosine excretion and risk of postmenopausal breast cancer: nested case-control study. Cancer Epidemiol Biomarkers Prev 2013;22:1289–96. https://doi.org/10.1158/1055-9965.EPI-13-0229.

[27] Lignitto L, LeBoeuf SE, Homer H, Jiang S, Askenazi M, Karakousi TR, et al. Nrf2 activation promotes lung cancer metastasis by inhibiting the degradation of Bach1. Cell 2019;178:316. https://doi.org/10.1016/J.CELL.2019.06.003.

[28] Panieri E, Buha A, Telkoparan-akillilar P, Cevik D, Kouretas D, Veskoukis A, et al. Potential applications of NRF2 modulators in cancer therapy. Antioxidants 2020;9. https://doi.org/10.3390/ANTIOX9030193.

[29] Nguyen NH, Tran GB, Nguyen CT. Anti-oxidative effects of superoxide dismutase 3 on inflammatory diseases. J Mol Med (Berl) 2020;98:59–69. https://doi.org/10.1007/S00109-019-01845-2.

[30] Misra HP, Fridovich I. The role of superoxide anion in the autoxidation of epinephrine and a simple assay for superoxide dismutase. J Biol Chem 1972;247:3170–5. https://doi.org/10.1016/s0021-9258(19)45228-9.

[31] Glorieux C, Calderon PB. Catalase, a remarkable enzyme: targeting the oldest antioxidant enzyme to find a new cancer treatment approach. Biol Chem 2017;398:1095–108. https://doi.org/10.1515/HSZ-2017-0131/PDF.

[32] Sies H. Hydrogen peroxide as a central redox signaling molecule in physiological oxidative stress: oxidative eustress. Redox Biol 2017;11:613–9. https://doi.org/10.1016/j.redox.2016.12.035.

[33] Aebi M. Catalase. In: Methods of enzymatic analysis, vol 2. NY, USA: Verlag Chemie-Academic Press; 1974.

[34] Margis R, Dunand C, Teixeira FK, Margis-Pinheiro M. Glutathione peroxidase family - an evolutionary overview. FEBS J 2008;275:3959–70. https://doi.org/10.1111/j.1742-4658.2008.06542.x.

[35] Flohé L, Günzler WA. Assays of glutathione peroxidase. Methods Enzymol 1984;105:114–20. https://doi.org/10.1016/S0076-6879(84)05015-1.

[36] Ulker S, McKeown P, Bayraktutan U. Vitamins reverse endothelial dysfunction through regulation of eNOS and NAD(P)H oxidase activities. Hypertension 2003;41:534–9. https://doi.org/10.1161/01.HYP.0000057421.28533.37.

[37] Newaz MA, Yousefipour Z, Nawal NNA. Modulation of nitric oxide synthase activity in brain, liver, and blood vessels of spontaneously hypertensive rats by ascorbic acid: protection from free radical injury. Clin Exp Hypertens 2005;27:497–508. https://doi.org/10.1081/CEH-200067681.

[38] Cárcamo JM, Pedraza A, Bórquez-Ojeda O, Golde DW. Vitamin C suppresses TNFα-induced NFκB activation by inhibiting IκBα phosphorylation. Biochemistry 2002;41:12995–3002. https://doi.org/10.1021/bi0263210.

[39] Roe JH, Kuether CA. A color reaction for dehydroascorbic acid useful in the determination of vitamin C. Science 1942;95:77. https://doi.org/10.1126/SCIENCE.95.2455.77.

[40] Burton GW, Ingold KU. Vitamin E as an in vitro and in vivo antioxidant. Ann N Y Acad Sci 1989;570:7–22. https://doi.org/10.1111/J.1749-6632.1989.TB14904.X.

[41] Teissier E, Walters-Laporte E, Duhem C, Luc G, Fruchart JC, Duriez P. Rapid quantification of alpha-tocopherol in plasma and low- and high-density lipoproteins. Clin Chem 1996;42:430–5. https://doi.org/10.1093/CLINCHEM/42.3.430.

[42] Forman HJ, Zhang H, Rinna A. Glutathione: overview of its protective roles, measurement, and biosynthesis. Mol Aspect Med 2009;30:1–12. https://doi.org/10.1016/J.MAM.2008.08.006.

[43] Hissin PJ, Hilf R. A fluorometric method for determination of oxidized and reduced glutathione in tissues. Anal Biochem 1976;74:214–26. https://doi.org/10.1016/0003-2697(76)90326-2.

[44] Benzie IFF, Strain JJ. The ferric reducing ability of plasma (FRAP) as a measure of "antioxidant power": the FRAP assay. Anal Biochem 1996;239:70–6. https://doi.org/10.1006/ABIO.1996.0292.

[45] Gulcin İ. Antioxidants and antioxidant methods: an updated overview. Arch Toxicol 2020;94:651–715. https://doi.org/10.1007/S00204-020-02689-3.

[46] Sambiagio N, Berthet A, Wild P, Sauvain JJ, Auer R, Schoeni A, et al. Associations between urinary biomarkers of oxidative stress and biomarkers of tobacco smoke exposure in smokers. Sci Total Environ 2022;852. https://doi.org/10.1016/J.SCITOTENV.2022.158361.

[47] Brouwers S, Sudano I, Kokubo Y, Sulaica E. Arterial hypertension. Lancet (London, England) 2021;398:249–61. https://doi.org/10.1016/S0140-6736(21)00221-X.

[48] NCD Risk Factor Collaboration (NCD-RisC). Worldwide trends in hypertension prevalence and progress in treatment and control from 1990 to 2019: a pooled analysis of 1201 population-representative studies with 104 million participants. Lancet 2021;398:957–80. https://doi.org/10.1016/S0140-6736(21)01330-1.

[49] Kovacic JC, Moreno P, Hachinski V, Nabel EG, Fuster V. Cellular senescence, vascular disease, and aging. Circulation 2011;123:1650–60. https://doi.org/10.1161/CIRCULATIONAHA.110.007021.

[50] Zepeda RJ, Castillo R, Rodrigo R, Prieto JC, Aramburu I, Brugere S, et al. Effect of carvedilol and nebivolol on oxidative stress-related parameters and endothelial function in patients with essential hypertension. Basic Clin Pharmacol Toxicol 2012;111:309–16. https://doi.org/10.1111/J.1742-7843.2012.00911.X.

[51] Montezano AC, Dulak-Lis M, Tsiropoulou S, Harvey A, Briones AM, Touyz RM. Oxidative stress and human hypertension: vascular mechanisms, biomarkers, and novel therapies. Can J Cardiol 2015;31:631–41. https://doi.org/10.1016/J.CJCA.2015.02.008.

[52] Xiao L, Liu Y, Wang N. New paradigms in inflammatory signaling in vascular endothelial cells. Am J Physiol Heart Circ Physiol 2014;306. https://doi.org/10.1152/AJPHEART.00182.2013.

[53] Rodrigo R, Prat H, Passalacqua W, Araya J, Guichard C, Bächler JP. Relationship between oxidative stress and essential hypertension. Hypertens Res 2007;30:1159–67. https://doi.org/10.1291/hypres.30.1159.

[54] Sinha N, Dabla P. Oxidative stress and antioxidants in hypertension—a current review. Curr Hypertens Rev 2015;11:132–42. https://doi.org/10.2174/1573402111666150529130922.

[55] Guzik TJ, Touyz RM. Oxidative stress, inflammation, and vascular aging in hypertension. Hypertension 2017;70:660–7. https://doi.org/10.1161/HYPERTENSIONAHA.117.07802.

[56] P. Pantelidis, M. Sideris, et al, undefined 2018, The mechanisms of actions of aldosterone and its antagonists in cardiovascular disease, Ingentaconnect.Com. (n.d.). https://www.ingentaconnect.com/content/ben/cpd/2018/00000024/00000046/art00003 (accessed July 25, 2022).

[57] McCurley A, Pires P, Bender S, Medicine MA-N. Direct regulation of blood pressure by smooth muscle cell mineralocorticoid receptors. Nat Commun 2012;18:1429–33.

[58] Virdis A, Neves MF, Amiri F, Viel E, Touyz RM, Schiffrin EL. Spironolactone improves angiotensin-induced vascular changes and oxidative stress. Hypertension 2002;40:504–10. https://doi.org/10.1161/01.HYP.0000034738.79310.06.

[59] Bienvenu L, Morgan J, Rickard A, et al. Macrophage mineralocorticoid receptor signaling plays a key role in aldosterone-independent cardiac fibrosis. Endocrinology 2012;153:3416–25.

[60] Ahokas RA, Warrington KJ, Gerling IC, Sun Y, Wodi LA, Herring PA, et al. Aldosteronism and peripheral blood mononuclear cell activation. Circ Res 2003;93. https://doi.org/10.1161/01.RES.0000102404.81461.25.

[61] Derhaschnig U, Testori C, Riedmueller E, Aschauer S, Wolzt M, Jilma B. Hypertensive emergencies are associated with elevated markers of inflammation, coagulation, platelet activation and fibrinolysis. J Hum Hypertens 2012;27:368–73. https://doi.org/10.1038/JHH.2012.53.

[62] Dawes M, Brett SE, Chowjenczyk PJ, Mant TGK, Ritter JM. The vasodilator action of nebivolol in forearm vasculature of subjects with essential hypertension. Br J Clin Pharmacol 1999;48:460–3. https://doi.org/10.1046/J.1365-2125.1999.00037.X.

[63] Dandona P, Ghanim H, Brooks DP. Antioxidant activity of carvedilol in cardiovascular disease. J Hypertens 2007;25:731–41. https://doi.org/10.1097/HJH.0B013E3280127948.

[64] Burton GJ, Jauniaux E. Oxidative stress. Best Pract Res Clin Obstet Gynaecol 2011;25:287–99. https://doi.org/10.1016/J.BPOBGYN.2010.10.016.

[65] Rani N, Dhingra R, Arya DS, Kalaivani M, Bhatla N, Kumar R. Role of oxidative stress markers and antioxidants in the placenta of

preeclamptic patients. J Obstet Gynaecol Res 2010;36:1189–94. https://doi.org/10.1111/J.1447-0756.2010.01303.X.

[66] Visintin C, Mugglestone MA, Almerie MQ, Nherera LM, James D, Walkinshaw S. Management of hypertensive disorders during pregnancy: summary of NICE guidance. BMJ 2010;341:499–501. https://doi.org/10.1136/BMJ.C2207.

[67] Magee LA, Helewa M, Mb W, Rey E, Von Dadelszen P, Audibert F, et al. Diagnosis, evaluation, and management of the hypertensive disorders of pregnancy: executive summary. 2014. http://www.pregnancyhypertension.org/article/S2210-. [Accessed 30 July 2022].

[68] Yang Y, Jin H, Qiu Y, Liu Y, Wen L, Fu Y, et al. Reactive oxygen species are essential for placental angiogenesis during early gestation. Oxid Med Cell Longev 2022;2022:1–14. https://doi.org/10.1155/2022/4290922.

[69] Hamad RR, Larsson A, Pernow J, Bremme K, Eriksson MJ. Assessment of left ventricular structure and function in preeclampsia by echocardiography and cardiovascular biomarkers. J Hypertens 2009;27:2257–64. https://doi.org/10.1097/HJH.0B013E3283300541.

[70] Santoyo JM, Noguera JA, Avilés F, Delgado JL, de Paco-Matallana C, Pérez V, et al. Factors involved in endothelial dysfunction related to angiogenic disbalance and oxidative stress, in Women at High Risk of Term Pre-Eclampsia. Antioxidants (Basel, Switzerland) 2022;11:1409. https://doi.org/10.3390/ANTIOX11071409.

[71] Karrar SA, Hong PL. Preeclampsia, StatPearls. 2022. https://www-ncbi-nlm-nih-gov.uchile.idm.oclc.org/books/NBK570611/. [Accessed 31 July 2022].

[72] Dap M, Romiti J, Dolenc B, Morel O. Thrombotic thrombocytopenic purpura and severe preeclampsia: a clinical overlap during pregnancy and a possible coexistence. J Gynecol Obstet Hum Reprod 2022;51:102422. https://doi.org/10.1016/J.JOGOH.2022.102422.

[73] Lam C, Lim KH, Kang DH, Karumanchi SA. Uric acid and pre-eclampsia. Semin Nephrol 2005;25:56–60. https://doi.org/10.1016/J.SEMNEPHROL.2004.09.009.

[74] Wei W, Wang X, Zhou Y, Shang X, Yu H. The genetic risk factors for pregnancy-induced hypertension: evidence from genetic polymorphisms. Faseb J 2022;36. https://doi.org/10.1096/FJ.202101853RR.

[75] Zaugg J, Solenthaler F, Albrecht C. Materno-fetal iron transfer and the emerging role of ferroptosis pathways. Biochem Pharmacol 2022;202:115141. https://doi.org/10.1016/J.BCP.2022.115141.

[76] Dai D-F, Chiao YA, Marcinek DJ, Szeto HH, Rabinovitch PS. Mitochondrial oxidative stress in aging and healthspan. Longev Heal 2014;3. https://doi.org/10.1186/2046-2395-3-6.

[77] Kelso GF, Porteous CM, Coulter CV, Hughes G, Porteous WK, Ledgerwood EC, et al. Selective targeting of a redox-active ubiquinone to mitochondria within cells: antioxidant and antiapoptotic properties. J Biol Chem 2001;276:4588–96. https://doi.org/10.1074/JBC.M009093200.

[78] Torres M. Mitogen-activated protein kinase pathways in redox signaling. Front Biosci 2003;8. https://doi.org/10.2741/999.

[79] Myatt L, Cui X. Oxidative stress in the placenta. Histochem Cell Biol 2004;122:369–82. https://doi.org/10.1007/S00418-004-0677-X.

[80] Schoofs K, Grittner U, Engels T, Pape J, Denk B, Henrich W, et al. The importance of repeated measurements of the sFlt-1/PlGF ratio for the prediction of preeclampsia and intrauterine growth restriction. J Perinat Med 2014;42:61–8. https://doi.org/10.1515/JPM-2013-0074.

[81] Aydin S, Benian A, Madazli R, Uludağ S, Uzun H, Kaya S. Plasma malondialdehyde, superoxide dismutase, sE-selectin, fibronectin, endothelin-1 and nitric oxide levels in women with preeclampsia. Eur J Obstet Gynecol Reprod Biol 2004;113:21–5. https://doi.org/10.1016/S0301-2115(03)00368-3.

[82] Mutlu-Türkoğlu Ü, Ademoğlu E, Ibrahimoğlu L, Aykąç-Toker G, Uysal M. Imbalance between lipid peroxidation and antioxidant status in preeclampsia. Gynecol Obstet Invest 1998;46:37–40. https://doi.org/10.1159/000009994.

[83] Halladin NL. Oxidative and inflammatory biomarkers of ischemia and reperfusion injuries. Dan Med J 2014;62:B5054.

[84] Wu M, Yiang G, Liao W, Tsai A, Cheng Y, Cheng P, et al. Current mechanistic concepts in ischemia and reperfusion injury. Cell Physiol Biochem 2018;46:1650–67. https://doi.org/10.1159/000489241.

[85] Paravicini TM, Touyz RM. NADPH oxidases, reactive oxygen species, and hypertension: clinical implications and therapeutic possibilities. Diabetes Care 2008;31(Suppl. 2). https://doi.org/10.2337/DC08-S247.

[86] Brandes RP, Weissmann N, Schröder K. Redox-mediated signal transduction by cardiovascular Nox NADPH oxidases. J Mol Cell Cardiol 2014;73:70–9. https://doi.org/10.1016/J.YJMCC.2014.02.006.

[87] Chung H, Baek B, Song S, Kim M, Huh J, Shim K, et al. Xanthine dehydrogenase/xanthine oxidase and oxidative stress. Age 1997;20:127–40. https://doi.org/10.1007/S11357-997-0012-2.

[88] Lee M, Velayutham M, Komatsu T, Hille R, Zweier J. Measurement and characterization of superoxide generation from xanthine dehydrogenase: a redox-regulated pathway of radical generation in ischemic tissues. Biochemistry 2014;53:6615–23. https://doi.org/10.1021/BI500582R.

[89] Förstermann U, Sessa W. Nitric oxide synthases: regulation and function. Eur Heart J 2012;33. https://doi.org/10.1093/EURHEARTJ/EHR304.

[90] Alkaitis M, Crabtree M. Recoupling the cardiac nitric oxide synthases: tetrahydrobiopterin synthesis and recycling. Curr Heart Fail Rep 2012;9:200–10. https://doi.org/10.1007/S11897-012-0097-5.

[91] World Health Organization. Cardiovascular diseases (CVDs). 2021. https://www.who.int/news-room/fact-sheets/detail/cardiovascular-diseases-(cvds). [Accessed 1 October 2022].

[92] Rodrigo R, Prieto JC, Aguayo R, Ramos C, Puentes Á, Gajardo A, et al. Joint cardioprotective effect of vitamin C and other antioxidants against reperfusion injury in patients with acute myocardial infarction undergoing percutaneous coronary intervention. Molecules 2021;26. https://doi.org/10.3390/MOLECULES26185702.

[93] Lu Y, Li S, Lou H. Patchouli alcohol protects against myocardial ischaemia-reperfusion injury by regulating the Notch1/Hes1 pathway. Pharm Biol 2022;60:949–57. https://doi.org/10.1080/13880209.2022.2064881.

[94] Yellon DM, Hausenloy DJ. Myocardial reperfusion injury. N Engl J Med 2007;357:1121–35. https://doi.org/10.1056/NEJMRA071667.

[95] Zou R, Shi W, Qiu J, Zhou N, Du N, Zhou H, et al. Empagliflozin attenuates cardiac microvascular ischemia/reperfusion injury through improving mitochondrial homeostasis. Cardiovasc Diabetol 2022;21. https://doi.org/10.1186/S12933-022-01532-6.

[96] Peng JR, Lu TT, Chang HT, Ge X, Huang B, Li WM. Elevated levels of plasma superoxide dismutases 1 and 2 in patients with coronary artery disease. BioMed Res Int 2016;2016. https://doi.org/10.1155/2016/3708905.

[97] Nepal M, Jaisawal S, Guragain M, Kafle P, Mukkera S, Ghimire RK, et al. Ischemic modified albumin (IMA) as a novel marker for ischemic heart disease and surrogate marker for other high oxidative-ischemic conditions. J Cardiovasc Dis Res 2017;8:112–6. https://doi.org/10.5530/JCDR.2017.4.26.
[98] Dare AJ, Bolton EA, Pettigrew GJ, Bradley JA, Saeb-Parsy K, Murphy MP. Protection against renal ischemia-reperfusion injury in vivo by the mitochondria targeted antioxidant MitoQ. Redox Biol 2015;5:163–8. https://doi.org/10.1016/J.REDOX.2015.04.008.
[99] Gottwald EM, Duss M, Bugarski M, Haenni D, Schuh CD, Landau EM, et al. The targeted anti-oxidant MitoQ causes mitochondrial swelling and depolarization in kidney tissue. Phys Rep 2018;6. https://doi.org/10.14814/PHY2.13667.
[100] Castillo R, Rodrigo R, Perez F, Cereceda M, Asenjo R, Zamorano J, et al. Antioxidant therapy reduces oxidative and inflammatory tissue damage in patients subjected to cardiac surgery with extracorporeal circulation. Basic Clin Pharmacol Toxicol 2011;108:256–62. https://doi.org/10.1111/J.1742-7843.2010.00651.X.
[101] Orellana-Urzúa S, Rojas I, Líbano L, Rodrigo R. Pathophysiology of ischemic stroke: role of oxidative stress. Curr Pharmaceut Des 2020;26:4246–60. https://doi.org/10.2174/1381612826666200708133912.
[102] World Health Organization, Stroke, Cerebrovascular accident, (n.d.). http://www.emro.who.int/health-topics/stroke-cerebrovascular-accident/index.html (accessed November 3, 2021).
[103] Tsao CW, Aday AW, Almarzooq ZI, Alonso A, Beaton AZ, Bittencourt MS, et al. Heart disease and stroke statistics-2022 update: a report from the American heart association. Circulation 2022;145:e153–639. https://doi.org/10.1161/CIR.0000000000001052.
[104] Wang Z, Liu T, Gan L, Wang T, Yuan X, Zhang B, et al. Shikonin protects mouse brain against cerebral ischemia/reperfusion injury through its antioxidant activity. Eur J Pharmacol 2010;643:211–7. https://doi.org/10.1016/J.EJPHAR.2010.06.027.
[105] Muñoz Cimadevilla H. Nuevos métodos para la determinación de estrés oxidativo. Aplicación al acv isquémico - dialnet. Universidad de Oviedo; 2015. https://dialnet.unirioja.es/servlet/tesis?codigo=208104. [Accessed 1 August 2022].
[106] Kleinschnitz C, Grund H, Wingler K, Armitage ME, Jones E, Mittal M, et al. Post-stroke inhibition of induced NADPH oxidase type 4 prevents oxidative stress and neurodegeneration. PLoS Biol 2010;8:e1000479. https://doi.org/10.1371/JOURNAL.PBIO.1000479.
[107] Eom JW, Lee JM, Koh JY, Kim YH. AMP-activated protein kinase contributes to zinc-induced neuronal death via activation by LKB1 and induction of Bim in mouse cortical cultures. Mol Brain 2016;9. https://doi.org/10.1186/S13041-016-0194-6.
[108] Eom JW, Kim TY, Seo BR, Park H, Koh JY, Kim YH. Identifying new AMP-activated protein kinase inhibitors that protect against ischemic brain injury. ACS Chem Neurosci 2019;10:2345–54. https://doi.org/10.1021/ACSCHEMNEURO.8B00654.
[109] Dávila D, Jiménez-Mateos EM, Mooney CM, Velasco G, Henshall DC, Prehn JHM. Hsp27 binding to the 3'UTR of bim mRNA prevents neuronal death during oxidative stress-induced injury: a novel cytoprotective mechanism. Mol Biol Cell 2014;25:3413–23. https://doi.org/10.1091/MBC.E13-08-0495.
[110] O'Collins VE, Macleod MR, Donnan GA, Horky LL, Van Der Worp BH, Howells DW. 1,026 experimental treatments in acute stroke. Ann Neurol 2006;59:467–77. https://doi.org/10.1002/ANA.20741.
[111] Rodrigo R, Fernandez-Gajardo R, Gutierrez R, Matamala J, Carrasco R, Miranda-Merchak A, et al. Oxidative stress and pathophysiology of ischemic stroke: novel therapeutic opportunities. CNS Neurol Disord Drug Targets 2013;12:698–714. https://doi.org/10.2174/1871527311312050015.
[112] Kamat CD, Gadal S, Mhatre M, Williamson KS, Pye QN, Hensley K. Antioxidants in central nervous system diseases: preclinical promise and translational challenges. J Alzheimers Dis 2008;15:473. https://doi.org/10.3233/JAD-2008-15314.
[113] von Dessauer B, Bongain J, Molina V, Quilodrán J, Castillo R, Rodrigo R. Oxidative stress as a novel target in pediatric sepsis management. J Crit Care 2011;26:103.e1–7. https://doi.org/10.1016/J.JCRC.2010.05.001.
[114] Vera S, Martínez R, Gormaz JG, Gajardo A, Galleguillos F, Rodrigo R. Novel relationships between oxidative stress and angiogenesis-related factors in sepsis: new biomarkers and therapies. Ann Med 2015;47:289–300. https://doi.org/10.3109/07853890.2015.1029967.
[115] Di Meo S, Reed TT, Venditti P, Victor VM. Role of ROS and RNS sources in physiological and pathological conditions. Oxid Med Cell Longev 2016;2016. https://doi.org/10.1155/2016/1245049.
[116] Andrades MT, Morina A, Spasić S, Spasojević I. Bench-to-bedside review: sepsis - from the redox point of view. Crit Care 2011;15. https://doi.org/10.1186/CC10334.
[117] Liu L, Sun B. Neutrophil pyroptosis: new perspectives on sepsis. Cell Mol Life Sci 2019;76. https://doi.org/10.1007/S00018-019-03060-1.
[118] Molina V, von Dessauer B, Rodrigo R, Carvajal C. Oxidative stress biomarkers in pediatric sepsis: a prospective observational pilot study. Redox Rep 2017;22:330–7. https://doi.org/10.1080/13510002.2016.1239866.
[119] Basile DP, Anderson MD, Sutton TA. Pathophysiology of acute kidney injury. Compr Physiol 2012;2:1303–53. https://doi.org/10.1002/CPHY.C110041.
[120] Dennis JM, Witting PK. Protective role for antioxidants in acute kidney disease. Nutrients 2017;9. https://doi.org/10.3390/NU9070718.
[121] Aniort J, Heng AÉ, Deteix P, Souweine B, Lautrette A. Epidemiology of acute renal failure. Néphrol Thérapeutique 2019;15:63–9. https://doi.org/10.1016/J.NEPHRO.2018.11.002.
[122] Sharma R, Gaze DC, Pellerin D, Mehta RL, Gregson H, Streather CP, et al. Ischemia-modified albumin predicts mortality in ESRD. Am J Kidney Dis 2006;47:493–502. https://doi.org/10.1053/J.AJKD.2005.11.026.
[123] Himmelfarb J, McMonagle E, Freedman S, Klenzak J, McMenamin E, Le P, et al. Oxidative stress is increased in critically ill patients with acute renal failure. J Am Soc Nephrol 2004;15:2449–56. https://doi.org/10.1097/01.ASN.0000138232.68452.3B.
[124] Bellomo R, Kellum JA, Ronco C. Acute kidney injury. Lancet (London, England) 2012;380:756–66. https://doi.org/10.1016/S0140-6736(11)61454-2.
[125] Ahsan H. 3-Nitrotyrosine: a biomarker of nitrogen free radical species modified proteins in systemic autoimmunogenic conditions. Hum Immunol 2013;74:1392–9. https://doi.org/10.1016/J.HUMIMM.2013.06.009.
[126] Gallo G, Sprovieri P, Martino G. 4-hydroxynonenal and oxidative stress in several organelles and its damaging effects on cell functions. J Physiol Pharmacol 2020;71. https://doi.org/10.26402/JPP.2020.1.07.

[127] Ellis EM. Reactive carbonyls and oxidative stress: potential for therapeutic intervention. Pharmacol Ther 2007;115:13–24. https://doi.org/10.1016/J.PHARMTHERA.2007.03.015.

[128] El Assar M, Angulo J, Rodríguez-Mañas L. Oxidative stress and vascular inflammation in aging. Free Radic Biol Med 2013;65:380–401. https://doi.org/10.1016/J.FREERADBIOMED.2013.07.003.

[129] Nikolaidis MG, Kyparos A, Vrabas IS. F2-isoprostane formation, measurement and interpretation: the role of exercise. Prog Lipid Res 2011;50:89–103. https://doi.org/10.1016/J.PLIPRES.2010.10.002.

[130] Tsikas D. Assessment of lipid peroxidation by measuring malondialdehyde (MDA) and relatives in biological samples: analytical and biological challenges. Anal Biochem 2017;524:13–30. https://doi.org/10.1016/J.AB.2016.10.021.

[131] Bryk D, Olejarz W, Zapolska-Downar D. The role of oxidative stress and NADPH oxidase in the pathogenesis of atherosclerosis. Adv Hyg Exp Med 2017;71:57–68. https://doi.org/10.5604/01.3001.0010.3790.

[132] Glantzounis G, Tsimoyiannis E, Kappas A, Galaris D. Uric acid and oxidative stress. Curr Pharmaceut Des 2005;11:4145–51. https://doi.org/10.2174/138161205774913255.

[133] Lubos E, Loscalzo J, Handy DE. Glutathione peroxidase-1 in health and disease: from molecular mechanisms to therapeutic opportunities. Antioxidants Redox Signal 2011;15:1957. https://doi.org/10.1089/ARS.2010.3586.

[134] Nozik-Grayck E, Suliman HB, Piantadosi CA. Extracellular superoxide dismutase. Int J Biochem Cell Biol 2005;37:2466–71. https://doi.org/10.1016/J.BIOCEL.2005.06.012.

Chapter 9

Modulation of the antioxidant defense system against pathophysiological redox imbalance in cardiovascular diseases

José Lillo-Moya, Catalina Rojas-Solé and Ramón Rodrigo
Molecular and Clinical Pharmacology Program, Institute of Biomedical Sciences, Faculty of Medicine, University of Chile, Santiago, Chile

Introduction

We are currently undergoing an epidemiological transition due to the increase in life expectancy and along with this, the increase in noncommunicable diseases, which kill 41 million people each year equivalent to 71% of all deaths globally. Within this group, cardiovascular diseases constitute the majority of deaths from noncommunicable diseases, resulting in 18.6 million deaths per year. It has many causes, such as smoking, diabetes, sedentary lifestyle, dyslipidemia, high blood pressure, obesity, air pollution, and less common conditions such as Chagas disease and cardiac amyloidosis [1,2].

Oxidative stress is an unbalance between the abundance of pro-oxidant and antioxidant agents in favor of the first, and their responses can have important repercussions on cardiac tissue that cause the development of pathologies, leading to heart failure as the final event. It should be noted that oxidative stress is a common theme in the pathophysiology of ischemic and nonischemic cardiomyopathy. However, there are many changes that precede heart failure such as cardiac hypertrophy and impairing remodeling which depends on homeostatic alterations occurring in oxidative and nitrosative stresses.

This is why early treatment or intervention in the oxidative stress process can have very important therapeutic implications with great benefits in cardiovascular morbidity and mortality, especially in the management of heart failure. Indeed, various antioxidant drugs as well as preconditioning therapies have been studied to prevent the damage caused by reactive oxygen species (ROS) and reactive nitrogen species (RNS), thus maintaining adequate pro-oxidant and antioxidant homeostasis. Furthermore, indirect and endogenous modulation of antioxidant systems can also be a therapeutic target [3–5].

This chapter presents a perspective of the mechanisms of several cardiac diseases that are involved in the maintenance of the pro- and antioxidant homeostasis and the protective effect of dietary and pharmacological agents capable of modulating these injurious mechanisms through an enhancement of the antioxidant defense system.

Modulation of the antioxidant defense system components

The antioxidant system is a fundamental part of our cells. It is responsible for combating those states where the oxidative component begins to increase. This is made up of an enzymatic part, where we find superoxide dismutase (SOD), catalase (CAT), peroxiredoxins, thioredoxins, glutaredoxins, and glutathione peroxidases (GPX), as well as a nonenzymatic part, within which we have reduced glutathione, NADPH, and exogenous molecules including vitamin C, vitamin E, carotenoids, flavonoids, and polyphenols, among others [6]. All this machinery is present in the cell to be able to respond to oxidative stress. However, under certain circumstances, such as some cardiovascular pathologies, the activity of this system is diminished, making it more vulnerable to oxidative damage. In addition, there are pathologies where oxidative stress is fundamental in its pathogenesis, causing the antioxidant response to be insufficient to provide a response that mitigates the damage. Due to this, various pharmacological strategies have been developed to modulate this antioxidant system and thus be able to respond to various diseases related to oxidative stress.

Modulation of Oxidative Stress. https://doi.org/10.1016/B978-0-443-19247-0.00009-6

Antioxidant enzymes modulation

Antioxidant enzymes play a fundamental role in the response against oxidative stress, with SOD, CAT, and GPX enzymes being the first line of cellular defense (Fig. 9.1). In general, the role of SOD is to reduce the superoxide anion radical ($O_2^{\cdot-}$) to hydrogen peroxide (H_2O_2). SOD has three isoforms in mammalian cells: cytosolic or Cu/ZnSOD, mitochondrial or MnSOD, and extracellular SOD. The latter is particularly found in the walls of vascular tissue, being synthesized mainly by smooth muscle cells [7,8]. The $O_2^{\cdot-}$ is produced physiologically at the vascular level as a product of cellular metabolism. It is a precursor in the generation of H_2O_2 and peroxynitrite ($ONOO^-$) and has a role in the modulation of the tone of blood vessels, so that alterations in SOD have been reflected in cardiovascular-related pathologies, such as hypertension and atherosclerosis [9]. A decrease in extracellular SOD has also been associated with remodeling of the cardiac left ventricle, which could indicate a link between extracellular SOD and heart failure [10]. CAT reduces H_2O_2 to water (H_2O), as does GPX, where the latter is also capable of reducing organic hydroperoxides by oxidizing reduced glutathione. It has been reported that increased expression of SOD or CAT inhibited the development of atherosclerosis in apolipoprotein E knockout mice [11]. On the other hand, alterations in GPX levels have also been associated with various cardiovascular diseases. In mammalian cells, there are different isoforms of GPX (GPX-1, GPX-2, GPX-3, and GPX-4). Regarding GPX-1, it has been reported that a higher activity of this enzyme allows preserving cardiac function after an IR process, as well as their activity is fundamental to maintain endothelial function [12].

Finally, many of the cardiovascular pathologies include the formation of high levels of ROS and oxidative stress at

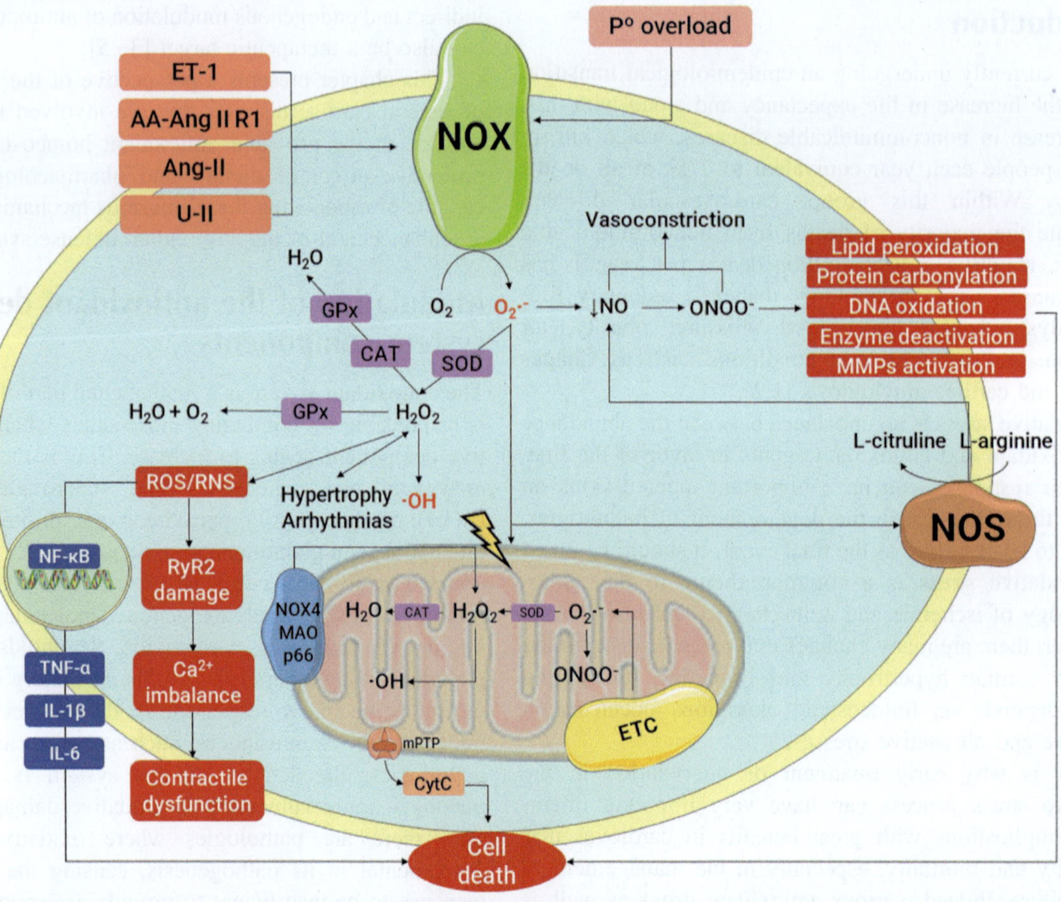

FIGURE 9.1 Molecular mechanisms of oxidative stress-induced injury and inflammation in cardiomyocytes and the central role of the mitochondria. *AA-Ang II R1*, agonistic autoantibodies to type 1 angiotensin II receptor; *Ang-II*, angiotensin II; Ca^{2+}, calcium; *CAT*, catalase; *CytC*: Cytochrome C; *DNA*, deoxyribonucleic acid; *ET-1*, endothelin 1; *ETC*, electron transport chain; *GPx*, glutathione peroxidase; H_2O, water; H_2O_2, hydrogen peroxide; $HO^{\cdot}$, hydroxyl radical; *IL-1β*, interleukin 1 beta; *IL-6*, interleukin 6; *MMPs*, extracellular matrix metalloproteinases; *mPTP*, mitochondrial permeability transition pore; *NF-κB*, nuclear factor kappa-light-chain-enhancer of the activated B cells; *NO*, nitric oxide; *NOS*, nitric oxide synthase; *NOX*, NADPH oxidase; O_2, oxygen; $O_2^{\cdot-}$, superoxide anion; $ONOO^-$, peroxynitrite; *ROS*, reactive oxygen species; *RNS*, reactive nitrogen species; *RyR2*, ryanodine receptor 2; *SOD*, superoxide dismutase; *TNF-α*, tumor necrosis factor alpha; *U-II*, urotensin II.

the level of the vascular walls, such as atherosclerosis, diabetes, hypertension, thrombosis, or myocardial ischemia/reperfusion [13], thus enhancing the activity and formation of antioxidant enzymes become relevant as a possible pharmacological and therapeutic target.

Exogenous direct antioxidants

Vitamin C

Vitamin C or ascorbic acid is a water-soluble antioxidant compound, which reduces free radicals by donating electrons and oxidizing to dehydroascorbate. This compound can be acquired through foods such as fruits or vegetables or as supplements orally or intravenously since our cells do not synthesize this molecule. Although the best known mechanism of action of vitamin C is that of ROS scavenger, it has also been shown to be able to modulate enzymes and thus indirectly reduce the formation of ROS (Fig. 9.2). Within these modulations, it has been reported that vitamin C can decrease the expression of the NADPH oxidase enzyme (NOX) [14], inhibit the activation of NF-κB pathway [15], prevent the uncoupling of endothelial NOS (eNOS) enzyme through the stabilization of BH4 (prevents its oxidation) and improve the generation of nitric oxide (NO), increasing the vasodilation [16,17], as well as is responsible for recycling vitamin E in the interphase of lipid-aqueous compartments [18], lipid bilayer [19], and erythrocytes [20] (Fig. 9.2).

The use of vitamin C in the context of cardiovascular diseases has long been discussed, where the results in the various studies that have been carried out are discordant. Within these studies, at the level of prevention of cardiovascular diseases, a meta-analysis has concluded that observational cohort studies, clinical trials and other meta-analyses have not shown a clear tendency for vitamin C supplementation to have cardiovascular benefits [21]. However, they highlight that observational cohort studies report that a higher concentration of vitamin C in plasma could be related to a lower risk of heart disease [21–23]. On the other hand, regarding vitamin C as a treatment, its use is still under discussion. In pathologies such as hypertension, previous clinical trials have shown that the administration of vitamin C lowers blood pressure [24,25], as well as recently it has been shown that vitamin C supplementation generates a significant vasodilator effect in patients with essential hypertension [6,26]. As for its use in myocardial IRI after angioplasty in patients with acute myocardial infarction, this has been widely discussed, where some studies actually show a decrease in oxidative stress parameters but that ultimately do not correlate with a lower infarct size, as well as a trend toward improvements in cardiac functional parameters [27].

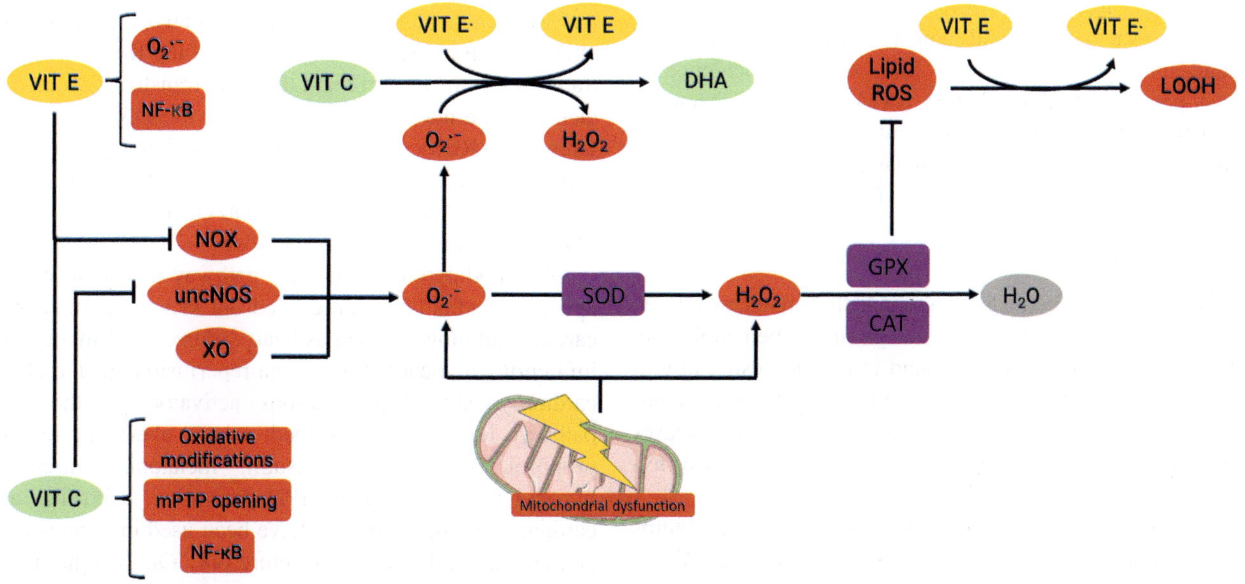

FIGURE 9.2 Molecular mechanisms of antioxidant activity of enzymes and vitamin C and E. Oxidizing enzymes such as NADPH oxidase (NOX), uncoupled nitric oxide synthase (uncNOS), and xanthine oxidase (XO), as well as mitochondria, generate reactive oxygen species (ROS) such as hydrogen peroxide and superoxide anion radical. The former is reduced by the enzyme superoxide dismutase (SOD) to hydrogen peroxide. However, vitamin C and E can also reduce it. Hydrogen peroxide can subsequently be reduced to water by both the enzyme catalase (CAT) and glutathione peroxidase (GPX). In addition, glutathione peroxidase and vitamin E can reduce lipid organic radicals in alcoholic lipids and thus reduce damage to biological membranes due to oxidation. Other functions of vitamin E correspond to the decrease in NOX activity and the down-regulation of the NF-κB pathway, just like vitamin C, but in addition, vitamin C manages to recycle vitamin E and thereby continue reducing ROS, as well. It also manages to reduce other types of oxidative modifications and prevent the opening of the mPTP in the event of an increase in calcium, as can occur in cardiac ischemia-reperfusion damage.

Finally, Lykkedsfeldt and Tveden-Nyborg concluded that there has been a lack of understanding regarding the pharmacokinetics of vitamin C, which has led to suboptimal designs, misinterpretations, and erroneous conclusions in clinical trials [28]. This finally makes it difficult to compare the results between different studies in such a way as to conclude the true pharmacological properties that vitamin C possesses in human health and disease.

Vitamin E

Vitamin E or alpha-tocopherol is a lipid-soluble molecule with antioxidant and anti-inflammatory capacity (Fig. 9.2). This can act directly as an ROS scavenger, as well as being able to modulate enzymes such as eNOS to prevent its uncoupling and reduce NOX activity [29]. Epidemiological data have reported that a high intake of vitamin E could be associated with a lower incidence of cardiovascular disease [30,31], as well as a reduced risk of coronary pathology in men [32], but this is still a matter of discussion since other studies have not been able to demonstrate this protective effect of vitamin E [33]. Regarding the treatment of hypertension, the use of vitamin E by itself has not shown benefits, but its association with vitamin C in a randomized double-blind placebo-controlled clinical trial has managed to reduce both the systolic and diastolic pressure of patients [34]. Regarding its use to reduce damage due to myocardial reperfusion, different results have been obtained that are not conclusive. However, when used in combination with vitamin C, it was shown in a clinical trial to decrease oxidative stress levels and improve cardiac function in patients undergoing angioplasty [35]. A lower incidence of postoperative atrial fibrillation (POAF) has also been reported when using vitamin E in combination with other direct antioxidants such as vitamin C and indirect antioxidants such as n-3 polyunsaturated fatty acids (PUFAs) [33,36].

Polyphenols

Polyphenols are chemical compounds that are characterized by having more than one phenol group in their molecule. They are common nutrients found in the diet, especially in vegetables, and are substances with great antioxidant power, especially used in the study of cardiovascular diseases such as atherosclerosis-related ischemic heart disease, hypertension, and stroke [37,38].

In this group, there are flavonoids, quercetin, lignins and lignans, kampferol, and catechins, among others. Polyphenols increase eNOS activity, inhibit oxidases such as NOX and xanthine oxidase (XO), and consequently reduce ROS production along with enhancing mitochondrial oxidative stress. In addition, antiatherogenic, antithrombotic, anti-inflammatory, and metal chelators effects have been described [39,40]. Indeed, these compounds act as a cardioprotector by improving endothelial function through acting as ROS scavengers and increasing NO bioavailability [41,42]. In addition, it has been described that multiple polyphenols have the ability to be activators of the nuclear factor erythroid 2-related factor 2 (Nrf2) pathway, which increases the endogenous antioxidant response by translocating to the nucleus, as will be explained later in this chapter [43] (Fig. 9.3). The anti-inflammatory effect is due to the down-regulation of the genomic pathway of NF-κB and the modulation several regulators of inflammatory response such as the inhibition of cytokines (TNF-α, IL-1-β, and IL-6) [44,45] and arachidonic acid pathways by their function to inhibit cellular enzymes, such as PLA2, COX, and LOX [46,47] (Fig. 9.3), producing beneficial effects in the progression of chronic diseases [44].

However, more research is still needed to determine dosage, long-term use, pharmacokinetic, and toxicological profile [33].

Indirect antioxidants

Indirect antioxidants are those that do not act directly on ROS or RNS but instead activate signaling pathways such as the Nrf2, which is capable of generating an antioxidant response at the genomic level. One of the ways to modulate this system corresponds to the use of polyunsaturated fatty acids, which induce the formation of ROS but at sub-lethal levels, in such a way as to give a stimulus from this nonhypoxic preconditioning to the cell by activating the Nrf2 pathway. This pathway is activated by exposure to oxidative or electrophilic stress, which induce the dissociation of the Keap1 from the transcription factor Nrf2 and the latter translocate to the nucleus. In the nucleus, it binds to specific DNA sequences known as ARE located in the promoter region of target genes, increasing the expression of components of the antioxidant system, both enzymatic and nonenzymatic, such as CAT, SOD, GPX, and reduced glutathione.

The modulation of the Nrf2 pathway in search of therapeutic benefits has been carried out in various models of cardiac pathologies, such as heart failure, acute myocardial infarction, myocardial ischemia-reperfusion, and diabetic cardiomyopathy [48]. Various activators of the Nrf2 pathway have been described, where obestatin, relaxin, propofol, sulforaphane, fasudil, melatonin, curcumin, nitronyl nitroxide radical-HPN derivative, quercetin, and cardamonin, among others, have been used in various cells and animal models of heart failure [48]. On the other hand, in studies on POAF, it has been mentioned that a possible way through which the use of n3-PUFAs could generate a benefit by reducing the incidence of POAF would be through the activation of Nrf2 pathway, which would increase the response of the system antioxidant and thereby reduce the damage caused by IR during surgery [36] (Fig. 9.4).

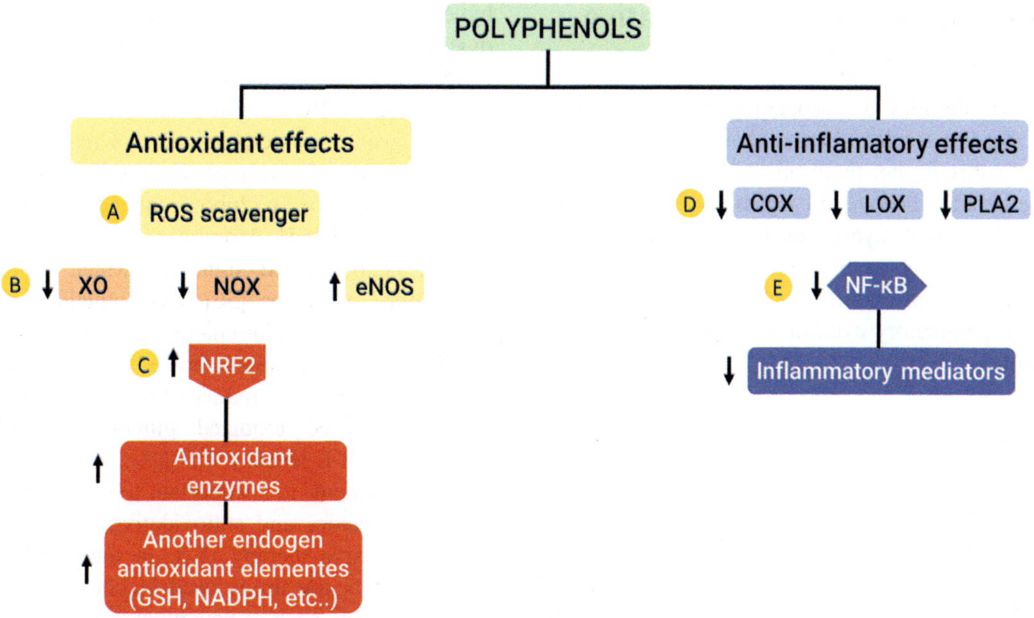

FIGURE 9.3 Diagram of antioxidant and anti-inflammatory effects of polyphenols. Polyphenols have various effects at the cellular level, highlighting those antioxidants and anti-inflammatory. On the one hand, at the antioxidant level, polyphenols have the ability to be (A) ROS scavenger, (B) reduce the activity of certain oxidizing enzymes such as xanthine oxidase (XO) and NADPH oxidase (NOX) as well as increase the activity of the enzyme eNOS allowing to maintain the bioavailability of NO and finally also activates the Nrf2 pathway and thereby promotes the transcription of antioxidant enzymes such as SOD, CAT, GR, GPX along with other elements of the endogenous antioxidant system. On the other hand, at an anti-inflammatory level, polyphenols (D) decrease the activity of enzymes such as cyclooxygenase (COX), lipoxygenase (LOX) and phospholipase A2 (PLA2), as well as (E) promote the downregulation of the transcription factor NFκB, causing a decrease in the transcription of inflammatory mediators such as TNF-α, IL-1-β, and IL-6.

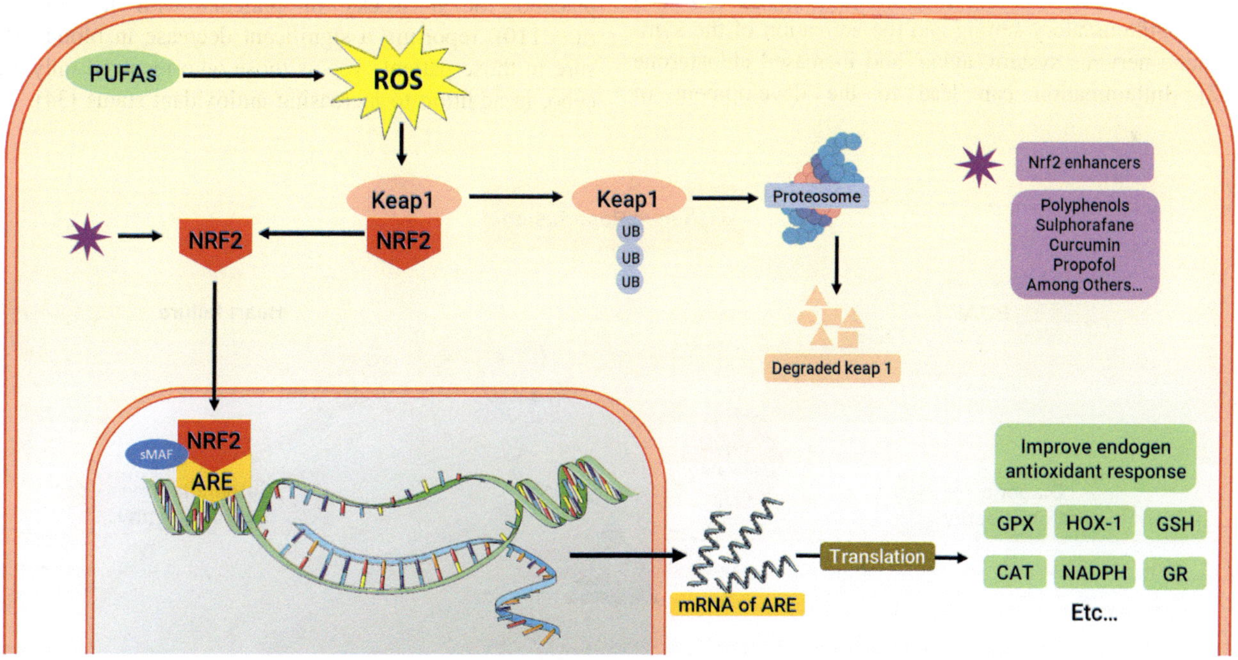

FIGURE 9.4 Molecular mechanism of Nrf2 pathway and its activators. One of the various roles that reactive oxygen species (ROS) have corresponds to being regulators of certain intracellular pathways, which can be protective or harmful for cell survival. One of these protective pathways is that of Nrf2. When ROS are in certain physiological ranges (H_2O_2 between 1 and 10 nM), they allow the endogenous antioxidant system to be activated through this pathway. ROS produce the oxidation of keap1 and thereby prevent its binding to Nrf2 and its subsequent degradation. As it is not degraded, its concentration increases and it begins to translocate to the nucleus, joining the sMAF protein and the antioxidant response element (ARE) binding site, promoting the transcription of antioxidant enzymes, among other antioxidant molecules, which allow responding to an increase of ROS and preventing the damage they produce at the cellular and molecular level.

Cardiovascular diseases and oxidative stress-related settings

During the last decades, an association between oxidative stress and cardiovascular diseases has been established (Fig. 9.5). In this group, there are numerous pathologies that will be detailed below, and which include endothelial dysfunction, increased myocardial mass, extracellular matrix, and apoptosis due to different stimuli such as neurohumoral and its mediators such as angiotensin II, endothelin, inflammatory cytokines, ROS, NO, and adhesion molecules.

Hypertension

Hypertension is one of the major risk factors for cardiovascular disease and is the leading preventable cause of premature death worldwide, and its incidence is growing. ROS play an important role in the development of hypertension, specifically on the vasculature which is a major source of NOX and is involved in systemic and vascular damage. Increase oxidative stress factors such $O_2^{\cdot -}$, macromolecules damage, higher lipid peroxidation, activation of metalloproteinases, reduced NO, formation of $ONOO^-$ and uncoupled nitric oxide synthase (uncNOS) produced changes in endothelial function and its remodeling, together with inflammation, hypertrophy, cell death, fibrosis, and angiogenesis [49–51].

Other factors are involved in the pathophysiology such as pro-inflammatory setting and the activation of the sympathetic nervous system, aging, and increased aldosterone [52]. Inflammation can lead to the development of hypertension and that oxidative stress and endothelial dysfunction are involved in the inflammatory cascade [53]. NOX is also the major ROS source in innate immune cells which produce ROS to kill pathogens, especially $O_2^{\cdot -}$ and H_2O_2, causing an overproduction of reactive species [54]. When Ang-II induced hypertension, T cells express higher levels of p47phox, p22phox, and NOX2, components of NOX2 oxidase [55]. Moreover, oxidative stress activates nuclear factor NF-κB signaling, which increases the inflammatory processes [56]. Sympathetic nervous system also increases the inflammatory response [57].

Hypertensive patients showed a decreased antioxidant system manifested as reduced total plasma antioxidant capacity, increased oxidized glutathione, and decreased vitamin C and E levels [58,59].

For treatment, it is important to consider the benefit of anti-inflammatory and antioxidative drugs and statins for antihypertensive therapy [52]. In this sense, it has been described that the drugs used in conventional antihypertensive therapy, such as beta blockers, angiotensin receptor inhibitors, calcium channel blockers and angiotensinogen converting enzyme inhibitors, in addition to lowering the blood pressure, also induce a decrease in oxidative stress levels, so the paradigm of using oxidative stress as a target to treat hypertension has been described as plausible for a long time [60]. Even in our laboratory, a randomized clinical trial was carried out using vitamin C + E [vitamin C (1 g/day) plus vitamin E (400 international units/day)] or placebo for 8 weeks in patients with hypertension ($n = 110$), reporting a significant decrease in blood pressure in those patients versus those who received only placebo, in addition to increasing antioxidant status [34].

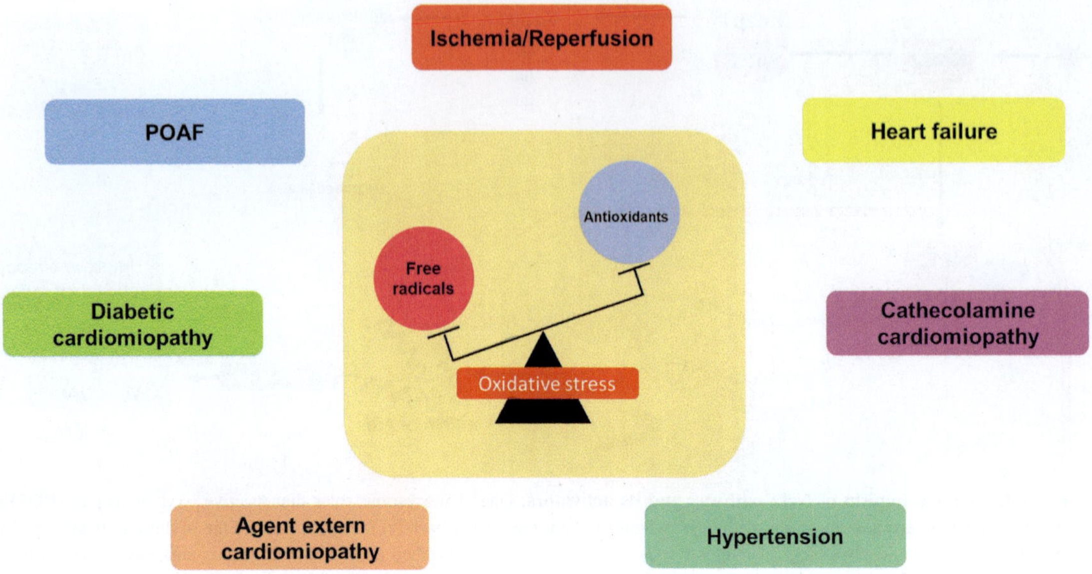

FIGURE 9.5 Diagram that summarizes the different cardiovascular pathologies where oxidative stress plays an important role in their pathophysiology and therefore could be a target to modulate within therapeutic strategies for these diseases.

Ischemia/reperfusion injury

Acute myocardial infarction is a leading cause of morbidity and mortality [61]. This ischemic event occurs after a thrombotic process derived from atherosclerotic plaques in the coronary arteries that produces complete reduction of local blood flow. Reperfusion often results in pathological sequelae leading to elevated ischemic damage [62]. Indeed, myocardial ischemia-reperfusion (IR) injury (IRI) is defined as the adverse effect produced by restoring blood flow. However, it can be responsible for up to 50% of the final infarct size [63]. The restoration of blood flow mainly by percutaneous coronary angioplasty is accompanied by the release of ROS, accumulation of intracellular calcium due to its reentry, alteration in cellular metabolism, leukocyte entrapment, changes in ion channels, excitation-contraction uncoupling, endothelial dysfunction, inflammatory processes, cardiomyocytes death, mitochondrial ROS, and mitochondrial impairment [64,65].

The essential pathway Nrf2/Keap1/ARE can decrease myocardial infarct size and preserve cardiac function after myocardial IRI. This genomic signaling confers cardioprotection due the up-regulation of antioxidant, anti-inflammatory, and autophagy mechanisms. Moreover, ischemic preconditioning and postconditioning might add a protective effect on myocardial IRI [62].

The heart requires significant amounts of high energy to maintain the contractile and metabolic function. The cardiomyocytes have several mitochondria and more than 95% of ATP is produced within mitochondria by oxidative substrate utilization [66]. The main ROS source in cardiomyocytes produced by IRI is succinate accumulation and $O_2^{\cdot-}$ production by electron transport chain (ETC) complexes [67,68] and under oxidative stress, ROS induced the opening of the mPTP, leading to CytC liberation, which has proapoptotic functions [69]. Mitochondrial oxidative stress is mild during ischemia itself but is much more severe during the reperfusion, following the onset of ROS [70].

Reactive oxygen species at ETC are the main source but not the only one [71]. Other mechanisms increasing ROS generation during IR, including monoamines oxidases, flavoproteins localized on the outer mitochondrial membrane, producing H_2O_2, lipid peroxidation, cell death, mitochondrial ultrastructural defects due aldehyde intermediates and ATP depletion [72,73]. Protein p66Shc is preferentially expressed within cardiomyocytes in numerous organelles. p66Shc increases in response to oxidative stress and oxidizes CytC [74]. Moreover, inhibition of transcriptional up-regulation of antioxidant enzymes [75] and NOX activation that generate $O_2^{\cdot-}$. NOX type 4 (NOX4) is located in the outer membrane of mitochondria and is involved in the myocardial IRI as well as NOX type 2. NOX4 increases ROS production and increases cardiac infarct size after IR [76] (Fig. 9.1). Other studies have shown a decrease in antioxidant systems and an increase in RNS. NO increase during ischemia together with $O_2^{\cdot-}$ and $ONOO^-$, which can oxidize mitochondrial proteins and lipids and aggravate the final infarct size and the myocardial IRI [77,78]. Cellular ROS Ca^{2+} overload produces changes in mitochondrial structure producing fission which are related to myocardial IRI [79]. Finally, mitophagy is the selective autophagy of mitochondria in response to mitochondrial damage. This mechanism plays a protective role during IR due to remotion of damaged mitochondria and attenuation of their detrimental consequences for the cardiomyocyte, including excessive ROS production [80].

One of the important points of this pathological model is that despite considerable research effort devoted to the prevention of tissue damage there is currently no established therapy to be able to reduce myocardial IRI after submitting patients to angioplasty to restore cardiac blood flow. One of the most promising advances is based on the idea of proposing acute myocardial infarction as a multifactorial pathological model, in which a multitarget therapeutic strategy is needed involving multiple drugs that exert an additive or synergistic infarct effect in order to achieve the objective of decrease the myocardial IRI and thus the final size [81]. Along these same lines, our laboratory is currently carrying out a randomized double-blind controlled clinical trial to be able to reduce the size of the infarct through a multitarget therapy composed of vitamin C, N-acetylcysteine and deferoxamine, so that in the next years we will be able to report the results obtained from this strategy.

Postoperative atrial fibrillation

Postoperative atrial fibrillation is the most common arrhythmia and complication of cardiac surgery that occurs in up to 60% of patients and is associated with elevated mortality and heart failure. The pathophysiological development is based on oxidative stress and inflammation, in which several redox signaling pathways have been involved. Both alterations are caused by IR. As a consequence, atrial electrophysiological and structural abnormalities occurs [82]. Respect to oxidative stress, increased nitrotyrosine and protein carbonyls formation have been reported [83] as well calcium accumulation provoking a decrease in tissue levels of vitamin C and reduced glutathione [84,85].

Morphometric analysis showed that cardiomyocyte hypertrophy, myolytic damage, and interstitial fibrosis occur together with oxidative stress and inflammation [86].

The main ROS source involved in this pathology is NOX. Other sources of ROS are XO, uncNOS, mitochondrial dysfunction, myeloperoxidase (MPO), and monoamine oxidase [87]. NOX leads to fibrosis through upregulation of connective tissue growth factor expression induced by angiotensin II and MPO activity [88,89]. MPO produces ROS such as hypochlorous acid which affects intracellular signaling and deposition of atrial collagen [90]. Moreover O_2^- and $ONOO^-$ are associated with increased risk of POAF [91].

In clinical settings, several drugs with pleiotropic effects, including antioxidant and anti-inflammatory have been tested in POAF with variable results. However, due to the multifactorial causes behind the cardiovascular diseases, the best choice is point to an associated and multi-target therapy [33,92–95].

Diabetic cardiomyopathy

Diabetes mellitus is a metabolic disease characterized by impaired glucose regulation. Patients with type 2 diabetes mellitus are at increased risk of developing heart failure, which is a complication that includes changes in myocardial structure and function, together with cardiomyocyte fibrosis and apoptosis, diastolic and systolic dysfunction, reductions in heart rate, left ventricular ejection fraction, stroke work, cardiac output, and left ventricular end-systolic volume [96,97].

Moreover, there is oxidative stress, activation of multiple inflammatory pathways involved in cellular injury, endoplasmic reticulum stress, aberrant insulin signaling, accumulation of advanced glycated end-products, altered autophagy, changes in myocardial substrate metabolism and mitochondrial bioenergetics, lipotoxicity, and altered signal transduction. In addition, an increase to supra-physiological levels in catecholamine levels has been reported [98]. This situation causes catecholamines that are not metabolized by the monoamine oxidase enzyme, producing other types of molecules such as quinones due to their oxidation, which is accompanied by the generation of ROS, such as hydroxyl radical, superoxide anion radical, and hydrogen peroxide. Therefore, the increase in catecholamine levels is another important component to consider as a producer of oxidative stress in diabetic cardiomyopathy.

Successful pharmacological targets of these pathways have shown effectiveness in reducing the clinical repercussions of hyperglycemia and heart failure as anti-fibrotic agents, anti-inflammatory agents, statins, and antioxidants [97,99,100].

Focusing on oxidative stress, diabetes is related to elevated markers of ROS such as 15-F2t-isoprostane, SOD, malondialdehyde, gp91phox, Cyt-Cyto C, enhanced cell apoptosis and autophagy (Bax/Bcl-2, Cleaved caspase-3, TUNEL-positive cells) and increased Foxo1 (transcription factor) acetylation, being the cellular and mitochondrial NOX enzyme the main source of free radicals in the diabetic heart [101]. On the other hand, there exists a reduced Akt phosphorylation and reduced expression of Nrf2, heme oxygenase-1, and Keap1 [96].

Other drugs, such as empagliflozin and allopurinol, activate the Nrf2/Keap1/ARE signal following the disassociation with its repressor Keap1 under oxidative stress can maintain inner redox homeostasis and attenuate diabetes cardiac injury with concomitant attenuation of autophagy [96,102]. Also, Tan et al. [101] proposes zinc and sulforaphane as possible agents to modulate the oxidative stress behind diabetes mellitus and thus prevent diabetic heart disease, where sulforaphane promotes the activation of the Nrf2 pathway [103], reporting in a randomized and controlled clinical study that sulforaphane improves fasting glucose and HbA1c in obese patients with dysregulated type 2 diabetes mellitus, in addition to reducing the glucose production through activation of the Nrf2 pathway and decreased expression of key gluconeogenic enzymes [104]. However, in the case of zinc, it is not yet clear how its supplementation improves the parameters in patients with and without diabetes, but it is believed that it could be linked to the function of metallothionein [101].

Catecholamine cardiomyopathy

Cardiomyopathies due to adrenal hormone excess such as catecholamines are an interesting and unexplored clinical setting.

Stress cardiomyopathy, or Takotsubo syndrome, is an acute and reversible cardiac dysfunction presenting with characteristic apical left ventricular ballooning precipitated by acute emotional or physical stress. In this event, plasma catecholamine levels are markedly elevated compared with AMI. Indeed, sympathetic activation is suspected as one of its pathophysiology [105,106].

The newest macroscopic and microscopic cardiac features evidence is vital to understand the pathophysiology and its detrimental effects in direct and indirect ways of the signaling and the structural alteration of cardiomyocytes.

Exposure to catecholamines and beta-receptor agonists can precipitate the features of stress cardiomyopathy, including cardiac isoenzyme elevation, QTc interval prolongation, and rapidly reversible cardiac dysfunction [107]. Endomyocardial biopsy samples also support these results since contraction band necrosis, a unique and peculiar form of myocyte injury observed in clinical states of catecholamine excess, has been demonstrated [105]. Microscopically, edema and a modest loss of striations and interstitial fibrosis in cardiomyocytes may also occur. The oxidation products of catecholamines, such as aminochrome and oxyradicals cause a toxic effect on the myocardium. This can lead to calcium overload in cardiomyocytes, metabolic unbalance, Ca^{2+}-handling abnormalities, activation of proteases, changes in myocardial gene expression, ROS damage, and mitochondrial dysfunction, which causes coronary artery spasm, arrhythmias, cardiac dysfunction, and cardiac hypertrophy [108–110]. In these last cases, stimulated myocytes induce adaptive mechanisms, including β-receptor internalization and subsequent desensitization, provoking the detrimental consequences mentioned before [108]. Regarding the dysfunction of the microvasculature present in the pathophysiology of takotsubo cardiomyopathy, there is evidence suggesting that inflammation and oxidative stress would have a central role, where the increase in the concentration of catecholamines produces an increase in the formation of ROS through adrenergic stimulation and activation of NOX [111]. In addition, it has been described in in vitro and in vivo studies that the increase in catecholamines induce lipid peroxidation and increased levels of GSSG (both markers of oxidative stress). Also, in female patients suffering from takotsubo syndrome, an increase in the activation of genes induced by Nrf2 was reported [112].

Generally, stress-induced cardiomyopathy is self-limiting. However, in particular cases, patients may require nonadrenergic inotropes treatment or angiotensin converting enzyme blockers and β-adrenergic receptors blockers [113]. In addition, treatment with vitamin E reduces the incidence of catecholamine-induced cardiac arrhythmias [114].

Drug- or external agent-induced cardiomyopathy

Toxic cardiomyopathy can be a direct result of toxic exposure to a variety of agents, most notably alcohol and medications (particularly chemotherapeutic drugs). This is a complex and multifactorial mechanism which includes mishandling of cellular energy and calcium homeostasis, together with ROS generation, neurohormonal stress, and induction of apoptosis. Nevertheless, it is difficult to establish which components of heart failure are due to the toxicity itself [111]. In the following paragraphs, we will include some examples of these interactions between drugs and ROS.

Anticancer drugs produce cardiomyopathy, as has been reported when paclitaxel is combined with doxorubicin, a heart failure that has been developed in up to 20% of patients treated with paclitaxel and doxorubicin [115]. Antiretroviral drugs such as azidothymidine are cardiotoxic due to energy depletion produced by mitochondrial toxicity and also increases the production of mitochondrial ROS and reduces mitochondrial DNA. The damage is prevented by SOD and CAT as well as the use of polyphenols [116,117]. Ethanol cardiotoxicity is multifactorial, and it involves apoptosis, alterations of the excitation–contraction coupling in cardiac myocytes, structural impairment of the mitochondria and sarcoplasmic reticulum, changes in calcium homeostasis flows, alterations of mitochondrial oxidation, lipid peroxidation, deregulation of protein synthesis, decrease of contractile proteins and changes in the regulation of myosin ATPase, and other ion channels as well as an increased of oxidative stress. Moreover, increase of XO activity, enhance of the $O_2^{\cdot-}$ formation, elevation of lactate dehydrogenase and creatine phosphokinase activities, and decrease in antioxidant capacity of the heart were reported in ethanol-induced oxidative stress and cardiomyopathy [111,118].

In the case of heart damage caused by anthracyclines, various therapies capable of modulating the cellular redox balance have been tested over the years. One of these drugs is dexraxozane, which is the only drug approved by the FDA to prevent anthracycline cardiotoxicity. Three multicenter studies concluded that the use of dexrazoxane provides cardioprotection after the administration of chemotherapy containing doxorubicin [119–121]. However, its use is quite limited as it is only approved for women with metastatic breast cancer who have a cumulative dose of 300 mg/m^2 of chemotherapy [122,123]. Its mechanism of action is based on chelating labile iron to form a complex when binding to anthracycline, thus preventing the formation of hydroxyl radicals mediated by the Fenton reaction. However, other iron chelating agents (deferasirox or ICRF-161) have failed to confer cardioprotection [122,124,125].

On the other hand, randomized clinical trials attempting to determine the efficacy of N-acetylcysteine to prevent heart damage caused by doxorubicin have concluded that this compound does not have protective effects compared to the placebo group after chemotherapy [126,127]. In addition, attempts have been made to demonstrate the efficacy of various antihypertensive drugs to prevent the cardiotoxicity of anthracyclines, such as beta blockers [128–131], ARB's [132,133], ACE inhibitors [134], or RAAS [135], with carvedilol being one of the most studied. A meta-analysis performed in 2018 concluded that carvedilol manages to preserve cardiac function (LVEF) in patients who were administered carvedilol preventively to chemotherapy with anthracyclines [136]. However, this conclusion is limited to the analysis of 8 randomized and controlled clinical trials, where the vast majority of those that show benefits are with a small sample size and the CECCY trial [131] being the one with the largest sample size and the one that did not report benefits using carvedilol preventively compared to the placebo group.

Heart failure

Heart failure (HF) is defined as the inability of the heart to pump enough blood to the peripheral tissues according to their metabolic demands [137]. This decreased cardiac output occurs due to various pathophysiological events occurring in cardiac tissue. Some of them correspond to architectural changes at the microstructural level such as hypertrophy, apoptosis, necrosis, and autophagy of cardiomyocytes, changes at the macrostructural level such as left ventricular hypertrophy, ventricular dilation, and increased left ventricular stiffness, as well as interstitial fibrosis [137]. Other pathophysiological events correspond to the activation of the neurohumoral system, inflammation processes, biochemical changes, and oxidative stress [138]. Each one of these changes ultimately leads to a malfunction of the heart, expressing itself in a clinical syndrome characterized by symptoms such as dyspnea, orthopnea, and paroxysmal nocturnal dyspnea as a result of the pulmonary congestion present in these patients as the main causal factor, peripheral edema, elevated jugular venous pressure, Cheyne-Stokes respiration in advanced HF, and gastrointestinal symptoms, among others [137].

Oxidative stress in the context of HF is one of the pathophysiological pillars, where if we propose a timeline, oxidative stress plays an important role in various stages of HF development. We have a starting point in which the increase in oxidative stress has been associated with the main risk factors for developing cardiovascular diseases, such as hypertension, diabetes, obesity, advanced age, dyslipidemia, and chronic kidney disease [137,139]. Likewise, oxidative stress would be related to the pathological remodeling that occurs during the development of HF, as reported by studies where the increase in oxidative stress is associated with the activation of signaling pathways, such as MAP kinases and transcription factor NF-κB involved in cardiomyocyte hypertrophy [137,140]. As well as in other processes such as fibrosis, reorganization of the extracellular matrix by activation of MMP, inflammation, and finally with the death of cardiomyocytes (apoptosis, necrosis, autophagy), further weakening the heart tissue [137,138,141].

The unbalance in the cellular redox state mentioned previously is based on measurements of oxidative stress parameters in both humans and animals, where it has been described that those subjects suffering from HF have low levels of GSH and NADH [142]. Furthermore, several studies have reported the decrease in the activity of the antioxidant enzymes CAT, SOD, and GPX in animal models of HF subsequent to acute myocardial infarction [143,144], added to a decrease in the expression of the enzymes CAT and SOD at the mRNA level in the same animal model [145]. On the other hand, when talking about biomarkers in HF, troponins and natriuretic peptides are currently the most used in the clinic. However, Lubrano and Balzan discussed the existence of other biomarkers related to oxidative stress, to diagnose, monitor, or treat the patient with HF, these correspond to: galactin-3 (GAL-3), α1-antitrypsin (AAT) and lectin-like oxidized low-density-lipoprotein receptor-1 (LOX-1), concluding that AAT and LOX-1 present the most robust evidence for their use, unlike GAL-3, which presents studies with contradictory conclusions, so its evidence must continue to be deepened [139].

Over the years, various pharmacological strategies that modulate the redox balance have been studied as a treatment in HF, some increasing the antioxidant capacity through drugs such as NAC that increase the endogenous antioxidant capacity or the supplementation of exogenous antioxidants (vitamins C or E) that act directly as ROS scavengers, as well as others that inhibit the production of agents that increase oxidative stress (hypouricements or inhibitors of NOS uncoupling). However, the results of these studies have not been conclusive, with some drugs having a higher level of therapeutic evidence than others. It is important to mention that various drugs currently recommended for the management of HF, such as angiotensin-converting enzyme inhibitors, beta-blockers or statins, have an antioxidant effect. However, the therapeutic efficacy of the oxidative stress-reducing effect of these drugs has yet to be proven [138].

The administration of exogenous antioxidants, such as ascorbic acid, alpha tocopherol, retinol, or folic acid in patients with HF has been studied in various clinical settings, based on the assumption that exogenously replacing and increasing their plasma levels should enhance the antioxidant component and thus address the oxidative unbalance suffered by subjects with HF by acting directly as ROS scavengers, in addition to the fact that several studies have reported a decrease in plasma levels of vitamin C and E in these subjects. However, the evidence reported for this hypothesis in randomized clinical trials has not been very encouraging. One small uncontrolled study ($n = 20$) reported reduced oxidative stress biomarkers in HF patients (malondialdehyde and superoxide anion levels) but had no statistically significant effects on antioxidant enzymes (SOD, CAT, and GR) [146]. Another study ($n = 56$) enrolled patients with advanced HF (NYHA class III and IV) and supplemented them with 2 capsules of 500 IU of vitamin E per day for 12 weeks, finally reporting that although plasma levels of vitamin E increased in supplemented patients, both oxidative stress parameters and quality of life did not vary or were significantly better than the placebo group [147]. It should be mentioned that plasma vitamin E levels do not necessarily reflect the vitamin E homeostasis. Tousoulis reported that although the use of atorvastatin improves endothelial function and reduces inflammatory parameters in patients with ischemic HF, supplementing therapy with vitamin E produces a decrease in this effect [148], and Khan in a systematic review suggested that vitamin E would be associated with a significant but small increase in the risk of hospitalization for HF [149].

High levels of serum uric acid have been described in patients with HF, along with being an incident HF prognosis marker in patient with hypertension, stable coronary arterial disease, and after suffering an acute myocardial infarction [138,150,151]. Therefore, uric acid has been raised as a possible target to treat different outcomes in relation to HF, obtaining different results in clinical trials. A randomized clinical trial that contemplated 405 patients suggested that oxypurinol decreases uric acid levels and improves symptoms specifically in a subgroup of patients with HF and hyperuricemia but not in patients without hyperuricemia [152]. On the other hand, another study reported that allopurinol decreases uric acid levels in patients with reduced ejection fraction HF and high uric acid levels but without improving clinical status, exercise capacity, quality of life or right ventricular ejection fraction after 24 weeks [153].

Another antioxidant drug that has been studied over the years corresponds to coenzyme Q10, where the randomized controlled multicenter trial Q-SYMBIO evaluated its use as an adjuvant to standard therapy for patients with HF, reporting that coenzyme Q10 improves symptoms, reduces major cardiovascular adverse events, and is safe [154]. In addition, in 2019, a subgroup of European patients from the Q-SYMBIO study was analyzed, confirming the beneficial effects of the use of coenzyme Q10 with standard therapy, also showing that it improves LVEF and NYHA classification, which had not been reported in the initial study [155]. On the other hand, a systematic review carried out in 2021 reported that the consumption of coenzyme Q10 is associated with lower all-cause mortality in patients with HF but without an improvement in the NYHA classification or in the LVEF [149]. However, there is currently a discussion regarding the results. On the one hand, some researchers such as Filipiak et al. discuss why the international clinical guidelines do not include the evidence provided by this study regarding the use of coenzyme Q10 in the treatment of patients with HF, while other studies with similar numbers of enrolled participants did manage to change the clinical guidelines [156]. On the other hand, Khan et al. refer that the validity of the results reported in their systematic review regarding coenzyme Q10 and the risk of mortality is debatable, where if the Q-SYMBIO study is excluded from the evidence, the results in terms of mortality, they are not significant, so it is necessary to carry out more randomized clinical trials and increase their statistical power to be able to consider the use of coenzyme Q10 in the treatment of HF [149].

Concluding remarks

In conclusion, the relevance of oxidative stress-related biomarkers is supported by the key role of this metabolic derangement in the functions of the cardiovascular system and its remodeling. The growing evidence on the multiple sources of ROS and RNS in cardiac tissue and their relevant intervention may have important therapeutic implications with great benefits in cardiovascular morbidity and mortality, especially in the management of heart failure due to the process of hypertrophy and intra- and extracellular damage. However, numerous systems are involved in the pathophysiology of heart failure, which makes it difficult to determine the origin of the damage, perpetuating a vicious circle. Thus causes an unbalance in redox state, ion and tissue homeostasis which all lead to hemodynamic overload. This fact initiates a compensatory response that activates neuroendocrine systems such as the adrenergic system, the renin-angiotensin system and the endothelins, all of which causes an increase in ROS generators such as NOX, XO, or uncNOS. Indeed, heart failure is a severe clinical syndrome, and the death of patients is mainly caused by the repetitive dysfunction of these systems that increases the stress of the wall due to hypertrophy and leads to subendocardial ischemia that can trigger the death of cardiomyocytes and cardiac arrhythmias. The available pharmacological treatment of the pathologies mentioned in this chapter is still not optimal due to the variety of underlying causes; however, benefits of antioxidants, anti-inflammatories, inhibitors of the renin angiotensin system, aldosterone antagonists, and β-adrenergic blockers have been reported. Based on the above, a new paradigm has been proposed for some time which has begun to take a promising role in terms of therapeutic strategies. This emphasizes analyzing the disease as a multifactorial process, as can be seen in the description of the diseases that were analyzed in this chapter. Therefore, the treatment must be with a multitarget approach, simultaneously using drugs that attack the different pathophysiological processes involved in its pathogenesis, as well as acting at different levels of the same pathophysiological process, in such a way as to exert a therapeutic effect that is additive or synergistic. Finally, further research in this area will test the added value of incorporation of new pharmacological therapy and multiple biomarkers with a special focus on cardiovascular diseases that can maximize prevention and early diagnosis.

Acknowledgments

This study was supported by the Agencia Nacional de Investigación y Desarrollo (ANID) to a project of the Fondo Nacional de Desarrollo Científico y Tecnológico (FONDECYT, grant number 1211850).

References

[1] Pan American Health Organization. World heart day 2021—PAHO/WHO. Pan American Health Organization; 2021. https://www.paho.org/en/campaigns/world-heart-day-2021. [Accessed 3 January 2022].

[2] World Heart Organization. Noncommunicable diseases. 2022. https://www.who.int/news-room/fact-sheets/detail/noncommunicable-diseases; 2022. [Accessed 3 January 2022].

[3] dos Santos JL, de Quadros AS, Weschenfelder C, Garofallo SB, Marcadenti A. Oxidative stress biomarkers, nut-related antioxidants, and cardiovascular disease. Nutrients 2020;12. https://doi.org/10.3390/NU12030682.

[4] Steven S, Frenis K, Oelze M, Kalinovic S, Kuntic M, Jimenez MTB, et al. Vascular inflammation and oxidative stress: major triggers for cardiovascular disease. Oxid Med Cell Longev 2019;2019. https://doi.org/10.1155/2019/7092151.

[5] Pignatelli P, Menichelli D, Pastori D, Violi F. Oxidative stress and cardiovascular disease: new insights. Kardiol Pol 2018;76:713–22. https://doi.org/10.5603/KP.A2018.0071.

[6] Rodrigo R, Prieto JC, Castillo R. Cardioprotection against ischaemia/reperfusion by vitamins C and E plus n-3 fatty acids: molecular mechanisms and potential clinical applications. Clin Sci 2013;124:1–15. https://doi.org/10.1042/CS20110663.

[7] Strålin P, Karlsson K, Johansson BO, Marklund SL. The interstitium of the human arterial wall contains very large amounts of extracellular superoxide dismutase. Arterioscler Thromb Vasc Biol 1995;15:2032–6. https://doi.org/10.1161/01.ATV.15.11.2032.

[8] Fukai T, Folz RJ, Landmesser U, Harrison DG. Extracellular superoxide dismutase and cardiovascular disease. Cardiovasc Res 2002;55:239–49. https://doi.org/10.1016/S0008-6363(02)00328-0.

[9] Fukai T, Ushio-Fukai M. Superoxide dismutases: role in redox signaling, vascular function, and diseases. Antioxid Redox Signal 2011;15:1583–606. https://doi.org/10.1089/ars.2011.3999.

[10] Li X, Lin Y, Wang S, Zhou S, Ju J, Wang X, et al. Extracellular superoxide dismutase is associated with left ventricular geometry and heart failure in patients with cardiovascular disease. J Am Heart Assoc 2020;9. https://doi.org/10.1161/JAHA.120.016862.

[11] Maksimenko AV, Vavaev AV. Antioxidant enzymes as potential targets in cardioprotection and treatment of cardiovascular diseases. Enzyme antioxidants: the next stage of pharmacological counterwork to the oxidative stress. Heart Int 2012;7:14–9. https://doi.org/10.4081/HI.2012.E3.

[12] Lubos E, Loscalzo J, Handy DE. Glutathione peroxidase-1 in health and disease: from molecular mechanisms to therapeutic opportunities. Antioxid Redox Signal 2011;15:1957–97. https://doi.org/10.1089/ars.2010.3586.

[13] Muzykantov VR. Targeting of superoxide dismutase and catalase to vascular endothelium. J Contr Release 2001;71:1–21. https://doi.org/10.1016/S0168-3659(01)00215-2.

[14] Ulker S, McKeown P, Bayraktutan U. Vitamins reverse endothelial dysfunction through regulation of eNOS and NAD(P)H oxidase activities. Hypertension 2003;41:534–9. https://doi.org/10.1161/01.HYP.0000057421.28533.37.

[15] Cárcamo J, Pedraza A, Bórquez-Ojeda O, Golde D. Vitamin C suppresses TNF alpha-induced NF kappa B activation by inhibiting I kappa B alpha phosphorylation. Biochemistry 2002;41:12995–3002. https://doi.org/10.1021/BI0263210.

[16] Newaz MA, Yousefipour Z, Nawal NNA. Modulation of nitric oxide synthase activity in brain, liver, and blood vessels of spontaneously hypertensive rats by ascorbic acid: protection from free radical injury. Clin Exp Hypertens 2005;27:497–508. https://doi.org/10.1081/CEH-200067681.

[17] d'Uscio LV, Milstien S, Richardson D, Smith L, Katusic ZS. Long-term vitamin C treatment increases vascular tetrahydrobiopterin levels and nitric oxide synthase activity. Circ Res 2003;92:88–95. https://doi.org/10.1161/01.RES.0000049166.33035.62.

[18] Packer JE, Slater TF, Willson RL. Direct observation of a free radical interaction between vitamin E and vitamin C. Nature 1979;278:737–8. https://doi.org/10.1038/278737A0.

[19] Niki E, Noguchi N, Tsuchihashi H, Gotoh N. Interaction among vitamin C, vitamin E, and beta-carotene. Am J Clin Nutr 1995;62. https://doi.org/10.1093/AJCN/62.6.1322S.

[20] May J, Qu Z, Mendiratta S. Protection and recycling of alpha-tocopherol in human erythrocytes by intracellular ascorbic acid. Arch Biochem Biophys 1998;349:281–9. https://doi.org/10.1006/ABBI.1997.0473.

[21] Moser MA, Chun OK. Vitamin C and heart health: a review based on findings from epidemiologic studies. Int J Mol Sci 2016;17. https://doi.org/10.3390/IJMS17081328.

[22] Pfister R, Sharp SJ, Luben R, Wareham NJ, Khaw KT. Plasma vitamin C predicts incident heart failure in men and women in European Prospective Investigation into Cancer and Nutrition-Norfolk prospective study. Am Heart J 2011;162:246–53. https://doi.org/10.1016/j.ahj.2011.05.007.

[23] Khaw K, Bingham S, Welch A, Luben R. Relation between plasma ascorbic acid and mortality in men and women in EPIC. Lancet 2001;357:657–63.

[24] Duffy SJ, Gokce N, Holbrook M, Huang A, Frei B, Keaney JF, Vita JA. Treatment of hypertension with ascorbic acid. Lancet 1999;354:2048–9. https://doi.org/10.1016/S0140-6736(99)04410-4.

[25] Bates CJ, Walmsley CM, Prentice A, Finch S. Does vitamin C reduce blood pressure? Results of a large study of people aged 65 or older. J Hypertens 1998;16:925–32. https://doi.org/10.1097/00004872-199816070-00005.

[26] Guan Y, Dai P, Wang H, Wane D. Effects of vitamin C supplementation on essential hypertension: a systematic review and meta-analysis. Medicine 2020;99. https://doi.org/10.1097/MD.0000000000019274.

[27] Rodrigo R, Prieto JC, Aguayo R, Ramos C, Puentes Á, Gajardo A, et al. Joint cardioprotective effect of vitamin c and other antioxidants against reperfusion injury in patients with acute myocardial infarction undergoing percutaneous coronary intervention. Molecules 2021;26:1–27. https://doi.org/10.3390/molecules26185702.

[28] Lykkesfeldt J, Tveden-Nyborg P. The pharmacokinetics of vitamin C. Nutrients 2019;11. https://doi.org/10.3390/nu11102412.

[29] Llorens C, Báez M del C, Tarán M, Campana V, Fonseca I, Oyola E, et al. Papel antioxidante de la vitamina E en la aterogénesis inducida por hiperfibrinogenemia. Rev Argent Cardiol 2010:405–10. http://www.scielo.org.ar/scielo.php?script=sci_arttext&pid=S1850-37482010000500006. [Accessed 2 February 2022].

[30] Kuwabara A, Nakade M, Tamai H, Tsuboyama-Kasaoka N, Tanaka K. The association between vitamin E intake and hypertension: results from the re-analysis of the National Health and Nutrition Survey. J Nutr Sci Vitaminol 2014;60:239–45. https://doi.org/10.3177/JNSV.60.239.

[31] Meydani M. Vitamin E modulation of cardiovascular disease. Ann N Y Acad Sci 2004;1031:271–9. https://doi.org/10.1196/ANNALS.1331.027.

[32] Rimm EB, Stampfer MJ, Ascherio A, Giovannucci E, Colditz GA, Willett WC. Vitamin E consumption and the risk of coronary heart disease in men. N Engl J Med 1993;328:1450–6. https://doi.org/10.1056/NEJM199305203282004.

[33] Rodrigo R, González-Montero J, Sotomayor CG. Novel combined antioxidant strategy against hypertension, acute myocardial

infarction and postoperative atrial fibrillation. Biomedicines 2021;9:1–20. https://doi.org/10.3390/biomedicines9060620.

[34] Rodrigo R, Prat H, Passalacqua W, Araya J, Bächler JP. Decrease in oxidative stress through supplementation of vitamins C and E is associated with a reduction in blood pressure in patients with essential hypertension. Clin Sci 2008;114:625–34. https://doi.org/10.1042/CS20070343.

[35] Valls N, Gormaz JG, Aguayo R, González J, Brito R, Hasson D, et al. Amelioration of persistent left ventricular function impairment through increased plasma ascorbate levels following myocardial infarction. Redox Rep 2016;21:75–83. https://doi.org/10.1179/1351000215Y.0000000018.

[36] Rodrigo R, Korantzopoulos P, Cereceda M, Asenjo R, Zamorano J, Villalabeitia E, et al. A randomized controlled trial to prevent postoperative atrial fibrillation by antioxidant reinforcement. J Am Coll Cardiol 2013;62:1457–65. https://doi.org/10.1016/J.JACC.2013.07.014.

[37] Cheng YC, Sheen JM, Hu WL, Hung YC. Polyphenols and oxidative stress in atherosclerosis-related ischemic heart disease and stroke. Oxid Med Cell Longev 2017;2017. https://doi.org/10.1155/2017/8526438.

[38] Breuss JM, Atanasov AG, Uhrin P. Resveratrol and its effects on the vascular system. Int J Mol Sci 2019;20. https://doi.org/10.3390/IJMS20071523.

[39] Neveu V, Perez-Jiménez J, Vos F, Crespy V, du Chaffaut L, Mennen L, et al. Phenol-explorer: an online comprehensive database on polyphenol contents in foods. Database 2010;2010. https://doi.org/10.1093/DATABASE/BAP024.

[40] Snopek L, Mlcek J, Sochorova L, Baron M, Hlavacova I, Jurikova T, et al. Contribution of red wine consumption to human health protection. Molecules 2018;23:1–16. https://doi.org/10.3390/MOLECULES23071684.

[41] Kane MO, Etienne-Selloum N, Madeira SVF, Sarr M, Walter A, Dal-Ros S, et al. Endothelium-derived contracting factors mediate the Ang II-induced endothelial dysfunction in the rat aorta: preventive effect of red wine polyphenols. Pflugers Arch 2010;459:671–9. https://doi.org/10.1007/S00424-009-0759-7.

[42] Nijveldt RJ, van Nood E, van Hoorn DEC, Boelens PG, van Norren K, van Leeuwen PAM. Flavonoids: a review of probable mechanisms of action and potential applications. Am J Clin Nutr 2001;74:418–25. https://doi.org/10.1093/AJCN/74.4.418.

[43] Zhou Y, Jiang Z, Lu H, Xu Z, Tong R, Shi J, Jia G. Recent advances of natural polyphenols activators for keap1-Nrf2 signaling pathway. Chem Biodivers 2019;16. https://doi.org/10.1002/CBDV.201900400.

[44] Yahfoufi N, Alsadi N, Jambi M, Matar C. The immunomodulatory and anti-inflammatory role of polyphenols. Nutrients 2018;10. https://doi.org/10.3390/NU10111618.

[45] González R, Ballester I, López-Posadas R, Suárez MD, Zarzuelo A, Martínez-Augustin O, Sánchez de Medina F. Effects of flavonoids and other polyphenols on inflammation. Crit Rev Food Sci Nutr 2011;51:331–62. https://doi.org/10.1080/10408390903584094.

[46] Yoon JH, Baek SJ. Molecular targets of dietary polyphenols with anti-inflammatory properties. Yonsei Med J 2005;46:585–96. https://doi.org/10.3349/YMJ.2005.46.5.585.

[47] Kim HP, Son KH, Chang HW, Kang SS. Anti-inflammatory plant flavonoids and cellular action mechanisms. J Pharmacol Sci 2004;96:229–45. https://doi.org/10.1254/JPHS.CRJ04003X.

[48] Vashi R, Patel BM. NRF2 in cardiovascular diseases: a ray of hope! J Cardiovasc Transl Res 2021;14:573–86. https://doi.org/10.1007/s12265-020-10083-8.

[49] Pinzón-Díaz CE, Calderón-Salinas JV, Rosas-Flores MM, Hernández G, López-Betancourt A, Quintanar-Escorza MA. Eryptosis and oxidative damage in hypertensive and dyslipidemic patients. Mol Cell Biochem 2018;440:105–13. https://doi.org/10.1007/S11010-017-3159-X/TABLES/3.

[50] Montezano AC, Nguyen Dinh Cat A, Rios FJ, Touyz RM. Angiotensin II and vascular injury. Curr Hypertens Rep 2014;16. https://doi.org/10.1007/S11906-014-0431-2.

[51] Castro MM, Tanus-Santos JE. Inhibition of matrix metalloproteinases (MMPs) as a potential strategy to ameliorate hypertension-induced cardiovascular alterations. Curr Drug Targets 2013;14:335–43. https://doi.org/10.2174/1389450111314030005.

[52] Dinh QN, Drummond GR, Sobey CG, Chrissobolis S. Roles of inflammation, oxidative stress, and vascular dysfunction in hypertension. BioMed Res Int 2014;2014. https://doi.org/10.1155/2014/406960.

[53] Crowley SD. The cooperative roles of inflammation and oxidative stress in the pathogenesis of hypertension. Antioxid Redox Signal 2014;20:102. https://doi.org/10.1089/ARS.2013.5258.

[54] Drummond GR, Selemidis S, Griendling KK, Sobey CG. Combating oxidative stress in vascular disease: NADPH oxidases as therapeutic targets. Nat Rev Drug Discov 2011;10:453–71. https://doi.org/10.1038/NRD3403.

[55] Guzik TJ, Hoch NE, Brown KA, McCann LA, Rahman A, Dikalov S, et al. Role of the T cell in the genesis of angiotensin II–induced hypertension and vascular dysfunction. J Exp Med 2007;204:2449. https://doi.org/10.1084/JEM.20070657.

[56] Canty TG, Boyle EM, Farr A, Morgan EN, Verrier ED, Pohlman TH. Oxidative stress induces NF-kappaB nuclear translocation without degradation of IkappaBalpha. Circulation 1999;100:II-361–II–364. https://doi.org/10.1161/01.CIR.100.-SUPPL_2.II-361.

[57] Lob HE, Marvar PJ, Guzik TJ, Sharma S, McCann LA, Weyand C, et al. Induction of hypertension and peripheral inflammation by reduction of extracellular superoxide dismutase in the central nervous system. Hypertension 2010;55:277–83. https://doi.org/10.1161/HYPERTENSIONAHA.109.142646.

[58] Redón J, Oliva MR, Tormos C, Giner V, Chaves J, Iradi A, Sáez GT. Antioxidant activities and oxidative stress byproducts in human hypertension. Hypertension 2003;41:1096–101. https://doi.org/10.1161/01.HYP.0000068370.21009.38.

[59] Rodrigo R, Prat H, Passalacqua W, Araya J, Guichard C, Bächler JP. Relationship between oxidative stress and essential hypertension. Hypertens Res 2007;30:1159–67. https://doi.org/10.1291/HYPRES.30.1159.

[60] Ward NC, Croft KD. Hypertension and oxidative stress. Clin Exp Pharmacol Physiol 2006;33:872–6. https://doi.org/10.1111/J.1440-1681.2006.04457.X.

[61] White HD, Chew DP. Acute myocardial infarction. Lancet 2008;372:570–84. https://doi.org/10.1016/S0140-6736(08)61237-4.

[62] Shen Y, Liu X, Shi J, Wu X. Involvement of Nrf2 in myocardial ischemia and reperfusion injury. Int J Biol Macromol 2019;125:496–502. https://doi.org/10.1016/J.IJBIOMAC.2018.11.190.

[63] Yellon DM, Hausenloy DJ. Myocardial reperfusion injury. N Engl J Med 2007;357:1121–35. https://doi.org/10.1056/NEJMRA071667.

[64] Yang M, Linn BS, Zhang Y, Ren J. Mitophagy and mitochondrial integrity in cardiac ischemia-reperfusion injury. Biochim Biophys Acta Mol Basis Dis 2019;1865:2293–302. https://doi.org/10.1016/J.BBADIS.2019.05.007.

[65] Lillo-Moya J, Rojas-Solé C, Muñoz-Salamanca D, Panieri E, Saso L, Rodrigo R. Targeting ferroptosis against ischemia/reperfusion cardiac injury. Antioxidants 2021;10. https://doi.org/10.3390/antiox10050667.

[66] Barth E, Stämmler G, Speiser B, Schaper J. Ultrastructural quantitation of mitochondria and myofilaments in cardiac muscle from 10 different animal species including man. J Mol Cell Cardiol 1992;24:669–81. https://doi.org/10.1016/0022-2828(92)93381-S.

[67] Chouchani ET, Pell VR, Gaude E, Aksentijević D, Sundier SY, Robb EL, et al. Ischaemic accumulation of succinate controls reperfusion injury through mitochondrial ROS. Nature 2014;515:431–5. https://doi.org/10.1038/NATURE13909.

[68] Zhang J, Wang YT, Miller JH, Day MM, Munger JC, Brookes PS. Accumulation of succinate in cardiac ischemia primarily occurs via canonical Krebs cycle activity. Cell Rep 2018;23:2617–28. https://doi.org/10.1016/J.CELREP.2018.04.104.

[69] Pasdois P, Parker JE, Griffiths EJ, Halestrap AP. The role of oxidized cytochrome c in regulating mitochondrial reactive oxygen species production and its perturbation in ischaemia. Biochem J 2011;436:493–505. https://doi.org/10.1042/BJ20101957.

[70] Petrosillo G, Ruggiero FM, di Venosa N, Paradies G. Decreased complex III activity in mitochondria isolated from rat heart subjected to ischemia and reperfusion: role of reactive oxygen species and cardiolipin. FASEB J 2003;17:714–6. https://doi.org/10.1096/FJ.02-0729FJE.

[71] Bugger H, Pfeil K. Mitochondrial ROS in myocardial ischemia reperfusion and remodeling. Biochim Biophys Acta Mol Basis Dis 2020;1866. https://doi.org/10.1016/J.BBADIS.2020.165768.

[72] Kaludercic N, Mialet-Perez J, Paolocci N, Parini A, di Lisa F. Monoamine oxidases as sources of oxidants in the heart. J Mol Cell Cardiol 2014;73:34–42. https://doi.org/10.1016/J.YJMCC.2013.12.032.

[73] Kaludercic N, Carpi A, Nagayama T, Sivakumaran V, Zhu G, Lai EW, et al. Monoamine oxidase B prompts mitochondrial and cardiac dysfunction in pressure overloaded hearts. Antioxid Redox Signal 2014;20:267–80. https://doi.org/10.1089/ARS.2012.4616.

[74] Giorgio M, Migliaccio E, Orsini F, Paolucci D, Moroni M, Contursi C, et al. Electron transfer between cytochrome c and p66Shc generates reactive oxygen species that trigger mitochondrial apoptosis. Cell 2005;122:221–33. https://doi.org/10.1016/J.CELL.2005.05.011.

[75] Nemoto S, Finkel T. Redox regulation of forkhead proteins through a p66shc-dependent signaling pathway. Science 2002;295:2450–2. https://doi.org/10.1126/SCIENCE.1069004.

[76] Matsushima S, Kuroda J, Ago T, Zhai P, Ikeda Y, Oka S, et al. Broad suppression of NADPH oxidase activity exacerbates ischemia/reperfusion injury through inadvertent downregulation of hypoxia-inducible factor-1α and upregulation of peroxisome proliferator-activated receptor-α. Circ Res 2013;112:1135–49. https://doi.org/10.1161/CIRCRESAHA.111.300171.

[77] MacMillan-Crow LA, Crow JP, Thompson JA. Peroxynitrite-mediated inactivation of manganese superoxide dismutase involves nitration and oxidation of critical tyrosine residues. Biochemistry 1998;37:1613–22. https://doi.org/10.1021/BI971894B.

[78] Liu B, Tewari AK, Zhang L, Green-Church KB, Zweier JL, Chen YR, He G. Proteomic analysis of protein tyrosine nitration after ischemia reperfusion injury: mitochondria as the major target. Biochim Biophys Acta 2009;1794:476–85. https://doi.org/10.1016/J.BBAPAP.2008.12.008.

[79] Ong SB, Subrayan S, Lim SY, Yellon DM, Davidson SM, Hausenloy DJ. Inhibiting mitochondrial fission protects the heart against ischemia/reperfusion injury. Circulation 2010;121:2012–22. https://doi.org/10.1161/CIRCULATIONAHA.109.906610.

[80] Zhou H, Zhu P, Wang J, Zhu H, Ren J, Chen Y. Pathogenesis of cardiac ischemia reperfusion injury is associated with CK2α-disturbed mitochondrial homeostasis via suppression of FUNDC1-related mitophagy. Cell Death Differ 2018;25:1080–93. https://doi.org/10.1038/S41418-018-0086-7.

[81] Davidson SM, Ferdinandy P, Andreadou I, Bøtker HE, Heusch G, Ibáñez B, et al. Multitarget strategies to reduce myocardial ischemia/reperfusion injury: JACC review topic of the week. J Am Coll Cardiol 2019;73:89–99. https://doi.org/10.1016/J.JACC.2018.09.086.

[82] Wolke C, Bukowska A, Goette A, Lendeckel U. Redox control of cardiac remodeling in atrial fibrillation. Biochim Biophys Acta 2015;1850:1555–65. https://doi.org/10.1016/J.BBAGEN.2014.12.012.

[83] Mihm MJ, Yu F, Carnes CA, Reiser PJ, McCarthy PM, van Wagoner DR, Bauer JA. Impaired myofibrillar energetics and oxidative injury during human atrial fibrillation. Circulation 2001;104:174–80. https://doi.org/10.1161/01.CIR.104.2.174.

[84] Carnes CA, Chung MK, Nakayama T, Nakayama H, Baliga RS, Piao S, et al. Ascorbate attenuates atrial pacing-induced peroxynitrite formation and electrical remodeling and decreases the incidence of postoperative atrial fibrillation. Circ Res 2001;89. https://doi.org/10.1161/HH1801.097644.

[85] Korantzopoulos P, Kolettis TM, Galaris D, Goudevenos JA. The role of oxidative stress in the pathogenesis and perpetuation of atrial fibrillation. Int J Cardiol 2007;115:135–43. https://doi.org/10.1016/J.IJCARD.2006.04.026.

[86] Corradi D, Callegari S, Manotti L, Ferrara D, Goldoni M, Alinovi R, et al. Persistent lone atrial fibrillation: clinicopathologic study of 19 cases. Heart Rhythm 2014;11:1250–8. https://doi.org/10.1016/J.HRTHM.2014.02.008.

[87] Kim Y, Guzik T, Zhang Y, Zhang M, Kattach H, Ratnatunga C, et al. A myocardial Nox2 containing NAD(P)H oxidase contributes to oxidative stress in human atrial fibrillation. Circ Res 2005;97(7):629–36. https://doi.org/10.1161/01.RES.0000183735.09871.61.

[88] Adam O, Lavall D, Theobald K, Hohl M, Grube M, Ameling S, et al. Rac1-induced connective tissue growth factor regulates connexin 43 and N-cadherin expression in atrial fibrillation. J Am Coll Cardiol 2010;55:469–80. https://doi.org/10.1016/J.JACC.2009.08.064.

[89] Friedrichs K, Baldus S, Klinke A. Fibrosis in atrial fibrillation—role of reactive species and MPO. Front Physiol 2012;3. https://doi.org/10.3389/FPHYS.2012.00214.

[90] Rudolph V, Andrié RP, Rudolph TK, Friedrichs K, Klinke A, Hirsch-Hoffmann B, et al. Myeloperoxidase acts as a profibrotic mediator of atrial fibrillation. Nat Med 2010;16:470–4. https://doi.org/10.1038/NM.2124.

[91] Antoniades C, Demosthenous M, Reilly S, Margaritis M, Zhang MH, Antonopoulos A, et al. Myocardial redox state predicts in-hospital clinical outcome after cardiac surgery effects of short-term pre-operative statin treatment. J Am Coll Cardiol 2012;59:60–70. https://doi.org/10.1016/J.JACC.2011.08.062.

[92] Rodrigo R. Prevention of postoperative atrial fibrillation: novel and safe strategy based on the modulation of the antioxidant system. Front Physiol 2012;3. https://doi.org/10.3389/FPHYS.2012.00093.

[93] Harling L, Rasoli S, Vecht JA, Ashrafian H, Kourliouros A, Athanasiou T. Do antioxidant vitamins have an anti-arrhythmic effect following cardiac surgery? A meta-analysis of randomised controlled trials. Heart 2011;97:1636−42. https://doi.org/10.1136/HEARTJNL-2011-300245.

[94] Ozaydin M, Peker O, Erdogan D, Kapan S, Turker Y, Varol E, et al. N-acetylcysteine for the prevention of postoperative atrial fibrillation: a prospective, randomized, placebo-controlled pilot study. Eur Heart J 2008;29:625−31. https://doi.org/10.1093/EURHEARTJ/EHN011.

[95] Mirmiran P, Hosseini-Esfahani F, Esfandiar Z, Hosseinpour-Niazi S, Azizi F. Associations between dietary antioxidant intakes and cardiovascular disease. Sci Rep 2022;12:1504. https://doi.org/10.1038/S41598-022-05632-X.

[96] Luo J, Yan D, Li S, Liu S, Zeng F, Cheung CW, et al. Allopurinol reduces oxidative stress and activates Nrf2/p62 to attenuate diabetic cardiomyopathy in rats. J Cell Mol Med 2020;24:1760−73. https://doi.org/10.1111/JCMM.14870.

[97] Kenny HC, Abel ED. Heart failure in type 2 diabetes mellitus. Circ Res 2019;124:121−41. https://doi.org/10.1161/CIRCRESAHA.118.311371.

[98] Dhalla NS, Ganguly PK, Bhullar SK, Tappia PS. Role of catecholamines in the pathogenesis of diabetic cardiomyopathy. Can J Physiol Pharmacol 2019;97:815−9. www.nrcresearchpress.com.

[99] Ritchie RH, Dale Abel E. Basic mechanisms of diabetic heart disease. Circ Res 2020;126:1501−25. https://doi.org/10.1161/CIRCRESAHA.120.315913.

[100] Henning RJ. Type-2 diabetes mellitus and cardiovascular disease. Future Cardiol 2018;14:491−509. https://doi.org/10.2217/FCA-2018-0045.

[101] Tan Y, Zhang Z, Zheng C, Wintergerst KA, Keller BB, Cai L. Mechanisms of diabetic cardiomyopathy and potential therapeutic strategies: preclinical and clinical evidence. Nat Rev Cardiol 2020;17:585−607. https://doi.org/10.1038/S41569-020-0339-2.

[102] Li C, Zhang J, Xue M, Li X, Han F, Liu X, et al. SGLT2 inhibition with empagliflozin attenuates myocardial oxidative stress and fibrosis in diabetic mice heart. Cardiovasc Diabetol 2019;18. https://doi.org/10.1186/S12933-019-0816-2.

[103] Fahey JW, Talalay P. Antioxidant functions of sulforaphane: a potent inducer of phase II detoxication enzymes. Food Chem Toxicol 1999;37:973−9. https://doi.org/10.1016/S0278-6915(99)00082-4.

[104] Axelsson AS, Tubbs E, Mecham B, Chacko S, Nenonen HA, Tang Y, et al. Sulforaphane reduces hepatic glucose production and improves glucose control in patients with type 2 diabetes. Sci Transl Med 2017;9. https://doi.org/10.1126/SCITRANSLMED.AAH4477.

[105] Wittstein IS, Thiemann DR, Lima JAC, Baughman KL, Schulman SP, Gerstenblith G, et al. Neurohumoral features of myocardial stunning due to sudden emotional stress. N Engl J Med 2005;352:539−48. https://doi.org/10.1056/NEJMOA043046.

[106] Ghadri JR, Wittstein IS, Prasad A, Sharkey S, Dote K, Akashi YJ, et al. International expert consensus document on takotsubo syndrome (part I): clinical characteristics, diagnostic criteria, and pathophysiology. Eur Heart J 2018;39:2032−46. https://doi.org/10.1093/EURHEARTJ/EHY076.

[107] Abraham J, Mudd JO, Kapur N, Klein K, Champion HC, Wittstein IS. Stress cardiomyopathy after intravenous administration of catecholamines and beta-receptor agonists. J Am Coll Cardiol 2009;53:1320−5. https://doi.org/10.1016/J.JACC.2009.02.020.

[108] Batisse-Lignier M, Pereira B, Motreff P, Pierrard R, Burnot C, Vorilhon C, et al. Acute and chronic pheochromocytoma-induced cardiomyopathies: different prognoses? A systematic analytical review. Medicine 2015;94. https://doi.org/10.1097/MD.0000000000002198.

[109] Han L, Luo JG, Chen X, Hu WZ, Chen LW, Xin XM, et al. Left ventricular noncompaction combined with epinephrine-secreted pheochromocytoma inducing heart failure. Int Heart J 2016;57:254−7. https://doi.org/10.1536/IHJ.15-311.

[110] de Miguel V, Arias A, Paissan A, de Arenaza DP, Pietrani M, Jurado A, et al. Catecholamine-induced myocarditis in pheochromocytoma. Circulation 2014;129:1348−9. https://doi.org/10.1161/CIRCULATIONAHA.113.002762.

[111] Hantson P. Mechanisms of toxic cardiomyopathy. Clin Toxicol 2019;57:1−9. https://doi.org/10.1080/15563650.2018.1497172.

[112] Nef HM, Möllmann H, Troidl C, Kostin S, Böttger T, Voss S, et al. Expression profiling of cardiac genes in Tako-Tsubo cardiomyopathy: insight into a new cardiac entity. J Mol Cell Cardiol 2008;44:395−404. https://doi.org/10.1016/J.YJMCC.2007.10.015.

[113] Kassim TA, Clarke DD, Mai VQ, Clyde PW, Shakir KMM. Catecholamine-induced cardiomyopathy. Endocr Pract 2008;14:1137−49. https://doi.org/10.4158/EP.14.9.1137.

[114] Singal PK, Kapur N, Dhillon KS, Beamish RE, Dhalla NS. Role of free radicals in catecholamine-induced cardiomyopathy. Can J Physiol Pharmacol 1982;60:1390−7. https://doi.org/10.1139/Y82-207.

[115] Gehl J, Boesgaard M, Paaske T, Vittrup Jensen B, Dombernowsky P. Combined doxorubicin and paclitaxel in advanced breast cancer: effective and cardiotoxic. Ann Oncol 1996;7:687−93. https://doi.org/10.1093/OXFORDJOURNALS.ANNONC.A010717.

[116] Gao RY, Mukhopadhyay P, Mohanraj R, Wang H, Horváth B, Yin S, Pacher P. Resveratrol attenuates azidothymidine-induced cardiotoxicity by decreasing mitochondrial reactive oxygen species generation in human cardiomyocytes. Mol Med Rep 2011;4:151−5. https://doi.org/10.3892/MMR.2010.390.

[117] Kohler JJ, Cucoranu I, Fields E, Green E, He S, Hoying A, et al. Transgenic mitochondrial superoxide dismutase and mitochondrially targeted catalase prevent antiretroviral-induced oxidative stress and cardiomyopathy. Lab Invest 2009;89:782−90. https://doi.org/10.1038/LABINVEST.2009.39.

[118] Saravanan R, Pugalendi V. Impact of ursolic acid on chronic ethanol-induced oxidative stress in the rat heart. Pharmacol Rep 2006;58:41−7.

[119] Venturini M, Michelotti A, del Mastro L, Gallo L, Carnino F, Garrone O, et al. Multicenter randomized controlled clinical trial to evaluate cardioprotection of dexrazoxane versus no cardioprotection in women receiving epirubicin chemotherapy for advanced breast cancer. J Clin Oncol 1996;14:3112−20. https://doi.org/10.1200/JCO.1996.14.12.3112.

[120] Swain SM, Whaley FS, Gerber MC, Ewer MS, Bianchine JR, Gams RA. Delayed administration of dexrazoxane provides cardioprotection for patients with advanced breast cancer treated with doxorubicin-containing therapy. J Clin Oncol 1997;15:1333−40. https://doi.org/10.1200/JCO.1997.15.4.1333.

[121] Swain SM, Whaley FS, Gerber MC, Weisberg S, York M, Spicer D, et al. Cardioprotection with dexrazoxane for doxorubicin-containing therapy in advanced breast cancer. J Clin Oncol 1997;15:1318–32. https://doi.org/10.1200/JCO.1997.15.4.1318.

[122] Vejpongsa P, Yeh ETH. Prevention of anthracycline-induced cardiotoxicity: challenges and opportunities. J Am Coll Cardiol 2014;64:938–45. https://doi.org/10.1016/J.JACC.2014.06.1167.

[123] US Food and Drugs Administration. Drug safety and availability. FDA statement on dexrazoxane; 2011.

[124] Hasinoff BB, Patel D, Wu X. The oral iron chelator ICL670A (deferasirox) does not protect myocytes against doxorubicin. Free Radic Biol Med 2003;35:1469–79. https://doi.org/10.1016/j.freeradbiomed.2003.08.005.

[125] Martin E, Thougaard AV, Grauslund M, Jensen PB, Bjorkling F, Hasinoff BB, et al. Evaluation of the topoisomerase II-inactive bisdioxopiperazine ICRF-161 as a protectant against doxorubicin-induced cardiomyopathy. Toxicology 2009;255:72–9. https://doi.org/10.1016/J.TOX.2008.10.011.

[126] Unverferth Dv, Jagadeesh JM, Unverferth BJ, Magorien RD, Leier Cv, Balcerzak SP. Attempt to prevent doxorubicin-induced acute human myocardial morphologic damage with acetylcysteine. JNCI 1983;71:917–20. https://doi.org/10.1093/JNCI/71.5.917.

[127] Dresdale AR, Barr LH, Bonow RO, Mathisen DJ, Myers CE, Schwartz DE, et al. Prospective randomized study of the role of N-acetyl cysteine in reversing doxorubicin-induced cardiomyopathy. Am J Clin Oncol 1982;5:657–63. https://doi.org/10.1097/00000421-198212000-00015.

[128] Kalay N, Basar E, Ozdogru I, Er O, Cetinkaya Y, Dogan A, et al. Protective effects of carvedilol against anthracycline-induced cardiomyopathy. J Am Coll Cardiol 2006;48:2258–62. https://doi.org/10.1016/J.JACC.2006.07.052.

[129] Kaya MG, Ozkan M, Gunebakmaz O, Akkaya H, Kaya EG, Akpek M, et al. Protective effects of nebivolol against anthracycline-induced cardiomyopathy: a randomized control study. Int J Cardiol 2013;167:2306–10. https://doi.org/10.1016/J.IJCARD.2012.06.023.

[130] Abuosa AM, Elshiekh AH, Qureshi K, Abrar MB, Kholeif MA, Kinsara AJ, et al. Prophylactic use of carvedilol to prevent ventricular dysfunction in patients with cancer treated with doxorubicin. Indian Heart J 2018;70(Suppl. 3):S96–100. https://doi.org/10.1016/J.IHJ.2018.06.011.

[131] Avila MS, Ayub-Ferreira SM, de Barros Wanderley MR, das Dores Cruz F, Gonçalves Brandão SM, Rigaud VOC, et al. Carvedilol for prevention of chemotherapy-related cardiotoxicity: the CECCY trial. J Am Coll Cardiol 2018;71:2281–90. https://doi.org/10.1016/J.JACC.2018.02.049.

[132] Lee M, Chung WB, eun Lee J, Park CS, Park WC, Song BJ, Youn HJ. Candesartan and carvedilol for primary prevention of subclinical cardiotoxicity in breast cancer patients without a cardiovascular risk treated with doxorubicin. Cancer Med 2021;10:3964–73. https://doi.org/10.1002/CAM4.3956.

[133] Heck SL, Mecinaj A, Ree AH, Hoffmann P, Schulz-Menger J, Fagerland MW, et al. Prevention of cardiac dysfunction during adjuvant breast cancer therapy (PRADA): extended follow-up of a 2 × 2 factorial, randomized, placebo-controlled, double-blind clinical trial of candesartan and metoprolol. Circulation 2021;143:2431–40. https://doi.org/10.1161/CIRCULATIONAHA.121.054698.

[134] Janbabai G, Nabati M, Faghihinia M, Azizi S, Borhani S, Yazdani J. Effect of enalapril on preventing anthracycline-induced cardiomyopathy. Cardiovasc Toxicol 2017;17:130–9. https://doi.org/10.1007/S12012-016-9365-Z.

[135] Akpek M, Ozdogru I, Sahin O, Inanc M, Dogan A, Yazici C, et al. Protective effects of spironolactone against anthracycline-induced cardiomyopathy. Eur J Heart Fail 2015;17:81–9. https://doi.org/10.1002/EJHF.196.

[136] Kheiri B, Abdalla A, Osman M, Haykal T, Chahine A, Ahmed S, et al. Meta-analysis of carvedilol for the prevention of anthracycline-induced cardiotoxicity. Am J Cardiol 2018;122:1959–64. https://doi.org/10.1016/J.AMJCARD.2018.08.039.

[137] Tanai E, Frantz S. Pathophysiology of heart failure. Compr Physiol 2016;6:187–214. https://doi.org/10.1002/cphy.c140055.

[138] Aimo A, Castiglione V, Borrelli C, Saccaro LF, Franzini M, Masi S, et al. Oxidative stress and inflammation in the evolution of heart failure: from pathophysiology to therapeutic strategies. Eur J Prev Cardiol 2020;27:494–510. https://doi.org/10.1177/2047487319870344.

[139] Lubrano V, Balzan S. Role of oxidative stress-related biomarkers in heart failure: galectin 3, α1-antitrypsin and LOX-1: new therapeutic perspective? Mol Cell Biochem 2020;464:143–52. https://doi.org/10.1007/s11010-019-03656-y.

[140] Takimoto E, Kass DA. Role of oxidative stress in cardiac hypertrophy and remodeling. Hypertension 2007;49:241–8. https://doi.org/10.1161/01.HYP.0000254415.31362.A7.

[141] Spinale FG, Coker ML, Thomas Cv, Walker JD, Mukherjee R, Hebbar L. Time-dependent changes in matrix metalloproteinase activity and expression during the progression of congestive heart failure: relation to ventricular and myocyte function. Circ Res 1998;82:482–95. https://doi.org/10.1161/01.RES.82.4.482.

[142] van der Pol A, van Gilst WH, Voors AA, van der Meer P. Treating oxidative stress in heart failure: past, present and future. Eur J Heart Fail 2019;21:425–35. https://doi.org/10.1002/ejhf.1320.

[143] Hill MF, Singal PK. Antioxidant and oxidative stress changes during heart failure subsequent to myocardial infarction in rats. Am J Pathol 1996;148:291–300.

[144] Khaper N, Singal PK. Effects of afterload-reducing drugs on pathogenesis of antioxidant changes and congestive heart failure in rats. J Am Coll Cardiol 1997;29:856–61. https://doi.org/10.1016/S0735-1097(96)00574-8.

[145] Khaper N, Kaur K, Li T, Farahmand F, Singal PK. Antioxidant enzyme gene expression in congestive heart failure following myocardial infarction. Biochem Hypertrophy Heart Fail 2003:9–15. https://doi.org/10.1007/978-1-4419-9238-3_2.

[146] Ghatak A, Brar MJS, Agarwal A, Goel N, Rastogi AK, Vaish AK, et al. Oxy free radical system in heart failure and therapeutic role of oral vitamin E. Int J Cardiol 1996;57:119–27. https://doi.org/10.1016/S0167-5273(96)02787-8.

[147] Keith ME, Jeejeebhoy KN, Langer A, Kurian R, Barr A, O'Kelly B, Sole MJ. A controlled clinical trial of vitamin E supplementation in patients with congestive heart failure. Am J Clin Nutr 2001;73:219–24. https://doi.org/10.1093/AJCN/73.2.219.

[148] Tousoulis D, Antoniades C, Vassiliadou C, Toutouza M, Pitsavos C, Tentolouris C, et al. Effects of combined administration of low dose atorvastatin and vitamin E on inflammatory markers and endothelial function in patients with heart failure. Eur J Heart Fail 2005;7:1126–32. https://doi.org/10.1016/J.EJHEART.2005.03.007.

[149] Khan MS, Khan F, Fonarow GC, Sreenivasan J, Greene SJ, Khan SU, et al. Dietary interventions and nutritional supplements for heart failure: a systematic appraisal and evidence map. Eur J Heart Fail 2021;23:1468–76. https://doi.org/10.1002/EJHF.2278.

[150] Hamaguchi S, Furumoto T, Tsuchihashi-Makaya M, Goto K, Goto D, Yokota T, et al. Hyperuricemia predicts adverse outcomes in patients with heart failure. Int J Cardiol 2011;151:143–7. https://doi.org/10.1016/J.IJCARD.2010.05.002.

[151] von Lueder TG, Girerd N, Atar D, Agewall S, Lamiral Z, Kanbay M, et al. Serum uric acid is associated with mortality and heart failure hospitalizations in patients with complicated myocardial infarction: findings from the High-Risk Myocardial Infarction Database Initiative. Eur J Heart Fail 2015;17:1144–51. https://doi.org/10.1002/EJHF.419.

[152] Hare JM, Mangal B, Brown J, Fisher C, Freudenberger R, Colucci WS, et al. Impact of oxypurinol in patients with symptomatic heart failure: results of the OPT-CHF study. J Am Coll Cardiol 2008;51:2301–9. https://doi.org/10.1016/J.JACC.2008.01.068.

[153] Givertz MM, Anstrom KJ, Redfield MM, Deswal A, Haddad H, Butler J, et al. Effects of xanthine oxidase inhibition in hyperuricemic heart failure patients: the xanthine oxidase inhibition for hyperuricemic heart failure patients (EXACT-HF) study. Circulation 2015;131:1763–71. https://doi.org/10.1161/CIRCULATIONAHA.114.014536/FORMAT/EPUB.

[154] Mortensen SA, Rosenfeldt F, Kumar A, Dolliner P, Filipiak KJ, Pella D, et al. The effect of coenzyme Q10 on morbidity and mortality in chronic heart failure: results from Q-SYMBIO: a randomized double-blind trial. JACC Heart Fail 2014;2:641–9. https://doi.org/10.1016/J.JCHF.2014.06.008.

[155] Mortensen AL, Rosenfeldt F, Filipiak KJ. Effect of coenzyme Q10 in Europeans with chronic heart failure: a sub-group analysis of the Q-SYMBIO randomized double-blind trial. Cardiol J 2019;26:147–56. https://doi.org/10.5603/CJ.A2019.0022.

[156] Filipiak KJ, Surma S, Romańczyk M, Okopień B. Heart failure—do we need new drugs or have them already? A case of coenzyme Q10. J Cardiovasc Dev Dis 2022;9:161. https://doi.org/10.3390/JCDD9050161.

Chapter 10

Modulation of cancer cell proliferation by interfering with metabolic ROS production

Fabio Ciccarone[1,2] and Maria Rosa Ciriolo[1,2]
[1]Department of Biology, University of Rome "Tor Vergata", Rome, Italy; [2]IRCCS San Raffaele Roma, Rome, Italy

Key takeaways

- Reactive oxygen species (ROS) increase in cancer cells promotes multiple cancer hallmarks
- Metabolic rearrangements in cancer cells contribute to ROS production
- Cancer cell homeostasis is drawn by ROS-mediated signaling
- Buffering ROS production impact cancer cell proliferation
- Boosting metabolic ROS production may exert cytotoxic effects

Introduction

The augmented reactive oxygen species (ROS) production has been ever considered an inevitable aspect of cancer cells, affecting most, if not all, cancer hallmarks, primarily replicative immortality, metabolic rewiring, cell death resistance, and metastasis formation. The increased metabolic rate of highly proliferating cells could represent a confounding factor in assessing ROS levels when comparing cancer cells to differentiated slow-cycling or growth-arrested cells. However, the use of genetically controlled cell lines bearing only a specific oncogenic variant (e.g., Ras or Bcr-Abl) definitely proved that increased ROS burst is an event that accompanies cellular transformation [1,2]. Freely cycling cancer cells evidence a progressive increase of ROS production as cells proceed from the G1 phase to G2 and mitosis. In contrast, the peak of oxidative damage to proteins and nucleotides occurs specifically in mitotic cells. Both events are exacerbated by antimitotic drugs, such as docetaxel and nocodazole [3]. These results suggest ROS and biomolecule oxidation during cell cycle phases may imprint a signal necessary for mitotic progression.

ROS sources in a cell are multiple but can be clustered in metabolic or signaling-linked sources. The increased metabolic activity typical of cancer cells accounts for ROS production due to enhancement of oxidative metabolism or accumulation of dysfunctional mitochondria, overactivation of the peroxisomal activity, or stimulation of oxidases and oxygenases. On the other hand, growth factors and cytokines, released by infiltrating immune cells or in an autocrine way by cancer cells, can overstimulate cellular receptor signaling coupled with ROS sources, such as NADPH oxidase or enzymes producing oxygenated metabolites (e.g., lipoxygenases) [4]. The sites of ROS production in a cell are depicted in Fig. 10.1.

Genetic alterations and metabolic perturbations enhancing mitochondrial oxidation of energetic fuels can actively impact ROS production in cancer. This was shown to yield both deleterious and beneficial effects on tumor growth depending on the basal metabolism of the cell, the tolerance to the new metabolic setting, and the ability to mount an efficient antioxidant response or to activate restorative mechanisms that go from DNA repair to autophagy [5].

Redox signaling processes activate the expression of antioxidant enzymes and channel metabolic fluxes toward pathways that maintain intracellular redox balance to limit the accumulation of harmful ROS as metabolic by-products. A high NADPH/NADP$^+$ ratio is fundamental for the efficiency of antioxidant systems as NADPH provides reducing equivalents to maintain active catalase or regenerate thioredoxin and glutathione (GSH). These latter are directly or indirectly used by most enzymatic antioxidant systems, including glutaredoxins, peroxiredoxins, and glutathione peroxidases, to neutralize ROS or recover oxidized macromolecules. The fine-tuning of ROS flux in cancer cells is frequently achieved by altering the regulation of molecular sensors of prooxidant conditions, primarily the master regulator of antioxidant response nuclear factor erythroid 2 (NF-E2)-related factor 2 (NRF2). Deletion/mutation of Kelch-like ECH-associated protein 1 (KEAP1) and Cullin 3 (Cul3), which are involved in the ubiquitination-mediated

Modulation of Oxidative Stress. https://doi.org/10.1016/B978-0-443-19247-0.00017-5

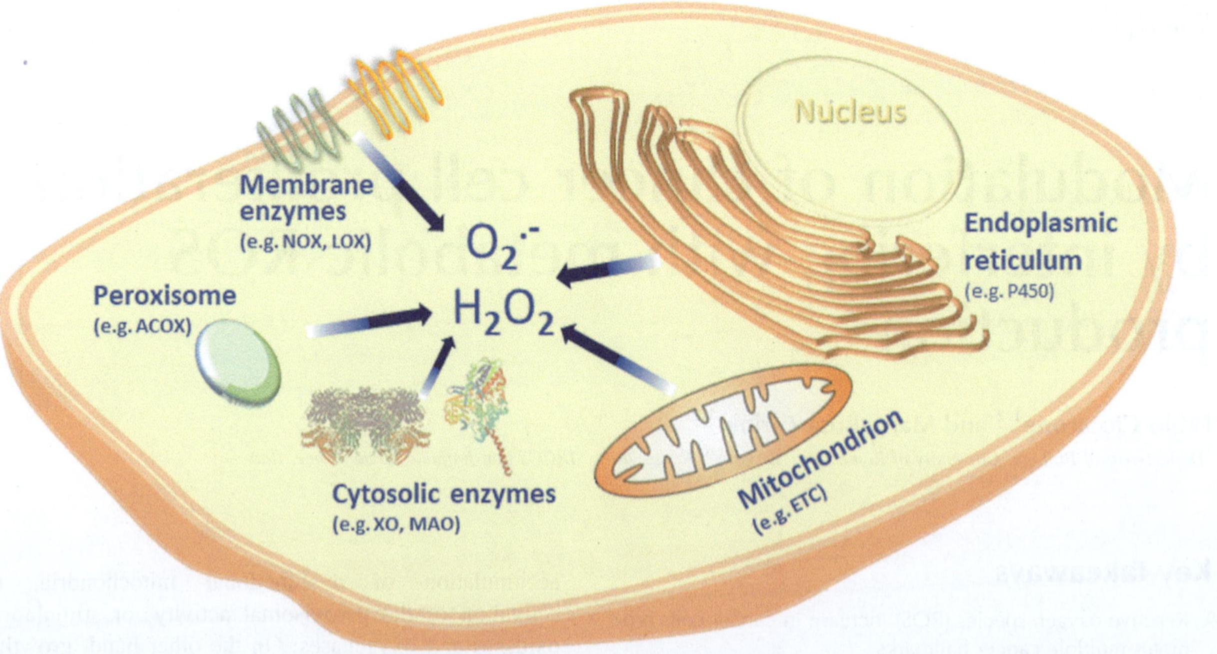

FIGURE 10.1 Endogenous reactive oxygen species (ROS) sources in the cell. Sites of production of the main ROS sources inside a mammalian cell. *ACOX*, acyl-coenzyme A oxidase; *ETC*, electron transport chain; *LOX*, lipoxygenase; *MAO*, monoamine oxidase; *NOX*, NADPH oxidase; *P450*, cytochrome P450; *XO*, xanthine oxidase.

degradation of NRF2 in unstressed conditions, or amplification of the genomic locus bearing NRF2-encoding gene contribute to the constitutive activation of NRF2 pathway in cancer. In this way, cancer cells are sheltered from the deleterious accumulation of damages deriving from electrophilic, metabolic, and oxidative stress [6,7].

A deep characterization of the origin and the function of ROS flux in cancer is ongoing to design therapeutic interventions that can hinder ROS protumorigenic functions or foster ROS cytotoxicity by overcoming the protective threshold of endogenous antioxidants.

Metabolic sources of ROS in cancer

Mitochondrial ROS as by-products of the electron transport chain

Mitochondrial respiration represents the primary metabolic source of ROS. Under normal conditions, mitochondrial ROS are physiologically produced by the electron transport chain (ETC) complexes in the form of superoxide anion radical ($O_2^{\cdot -}$) and released into the intermembrane space and mitochondrial matrix. Mitochondrial ROS passively flow out from the mitochondria generally as hydrogen peroxide (H_2O_2) upon dismutation of $O_2^{\cdot -}$ by Cu/Zn superoxide dismutase (SOD1) in the intermembrane space or by MnSOD (SOD2) in the mitochondrial matrix. However, the leakage of $O_2^{\cdot -}$ into the cytoplasm may rarely occur via the mitochondrial permeability transition pore [8].

One of the most intriguing findings about the production of mitochondrial ROS lies in their capacity to modulate different hallmarks of cancer cells acting on processes held in any cell compartment. For instance, mitochondrial ROS are coupled with DNA replication through direct oxidation of cyclin-dependent kinase 2 (CDK2) [9] and with the activation of metabolic pathways that sustain uncontrolled cell division and survival in stressful conditions.

The production of mitochondrial ROS is dramatically enhanced when ETC complexes exhibit genetic or acquired mutations or when metabolic perturbations increase the NADH/NAD^+ ratio or the proton motive force and the pool of reduced coenzyme Q (UQH_2) in conditions of low ATP demand. The principal ROS sources in the respiratory chain are the NADH:ubiquinone oxidoreductase (complex I), the succinate dehydrogenase complex (complex II), and the ubiquinol-cytochrome c oxidoreductase complex (complex III). Electron leak and $O_2^{\cdot -}$ formation typically occur at the flavin mononucleotide (FMN) site and Q binding site of complex I, at the FAD site of complex II, and at the inner or outer Q site of complex III consequently to the autooxidation of ubisemiquinone. In addition, complex I can produce ROS via reverse electron transfer (RET) when reduced coenzyme Q is overproduced and electrons are transferred back, reducing NAD^+ to NADH [10].

Genomic profiling of multiple tumor types has identified a high frequency of mutational events in mitochondrial DNA (mtDNA) with a preference for the replicative strand and coding regions. This indicates that mtDNA mutations in cancer mainly originate from endogenous mutational mechanisms dependent on replication [11,12]. More importantly, those mutational events may directly support cancer growth and/or progression affecting ROS generation [13]. For instance, G13997A and 13885insC mutations in the *ND6* subunit of complex I promoted a metastatic phenotype due to ROS overproduction [14]. Production of mitochondrial ROS by dysfunctional respiratory complexes is also caused by the mutation of nuclear-encoded subunits of ETC, as demonstrated for the four subunits (SDHA, B, C, and D) of the succinate dehydrogenase complex. SDH germline mutations are responsible for developing different types of tumors, more frequently pheochromocytoma and paraganglioma. In the presence of high succinate concentrations, complex II indirectly produces ROS forcing RET onto complex I [15]. Consistently, genetic alterations of all subunits lead to succinate accumulation and generate ROS, even though to a different extent [16]. SDHB depletion increases ROS production more than SDHA or D, which is also a consequence of changes in cell metabolism and iron homeostasis [17,18]. Moreover, the induction of mesenchymal markers typical of metastatic cells in the absence of SDHB is consistent with the fact that paragangliomas bearing mutations in the *SDHB* gene have a more aggressive phenotype. Different therapeutic approaches were tested to exacerbate oxidative stress in *SDHB*-mutated tumors. High doses of ascorbate were demonstrated to induce cytotoxicity by exploiting iron pro-oxidant activity via the Fenton reaction [18,19]. Inhibition of the NRF2 was an alternative strategy to dampen cell proliferation/survival and liver metastasis in a preclinical mouse model of *SDHB*-defective tumors [20].

Direct and indirect ROS generation by metabolic enzymes

In addition to ETC complexes, different mitochondrial enzymes produce ROS as by-products in their enzymatic reaction. They can be subcategorized into two classes according to the electron donating groups involved in ROS generation, the isopotential groups NADH/NAD^+ and UQH_2/UQ. Relevant enzymes that may aberrantly produce ROS from NADH are pyruvate dehydrogenase (PDH), which oxidizes pyruvate into acetyl-CoA, and α-ketoglutarate dehydrogenase (α-KGDH), which produces succinyl-CoA from α-KG in the Krebs cycle. Enzymes that utilize UQ as a co-substrate include the electron transfer flavoprotein:ubiquinone oxidoreductase (ETF-QO), which couples electrons derived from β-oxidation of fatty acids to the UQH_2 pool, and the dihydroorotate dehydrogenase (DHODH), which is involved in pyrimidine biosynthesis converting dihydroorotate to orotate [21]. The contribution of these enzymes to ROS generation in vivo is difficult to discern from other mitochondrial ROS sources as they mainly produce ROS via RET from ETC complexes. Nevertheless, their involvement in ROS increase in cancer can be envisaged as they belong to metabolic pathways extensively modulated in different tumor types and environmental conditions.

Conversely, other metabolic enzymes generating ROS directly from their enzymatic reaction have been connected to cancer ROS production. For instance, monoamine oxidase A (MAOA) catalyzes the oxidative deamination of endogenous and dietary amines producing H_2O_2. MAOA upregulation in prostate cancer promotes epithelial-to-mesenchymal transition and, thus, metastasis formation via ROS-mediated signaling [22]. Moreover, xanthine oxidase (XO), which is involved in the catabolism of purines, was shown to be activated by several antitumoral compounds. The consequent production of ROS triggers cell death [23,24]. This indicates that XO-mediated ROS have beneficial effects in chemotherapy and may justify why XO is frequently decreased in several tumor types [25].

Signaling-linked sources of ROS in cancer

NADPH oxidase

The NADPH oxidase (NOX) family is composed of transmembrane enzymes of which five NOX isoforms (NOX1−5) and two dual oxidase isoforms (DUOX1 and 2). Their enzymatic function produces ROS, transferring electrons from NADPH to molecular oxygen. NOX/DUOX enzymes are extensively upregulated in cancer and involved in most redox-signaling pathways linked to tumor proliferation and aggressiveness. For instance, NOX1, 2, 4, and DUOX2 promote angiogenesis and metastasis formation inducing the expression of vascular endothelial growth factor (VEGF) and matrix metalloproteinases by activating ERK-dependent signaling and redox-sensitive transcription factors [26]. NOX1 activation following WNT stimulation favors cell growth by stabilizing β-catenin through the oxidation of the negative regulator thioredoxin-like protein nucleoredoxin (NRX) [27]. NOX4-mediated ROS signaling is involved in epithelial-to-mesenchymal transition induced by TGF-β by oxidizing and inhibiting the phosphatase PTP1B in pancreatic cancer [28].

The protumorigenic activity of NOX/DUOX enzymes is a consequence of their overexpression in response to diverse oncogenic pathways, including insulin and platelet-derived growth factor (PDGF) signaling [26]. Conversely, the basal activity of NOX/DUOX enzymes has physiological effects and is required to maintain cellular homeostasis. For instance, the genetic deletion of NOX4 enhances carcinogen-induced tumorigenesis in mice models because constitutive low levels of ROS produced by NOX4 oxidize and inhibit AKT preserving genomic stability [29].

Cyclooxygenases and lipoxygenases

Cancer development and progression are frequently associated with enhanced production of signaling mediators with mitogenic effects or prosurvival properties. These include eicosanoids, which are lipid mediators deriving from polyunsaturated fatty acids (PUFA). The relevance of this class of molecules in cancer also depends on the enzymatic steps of their biosynthetic pathway catalyzed by cyclooxygenases (COX) or lipoxygenases (LOX), which contribute to ROS production.

The COX pathway produces prostaglandins (PG) and thromboxanes (TX) [30]. COX2 gene is particularly inducible and overexpressed in several cancer types following inflammatory stimuli and growth factors. Moreover, COX2 is a target of several oncogenic factors. Constitutively active mutant K-Ras(G12V) promotes COX2-dependent ROS production and consequent DNA damage that contribute to lung cell transformation [31].

The LOX pathway mainly produces leukotrienes (LT) and lipoxins. Some LOX enzymes can oxidze PUFA when still incorporated into membrane phospholipids. Thus their activity has been linked to lipid peroxidation-dependent ferroptotic cell death, as demonstrated in oncogenic Ras-expressing cancer cells [32]. Activation of LOX activity was observed in anaplastic large-cell lymphomas (ALCLs) bearing the oncogenic NPM-ALK chimeric protein. LOX-derived ROS were responsible for activating AKT, STAT3 and ERK1/2 signaling pathways, which are involved in the antiapoptotic and promitogenic effects of NPM−ALK [33]. Moreover, extracellular matrix proteins promote pancreatic cancer cell survival by activating 5-LOX, which is, directly and indirectly, responsible for ROS production by stimulating NOX activity [34]. LOX-derived eicosanoids can also stimulate the activity of NOX enzymes linked to their receptors on target cells. For instance, the leukotriene B(4) receptor BLT2 promotes NOX1/4-dependent ROS to facilitate NF-kB-mediated invasiveness in bladder cancer [35].

ROS and glucose metabolism in cancer

The enhancement of glucose metabolism and its atypical utilization in cancer cells is undoubtedly the most known mechanism related to cancer metabolic reprogramming. Cancer cells preferentially convert glucose-derived pyruvate into lactate even in aerobic conditions instead of directing it inside mitochondria. This phenomenon, called aerobic glycolysis or "the Warburg effect," was historically believed to depend on defects in oxidative metabolism due to dysfunctional mitochondria. While this can be considered valid for those examples of tumors originating from mutations in key mitochondrial components of the Krebs cycle or ETC, during the last decades, mitochondrial metabolism has been proven to work even in the presence of the Warburg effect. The necessity to limit mitochondrial respiration and the consequent ROS production is another possible explanation of the origin of the Warburg effect. Conversely, ROS triggered by microenvironmental fluctuations were also shown to be responsible for the Warburg effect [36]. ROS are critical regulators of cancer metabolic plasticity that satisfies bioenergetic and anabolic requirements in any specific genetic and environmental condition.

Nutrient deprivation and hypoxia typically occur in solid tumors due to limited blood supply, especially in the inner tumor mass. Mitochondrial ROS production is augmented by serum and amino acid withdrawal to promote the Warburg effect as an antiapoptotic and compensatory mechanism. This metabolic switch is achieved by ROS-mediated activation of AMP-activated protein kinase (AMPK) and consequent stimulation of pyruvate dehydrogenase kinase (PDK) activity. This enzyme is responsible for inhibiting PDH complex impeding pyruvate oxidation inside mitochondria while favoring lactate production by lactate dehydrogenase (LDH) and the Warburg effect [37]. Beyond starvation, hypoxia is undoubtedly the most prominent condition that imposes the activation of glycolysis as mitochondrial ATP production is inevitably impaired upon oxygen shortage. The paradoxical increase of mitochondrial ROS production occurring under hypoxia is necessary for activating downstream adaptative pathways. Cells depleted of mtDNA and thus unable to respire do not generate ROS during hypoxia and fail to promote glycolytic metabolism [38]. In particular, the quinol oxidation site of complex III was considered the primary mitochondrial source of ROS in hypoxic conditions [39]. Among the other mechanisms, hypoxia-dependent ROS contribute to the activation of hypoxia-inducible factor-1α (HIF-1α), the master regulator of the hypoxic response. HIF-1α-mediated rewiring of glucose metabolism is achieved by the upregulation of most of the genes involved in the glycolytic pathways (e.g., PGK and LDH), in addition to glucose transporters (e.g., GLUT1 and 3) and regulatory enzymes of glycolytic flux (e.g., PDK) [40]. A schematic of the regulation of HIF-1α activity on the switch between glycolytic and oxidative metabolism is reported in Fig. 10.2.

In normoxia, HIF-1α is efficiently hydroxylated by iron/α-KG dependent PHD enzymes, recognized by the von Hippel Lindau (VHL) E3 ubiquitin ligase and thus degraded via the proteasome [41,42]. In this context, ROS inhibits the PHD hydroxylase activity assuring HIF-1α stabilization in hypoxia [39]. Moreover, other players can promote ROS-mediated activation of HIF-1α, including the p38 MAPK [43] or the AMPK signaling [44], but the mechanisms of action, whether direct or indirect, have not been clarified yet.

Over the years, an alternative hypothesis on the role of mitochondria in HIF-1α stabilization has been proposed, independently of ROS production. In this model, mitochondrial respiration consumes residual oxygen content in hypoxic conditions, further decreasing cytosolic oxygen availability necessary for the activity of PHD enzymes [45,46]. While this is a reasonable possibility in low oxygen conditions, the role of mitochondria on HIF-1α stabilization is less questionable during "pseudohypoxia," which entails the activation of HIF-mediated hypoxic response in normoxia. Cancer metabolic rearrangements and ROS production frequently drive this condition.

The overexpression of G4776A mutated ND2 subunit of complex I, initially identified in human primary head and neck squamous cell carcinoma patients, induces the stabilization of HIF-1α in an ROS-dependent manner promoting

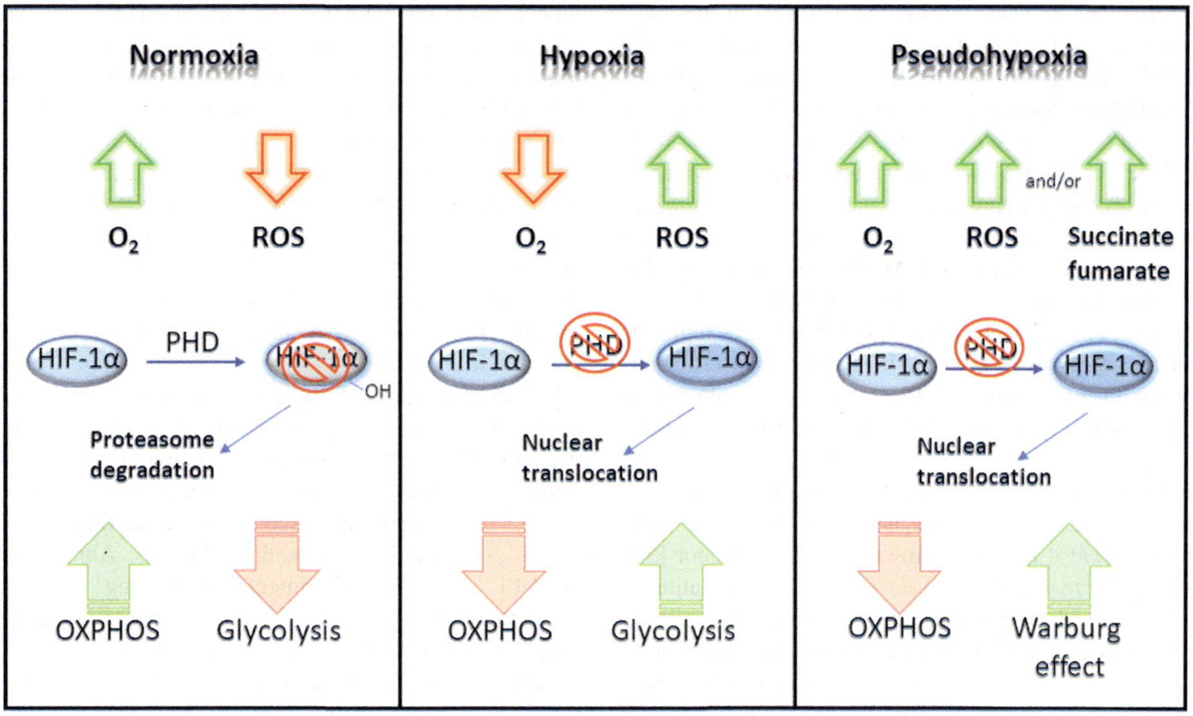

FIGURE 10.2 Regulation of HIF-1α in the switch between glycolysis and oxidative metabolism. Oxygen availability, reactive oxygen species (ROS) levels, and metabolic alterations influence the stability of HIF-1α permitting the choice between glycolysis and mitochondrial oxidative metabolism. *OXPHOS*, oxidative phosphorylation; *PHD*, prolyl hydroxylase.

a pseudohypoxic response and cell proliferation in different genetic backgrounds [47]. Pheochromocytoma and paraganglioma originating from any SDH mutant constantly develop a pseudohypoxic phenotype. This is mainly a consequence of succinate accumulation, which acts as an inhibitory factor of PHD enzymes leading to HIF stabilization [48]. However, high succinate levels are associated with ROS production by complex I via RET, and ROS-dependent contribution to pseudohypoxia was revealed upon SDHB downregulation [15,17]. Several mechanisms also determine the induction of HIF-1α in fumarate hydratase (FH)-deficient kidney cancer cells, which are characterized by defective mitochondrial metabolism and a shift toward aerobic glycolysis. As mentioned for succinate in SDH-mutated tumors, fumarate accumulation due to FH deficiency stabilizes HIF-1α by inhibiting PHDs and thus the ubiquitination by the VHL complex [49]. PHD enzymes were also shown to be inhibited by low intracellular iron levels due to reduced expression of the iron transporter DMT1 in FH-deficient tumors [49,50]. Moreover, ROS-mediated stabilization of HIF-1α was attributed to the activation of PKC serine/threonine kinases, which mediate glucose-dependent stimulation of NOX activity [51]. This latter result supports the evidence that ROS induce HIF-1α stabilization even though they do not derive from ETC. Several other examples of NOX-mediated upregulation of HIF-1α include NOX1 in colon cancer [52] or NOX5 in melanoma, lymphoma, and prostate cancer cells [53]. Notably, the mitochondrial NOX4 contributed to HIF-1α accumulation and consequent glycolytic activation, raising mitochondrial ROS levels in thyroid carcinomas exposed to hypoxic conditions [54].

Beyond modulation of mitochondrial enzymes or ROS-producing sources, pseudohypoxia can also be triggered by metabolic or pharmacological insults that lead to alteration of mitochondrial metabolism. Forced triglyceride hydrolysis in cervical cancer and the consequent increase in mitochondrial β-oxidation was responsible for ROS excess and mitochondrial damage. ROS-mediated activation of HIF-1α safeguarded cell survival by eliminating dysfunctional mitochondria via mitophagy and promoted cell proliferation by activating glycolysis [55]. Increased levels of ROS also account for HIF-1α activation in colorectal cancer cells resistant to 5-fluorouracil to foster the Warburg effect in the presence of dysfunctional mitochondria [56].

Pentose phosphate pathway

Enhanced glucose uptake and glycolysis in cancer cells also force glycolytic intermediates to enter accessory pathways. The pentose phosphate pathway (PPP) represents the most critical pathway involved in NADPH generation and is thus fundamental for redox homeostasis and anabolic requirements of cancer cells. Besides NADPH, cancer cells upregulate PPP to produce a high amount of ribose-5-phosphate, which is required for de novo nucleotide biosynthesis in proliferating cells. PPP is composed of an oxidative arm that diverges at the beginning of glycolysis from glucose-6-phosphate and a nonoxidative arm fueled by two downstream glycolytic intermediates, fructose-6-phosphate, and glyceraldehyde-3-

phosphate. The oxidative arm is the only critical for redox homeostasis as it entails two enzymatic reactions yielding NADPH. More specifically, glucose-6-phosphate dehydrogenase (G6PD) catalyzes the rate-limiting step of the pathway and produces the first molecule of NADPH converting glucose-6-phosphate (G6P) into 6-phosphogluconolactone, which is then hydrolyzed to 6-phosphogluconate. The latter is the substrate of 6-phosphogluconate dehydrogenase (6PGDH), which yields the second molecule of NADPH while producing ribulose-5-phosphate and, finally, ribose-5-phosphate [57].

Cancer cells frequently control glycolytic rate by replacing in the last step pyruvate kinase M1 (PKM1), which efficiently promotes glycolytic flux, with PKM2, the activity of which is highly regulated by posttranslational modifications to modulate the entry of glycolytic intermediates into diverging anabolic pathways. Phosphorylation and acetylation can decrease the activity of PKM2 and favor its nuclear translocation, where it acts as a transcriptional coregulator [58]. Moreover, increased ROS levels promote the oxidation of PKM2 cysteine 358 in human lung cancer cells to inhibit its enzymatic activity and favor glucose flux into the oxidative branch of PPP [59]. In this way, cellular metabolism is reprogrammed to augment NADPH production and GSH levels necessary for abrogating ROS toxicity. Analogously, cysteine oxidation of glyceraldehyde-3-phosphate dehydrogenase (GAPDH) accounts for enzyme inhibition and consequent enhancement of PPP flux. Nevertheless, the accumulation of upstream glycolytic intermediates is not considered the only mechanism that leads to rapid PPP activation following oxidative stress. Another possibility is that the inhibition of GAPDH allows fructose-6-phosphate and glyceraldehyde-3-phosphate produced by nonoxidative PPP to be converted back to glucose-6-phosphate following the gluconeogenetic direction and re-enter PPP for efficient NADPH production [60]. Notably, GAPDH oxidation is physiologically maintained by the activity of SOD1 to preserve redox homeostasis and antioxidant defense in aerobic conditions. Mechanistically, SOD1-mediated hydrogen peroxide production after the dismutation of superoxide anion oxidatively inactivates GAPDH to favor PPP metabolism and slow down downstream glycolytic flux [61]. The modulation of phosphofructokinase-1 (PFK-1), the rate-limiting enzyme of glycolysis, represents another mechanism involved in PPP activation in stressed cancer cells. PFK-1 can be inhibited by O-linked β-N-acetylglucosamine (O-GlcNAc) glycosylation during hypoxia or downregulated by Snail under starvation [62]. Alternatively, the direct upregulation of enzymes involved in the PPP is used for boosting NADPH production in cancer cells. In particular, G6PD, as also PGDH and enzymes of the nonoxidative branch, are targets of the NRF2, HIF-1α, and several other oncogenic signaling pathways [57].

ROS and lipid metabolism in cancer

Unlike glucose, which can be catabolized in aerobic or anaerobic conditions to yield ATP, fatty acids require mitochondria for oxidation and thus are necessarily catabolized in the presence of oxygen. This indicates that an intimate connection between lipid catabolism and ROS balance is fundamental for avoiding detrimental oxidative stress. Considering that cancer cells rely on higher baseline levels of ROS than nontransformed cells, well-tailored management of lipid catabolism is necessary for maintaining ROS below the cytotoxic threshold that can undermine cell viability [63]. How cancer cells adopt different strategies to regulate lipid metabolism and limit ROS toxicity or benefit from their proneoplastic effects is depicted in Fig. 10.3.

The upregulation of enzymes that promote lipid storage impeding fatty acid utilization inside mitochondria is one of the strategies used to mitigate oxidative stress. Glioblastoma upregulates diacylglycerol-acyltransferase 1 (DGAT1) to incorporate excess exogenous fatty acids inside triglycerides and, thus, lipid droplets. Abrogation of DGAT1 activity is detrimental increasing fatty acids oxidation and ROS levels that lead to apoptotic cell death [64]. Accumulation of lipid droplets is particularly enhanced during hypoxia when mitochondrial oxidative metabolism needs to be restrained and then reactivated upon oxygenation. HIF-1α promotes lipid droplet accumulation in hypoxia in multiple ways. It promotes the uptake and storage of exogenous lipids in breast cancer and glioblastoma cell lines upregulating FABP3/7 and PLIN2 in hypoxia-reoxygenation conditions, which resemble the abnormal vascularization of a developing tumor mass. The inhibition of lipid droplet biosynthesis is indeed accompanied by ROS accumulation and cell death [65]. These results are in accordance with the inhibitory effects that HIF-1α may exert on lipid catabolism. Hypoxia-inducible gene 2 (HIG2) is a direct inhibitor of adipose triglyceride lipase (ATGL), the rate-limiting enzyme of the lipolytic pathways involved in the breakdown of intracellular triglycerides. HIG2 upregulation during hypoxia contributes to cell survival by avoiding ROS production after mobilization and consequent oxidation of fatty acids released from lipid droplets [66]. Analogously, HIF-1α can decrease the expression of genes involved in fatty acid β-oxidation, including medium- and long-chain acyl-CoA dehydrogenases (MCAD and LCAD), reducing ROS levels while promoting lipid droplets accumulation and progression of hepatocellular carcinoma [67]. Therefore, the abrogation of lipid degrading pathways is an alternative way cancer cells exploit to accumulate lipid droplets and restrain ROS toxicity associated with fatty acid oxidation.

Proneoplastic functions of ROS deriving from lipid catabolism were demonstrated in co-culture experiments of cancer cells with adipocytes. In this condition, ovarian cancer cells upregulate the expression of FABP4 to promote the uptake of fatty acids released by adipocytes resulting in increased β-oxidation, ROS levels, and proliferation [68]. Conversely, prostate cancer cells do not oxidize exogenous fatty acids but accumulate them in lipid

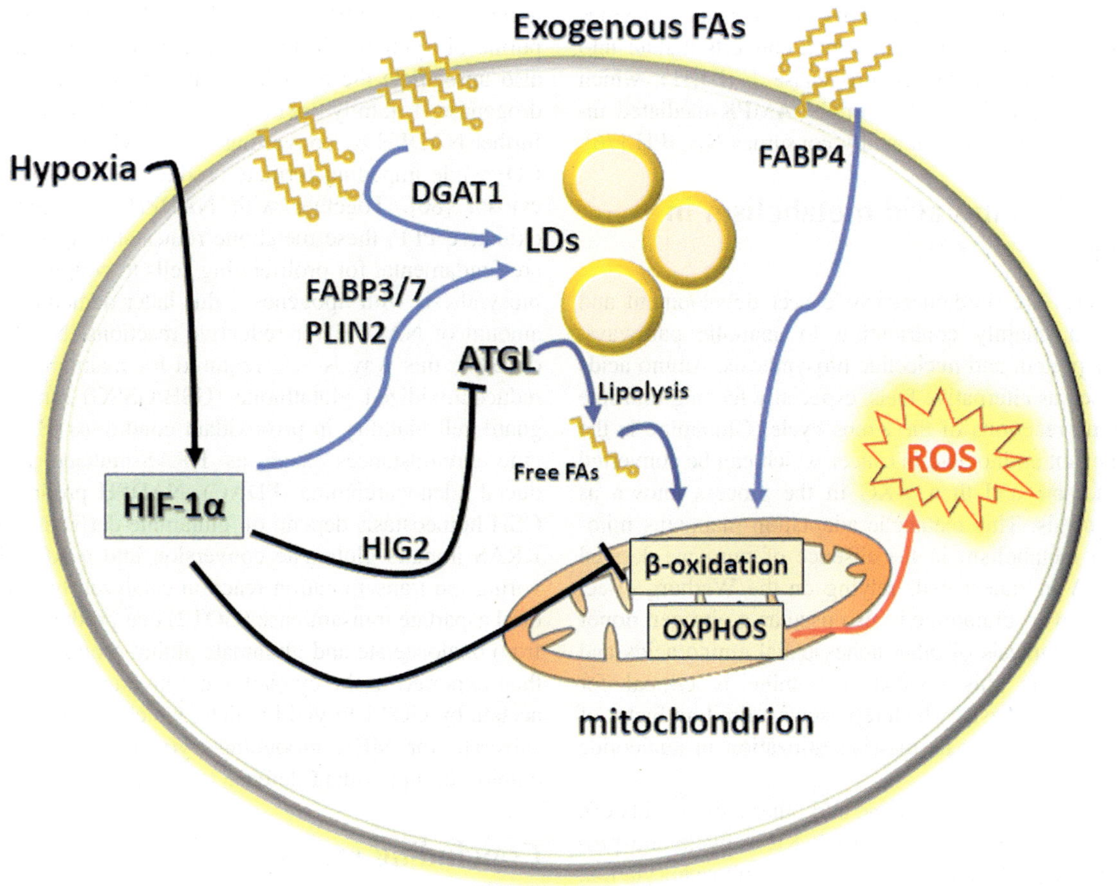

FIGURE 10.3 Modulation of lipid metabolism and effects on reactive oxygen species (ROS) production. The balance between lipid droplet formation and fatty acid oxidation regulates mitochondrial ROS production. *FAs*, fatty acids; *LDs*, lipid droplets; *OXPHOS*, oxidative phosphorylation.

droplets while upregulating NOX5 as the mediator of ROS burst and tumor aggressiveness [69]. Increased ROS levels and β-oxidation were also displayed in chemoresistant cells arising from cytarabine- or mitoxantrone-treated acute myeloid leukemia [70,71]. Analogously, cancer stem cells (CSCs), which are intrinsically characterized by a chemo-refractory phenotype, frequently depend on the metabolic and energetic advantage of operative fatty acid oxidation coupled with efficient quenching of harmful oxidative stress via the upregulation of antioxidant equipment [72,73]. Notably, the ability to mount an efficient adaptive antioxidant response also defines the impact of increased fatty acid oxidation on cancer cell proliferation. Forced lipid catabolism obtained by overexpressing the lipolytic enzyme ATGL was shown to reduce the proliferation of hepatocellular carcinoma cells without altering ROS levels while promoting ROS-mediated proliferation in cervical cancer cell lines [55,74]. To explain this cell type-specific response, hexanoic acid, a 6-carbon fatty acid that passively crosses mitochondrial membranes, was used to boost fatty acid oxidation. Cell lines that decrease their proliferation following hexanoic acid treatment were characterized by an enhancement of antioxidant enzymes, including catalase ad SOD1/2, that prevent ROS accumulation. On the other hand, accelerated proliferation and increased ROS levels were elicited by hexanoic acid because of reduced expression of enzymatic antioxidants. In this condition, cell survival was guaranteed by GSH-dependent antioxidant activities and the activation of mitophagy to limit mitochondrial ROS sources. Consistently, the inhibition of GSH synthesis induces the iron/ROS-dependent cell death mechanism known as ferroptosis, which represents an additional link between lipids and oxidative stress. Ferroptosis is triggered by an overwhelming accumulation of lethal lipid peroxides due to unrepaired (phospho)lipid peroxidation. This mainly occurs enzymatically by LOX activity or nonenzymatically via the Fenton reaction that produces the harmful hydroxyl radical in the presence of ferrous iron and hydrogen peroxide [75].

To assure a prompt antioxidant response, redox homeostasis needs to be tailored in response to lipid catabolism [63]. Consistently, NADPH-producing pathways are coupled to fatty acid oxidation, as demonstrated by the decrease of NADPH levels occurring upon inhibiting mitochondrial fatty acid oxidation in glioblastoma cells. On the other hand, increased levels of NADPH are guaranteed by AMPK when lipid catabolism is activated as a pro-survival mechanism upon glucose starvation. These conditions depend on the activity of cytosolic enzymes such as malic enzyme (ME1), which converts malate into pyruvate, and isocitrate dehydrogenase 1 (IDH1), which oxidizes isocitrate into α-KG, or the AMPK-mediated inhibition of lipogenesis that avidly consumes NADPH [76].

ROS and amino acid metabolism in cancer

Amino acids are fundamental to cancer development and progression, mainly contributing to anabolic pathways, primarily protein and nucleotide biosynthesis. Amino acids can be used as alternative fuels, especially feeding multiple anaplerotic reactions of the Krebs cycle. Glutamine is the most relevant amino acid in cancer which can be converted into glutamate and then α-KG in the process known as glutaminolysis. This metabolic adaptation maintains mitochondrial metabolism in the absence of pyruvate-derived acetyl-CoA in cancer cells relying on the Warburg effect [77]. Moreover, glutamine is also used as a nitrogen donor for the biosynthesis of other nonessential amino acids and nucleobases. In this context, glutamine is critical for aspartate biosynthesis, which represents a limiting factor of proliferating cells for its massive utilization in nucleotide biosynthesis [78].

The catabolism of glutamine and other amino acids can promote ROS levels by feeding the Krebs cycle and producing reduced equivalent for oxidative phosphorylation. Nevertheless, the contribution to redox homeostasis and antioxidant defences represents the most relevant aspects of amino acid metabolism in oxidative stress regulation.

GSH is the main nonenzymatic antioxidant. It is a tripeptide composed of glutamate, cysteine, and glycine. Glutamine addiction of cancer cells is frequently connected with GSH biosynthesis as glutamine-derived glutamate can be directly incorporated into GSH or secreted via the SLC7A11 (xCT) antiporter in exchange for cystine. Consistently, decreased GSH levels are associated with impaired cystine uptake following glutamine starvation. Cystine is the oxidized and predominant form of cysteine in the blood, necessary for satisfying cysteine intracellular need of cancer cells that the trans-sulfuration pathways cannot fulfill from methionine. The importance of the xCT transporter for GSH synthesis is also demonstrated by the ferroptosis induction due to GSH decrement upon its inhibition. The third amino acid glycine is generally not limiting for GSH biosynthesis as it is highly concentrated in the blood, and, even more, many cancer cells upregulate phosphoglycerate dehydrogenase (PHGDH) enzyme to diverge glycolytic intermediates toward serine biosynthesis, which ultimately can be converted to glycine by serine hydroxymethyltransferase (SHMT) enzymes [79].

To note, the serine biosynthetic pathway in proliferating cells is intimately connected with one-carbon metabolism (or folate cycle) to generate NADPH and 10-formyl-tetrahydrofolate (10-formyl-THF), which is employed in purine biosynthesis in the cytosol. Moreover, cancer cells also upregulate the mitochondrial enzyme aldehyde dehydrogenase 1 family member L2 (ALDHL2) to generate further NADPH by converting 10-formyl-THF in THF and CO_2 while impeding formate production and export in the cytosol [80]. Together with NADPH produced by the oxidative PPP, these metabolic routes starting from serine are fundamental for proliferating cells to couple nucleotide biosynthesis with lipogenesis, this latter demanding a high amount of NADPH for reductive reactions. NADPH produced in this way is also required for maintaining a high reduced/oxidized glutathione (GSH/GSSG) ratio to safeguard cell viability in pro-oxidant conditions [81]. In specific circumstances, such as KRAS-mutated pancreatic ductal adenocarcinoma (PDAC), NADPH production and GSH homeostasis depend on glutamine-derived glutamate. KRAS impairs glutamate conversion into α-KG while favoring the transamination reaction catalyzed by mitochondrial aspartate transaminase (GOT2) that produces aspartate from oxaloacetate and glutamate amino group. Aspartate is then exported to the cytosol and converted back to oxaloacetate by GOT1 to yield malate, which in turn becomes a substrate for ME1, producing pyruvate and NADPH to employ in antioxidant defense [82].

Concluding remarks

The evidence that the metabolic rewiring of cancer cells is also aimed at generating pro-neoplastic ROS production has offered during the years several hints for the design of new therapeutic strategies interfering with cancer redox homeostasis. Nevertheless, the effect of ROS modulation on cellular outcomes during chemotherapy is complex and difficult to be predicted. Together with ad hoc metabolic rearrangements and protective antioxidant response, cell survival mechanisms (e.g., autophagy) and cell death pathways (e.g., apoptosis) represent additional checkpoints that ROS orchestrate to promote cell proliferation. Currently, the most valuable therapeutic strategy is exacerbating oxidative stress above the cellular tolerability threshold. This seems to be mainly successful by modulating, genetically or pharmacologically, metabolic ROS production in a combinatory approach. In this way, mitochondrial ROS levels obtained from the stimulation of oxidative metabolism would be added to those generated by classical chemotherapeutic agents (e.g., cisplatin and doxorubicin). Alternatively, the accumulation of toxic ROS levels in the absence of exogenous damaging insults can be achieved by suppressing ROS detoxification systems. The most updated example is represented by ferroptosis induction, which is becoming an appealing mechanism for the identification of ROS-based antineoplastic strategies. Examples of clinical trials referred to drugs interfering with metabolic and redox pathways are reported in Table 10.1.

TABLE 10.1 Examples of completed or ongoing clinical trials of drugs interfering with redox homeostasis and metabolism.

Metabolic process	Drug	Target	Clinical trial ID	Cancer type	Combination strategy
Glucose metabolism	Dichloroacetate	Inhibition of glycolysis	NCT01386632	Stage III–IV squamous cell carcinoma of the head and neck	Cisplatin and radiotherapy
			NCT01029925	Recurrent and/or metastatic and pretreated breast and non-small-cell lung cancer	None
			NCT00540176	Malignant gliomas and glioblastome multiforme	None
	Metformin	Pleiotropic effects	NCT04559308	Breast cancer	Paclitaxel, doxorubicin, cyclophosphamide
			NCT02437656	Locally advanced rectal cancer	Neoadjuvant radiochemotherapy
			NCT02115464	Locally advanced non-small cell lung	Cisplatin and radiotherapy
			NCT01796028	Metastatic hormone-refractory prostate cancer	Docetaxel
			NCT01310231	Metastatic breast cancer	Anthracyclines, platinum, taxanes or capecitabine
Lipid metabolism	TVB-2640	Inhibition of fatty acid synthesis	NCT05118776	Recurrent glioblastoma	Bevacizumab
			NCT02980029	Colon cancer	None
			NCT03808558	KRAS mutant non-small cell lung	None
Amino acid metabolism	Sulfasalazine	Inhibition of cystine uptake	NCT04205357	Recurrent glioblastoma	Stereotactic radiosurgery
	CB-839	Inhibition of glutamine catabolism	NCT02771626	Clear cell renal cell carcinoma, melanoma, and non-small cell lung cancer	Nivolumab
			NCT03965845	Advanced or metastatic KRAS-mutated solid tumors	Palbociclib
			NCT03875313	Metastatic colorectal cancer	Talazoparib
			NCT03428217	Advanced or metastatic renal cell carcinoma	Cabozantinib
Redox homeostasis	Buthionine sulfoximine	Inhibition of GSH synthesis	NCT00005835	Resistant or recurrent neuroblastoma	Melphalan
			NCT00002730	Progressive neuroblastoma	Melphalan
	NOV-002	GSSG/GSH alteration	NCT00345540	Ovarian cancer resistant to carboplatin	Carboplatin
			NCT00499122	Stages IIB–IIIC breast cancer	Doxorubicin, cyclophosphamide, docetaxel
			NCT00347412	Advanced non-small-cell lung cancer	Paclitaxel and carboplatin

In conclusion, from the earliest associations of increased ROS production in cancer cells to date, significant advances have been made to dissect the mechanisms downstream of their increase. In this chapter, we have tried to summarize the evolution of the knowledge about the implication of ROS in the transformed cell by going along the milestones of this field of research and comprehending how they fit into a more general phenomenon. The scheme drawn indicates that ROS are not the principal players but *weighty protagonists* of the vast network governing cancerogenesis. Such an intricate and highly complex scenario strongly depends on the redox state of the cell where the enzymatic antioxidant defense, as a whole, concurs to modulate ROS concentration, thus regulating the function of a large number of redox-sensitive proteins implicated in the cell cycle regulation, proliferation, and cell death.

The remarkable progress accomplished in the last years allows asserting that, even though the pathways implicated in the production/induction of ROS have mainly remained unaltered during the years, many new "redox-dependent pieces" of the puzzle have been and are going to be added, thus rendering the redox signaling network downstream of ROS production of more general application and hopefully controlled at multiple levels.

Acknowledgments

This work was funded by Italian Association for Cancer Research (AIRC, IG 15403) and MIUR/PRIN 2017 (n. 2017A5TXC3).

References

[1] Sattler M, Verma S, Shrikhande G, Byrne CH, Pride YB, Winkler T, et al. The BCR/ABL tyrosine kinase induces production of reactive oxygen species in hematopoietic cells. J Biol Chem 2000;275:24273–8. https://doi.org/10.1074/jbc.M002094200.

[2] Trachootham D, Zhou Y, Zhang H, Demizu Y, Chen Z, Pelicano H, et al. Selective killing of oncogenically transformed cells through a ROS-mediated mechanism by beta-phenylethyl isothiocyanate. Cancer Cell 2006;10:241–52. https://doi.org/10.1016/j.ccr.2006.08.009.

[3] Patterson JC, Joughin BA, van de Kooij B, Lim DC, Lauffenburger DA, Yaffe MB. ROS and oxidative stress are elevated in mitosis during asynchronous cell cycle progression and are exacerbated by mitotic arrest. Cell Syst 2019;8:163–167.e2. https://doi.org/10.1016/j.cels.2019.01.005.

[4] Cheung EC, Vousden KH. The role of ROS in tumour development and progression. Nat Rev Cancer 2022;22:280–97. https://doi.org/10.1038/s41568-021-00435-0.

[5] Perillo B, Di Donato M, Pezone A, Di Zazzo E, Giovannelli P, Galasso G, et al. ROS in cancer therapy: the bright side of the moon. Exp Mol Med 2020;52:192–203. https://doi.org/10.1038/s12276-020-0384-2.

[6] He L, He T, Farrar S, Ji L, Liu T, Ma X. Antioxidants maintain cellular redox homeostasis by elimination of reactive oxygen species. Cell Physiol Biochem 2017;44:532–53. https://doi.org/10.1159/000485089.

[7] Rojo de la Vega M, Chapman E, Zhang DD. NRF2 and the hallmarks of cancer. Cancer Cell 2018;34:21–43. https://doi.org/10.1016/j.ccell.2018.03.022.

[8] Liou G-Y, Storz P. Reactive oxygen species in cancer. Free Radic Res 2010;44:479–96. https://doi.org/10.3109/10715761003667554.

[9] Kirova DG, Judasova K, Vorhauser J, Zerjatke T, Leung JK, Glauche I, et al. A ROS-dependent mechanism promotes CDK2 phosphorylation to drive progression through S phase. Dev Cell 2022;57:1712–1727.e9. https://doi.org/10.1016/j.devcel.2022.06.008.

[10] Murphy MP. How mitochondria produce reactive oxygen species. Biochem J 2009;417:1–13. https://doi.org/10.1042/BJ20081386.

[11] Ju YS, Alexandrov LB, Gerstung M, Martincorena I, Nik-Zainal S, Ramakrishna M, et al. Origins and functional consequences of somatic mitochondrial DNA mutations in human cancer. Elife 2014;3. https://doi.org/10.7554/eLife.02935.

[12] Stewart JB, Alaei-Mahabadi B, Sabarinathan R, Samuelsson T, Gorodkin J, Gustafsson CM, et al. Simultaneous DNA and RNA mapping of somatic mitochondrial mutations across diverse human cancers. PLoS Genet 2015;11:e1005333. https://doi.org/10.1371/journal.pgen.1005333.

[13] Hahn A, Zuryn S. Mitochondrial genome (mtDNA) mutations that generate reactive oxygen species. Antioxidants (Basel) 2019;8:E392. https://doi.org/10.3390/antiox8090392.

[14] Ishikawa K, Takenaga K, Akimoto M, Koshikawa N, Yamaguchi A, Imanishi H, et al. ROS-generating mitochondrial DNA mutations can regulate tumor cell metastasis. Science 2008;320:661–4. https://doi.org/10.1126/science.1156906.

[15] Hadrava Vanova K, Kraus M, Neuzil J, Rohlena J. Mitochondrial complex II and reactive oxygen species in disease and therapy. Redox Rep 2020;25:26–32. https://doi.org/10.1080/13510002.2020.1752002.

[16] Hadrava Vanova K, Yang C, Meuter L, Neuzil J, Pacak K. Reactive oxygen species: a promising therapeutic target for SDHx-mutated pheochromocytoma and paraganglioma. Cancers (Basel) 2021;13:3769. https://doi.org/10.3390/cancers13153769.

[17] Guzy RD, Sharma B, Bell E, Chandel NS, Schumacker PT. Loss of the SdhB, but Not the SdhA, subunit of complex II triggers reactive oxygen species-dependent hypoxia-inducible factor activation and tumorigenesis. Mol Cell Biol 2008;28:718–31. https://doi.org/10.1128/MCB.01338-07.

[18] Goncalves J, Moog S, Morin A, Gentric G, Müller S, Morrell AP, et al. Loss of SDHB promotes dysregulated iron homeostasis, oxidative stress, and sensitivity to ascorbate. Cancer Res 2021;81:3480–94. https://doi.org/10.1158/0008-5472.CAN-20-2936.

[19] Liu Y, Pang Y, Zhu B, Uher O, Caisova V, Huynh T-T, et al. Therapeutic targeting of SDHB-mutated pheochromocytoma/paraganglioma with pharmacologic ascorbic acid. Clin Cancer Res 2020;26:3868–80. https://doi.org/10.1158/1078-0432.CCR-19-2335.

[20] Liu Y, Pang Y, Caisova V, Ding J, Yu D, Zhou Y, et al. Targeting NRF2-governed glutathione synthesis for SDHB-mutated pheochromocytoma and paraganglioma. Cancers (Basel) 2020;12:E280. https://doi.org/10.3390/cancers12020280.

[21] Mailloux RJ, Jin X, Willmore WG. Redox regulation of mitochondrial function with emphasis on cysteine oxidation reactions. Redox Biol 2014;2:123–39. https://doi.org/10.1016/j.redox.2013.12.011.

[22] Wu JB, Shao C, Li X, Li Q, Hu P, Shi C, et al. Monoamine oxidase A mediates prostate tumorigenesis and cancer metastasis. J Clin Invest 2014;124:2891–908. https://doi.org/10.1172/JCI70982.

[23] Huang C-C, Lee C-C, Lin H-H, Chen M-C, Lin C-C, Chang J-Y. Autophagy-regulated ROS from xanthine oxidase acts as an early effector for triggering late mitochondria-dependent apoptosis in cathepsin S-targeted tumor cells. PLoS One 2015;10:e0128045. https://doi.org/10.1371/journal.pone.0128045.

[24] Xu H, Li C, Mozziconacci O, Zhu R, Xu Y, Tang Y, et al. Xanthine oxidase-mediated oxidative stress promotes cancer cell-specific apoptosis. Free Radic Biol Med 2019;139:70–9. https://doi.org/10.1016/j.freeradbiomed.2019.05.019.

[25] Chen M-M, Meng L-H. The double faced role of xanthine oxidoreductase in cancer. Acta Pharmacol Sin 2022;43:1623–32. https://doi.org/10.1038/s41401-021-00800-7.

[26] Konaté MM, Antony S, Doroshow JH. Inhibiting the activity of NADPH oxidase in cancer. Antioxid Redox Signal 2020;33:435–54. https://doi.org/10.1089/ars.2020.8046.

[27] Kajla S, Mondol AS, Nagasawa A, Zhang Y, Kato M, Matsuno K, et al. A crucial role for Nox 1 in redox-dependent regulation of Wnt-β-catenin signaling. FASEB J 2012;26:2049–59. https://doi.org/10.1096/fj.11-196360.

[28] Hiraga R, Kato M, Miyagawa S, Kamata T. Nox4-derived ROS signaling contributes to TGF-β-induced epithelial-mesenchymal transition in pancreatic cancer cells. Anticancer Res 2013;33:4431–8.

[29] Helfinger V, Freiherr von Gall F, Henke N, Kunze MM, Schmid T, Rezende F, et al. Genetic deletion of Nox4 enhances cancerogen-induced formation of solid tumors. Proc Natl Acad Sci USA 2021;118. https://doi.org/10.1073/pnas.2020152118. e2020152118.

[30] Fürstenberger G, Krieg P, Müller-Decker K, Habenicht AJR. What are cyclooxygenases and lipoxygenases doing in the driver's seat of carcinogenesis? Int J Cancer 2006;119:2247–54. https://doi.org/10.1002/ijc.22153.

[31] Maciag A, Sithanandam G, Anderson LM. Mutant K-rasV12 increases COX-2, peroxides and DNA damage in lung cells. Carcinogenesis 2004;25:2231–7. https://doi.org/10.1093/carcin/bgh245.

[32] Shintoku R, Takigawa Y, Yamada K, Kubota C, Yoshimoto Y, Takeuchi T, et al. Lipoxygenase-mediated generation of lipid peroxides enhances ferroptosis induced by erastin and RSL3. Cancer Sci 2017;108:2187–94. https://doi.org/10.1111/cas.13380.

[33] Thornber K, Colomba A, Ceccato L, Delsol G, Payrastre B, Gaits-Iacovoni F. Reactive oxygen species and lipoxygenases regulate the oncogenicity of NPM-ALK-positive anaplastic large cell lymphomas. Oncogene 2009;28:2690–6. https://doi.org/10.1038/onc.2009.125.

[34] Edderkaoui M, Hong P, Vaquero EC, Lee JK, Fischer L, Friess H, et al. Extracellular matrix stimulates reactive oxygen species production and increases pancreatic cancer cell survival through 5-lipoxygenase and NADPH oxidase. Am J Physiol Gastrointest Liver Physiol 2005;289:G1137–47. https://doi.org/10.1152/ajpgi.00197.2005.

[35] Kim E-Y, Seo J-M, Kim C, Lee J-E, Lee K-M, Kim J-H. BLT2 promotes the invasion and metastasis of aggressive bladder cancer cells through a reactive oxygen species-linked pathway. Free Radic Biol Med 2010;49:1072–81. https://doi.org/10.1016/j.freeradbiomed.2010.06.023.

[36] Vaupel P, Multhoff G. Revisiting the Warburg effect: historical dogma versus current understanding. J Physiol 2021;599:1745–57. https://doi.org/10.1113/JP278810.

[37] Wu C-A, Chao Y, Shiah S-G, Lin W-W. Nutrient deprivation induces the Warburg effect through ROS/AMPK-dependent activation of pyruvate dehydrogenase kinase. Biochim Biophys Acta 2013;1833:1147–56. https://doi.org/10.1016/j.bbamcr.2013.01.025.

[38] Chandel NS, Maltepe E, Goldwasser E, Mathieu CE, Simon MC, Schumacker PT. Mitochondrial reactive oxygen species trigger hypoxia-induced transcription. Proc Natl Acad Sci USA 1998;95:11715–20. https://doi.org/10.1073/pnas.95.20.11715.

[39] Bell EL, Klimova TA, Eisenbart J, Moraes CT, Murphy MP, Budinger GRS, et al. The Qo site of the mitochondrial complex III is required for the transduction of hypoxic signaling via reactive oxygen species production. J Cell Biol 2007;177:1029–36. https://doi.org/10.1083/jcb.200609074.

[40] Nagao A, Kobayashi M, Koyasu S, Chow CCT, Harada H. HIF-1-dependent reprogramming of glucose metabolic pathway of cancer cells and its therapeutic significance. Int J Mol Sci 2019;20:E238. https://doi.org/10.3390/ijms20020238.

[41] Ivan M, Kondo K, Yang H, Kim W, Valiando J, Ohh M, et al. HIFalpha targeted for VHL-mediated destruction by proline hydroxylation: implications for O2 sensing. Science 2001;292:464–8. https://doi.org/10.1126/science.1059817.

[42] Epstein AC, Gleadle JM, McNeill LA, Hewitson KS, O'Rourke J, Mole DR, et al. *C. elegans* EGL-9 and mammalian homologs define a family of dioxygenases that regulate HIF by prolyl hydroxylation. Cell 2001;107:43–54. https://doi.org/10.1016/s0092-8674(01)00507-4.

[43] Emerling BM, Platanias LC, Black E, Nebreda AR, Davis RJ, Chandel NS. Mitochondrial reactive oxygen species activation of p38 mitogen-activated protein kinase is required for hypoxia signaling. Mol Cell Biol 2005;25:4853–62. https://doi.org/10.1128/MCB.25.12.4853-4862.2005.

[44] Jung S-N, Yang WK, Kim J, Kim HS, Kim EJ, Yun H, et al. Reactive oxygen species stabilize hypoxia-inducible factor-1 alpha protein and stimulate transcriptional activity via AMP-activated protein kinase in DU145 human prostate cancer cells. Carcinogenesis 2008;29:713–21. https://doi.org/10.1093/carcin/bgn032.

[45] Kumar A, Vaish M, Karuppagounder SS, Gazaryan I, Cave JW, Starkov AA, et al. HIF1α stabilization in hypoxia is not oxidant-initiated. Elife 2021;10:e72873. https://doi.org/10.7554/eLife.72873.

[46] Chua YL, Dufour E, Dassa EP, Rustin P, Jacobs HT, Taylor CT, et al. Stabilization of hypoxia-inducible factor-1alpha protein in hypoxia occurs independently of mitochondrial reactive oxygen species production. J Biol Chem 2010;285:31277–84. https://doi.org/10.1074/jbc.M110.158485.

[47] Sun W, Zhou S, Chang SS, McFate T, Verma A, Califano JA. Mitochondrial mutations contribute to HIF1alpha accumulation via increased reactive oxygen species and up-regulated pyruvate dehydrogenease kinase 2 in head and neck squamous cell carcinoma. Clin Cancer Res 2009;15:476–84. https://doi.org/10.1158/1078-0432.CCR-08-0930.

[48] Selak MA, Armour SM, MacKenzie ED, Boulahbel H, Watson DG, Mansfield KD, et al. Succinate links TCA cycle dysfunction to oncogenesis by inhibiting HIF-alpha prolyl hydroxylase. Cancer Cell 2005;7:77–85. https://doi.org/10.1016/j.ccr.2004.11.022.

[49] Linehan WM, Rouault TA. Molecular pathways: fumarate hydratase-deficient kidney cancer—targeting the Warburg effect in cancer. Clin Cancer Res 2013;19:3345–52. https://doi.org/10.1158/1078-0432.CCR-13-0304.

[50] Tong W-H, Sourbier C, Kovtunovych G, Jeong SY, Vira M, Ghosh M, et al. The glycolytic shift in fumarate-hydratase-deficient

kidney cancer lowers AMPK levels, increases anabolic propensities and lowers cellular iron levels. Cancer Cell 2011;20:315–27. https://doi.org/10.1016/j.ccr.2011.07.018.

[51] Sudarshan S, Sourbier C, Kong H-S, Block K, Valera Romero VA, Yang Y, et al. Fumarate hydratase deficiency in renal cancer induces glycolytic addiction and hypoxia-inducible transcription factor 1alpha stabilization by glucose-dependent generation of reactive oxygen species. Mol Cell Biol 2009;29:4080–90. https://doi.org/10.1128/MCB.00483-09.

[52] Juhasz A, Markel S, Gaur S, Liu H, Lu J, Jiang G, et al. NADPH oxidase 1 supports proliferation of colon cancer cells by modulating reactive oxygen species-dependent signal transduction. J Biol Chem 2017;292:7866–87. https://doi.org/10.1074/jbc.M116.768283.

[53] Antony S, Jiang G, Wu Y, Meitzler JL, Makhlouf HR, Haines DC, et al. NADPH oxidase 5 (NOX5)-induced reactive oxygen signaling modulates normoxic HIF-1α and p27Kip1 expression in malignant melanoma and other human tumors. Mol Carcinog 2017;56:2643–62. https://doi.org/10.1002/mc.22708.

[54] Tang P, Dang H, Huang J, Xu T, Yuan P, Hu J, et al. NADPH oxidase NOX4 is a glycolytic regulator through mROS-HIF1α axis in thyroid carcinomas. Sci Rep 2018;8:15897. https://doi.org/10.1038/s41598-018-34154-8.

[55] Castelli S, Ciccarone F, Tavian D, Ciriolo MR. ROS-dependent HIF1α activation under forced lipid catabolism entails glycolysis and mitophagy as mediators of higher proliferation rate in cervical cancer cells. J Exp Clin Cancer Res 2021;40:94. https://doi.org/10.1186/s13046-021-01887-w.

[56] Dong S, Liang S, Cheng Z, Zhang X, Luo L, Li L, et al. ROS/PI3K/Akt and Wnt/β-catenin signalings activate HIF-1α-induced metabolic reprogramming to impart 5-fluorouracil resistance in colorectal cancer. J Exp Clin Cancer Res 2022;41:15. https://doi.org/10.1186/s13046-021-02229-6.

[57] Patra KC, Hay N. The pentose phosphate pathway and cancer. Trends Biochem Sci 2014;39:347–54. https://doi.org/10.1016/j.tibs.2014.06.005.

[58] Zahra K, Dey T, Ashish, Mishra SP, Pandey U. Pyruvate kinase M2 and cancer: the role of PKM2 in promoting tumorigenesis. Front Oncol 2020;10:159. https://doi.org/10.3389/fonc.2020.00159.

[59] Anastasiou D, Poulogiannis G, Asara JM, Boxer MB, Jiang J, Shen M, et al. Inhibition of pyruvate kinase M2 by reactive oxygen species contributes to cellular antioxidant responses. Science 2011;334:1278–83. https://doi.org/10.1126/science.1211485.

[60] Dick TP, Ralser M. Metabolic remodeling in times of stress: who shoots faster than his shadow? Mol Cell 2015;59:519–21. https://doi.org/10.1016/j.molcel.2015.08.002.

[61] Montllor-Albalate C, Kim H, Thompson AE, Jonke AP, Torres MP, Reddi AR. Sod1 integrates oxygen availability to redox regulate NADPH production and the thiol redoxome. Proc Natl Acad Sci USA 2022;119. https://doi.org/10.1073/pnas.2023328119. e2023328119.

[62] Cho ES, Cha YH, Kim HS, Kim NH, Yook JI. The pentose phosphate pathway as a potential target for cancer therapy. Biomol Ther (Seoul) 2018;26:29–38. https://doi.org/10.4062/biomolther.2017.179.

[63] Castelli S, De Falco P, Ciccarone F, Desideri E, Ciriolo MR. Lipid catabolism and ROS in cancer: a bidirectional liaison. Cancers (Basel) 2021;13:5484. https://doi.org/10.3390/cancers13215484.

[64] Cheng X, Geng F, Pan M, Wu X, Zhong Y, Wang C, et al. Targeting DGAT1 ameliorates glioblastoma by increasing fat catabolism and oxidative stress. Cell Metab 2020;32:229–242.e8. https://doi.org/10.1016/j.cmet.2020.06.002.

[65] Bensaad K, Favaro E, Lewis CA, Peck B, Lord S, Collins JM, et al. Fatty acid uptake and lipid storage induced by HIF-1α contribute to cell growth and survival after hypoxia-reoxygenation. Cell Rep 2014;9:349–65. https://doi.org/10.1016/j.celrep.2014.08.056.

[66] Zhang X, Saarinen AM, Hitosugi T, Wang Z, Wang L, Ho TH, et al. Inhibition of intracellular lipolysis promotes human cancer cell adaptation to hypoxia. Elife 2017;6:e31132. https://doi.org/10.7554/eLife.31132.

[67] Huang D, Li T, Li X, Zhang L, Sun L, He X, et al. HIF-1-mediated suppression of acyl-CoA dehydrogenases and fatty acid oxidation is critical for cancer progression. Cell Rep 2014;8:1930–42. https://doi.org/10.1016/j.celrep.2014.08.028.

[68] Mukherjee A, Chiang C-Y, Daifotis HA, Nieman KM, Fahrmann JF, Lastra RR, et al. Adipocyte-induced FABP4 expression in ovarian cancer cells promotes metastasis and mediates carboplatin resistance. Cancer Res 2020;80:1748–61. https://doi.org/10.1158/0008-5472.CAN-19-1999.

[69] Laurent V, Toulet A, Attané C, Milhas D, Dauvillier S, Zaidi F, et al. Periprostatic adipose tissue favors prostate cancer cell invasion in an obesity-dependent manner: role of oxidative stress. Mol Cancer Res 2019;17:821–35. https://doi.org/10.1158/1541-7786.MCR-18-0748.

[70] Salunkhe S, Mishra SV, Ghorai A, Hole A, Chandrani P, Dutt A, et al. Metabolic rewiring in drug resistant cells exhibit higher OXPHOS and fatty acids as preferred major source to cellular energetics. Biochim Biophys Acta Bioenerg 2020;1861:148300. https://doi.org/10.1016/j.bbabio.2020.148300.

[71] Farge T, Saland E, de Toni F, Aroua N, Hosseini M, Perry R, et al. Chemotherapy-resistant human acute myeloid leukemia cells are not enriched for leukemic stem cells but require oxidative metabolism. Cancer Discov 2017;7:716–35. https://doi.org/10.1158/2159-8290.CD-16-0441.

[72] Choi H-J, Jhe Y-L, Kim J, Lim JY, Lee JE, Shin M-K, et al. FoxM1-dependent and fatty acid oxidation-mediated ROS modulation is a cell-intrinsic drug resistance mechanism in cancer stem-like cells. Redox Biol 2020;36:101589. https://doi.org/10.1016/j.redox.2020.101589.

[73] Wang C, Shao L, Pan C, Ye J, Ding Z, Wu J, et al. Elevated level of mitochondrial reactive oxygen species via fatty acid β-oxidation in cancer stem cells promotes cancer metastasis by inducing epithelial-mesenchymal transition. Stem Cell Res Ther 2019;10:175. https://doi.org/10.1186/s13287-019-1265-2.

[74] Di Leo L, Vegliante R, Ciccarone F, Salvatori I, Scimeca M, Bonanno E, et al. Forcing ATGL expression in hepatocarcinoma cells imposes glycolytic rewiring through PPAR-α/p300-mediated acetylation of p53. Oncogene 2019;38:1860–75. https://doi.org/10.1038/s41388-018-0545-0.

[75] Li D, Li Y. The interaction between ferroptosis and lipid metabolism in cancer. Signal Transduct Target Ther 2020;5:108. https://doi.org/10.1038/s41392-020-00216-5.

[76] Qu Q, Zeng F, Liu X, Wang QJ, Deng F. Fatty acid oxidation and carnitine palmitoyltransferase I: emerging therapeutic targets in cancer. Cell Death Dis 2016;7:e2226. https://doi.org/10.1038/cddis.2016.132.

[77] DeBerardinis RJ, Mancuso A, Daikhin E, Nissim I, Yudkoff M, Wehrli S, et al. Beyond aerobic glycolysis: transformed cells can engage in glutamine metabolism that exceeds the requirement for protein and nucleotide synthesis. Proc Natl Acad Sci USA 2007;104:19345–50. https://doi.org/10.1073/pnas.0709747104.

[78] Gorgoglione R, Impedovo V, Riley CL, Fratantonio D, Tiziani S, Palmieri L, et al. Glutamine-derived aspartate biosynthesis in cancer

cells: role of mitochondrial transporters and new therapeutic perspectives. Cancers (Basel) 2022;14:245. https://doi.org/10.3390/cancers14010245.

[79] Wei Z, Liu X, Cheng C, Yu W, Yi P. Metabolism of amino acids in cancer. Front Cell Dev Biol 2020;8:603837. https://doi.org/10.3389/fcell.2020.603837.

[80] Vučetić M, Cormerais Y, Parks SK, Pouysségur J. The central role of amino acids in cancer redox homeostasis: vulnerability points of the cancer redox code. Front Oncol 2017;7:319. https://doi.org/10.3389/fonc.2017.00319.

[81] Fan J, Ye J, Kamphorst JJ, Shlomi T, Thompson CB, Rabinowitz JD. Quantitative flux analysis reveals folate-dependent NADPH production. Nature 2014;510:298–302. https://doi.org/10.1038/nature13236.

[82] Son J, Lyssiotis CA, Ying H, Wang X, Hua S, Ligorio M, et al. Glutamine supports pancreatic cancer growth through a KRAS-regulated metabolic pathway. Nature 2013;496:101–5. https://doi.org/10.1038/nature12040.

Chapter 11

Modulation of human hydrogen sulfide metabolism by physiological effectors

Karim Zuhra[1], Dalila G.F. Fernandes[2], Alessandro Giuffrè[3] and João B. Vicente[2]

[1]*University of Fribourg, Faculty of Science and Medicine, Department of Pharmacology, Fribourg, Switzerland;* [2]*Instituto de Tecnologia Química e Biológica António Xavier, NOVA University of Lisbon, Oeiras, Portugal;* [3]*Institute of Molecular Biology and Pathology, National Research Council, Rome, Italy*

Hydrogen sulfide in human pathophysiology

Hydrogen sulfide (H_2S), a gas commonly regarded as a foul-smelling toxic pollutant, has been shown to exert important signaling roles in biology and, particularly, in human (patho)physiology. The gaseous nature and signaling roles had H_2S entering the gallery of "gasotransmitters," alongside nitric oxide (NO) and carbon monoxide (CO). The discovery that specialized human enzymes are able to purposely synthesize and detoxify H_2S further emphasized its physiological relevance. Additional nonenzymatic sources and detoxifying pathways have since been unraveled. H_2S exerts multiple effects at molecular, cellular, and systemic (organs and tissues) levels, owing to its reactivity and ease of diffusion across all biological milieus. Due to its physicochemical properties and multitude of cellular targets, H_2S can act both as an antioxidant and pro-oxidant. Herein, we provide an overview of the human pathways involved in H_2S metabolism, their regulation highlighting the crosstalk between gasotransmitters, and how it impacts on oxidative stress in human (patho) physiology.

Sources of hydrogen sulfide in human physiology

Hydrogen sulfide (H_2S) can be produced in cells, tissues, and biological fluids both by enzymatic and nonenzymatic sources. Excellent reviews are available in the literature covering important details of H_2S metabolism (e.g., Refs. [1,2]).

One major nonenzymatic source consists of the decomposition of food-derived polysulfides (from foods rich in organosulfur compounds, such as, e.g., garlic) derived from diet that can result in H_2S production, mostly in the gastrointestinal tract, with implications for cardiovascular health [3]. Additionally, it has been demonstrated that in plasma, under physiological conditions, free cysteine can react directly with pyridoxal 5′-phosphate (PLP, vitamin B6) and iron (both in the form of free or heme-bound iron) to yield H_2S [4].

Regarding enzymatic sources relevant for human (mammalian) physiology, these can be divided between human and gut microbiota metabolic pathways. The main microbial H_2S-producing pathways in the human gut concern essentially the ubiquitous cysteine desulfurase enzyme present in various gut bacteria and the dissimilatory sulfate reduction (DSR) pathways from sulfate-reducing bacteria [5,6]. Cysteine desulfurase is a PLP-dependent enzyme that converts cysteine into alanine, resulting in a cysteine persulfide which subsequently decomposes into H_2S [7]. DSR involves multiple enzymes and auxiliary proteins, and H_2S production is mainly determined by the DsrAB complex and the DsrC protein [6]. Disturbed H_2S production by either microbial pathway has been linked to different human pathological conditions, particularly inflammatory bowel disorders (e.g., Ref. [8]).

Four human enzymes have been established as those mostly contributing to H_2S production (Fig. 11.1): cystathionine β-synthase (CBS), cystathionine γ-lyase (CSE), 3-mercaptopyruvate sulfurtransferase (MST) and, very recently, selenium-binding protein 1 (SELENBP1) [2,9]. CBS and CSE belong to the reverse transsulfuration pathway (RTP) that converts homocysteine derived from the methionine demethylation/remethylation cycle into cysteine. Both CBS and CSE are PLP-dependent, tetrameric enzymes in which the PLP moiety is covalently bound to a lysine residue. Each CBS monomer comprises a central catalytic domain flanked by two regulatory

Modulation of Oxidative Stress. https://doi.org/10.1016/B978-0-443-19247-0.00006-0

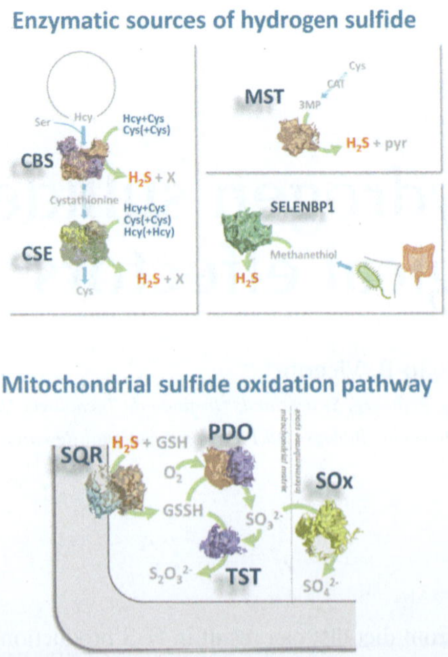

FIGURE 11.1 Human enzymatic pathways for hydrogen sulfide synthesis and consumption. *Top panel*, H_2S-producing enzymes. Dietary methionine (Met) is converted through the methionine cycle into homocysteine (Hcy). In the reverse transsulfuration pathway, cystathionine β-synthase (CBS) and cystathionine γ-lyase (CSE) catalyze Hcy conversion into cysteine (Cys). Both CBS and CSE catalyze alternative reactions using Cys and Hcy, or Cys alone, as substrates to produce hydrogen sulfide (H_2S). Cys is converted by cysteine aminotransferase (CAT) into 3-mercaptopyruvate (3MP), the substrate of 3-mercaptopyruvate sulfurtransferase (MST). The thiol group of 3MP is transferred to the MST active site Cys248, which becomes persulfidated, and pyruvate (Pyr) is released. The Cys248-SSH persulfide is then resolved e.g., by thioredoxin, and H_2S is produced. H_2S can also be produced by selenium-binding protein 1 (SELENBP1), which uses methanethiol derived from microbial metabolism in the gut, and converts it to H_2S, H_2O_2 and formaldehyde. *Bottom panel*, mitochondrial H_2S oxidation pathway. H_2S is oxidized by sulfide:quinone oxidoreductase (SQR), with glutathione (GSH) as co-substrate. The resulting glutathione persulfide (GSSH) follows two possible routes: oxidation into sulfite (SO_3^{-2}) by persulfide dioxygenase (PDO) with O_2 as co-substrate, and production of thiosulfate ($S_2O_3^{-2}$) by thiosulfate sulfurtransferase (TST), using PDO-derived sulfite as co-substrate. Sulfite can also be oxidized by sulfite oxidase (SOx), yielding sulfate (SO_4^{-2}). Protein-depicting cartoons generated with Pymol from PDB entries 4COO (CBS), 6NBA (CSE), 4JGT (MST), 6MP5 (SQR), 4CHL (PDO) and Alphafold models for TST and SOx.

domains [10,11]. The C-terminal regulatory domain binds *s*-adenosyl-L-methionine (AdoMet), while the N-terminal domain has two heme binding sites: the "canonical" one in the ordered part of this domain, and the recently described one in the intrinsically disordered segment corresponding to the first 40 residues [12]. While CBS and CSE were regarded historically for their role in the RTP, the discovery that they can catalyze H_2S production through alternative reactions brought them into the limelight. Indeed, like most PLP-dependent enzymes, CBS and CSE display a remarkable substrate versatility (or "promiscuity") that enables them to synthesize H_2S from (i) condensation of cysteine and homocysteine (the most effective combination), (ii) cysteine desulfuration or condensation of two cysteines, and (iii) homocysteine desulfuration or condensation of two homocysteines (exclusive to CSE) (reviewed e.g., in Ref. [13]). In addition, both CBS and CSE can convert cystine, the disulfide dimer of cysteine, into cysteine persulfides and polysulfides [14], small reactive sulfur species themselves endowed with numerous physiological signaling roles. The multitude of roles exerted by CBS and CSE places them at the interface of homocysteine, H_2S, and persulfides metabolism, along with cysteine and consequently glutathione.

Although both CBS and CSE are mainly localized in the cytosol, under certain (patho)physiological conditions they have been found in different subcellular compartments. For instance, under hypoxic conditions both CBS and CSE have been found in the mitochondria [15], while SUMOylated CBS has been found in the nucleus, where it interacts with the nuclear scaffold [16]. CBS is highly expressed in the central nervous system (mainly expressed in glia and astrocytes rather than neurons), liver and pancreas [17–19]. CSE is most abundantly detected in peripheral tissues such as cardiovascular and respiratory systems and liver, while its expression in the brain is lower as compared to CBS [20]. Extracellular circulating CBS and CSE have also been reported in plasma [21,22], although neither CBS nor CSE contain an N-terminal sequence that targets them for secretion, and most likely they are released from injured hepatocytes rather than active secretion [23].

MST is a monomeric enzyme of the sulfurtransferase/rhodanese family (reviewed in Ref. [24]). Each monomer is organized in two structurally related domains, possibly resulting from a gene duplication event. The 3-mercaptopyruvate (3MP) substrate is converted in the cysteine active site (Cys248) into pyruvate and a persulfidated Cys248-SSH. The sulfane sulfur from Cys248-SSH is resolved by thioredoxin or another acceptor, e.g., dihydrolipoic acid, to yield H_2S. MST function is tightly coupled to the enzymes that produce its 3MP substrate, particularly the PLP-dependent enzyme cysteine aminotransferase (CAT) (reviewed in Ref. [25]), which converts L-cysteine into 3MP. An additional pathway for 3MP production from D-cysteine by a D-amino acid oxidase has been reported [26]. Both CAT and MST localize to the mitochondria and to the cytosol with equal expression levels among the two fractions [27,28]. This notwithstanding, it has been shown that in rat, the CAT/MST pathway is more active (~3-fold higher) in the mitochondria than in the cytosol, possibly due to higher substrate availability (cysteine concentration is higher in the mitochondria than in the cytosol) [29]. In mouse, MST has a broader tissue distribution as compared to CBS and CSE, being nearly ubiquitous [30].

Recently, SELENBP1 has garnered attention as a H_2S-producing enzyme, by oxidizing methanethiol derived from gut microbial metabolism and converting it to H_2S, H_2O_2 and formaldehyde [9,31,32]. Raucci and co-workers carried out far-UV circular dichroism spectropolarimetry experiments and posited SELENBP1 to be an alpha-beta protein [33], consistently with the 3D model they generated, which was later confirmed by the structural model available from AlphaFold. Still, the structure and mechanistic details of SELENBP1 largely remain to be investigated. SELENBP1 is a cytoplasmatic protein mainly expressed in the large intestine and adipose tissue [34].

Sulfide detoxification in human physiology

In line with the potential toxicity of H_2S (described below), enzymatic mechanisms have evolved to cope with H_2S and even benefit from it in bioenergetics terms [35–37]. In mammalian physiology, a sulfide oxidation pathway is found in the mitochondria, composed of four enzymes (Fig. 11.1) [36,38]: sulfide:quinone oxidoreductase (SQR), persulfide dioxygenase (PDO), thiosulfate sulfurtransferase (TST, also known as rhodanese, Rhod), and sulfite oxidase (SOx). The importance of this detoxification system is attested by the cell/tissue distribution of these enzymes, which seems to be related to the degree of exposure to H_2S. Indeed, whereas colonocytes exhibit very high H_2S disposal capacity to cope with the high H_2S levels derived from the gut microbial metabolism, neurons are practically devoid of H_2S oxidation activity. The localization and expression of these enzymes in colorectal cancer cells appear to be sensitive to different stimuli, including hypoxic conditions [35,39]. The primary and committing H_2S-detoxifying step of this pathway is catalyzed by the membrane-associated SQR, a monomeric flavoenzyme that covalently binds flavin adenine dinucleotide (FAD) and contains a disulfide active site. Structural and mechanistic studies have been elucidative of the SQR reaction mechanism, showing that the enzyme resting state involves a cysteine trisulfide between Cys201 and Cys379, which is cleaved upon reaction with sulfide [40,41]. H_2S-derived electrons are transferred to quinone acceptors, namely coenzyme Q_{10}, and reduced glutathione is the preferred sulfane sulfur acceptor, generating glutathione persulfide (GSSH) [42,43]. GSSH is then metabolized, with O_2 as cosubstrate, by persulfide dioxygenase (PDO), yielding sulfite (SO_3^{2-}) and GSH. PDO is a homodimeric metalloprotein of the metallo β-lactamase family, harboring a catalytic mononuclear nonheme iron ion with two histidines, one carboxylate and three aquo/hydroxo ligands [44]. One cysteine residue of PDO, Cys247, is considered a "catalytic" residue for its role in the interaction with the GSSH substrate during the catalytic cycle. The next enzyme in the pathway, TST, catalyzes the transfer of a sulfane sulfur from GSSH to sulfite (derived from PDO) to generate GSH and thiosulfate [36]. TST is another member of the sulfurtransferase/rhodanese family, structurally and functionally similar to MST. Differences in the substrate binding sites justify the substrate preference of either enzyme, despite the marked overall structural similarities. Like MST, TST displays a cysteine residue, Cys247, as the active site. Sulfite can also be oxidized to sulfate by the multisubunit sulfite oxidase (SOx) in the intermembrane space. SOx bears a catalytic molybdenum-containing cofactor and a b_5-type heme that transfers electrons to cytochrome *c* [45].

The ability of SQR to reduce quinones establishes an important link with mitochondrial bioenergetics [46,47]. Indeed, at low physiological H_2S concentrations, H_2S stimulates cellular respiration by injecting sulfide-derived electron equivalents into the mitochondrial electron transfer chain, thereby contributing to ATP production. In addition, persulfidation of ATPase also enhances its enzymatic activity [48]. However, if H_2S levels progressively increase above the capacity of the sulfide oxidation pathway to dispose of it, H_2S becomes inhibitory toward cytochrome *c* oxidase (CcOx, detailed below), thereby halting cellular respiration and decreasing ATP production.

Other proteins are able to react with H_2S and thereby contribute to its metabolization. Besides heme proteins (described below), copper/zinc superoxide dismutase has been reported to oxidize in vitro H_2S to polysulfides [49]. In addition to the enzymatic systems, nonenzymatic H_2S-detoxifying reactions have been described, particularly the ability of coenzyme Q10 and other quinones to directly oxidize H_2S to polysulfide species and thiosulfate [50].

The expression levels and function of H_2S-synthesizing and H_2S-consuming enzymes have a wide and heterogeneous distribution across the different cell types and organs. Their roles are conditioned by several factors such as: the cellular redox state and overall redox environment, metabolic status, and availability of substrates, among others. Moreover, seemingly overlapping functions in terms of H_2S production may actually reflect different subtle roles for various physiological processes. One example is the reciprocal regulation of CBS and SELENBP1 underlying the spontaneous differentiation of the colorectal cancer cell line Caco-2 into colonocytes reported by Scheller and co-workers [51]. H_2S metabolism is inextricably linked to cysteine metabolism [52], and consequently to that of glutathione. Indeed, cysteine, while being generated from homocysteine by the RTP enzymes CBS and CSE, is also one of the prime substrates of both enzymes for H_2S production, as well as for CAT to generate 3MP for MST-catalyzed H_2S synthesis. CBS and CSE can further metabolize cystine, more prevalent in oxidative conditions. While the H_2S levels are unlikely per se to directly vary cysteine and/or glutathione levels and thereby the redox status, the subtle modulation of key cellular targets may suffice to shift the redox balance, as exemplified below.

Cellular targets of hydrogen sulfide

Hydrogen sulfide exerts its signaling function by targeting proteins according to two mechanisms, namely through (i) persulfidation of cysteine thiols and (ii) binding to heme moieties.

Protein persulfidation

Signaling by H_2S has been shown to occur mainly through a chemical modification of specific cysteine side chains in target proteins, designated as protein persulfidation. Persulfidation occurs when the targeted thiol residues (P-SH) are converted into their corresponding persulfides (P-SSH), with modulatory effects on the function of the modified protein. Such covalent post-translational modification of protein cysteine residues often involves low-molecular-weight (LMW) persulfides (RSSH), particularly cysteine persulfide (CysSSH) and glutathione persulfide (GSSH), or polysulfides (RS_nSH). Polysulfides, in addition to persulfides, have emerged as physiologically relevant cellular species, as reviewed elsewhere [53]. Of interest from a cellular perspective, protein persulfidation by H_2S and per/poly-sulfides represents an effective switching modification in that it can be reverted, regenerating the initial thiol moiety, by reaction of the protein persulfide with reduced glutathione (GSH) or the thioredoxin system. Protein persulfidation is presently considered as key in the regulation of many physiological processes. Thus, it is not surprising that several pathologies, including the neurodegenerative ones and those affecting the cardiovascular system, are associated to deficiency in persulfidated proteins [54,55]. Also, of relevance for redox biology, persulfidation was suggested to represent a protective mechanism to prevent irreversible protein damage linked to thiol hyperoxidation [56]. The propensity of a protein thiol to be persulfidated critically depends on the protein environment surrounding the cysteine residue, but also on the redox status of the cell and the availability of H_2S and free per/poly-sulfides to react with the target cysteine. From a chemical viewpoint, post-translational protein persulfidation can occur through several pathways. Protein cysteine residues in the reduced thiol state (−SH) cannot react directly with H_2S, but they can be persulfidated by reacting with the thyil radical $HS\cdot$, formed upon reaction of H_2S with metal centers, including protein heme iron in the oxidized state. Another way for protein persulfidation to occur is through reaction of reduced protein thiol with LMW persulfides (RSSH), such as GSSH or (homo)cysteine persulfide that can be produced enzymatically in the H_2S biosynthetic and catabolic pathways. The reaction of a protein cysteine thiol (P-SH) with $HS\cdot$ is expected to transiently produce a protein-$SSH\cdot^-$ radical derivative, eventually yielding the persulfidated derivative (P-SSH) and superoxide anion, upon reaction with O_2 [57,58]. Alternatively, protein persulfidation can result from reaction of H_2S with the target cysteine which was previously oxidized to either (i) a disulfide (−SS−) by reaction with oxidized glutathione (GSSG) or other oxidized sulfur-containing LMW species or to (ii) a sulfenic moiety (P-SOH) possibly produced by reaction with H_2O_2 [59].

Protein persulfidation was found to occur in mammals not only post-translationally, but also co-translationally via incorporation of cysteine persulfide or polysulfide into the polypeptide chain of a nascent protein by cysteinyl-tRNA synthetases (CARSs), particularly the mitochondrial isoform CARS2 [60]. These enzymes are currently recognized as major sources of CysSSH and $CysSS_{(n)}H$.

Despite the relative instability of persulfides, persulfidation at specific cysteine residues has been reported for numerous proteins and shown to play a role in the regulation of several physiological processes (reviewed in Refs. [61,62]), such as glycolysis [63], endoplasmic reticulum stress [64], apoptosis [65], vasorelaxation, and vasodilation [66]. Due to the relatively high reactivity of persulfides, protein persulfidation is still technically challenging to be detected in living cells. Yet, the setup of assays more specifically detecting persulfidated proteins coupled to proteomic approaches has been revealing a constantly increasing number of persulfidated proteins, and this number will likely increase further, unveiling yet unidentified signaling pathways.

Binding to heme proteins

As mentioned above, H_2S can exert its signaling action not only by promoting protein thiol persulfidation but also by reacting with protein-bound hemes (reviewed in Ref. [67]). The latter reaction critically depends on the redox and ligation state of the heme iron, the physicochemical properties of the residues in the heme pocket and the possible presence of reducing agents or O_2 in solution. H_2S can reversibly bind the oxidized heme iron (Fe(III)) as such or as HS^-. The Fe-HS^- and Fe-H_2S adducts are stabilized respectively by the presence in the heme pocket of either basic residues able to accept protons from bound H_2S or apolar residues promoting the ligand full protonation. After binding the heme iron, sulfide can slowly reduce the metal, and the resulting heme-Fe(II)-$HS\cdot$ radical adduct can lead to formation of thiosulfate or polysulfides, upon further reacting with O_2/H_2O or excess $HS^-/HS\cdot$, respectively. Therefore, any hemeprotein can in principle be a source of sulfane sulfur-containing species, but this ability largely varies from protein to protein. In some cases, the reaction of H_2S with hemeproteins was demonstrated to covalently and irreversibly modify the heme moiety due to incorporation of a sulfur atom into one of the porphyrin pyrroles rings. The sulfur atom incorporation leads to formation of the so-called "sulfheme", with impaired redox and ligand binding properties. The list of hemeproteins whose reaction with H_2S was documented is quite long. Among them, there are globins from a variety of different sources, terminal respiratory oxidases such as the mitochondrial CcOx, antioxidant enzymes such as catalases and different types of peroxidases, and proteins involved in the sensing of O_2, NO and CO.

The reaction of H_2S with human hemoglobin (Hb) was investigated in detail. Interestingly, this globin can work as a source of physiologically relevant sulfane sulfur species, namely thiosulfate and GSSH, which are emerging as signaling molecules themselves [68,69]. Hb can exert protective effects against sulfide toxicity, favoring the disposal of H_2S, or on the opposite it can mediate sulfide toxicity after conversion to sulfhemoglobin. As compared to the native protein, the green-colored sulfhemoglobin, resulting from irreversible covalent modification of the heme to the sulfheme derivative, displays lower O_2 affinity, causing a rare disease known as "sulfhemoglobinemia". Sulfide binds to the heme Fe in oxidized Hb (metHb) with relatively low affinity (K_D of 17 μM at pH 7.4 and 37°C) and a rate constant increasing at lower pH values. This points to H_2S rather than HS^- as the binding species, which then deprotonates upon Fe binding, as shown by the crystallographic structure of sulfide-bound Hb [68]. Following H_2S binding, metHb can slowly catalyze its oxidative degradation to a mixture of thiosulfate and polysulfides, a reaction that can be of physiological relevance in red blood cells which, being amitochondriate, are unable to detoxify H_2S via the mitochondrial sulfide oxidizing pathway. Notably, Hb-bound polysulfides can further react with GSH or cysteine, yielding GSSH or CysSSH that are eventually released into the solution, making Hb a source of species able to mediate protein persulfidation.

H_2S has long been known to inhibit mitochondrial respiration, targeting CcOX. The inhibition results from sulfide binding to the copper in the active site (Cu_B) of CcOX, followed by intramolecular transfer to the nearby ferric heme a_3 [70]. Inhibition by H_2S is fairly fast [70], potent ($K_i = 0.2$ μM at pH 7.4), independent of $[O_2]$ and reversible [71]. Susceptibility of CcOX to sulfide inhibition increases as the pH decreases, again pointing to H_2S rather than HS^- as the species binding to the enzyme. Following binding to the fully oxidized so-called "pulsed" state of CcOX, H_2S can slowly reduce the enzyme, leading to formation of oxidation products which have yet to be characterized. In prokaryotes, terminal respiratory oxidases can be of the heme-copper type, like the mitochondrial CcOX, or of the *bd*-type. The latter oxidases are not found in Eukaryotes. The *bd*-type oxidases lack copper, are preferentially expressed under microaerobic conditions, are cyanide-insensitive, confer resistance to oxidative and nitrosative stress, and promote bacterial virulence [72]. Notably, these oxidases were found to be insensitive to H_2S, allowing bacterial growth in the presence of sulfide [73]. It is still unclear if such insensitivity of *bd*-type oxidases to H_2S is physiologically relevant, but intriguingly in the well-known pathogen *Mycobacterium tuberculosis*, endogenously produced H_2S was recently found to modulate the metabolism and redox status of this bacterium, while enhancing bacterial O_2 respiration through the *bd* oxidase [74,75].

Modulation of oxidative stress by hydrogen sulfide

H_2S has proven to regulate several physiological functions and to act as a cytoprotectant mainly stimulating antioxidant and anti-inflammatory pathways [20,76]. As such, H_2S shows a wide pharmacological potential, being able to provide beneficial effects in a large panel of chronic multifactorial disorders characterized by the lack of a unique etiology, such as neurodegenerative, cardiovascular, and lipid metabolism diseases [77,78]. The broad-spectrum therapeutic potential of H_2S lies on its ability to counteract oxidative stress through various independent mechanisms, overall providing a multitarget cytoprotective effect, such as (i) direct scavenging of reactive oxygen species (ROS), (ii) persulfidation of target proteins, and (iii) activation of the Nrf2/Keap1 pathway and the antioxidant response (Fig. 11.2). All these mechanisms depend on the nucleophilic and reducing character of H_2S, leading to redox reactions involving a change of the oxidation state of the sulfur atoms. For a better understanding of the reactivity of sulfur compounds in a biological milieu it is worth mentioning some of its chemico-physical properties. Sulfur has 6 valence electrons and a vacant 3d orbital, thus enabling to adopt oxidation states between −2 and +6. In the form of H_2S, sulfur shows an oxidation state of −2; hence, it cannot be further reduced but, on the contrary, acts as a reducing agent. H_2S is a weak acid with a $pKa_1^{H_2S} = 7.05$ ($H_2S \rightleftharpoons HS^- + H^+$), meaning that at pH 7.4 and 20°C the percent distribution of H_2S:HS^- is approximately 30:70, respectively, while at 37°C, the equilibrium is almost completely shifted toward the anionic HS^- form, more reactive and more nucleophilic than H_2S due to the net negative charge [79]. Although sulfide (mainly in the form of HS^-) engages into one-electron and two-electron reactions with most of the biologically relevant ROS, the kinetics of these reactions is not outstanding and overall does not appear to be much different from other LMW thiols such as cysteine (Cys) and glutathione (GSH) (e.g., H_2S, Cys, and GSH engage into two-electron reduction of H_2O_2 with second-order rate constants in the same order of magnitude, namely, 0.73, 2.9, and 0.87 $M^{-1}{\bullet}s^{-1}$, respectively). This, together with the fact that in mammalian cells free cellular H_2S levels are in the range of

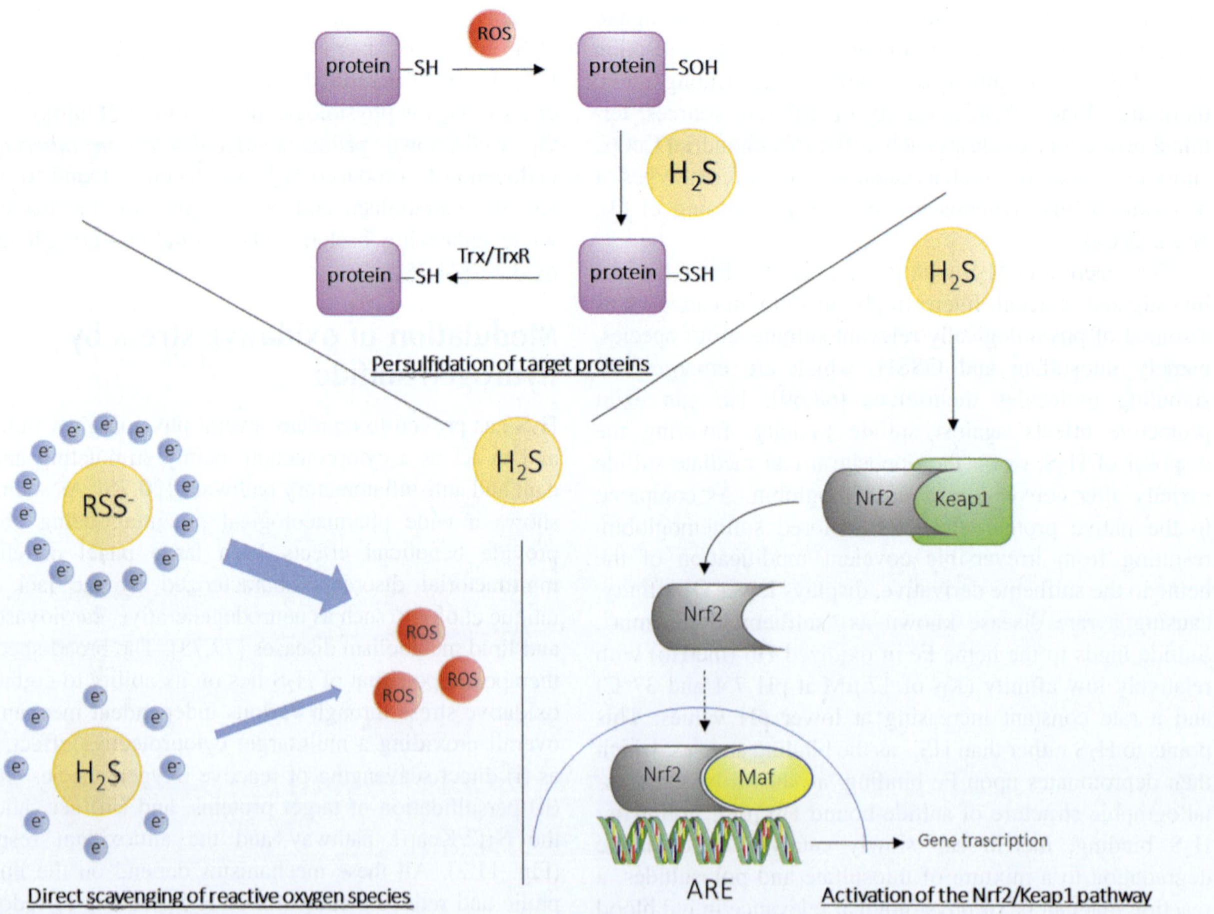

FIGURE 11.2 Cytoprotective and antioxidant mechanisms of H_2S. Hydrogen sulfide (H_2S)-mediated cytoprotection is accomplished by distinct mechanisms, some of which are illustrated above, to maintain the cellular redox balance. As a reductant, H_2S and related reactive species (such as hydropersulfides and polysulfides) exert an antioxidant effect by direct scavenging of reactive oxygen species (ROS). H_2S-mediated protein persulfidation at redox sensitive cysteine residues protects proteins from irreversible oxidation and overall has an anti-aging effect. Moreover, persulfidation of the Kelch-like ECH-associated protein 1 (Keap1) induces the release of the active form of the nuclear factor erythroid 2-related factor 2 (Nrf2), resulting in increased expression of antioxidant-response elements (AREs).

two-digits nanomolar concentrations and are almost negligible as compared to GSH levels (in the order of millimolar), makes it unlikely that sulfide as such has a direct protective role against oxidative stress in an in vivo context [80]. In more recent years, it has become increasingly clear that the pool of sulfur-containing species such as alkyl hydropersulfides and polysulfides (i.e., RSSH and RSS_nH, $n > 1$) might be the actual mediators of at least some of the biological signaling effects commonly ascribed to H_2S. Indeed RSSH (or RSS_nH) have been proposed to be hyperactivated thiols, meaning that all the chemical features associated to sulfide or thiols (i.e., nucleophilicity, reducing properties) are enhanced [57,81]. Similarly to sulfide, the nucleophilicity of the anion RSS^- arises from the net negative charge of the terminal sulfur and is potentiated by the so called α-effect (increase in reactivity of the terminal atom due to the presence of an adjacent α-atom with lone pair of electrons) [82]. Consistently, in the presence of oxidants such as H_2O_2, alkyl hydropersulfides are oxidized more rapidly than their thiolic cognate and overexpression of the persulfide-producing enzyme CSE prevents H_2O_2-mediated toxicity in mammalian cells (Fig. 11.2) [14]. Understanding the biological context in which alkyl hydropersulfides (which are precursors for polysulfides) are generated is of foremost importance for interpreting their physiological role. As mentioned above, one of the major pathways for hydropersulfide generation is the enzymatic conversion of cystine (Cys-SS-Cys) to cysteine persulfide (CysSSH) by CSE [14,37]. In turn, the formation of Cys-SS-Cys occurs by nonenzymatic oxidation of Cys by oxidants such as ROS. In general, the generation of an RSSH requires the oxidation of an R-SH. Thus, the formation of a hydropersulfide requires an initial oxidation event. The relevance of this information becomes even clearer when applied to the effect of oxidative stress on the modulation of pivotal cellular pathways. Among the numerous proteins shown to be persulfidated in various physiological contexts, glyceraldehyde-3-phosphate dehydrogenase (GAPDH), a central enzyme in glycolysis whose activity is sensitive to oxidative stress (i.e., its catalytic activity is negatively modulated in the presence of H_2O_2), has been shown to be positively modulated and protected from oxidative stress when one of its cysteine residues is persulfidated [61,63]. Although protein persulfidation has long been understudied due to its intrinsic instability and chemical reactivity, nowadays it is considered a major redox-switch protein post-translational modification, along with *s*-glutathionylation, *s*-nitrosation, and *s*-sulfenylation [83]. Even in the case of protein persulfidation, the initial event leading to the formation of a hydropersulfide is an oxidation. Indeed, protein persulfidation occurs through a nonenzymatic reaction between H_2S and oxidized cysteine residues, such as sulfenylated cysteine, likely generated in the presence of a source of ROS [14,84]. Protein cysteine residues are major cellular targets for ROS and get oxidized to sulfenic acid (P-SOH), which is a physiological post-translational modification involved in the regulation of important cellular processes, such as proliferation, differentiation, and apoptosis [85]. However, oxidation above the sulfenic acid state (sulfenylated cysteine can be further oxidized to sulfinic, P-SO_2H and sulfonic, P-SO_3H adducts) is often associated with irreversible structural and functional changes of target proteins, thus requiring de novo protein synthesis for regaining biological activity [85]. On the other hand, in the presence of H_2S, P-SOH readily reacts to form P-SSH which eventually (under normal reducing conditions) is reduced back to the correspondent P-SH by the thioredoxin/thioredoxin reductase system (Trx/TrxR), thus preserving structure and function of the target protein (Fig. 11.2) [86]. H_2S is not the only thiol compound able to preserve the redox state of protein cysteine residues. Glutathione has been reported to be reactive toward oxidized cysteine residues with which it readily reacts to generate *s*-glutathionylated proteins (P-SSG), which are then reconverted to P-SH by the Trx/TrxR system. Another mechanism of cytoprotection mediated by H_2S and RSSH has been reported to rely on the activation of the Nuclear factor erythroid 2-related factor 2 (Nrf2) signaling, a transcription factor which is considered a master regulator of the oxidative stress response (Fig. 11.2). Particularly, reactive sulfur species have been shown to inactivate Kelch-like ECH associated protein 1 (Keap1), a negative modulator of Nrf2, via persulfidation of redox sensitive cysteines, thus promoting the translocation of Nrf2 into the nucleus where it induces the expression of more than 250 genes involved in the oxidative stress response [78,87]. Nrf2 activation maintains the cellular redox balance by promoting the expression of ROS scavenging enzymes such as superoxide dismutase (SOD), NAD(P)H:quinone acceptor oxidoreductase 1 (NQO1), heme oxygenase-1 (HO-1), and glutathione peroxidase (GPx). Nrf2 activation stimulates GSH de novo biosynthesis and recycling by inducing the expression levels of glutamate–cysteine ligase (GCL) and glutathione reductase. The CBS- and CSE-encoding genes are among the ones whose expression is controlled by Nrf2, thus establishing a feedback loop whereby H_2S (and RSSH) activate Nrf2, which in turn enhances the expression levels of the reverse transsulfuration pathway enzymes. The latter is also the major source of endogenous Cys, thus feeding and sustaining the biosynthesis of GSH [78].

Hydrogen sulfide metabolism in human disease

Given the relevance of H_2S in protecting cells from oxidative stressors, it is not surprising that dysregulated H_2S metabolism has been reported for a consistent number of diseases, ranging from neurodegeneration to cancer, thus highlighting the wide implications that sulfur metabolism has in human (patho)physiology. Particularly, the physiological functions of H_2S are exerted within a narrow window of concentrations, H_2S being potentially toxic at lower levels (i.e., cellular redox imbalance) or higher than physiological levels (i.e., blocking of mitochondrial respiration through tight inhibition of CcOx) (Fig. 11.3). Therefore, steady-state levels of H_2S must be kept under tight control through a fine regulation of its biosynthesis and catabolism. Aging is a common thread through many of the diseases (or disorders) associated with reduced H_2S levels. Indeed, it has been observed in different animal models (e.g., *Caenorhabditis elegans*, mouse, rat) and humans that the expression levels of the three main H_2S-sythesizing enzymes, namely CBS, CSE, and MST, lower with age, with concomitant reduction of protein persulfides, thus leaving proteins vulnerable to oxidative damage [84]. In turn, aging is considered a risk factor for many neurodegenerative diseases (such as Parkinson's, Alzheimer's, Huntington's diseases, spinocerebellar ataxia, and amyotrophic lateral sclerosis) [83], cardiovascular diseases (such as hypertension and atherosclerosis) and lipid metabolism disorders [78,88]. For instance, in Alzheimer's disease (AD) impaired expression levels of CSE resulted in increased homocysteine plasma levels, depletion of cysteine and reduced protein persulfidation levels both in mice and postmortem AD patients' brains. On the other hand, administration of the slow-releasing H_2S donor GYY4137 to a rodent's model of AD ameliorated learning and memory and alleviated motor deficits [89]. Even in brain of humans with Huntington's disease (HD), it has been observed a significant decrease in CSE expression levels, particularly in the striatum, while moderate reduction to unaffected expression levels were observed respectively in the cerebral cortex and in the cerebellum, reflecting the

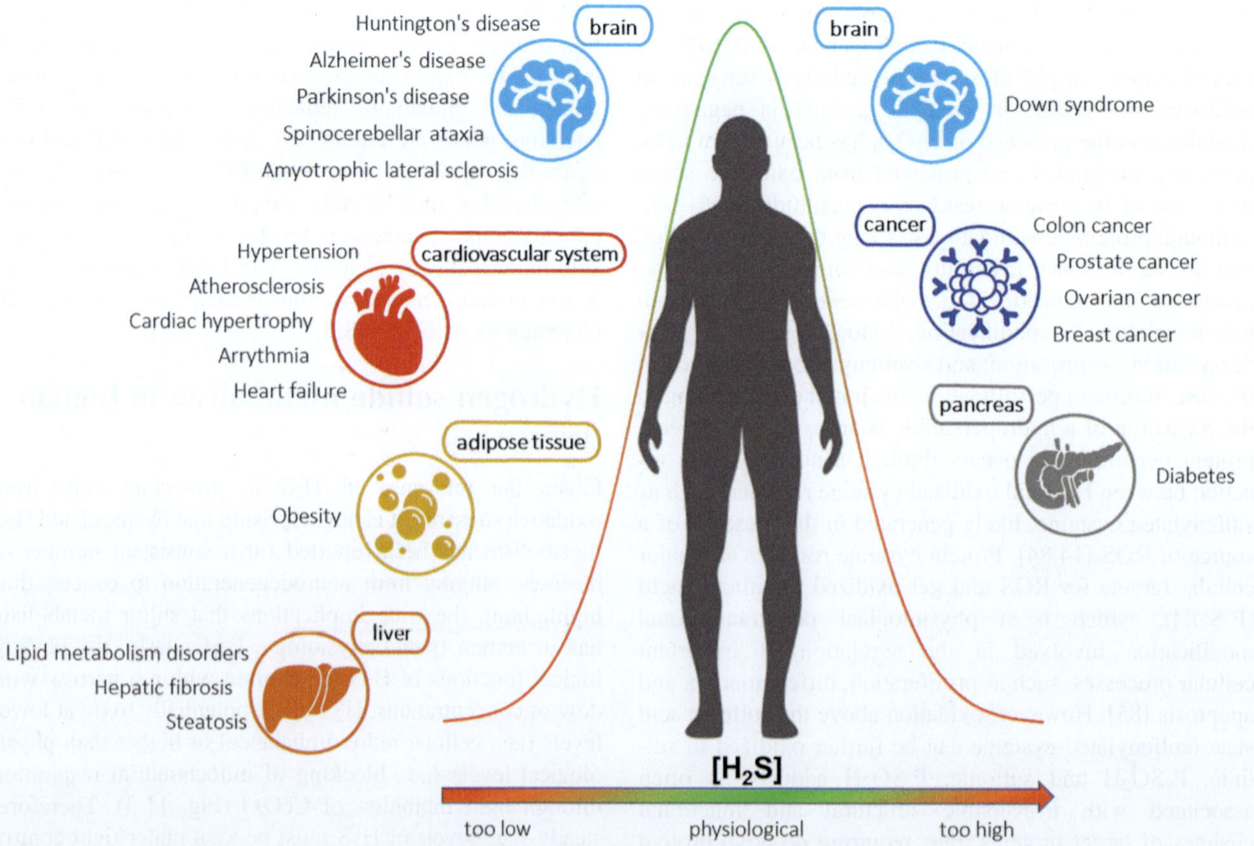

FIGURE 11.3 Correlation between altered H_2S metabolism and disease. Hydrogen sulfide (H_2S) signaling is accomplished within a narrow range of concentrations. Alteration of its metabolism, thus resulting in lower or higher than physiological concentrations, has been associated to a number of diseases. On the left and on the right side of the bell-shaped model are respectively represented some of the diseases (or disturbances) associated with decreased and increased levels of H_2S.

relative vulnerability of the aforementioned brain regions to damages due to HD. Most importantly, the progressive CSE depletion observed in postmortem patients at different stage of the disease, correlated with severity of the neurodegeneration. As shown in an HD mouse model, feeding animals with a cysteine-rich diet, together with supplementation of drinking water with *N*-acetyl-cysteine (a stable cysteine precursor) delayed the onset of motor disabilities [90]. In the cardiovascular system, the main enzyme involved in H_2S biosynthesis is CSE, expressed in cardiac myocytes, smooth muscle, and endothelial cells. Reduced H_2S levels have been associated with diseases such as atherosclerosis, which correlates with marked changes in persulfidation of a spectrum of endothelial proteins (most of them belonging to the integrins family), as shown in native and cultured human endothelial cells. Deficit of the RTP has been observed in human patients and mouse models affected by atherosclerosis, often correlating with increase of circulating levels of cystathionine due to decreased CSE activity. Treatment with the sulfide donor SG1002 in cultured cells or mice, as well as administration of methylsulfonylmethane in human patients, resulted in increased circulating polysulfide levels and significantly improved the flow-induced vasodilation [91]. Alteration of H_2S metabolism has been linked to lipid metabolism disorders and obesity, as witnessed by several lines of evidence accumulated both in vitro and in vivo. Indeed, CSE and MST deficiency correlated with lipid accumulation both in a mouse model and human subjects and particularly, MST deficiency was associated with diminished β-oxidation, Krebs cycle and oxidative phosphorylation, thus increasing lipid storage. Conversely, administration of sulfide donors such as SG1002 and Na_2S_3 both reduced weight gain in mice and improved metabolic health [92]. According to the hypothesized bell-shaped effect, toxicity is also observed at the other end of H_2S (and related reactive sulfur species) scale of concentration. Overexpression of CBS and CSE has been associated with a number of oncological diseases, the onset of diabetes and cognitive deficits related to Down syndrome (DS) [78,93,94]. The fact that the *cbs* gene is encoded on chromosome 21 led Prof. Kamoun to hypothesize that over expression of CBS may be responsible for some clinical aspects often associated with trisomy 21, such as marked increase of circulating levels of sulfhemoglobin, increased urinary excretion of thiosulfate, low circulating levels of homocysteine, and accumulation of Krebs cycle intermediates (suggestive of inhibition of mitochondrial respiration). Indeed, CBS overexpression has been shown in different tissues including the brain of mouse, rat and postmortem human subjects affected by DS [94]. The Kamoun hypothesis was later corroborated in vitro with dermal fibroblasts from healthy and DS subjects, in which it was observed that overproduction of H_2S (consequent to CBS overexpression) is responsible for impairment of mitochondrial oxidative phosphorylation due to inhibition of the CcOx [95]. In vivo studies on DS mouse and rat models demonstrated that animal treatment with inhibitors of CBS resulted in amelioration of electrophysiological and neurobehavioral alterations along with ability of the DS brain to generate ATP (ex vivo) [95,96]. Hyperactivation of the RTP has been observed in vitro, animal models and clinical specimens of various types of cancer, namely colon cancer, ovarian cancer, prostate cancer, and breast cancer, showing increased expression levels of CBS and increased amounts of H_2S as compared to the surrounding noncancerous tissues. Mechanistically, beyond the already mentioned role of sulfur species in protecting cells from oxidative stress, H_2S can stimulate cancer bioenergetic capacity, to meet the high ATP demand of its rapid proliferation and growth by (i) donating electrons to the electron transport chain (at the level of coenzyme Q via SQR), (ii) positively modulating the catalytic activity of ATPase, GAPDH and lactate dehydrogenase via persulfidation of redox sensitive cysteines, and (iii) by increasing levels of cyclic AMP. Although overexpression of CSE and MST has been also reported in various cancer cells, CBS seems to have a major role in supporting cancer development. Accordingly, in both in vitro and in vivo studies, downregulation or inhibition of CBS resulted in suppression of bioenergetics (both mitochondrial oxidative phosphorylation and glycolysis), depletion of intracellular levels of GSH and triggered the apoptotic cascade via modulation of nuclear factor-κB (NF-κB) and p53 pathways [93]. Interestingly, SELENBP1 appears to be repressed in several cancer types [33,97], highlighting that the H_2S-synthesizing enzymes may serve different functions in cancer etiology, despite their common role in sulfide production. Eventually, there are cases in which the antioxidant properties of H_2S are exploited to counteract metabolic dysfunctions, but an excessive and protracted overproduction of H_2S may lead to toxicity instead of being an advantage. This is the case, for instance, of diabetes, for which overproduction of intraislet H_2S, as a response to increased circulating glucose levels, has been associated with progressive pancreatic β-cells toxicity, thus supporting the onset of diabetes [78,98].

Overall in this section, we tried to summarize the major findings on the role of H_2S in pathology and clearly highlighted its double-faced character, depending on the H_2S concentrations. Strong experimental evidence suggests that for diseases associated with deficits of sulfur metabolism, the stimulation of the reverse transsulfuration pathway and/or pharmacological interventions using sulfide donors have the potential to repersulfidate target proteins and may be beneficial for counteracting oxidative stress, thus providing a strategy for alleviating symptoms associated to such diseases/disorders. On the other hand, the findings reported on DS, characterized by an overdosage of H_2S, may lead to the development of pharmacotherapies targeting CBS for the treatment of cognitive disabilities associated with DS. Of course, it would be naïve looking at a potential pharmacological treatment of DS as the solution. It should instead be considered an adjuvant therapy to be flanked by more traditional interventions such as speech, physical and occupational therapies. Although a consistent body of preclinical and clinical data have evidenced the pathogenic role of CBS in supporting different forms of cancer (and its correlation with DS), to date, in spite of the efforts done, a selective inhibitor against CBS is still lacking. Aminooxyacetic acid (AOAA), the gold-standard inhibitor for CBS lacks selectivity (i.e., interferes with the activity of at least 40 other PLP-dependent enzymes). It is therefore conceivable that the future drug screening campaigns will be focused on non-PLP-targeting compounds, such as the substrate access channel, in order to identify new classes of CBS-specific inhibitors, which would find their use in further research and potential clinical development [99].

Modulation of H_2S metabolism by physiological effectors

The importance of maintaining homeostatic H_2S levels is attested by the numerous regulatory mechanisms that control the enzymes catalyzing its production and consumption. Transcriptional control of the genes encoding H_2S metabolism enzymes involves intricate and multifactorial processes in many different cell types and (patho)physiological contexts and will not be addressed here. Instead, herein are described several posttranslational regulatory mechanisms at the protein level, involving direct interaction with and/or modification by physiological effectors. Whereas vast amounts of data result from in vitro studies on the isolated enzymes, several studies have demonstrated the importance of these regulatory mechanisms in relevant (patho)physiological contexts. Among the H_2S-synthesizing and H_2S-consuming enzymes, CBS and CSE are those for which more diverse lines of evidence of posttranslational regulatory control have been acquired (Fig. 11.4).

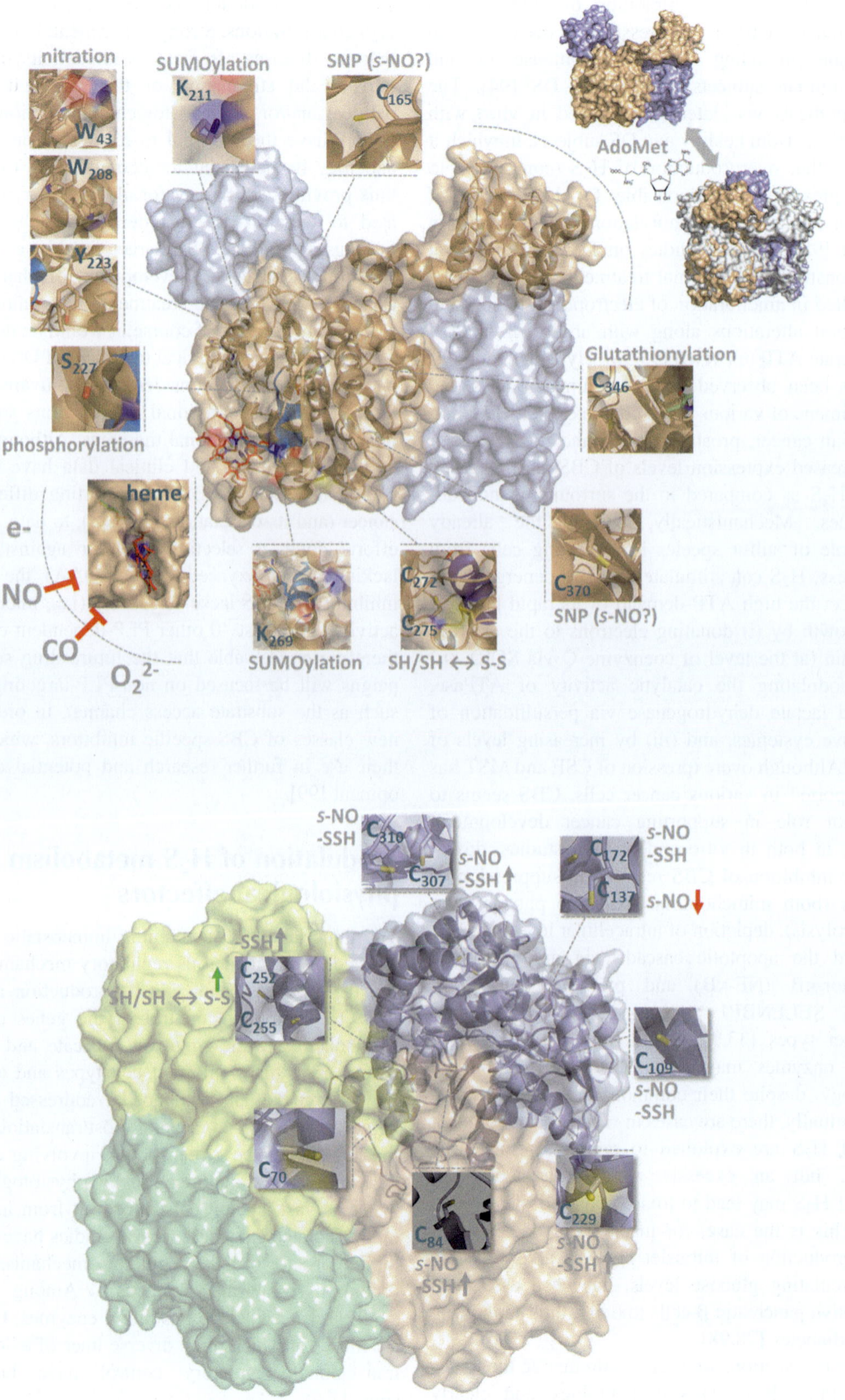

FIGURE 11.4 Modulation of human CBS and CSE by physiological effectors and post-translational modifications. *Top panel,* modulation of CBS upon binding of *s*-adenosyl-L-methionine (AdoMet) to the C-terminal domain, SUMOylation of K211 and K269, nitration of W43, W208 and Y223, phosphorylation of S227, by oxidative modification of cysteine residues (glutathionylation of C346, putative *s*-nitrosation of C165 and C370, and redox state of C272-C275 disulfide), and by the redox and ligation state of the regulatory heme. *Bottom panel,* modulation of CSE by persulfidation of C84, C229, C252 and C307, *s*-nitrosation of C137, redox state of the C252-C255 disulfide, and phosphorylation of S377.

Modulation of human CBS and CSE by physiological effectors and post-translational modifications

One of the most well studied regulatory mechanisms of CBS is its activation, or de-repression, upon interaction with *s*-adenosyl-L-methionine (AdoMet). In free CBS, the C-terminal regulatory domains "sit" on the substrate entrance in catalytic domain. Upon AdoMet binding, the C-terminal domains move away from the resting position and form a disc-like structure. This causes a release of the steric hindrance otherwise imposed on the substrates to access the active site and CBS becomes activated 2–5× [100]. The relevance of this control mechanism is attested by the number of *CBS* mutations identified in homocystinuric patients which generate variants with impaired AdoMet regulation [101]. On the N-terminal region, CBS contains a ~40 amino acid intrinsically disordered segment that is absent from all crystallographic structures thus far obtained. Interestingly, this peptide has been shown to be able to bind heme *b* with relatively high affinity. Surprisingly, deletion of this N-terminal disordered segment renders the enzyme less active [12] although the exact mechanism whereby it modulates enzymatic activity has not been elucidated. CBS has been shown to be a target of SUMOylation by SUMO-1 and Polycomb-2 at lysines 211 and 269 (both located near the PLP active site), promoting up to 70% enzyme inhibition [16,102]. Phosphorylation of CBS Ser227 mediated by the cGMP/PKG pathway has been demonstrated in human bladder samples and in the urothelial T24 cell line upon stimulation with carbachol [103].

Several redox modifications of particular cysteine residues have been reported for CBS. Glutathionylation of Cys346 has been shown to enhance 1.5–2× CBS activity depending on whether the enzyme has been "primed" with diamide or H_2O_2, although the modified enzyme lost the AdoMet activation [104,105]. This activity enhancement extends to 3× the basal activity in cells under oxidative stress [105]. Conversely, a redox switch located at the $C_{272}XXC_{275}$ motif has been reported to exert the opposite effect, i.e., enhance enzymatic activity in the reduced state. The importance of maintaining these residues dissociated to afford higher activity is confirmed by the increased enzymatic activity of cysteine-to-alanine single variants of either residue. The oxidized disulfide is thus likely to impose a structural constraint that propagates to the active site. Indeed, this motif is adjacent to an α-helical segment responsible for allosteric communication with the PLP site, first attributed in relation to the regulatory heme. By working on rat brain homogenates, Eto and Kimura reported on the CBS H_2S-synthesizing activity enhancement upon incubation with sodium nitroprusside (SNP) [106], a reactive nitrogen species donor that releases nitrosonium and may thereby induce *s*-nitrosation of cysteine residues. Four cysteine residues were identified as targets of SNP-derived *s*-nitrosation, two of which are conserved in human CBS, namely Cys165 and Cys370. It remains to be determined whether these residues are also *s*-nitrosated in human CBS.

Still within the realm of redox modifications, CBS has been reported to be inactivated by peroxynitrite [107], a potent physiological oxidant mainly resulting from the diffusion rate limited reaction between nitric oxide and superoxide anion. The calculated IC_{50} of 150 μM is far above (patho)physiological peroxynitrite levels. Still, the inhibitory mechanism has been investigated, revealing that the heme thiolate ligand is displaced and that residues Trp43, Trp208, and Tyr223 become nitrated.

The majority of the research efforts on CBS redox regulation have focused on the noncatalytic type-b heme bound to the N-terminal domain, with endogenous axial ligands Cys52 and His65. The enzyme is fully active when the heme iron remains in the ferric state. However, upon reduction with sodium dithionite, the enzyme becomes partially inactivated [108,109] and the heme progressively loses its thiolate ligand which becomes replaced by a yet undetermined ligand [110,111]. Despite the very low redox potential of this heme (−350 mV) rendering its physiological significance questionable [112], at least one human enzyme, namely methionine synthase reductase, has been shown to be able to reduce CBS at the expense of NADPH oxidation. Moreover, this enzyme was shown to enable formation of the CO-bound ferrous adduct of CBS [113,114]. Heme reduction can be quickly reversed by reaction with O_2 ($k = 1.1–1.3 \times 10^5\ M^{-1}{\bullet}s^{-1}$) through an outer-sphere mechanism, yielding superoxide anion [115,116]. In turn, superoxide anion reacts even faster with ferrous CBS ($k = 2–10 \times 10^6\ M^{-1}{\bullet}s^{-1}$), yielding hydrogen peroxide and leading to heme loss and consequent impaired activity [115].

Communication between the heme site and the PLP active site has been assigned to an α-helical segment that has Arg266 at one end and Thr257 and Thr260 at the other end. While Arg266 establishes electrostatic contacts with the Cys52 heme ligand, Thr257 and Thr260 bind to the phosphate moiety of the PLP cofactor. Therefore, redox changes in the heme environment are communicated to the active site. Likewise, the binding of endogenously generated ligands, particularly CO and NO, to the reduced CBS heme has also been extensively demonstrated and postulated to have pathophysiological significance. CO binds to the reduced heme in CBS with relatively high affinity, resulting in enzyme inhibition [109,116,117]. CO binding is limited by displacement of the endogenous Cys52 thiolate ligand and this movement is communicated through Arg266 to the active site, resulting in the conversion of the PLP moiety from its active ketoenamine form, into the inactive enolimine form [118,119]. The CO-bound adduct retains its His65 ligand, thereby maintaining hexa-coordination of the heme iron. The significance of this regulatory mechanism has been proposed for different pathophysiological processes (reviewed in Ref. [13]). In addition, we demonstrated increased affinity for CO in a pathogenic p.P49L variant of CBS identified in classical homocystinuric patients, supporting our proposal that enhanced sensitivity to CO or other inhibitory endogenous ligands may constitute a novel molecular basis of CBS deficiency. This would be particularly elucidative for variants displaying WT-like behavior in terms of activity, AdoMet regulation and protein stability. NO was found to bind >100× quicker and >100× tighter than CO to the reduced CBS heme, also resulting in enzyme inhibition [116,120]. Indeed, the estimated K_D of ≤ 230 nM is compatible with physiological NO levels. Differently from CO, NO displaces both endogenous ligands thereby generating a penta-coordinated heme [116,120]. However, NO binding does not seem limited by displacement of the Cys52 ligand, which suggests that NO initially binds on the His65 site, subsequently strongly decreasing the affinity of the endogenous Cys52 ligand [116,121]. Interestingly, a puzzling effect of AdoMet on CO/NO binding was reported. Despite the known stimulatory effect on enzymatic activity, AdoMet was shown to enhance CBS inhibition by CO, as well as its affinity for this ligand [117]. Both CO and NO also appeared to bind faster to AdoMet-incubated CBS. This apparently counter-intuitive regulatory mechanism actually affords a tight regulation and a quick response to varying cellular metabolic statuses, oxidative states, etc.

Human CSE contains an unusually high number of cysteine residues in its sequence which do not appear to spontaneously form disulfide bonds, as judged from the reported crystallographic structures (PDB IDs: 2NMP, 3ELP, 6NBA) [122,123], despite the existence of two CXXC motifs and the structural vicinity of other pairs of cysteine residues. This unusual disposition of cysteine residues, with varying degrees of solvent exposure and accessibility, renders their side chains as likely targets for oxidative modification. Indeed, our group and others have recently reported on such modifications of key cysteine residues in human CSE. Luo and colleagues have demonstrated the functional impact of persulfidation of cysteine residues of human CSE. Cys84, Cys109, Cys172, Cys229, Cys252, Cys307, and Cys310 were targets for persulfidation. While persulfidation of Cys84, Cys109, Cys229, Cys252, and Cys307 were deemed necessary to keep enzymatic activity, persulfidation of Cys172 and Cys310 did not seem relevant for CSE function [124].

In the same study, it was shown that enhanced nitration of CSE results in enzyme inhibition, although the target tyrosine residues were not identified. In our study [125], by working on recombinant human CSE, we have reported the ability of the physiological nitrosating agent *s*-nitrosoglutathione (GSNO) to inhibit CSE. HPLC-coupled mass spectrometry employing a dual derivatization strategy, allowed us to observe that GSNO promotes the *s*-nitrosation of seven Cys residues (Cys84, Cys109, Cys137, Cys172, Cys229, Cys307, Cys310). By generating conservative cysteine-to-serine variants of all cysteine residues, we observed that only *s*-nitrosation of Cys137 appears to contribute to CSE inhibition by GSNO. Recently, Wang and colleagues have shown that oxidation of the $Cys_{272}XXCys_{275}$ motif to a disulfide results in a ~2.5× increase in CSE enzymatic activity [126]. Furthermore, it was observed that H_2O_2-derived sulfenylation of Cys255 is crucial to establish the disulfide formation with Cys252. Notably, overall these observations show different levels of redox sensitivity of CSE in response to different oxidative stimuli. While some of its cysteines require to be persulfidated to sustain enzymatic activity, upon oxidation of the $Cys_{272}XXCys_{275}$ motif by H_2O_2, CSE is further activated, thereby stimulating H_2S production to counteract oxidative stress. This tight and sophisticated regulation allows CSE to quickly respond to oxidative conditions. Conversely, H_2S production appears to be halted by nitrosative conditions. In addition to oxidative modifications, the phosphorylation of Ser377 in human CSE has been proposed to result in decreased enzymatic activity, affecting persulfidation of human antigen R in a model of endothelial dysfunction as well as in atherosclerotic patient samples [127].

Modulation of other H_2S-producing and H_2S-consuming enzymes

Regarding the human MST and SELENBP1, there is a paucity of information concerning their post-translational regulation. As reviewed in Ref. [24], phosphorylation of MST Ser2 and Ser35 has been demonstrated and posited to negatively regulate the mitochondrial targeting and consequently the import of MST [128]. This may be relevant for conditions where MST activity is required in the cytosol, e.g., upon oxidative stress, and/or "undesired" at the mitochondria. Another layer of post-translational regulation concerns redox modifications at cysteine residues, particularly the cysteine active site. Cys248 can be oxidized by H_2O_2, resulting in enzyme inhibition. In this report, the Cys248 thiol was shown to be modified to a reversible sulfenate at low H_2O_2 concentrations and to an irreversibly damaged sulfonate at higher H_2O_2. Although the fairly high K_i value (120.5 μM) renders this inhibition mechanism unlikely [129], exogenous H_2O_2 was demonstrated to abolish 3MP-sustained mitochondrial respiration [130]. As for SELENBP1, little is known about post-translational modifications. In red blood cells from patients with refractory schizophrenia or patients with chronic kidney disease, SELENBP1 was identified as a highly accumulated argpyrimidine-modified protein [131]. This modification is an advanced glycation end-product possibly resulting from methylglyoxal reaction with arginine residues. Neatly, this highlights another mechanism whereby oxidative stress and hydrogen sulfide exhibit a crosstalk. The Cys57 residue in human SELENBP1 has been posited as the selenium binding site [33,132], and its degree of solvent accessibility and exposure suggests it may be a target for cysteine (oxidative) modifications.

Regarding the sulfide oxidation pathway, information about its post-translational regulation and modulation by effectors is even scarcer. Human PDO has been shown to be a target for protein persulfidation and polysulfidation and that its Cys247 is essential to polysulfidate the other Cys residues [133]. Cys247, a key residue for enzymatic activity and thereby often termed a "catalytic" residue, is thus both a target and a mediator of post-translational modifications. Despite the absence of evidence for other post-translational redox modifications of sulfide oxidation pathway enzymes, various proteomics studies have revealed the presence of lysine acetylations and serine phosphorylations in all four enzymes of the sulfide oxidation pathway. While lysine acetylation has been directly detected in human PDO (Lys66) and TST (Lys14) [134], this modification has been proposed for SQR Lys173, PDO Lys172, and TST Lys136, Lys163, Lys175, Lys224, Lys236, and Lys237, based on evidence for the modification of the homologous residues in the mouse enzyme counterparts [135,136]. Similarly, serine phosphorylation has been detected in PDO Ser19 and SOx Ser123 [128], while the SQR Ser343, PDO Ser14, and TST Ser38 may be phosphorylated like their mouse/rat homologs [135–137].

Crosstalk between gasotransmitters and impact on oxidative stress

The term "gasotransmitters" collectively designates the signaling molecules in mammalian physiology that are gaseous in nature and that freely diffuse across biological milieus due to their solubility both in aqueous environments and in membranes. Due to their reactivity and broadness of action toward cellular targets, their signaling roles largely depend on their concentration, since at higher levels, they become cytotoxic and eventually lethal. Gasotransmitters are also expected to be biologically produced in a regulated manner, i.e., enzymatically generated by cells and tissues using endogenous substrates. Thus far, the main gasotransmitters are NO, CO, and H_2S. In light of growing evidence in the literature, other molecules such as ammonia and cyanide are expected to acquire the same designation in the near future [138,139]. One example concerns the recently reported ability of cyanide at low physiological concentrations to stimulate oxygen respiration by the mitochondrial electron transfer chain, in stark contrast to its known ability to inhibit CcOx at high concentrations [140]. Another notable aspect of gasotransmitters physiology is the ability of each one in cross-regulating the others. This is done essentially by each gasotransmitter affecting the expression and/or function of the enzymes synthesizing or consuming the other gasotransmitters. This can occur both at transcriptional and post-translational levels. Regarding the latter, control may be exerted directly from the active species on the enzyme(s) or through activation/inactivation of signaling cascades and consequent indirect post-translational modification. While several studies have focused on these effects in vitro focusing on the direct effects of reactive species on their target proteins, several lines of evidence obtained in cell and animal models attest the relevance of this crosstalk, despite the inherent technical challenges in dealing with these transient regulatory mechanisms. As reviewed e.g., in Ref. [13], H_2S regulates CO and NO levels both by "indirect" effects on signaling/regulatory pathways controlling expression of NO synthases (NOS) and heme oxygenases (that synthesize CO), and also by "direct" effects on NO synthase. Conversely, as described above, CO and NO potently inhibit CBS and NO-derived species inhibit CSE, with consequences for different physiological processes. In this regard, myriad hybrid reactive sulfur/nitrogen species have also emerged as relevant players in signaling processes (e.g., in Ref. [141]). Altogether, the fact that these gasotransmitters regulate each other will likely have an impact on the oxidative stress response. Indeed, these reactive species and the cellular redox status are intimately connected, due to the ability of gasotransmitters in reacting with various redox-relevant players [142]. Overall, understanding the interconnectedness of H_2S metabolism and the oxidative status, including oxidative stress, is of paramount importance to understand human redox (patho)physiology. It is particularly important to appreciate how pharmacological interventions targeting H_2S metabolism may overall impact on the cellular redox state.

Abbreviations

3MP	3-Mercaptopyruvate
AD	Alzheimer's disease
AdoMet	*s*-adenosyl-L-methionine
AOAA	Aminooxyacetic acid
CARS	Cysteinyl-tRNA synthetase
CAT	Cysteine aminotransferase
CBS	Cystathionine β-synthase
CcOX	Cytochrome *c* oxidase
CO	Carbon monoxide
CSE	Cystathionine γ-lyase
Cys	Cysteine
Cys-SS-Cys	Cystine
CysSSH	Cysteine persulfide

DS	Down syndrome
DSR	Dissimilatory sulfate reduction
FAD	Flavin adenine dinucleotide
GAPDH	Glyceraldehyde-3-phosphate dehydrogenase
GCL	Glutamate−cysteine ligase
GPx	Glutathione peroxidase
GSH	Reduced glutathione
GSNO	*s*-nitrosoglutathione
GSSG	Oxidized glutathione
GSSH	Glutathione persulfide
H_2S	Hydrogen sulfide
Hb	Hemoglobin
HD	Huntington's disease
HO-1	Heme oxygenase-1
Keap1	Kelch-like ECH associated protein 1
LMW	Low molecular weight
metHb	Oxidized Hb
MST	3-Mercaptopyruvate sulfurtransferase
NF-κB	Nuclear factor-κB
NO	Nitric oxide
NOS	Nitric oxide synthases
NQO1	NAD(P)H:quinone acceptor oxidoreductase 1
Nrf2	Nuclear factor erythroid 2-related factor 2
P-SH	Protein-bound cysteine thiol
P-SO_2H	Protein-bound sulfinic moiety
P-SO_3H	Protein-bound sulfonic moiety
P-SOH	Protein-bound sulfenic moiety
P-SSH	Protein-bound persulfide
PDO	Persulfide dioxygenase
PLP	Pyridoxal 5′-phosphate
Pyr	Pyruvate
ROS	Reactive oxygen species
RS_nSH	Polysulfides
RSSH	Low molecular weight persulfides
RTP	Reverse transsulfuration pathway
$S_2O_3^{-2}$	Thiosulfate
SELENBP1	Selenium-binding protein 1
SNP	Sodium nitroprusside
SO_3^{2-}	Sulfite
SO_4^{-2}	Sulfate
SOD	Superoxide dismutase
SOx	Sulfite oxidase
SQR	Sulfide quinone oxidoreductase
Trx/TrxR	Thioredoxin/thioredoxin reductase system
TST	Thiosulfate sulfurtransferase (also known as rhodanese, Rhod)

References

[1] Rose P, Moore PK, Zhu YZ. H_2S biosynthesis and catabolism: new insights from molecular studies. Cell Mol Life Sci 2017;74:1391−412.

[2] Kabil O, Banerjee R. Enzymology of H_2S biogenesis, decay and signaling. Antioxid Redox Signal 2014;20:770−82.

[3] Benavides GA, Squadrito GL, Mills RW, Patel HD, Isbell TS, Patel RP, et al. Hydrogen sulfide mediates the vasoactivity of garlic. Proc Natl Acad Sci USA 2007;104:17977−82.

[4] Yang J, Minkler P, Grove D, Wang R, Willard B, Dweik R, Hine C. Non-enzymatic hydrogen sulfide production from cysteine in blood is catalyzed by iron and vitamin B6. Commun Biol 2019;2:194.

[5] Shen X, Carlstrom M, Borniquel S, Jadert C, Kevil CG, Lundberg JO. Microbial regulation of host hydrogen sulfide bioavailability and metabolism. Free Radic Biol Med 2013;60:195−200.

[6] Santos AA, Venceslau SS, Grein F, Leavitt WD, Dahl C, Johnston DT, Pereira IA. A protein trisulfide couples dissimilatory sulfate reduction to energy conservation. Science 2015;350:1541−5.

[7] Blachier F, Beaumont M, Kim E. Cysteine-derived hydrogen sulfide and gut health: a matter of endogenous or bacterial origin. Curr Opin Clin Nutr Metab Care 2019;22:68−75.

[8] Blachier F, Andriamihaja M, Larraufie P, Ahn E, Lan A, Kim E. Production of hydrogen sulfide by the intestinal microbiota and epithelial cells and consequences for the colonic and rectal mucosa. Am J Physiol Gastrointest Liver Physiol 2021;320:G125−35.

[9] Randi EB, Casili G, Jacquemai S, Szabo C. Selenium-binding protein 1 (SELENBP1) supports hydrogen sulfide biosynthesis and adipogenesis. Antioxidants (Basel) 2021;10:361.

[10] Ereno-Orbea J, Majtan T, Oyenarte I, Kraus JP, Martinez-Cruz LA. Structural basis of regulation and oligomerization of human cystathionine beta-synthase, the central enzyme of transsulfuration. Proc Natl Acad Sci USA 2013;110:E3790−9.

[11] Ereno-Orbea J, Majtan T, Oyenarte I, Kraus JP, Martinez-Cruz LA. Structural insight into the molecular mechanism of allosteric activation of human cystathionine beta-synthase by S-adenosylmethionine. Proc Natl Acad Sci USA 2014;111:E3845−52.

[12] Kumar A, Wissbrock A, Goradia N, Bellstedt P, Ramachandran R, Imhof D, Ohlenschlager O. Heme interaction of the intrinsically disordered N-terminal peptide segment of human cystathionine-beta-synthase. Sci Rep 2018;8:2474.

[13] Giuffre A, Vicente JB. Hydrogen sulfide biochemistry and interplay with other gaseous mediators in mammalian physiology. Oxid Med Cell Longev 2018;2018:6290931.

[14] Ida T, Sawa T, Ihara H, Tsuchiya Y, Watanabe Y, Kumagai Y, et al. Reactive cysteine persulfides and S-polythiolation regulate oxidative stress and redox signaling. Proc Natl Acad Sci USA 2014;111:7606−11.

[15] Teng H, Wu B, Zhao K, Yang G, Wu L, Wang R. Oxygen-sensitive mitochondrial accumulation of cystathionine beta-synthase mediated by Lon protease. Proc Natl Acad Sci U S A 2013;110:12679−84.

[16] Kabil O, Zhou Y, Banerjee R. Human cystathionine beta-synthase is a target for sumoylation. Biochemistry 2006;45:13528−36.

[17] Enokido Y, Suzuki E, Iwasawa K, Namekata K, Okazawa H, Kimura H. Cystathionine beta-synthase, a key enzyme for homocysteine metabolism, is preferentially expressed in the radial glia/astrocyte lineage of developing mouse CNS. FASEB J 2005;19:1854−6.

[18] Bao L, Vlcek C, Paces V, Kraus JP. Identification and tissue distribution of human cystathionine beta-synthase mRNA isoforms. Arch Biochem Biophys 1998;350:95−103.

[19] Kabil O, Vitvitsky V, Xie P, Banerjee R. The quantitative significance of the transsulfuration enzymes for H_2S production in murine tissues. Antioxid Redox Signal 2011;15:363−72.

[20] Wang R. Physiological implications of hydrogen sulfide: a whiff exploration that blossomed. Physiol Rev 2012;92:791−896.

[21] Bearden SE, Beard Jr RS, Pfau JC. Extracellular transsulfuration generates hydrogen sulfide from homocysteine and protects endothelium from redox stress. Am J Physiol Heart Circ Physiol 2010;299:H1568−76.

[22] Alcaide P, Krijt J, Ruiz-Sala P, Jesina P, Ugarte M, Kozich V, Merinero B. Enzymatic diagnosis of homocystinuria by determination of cystathionine-ss-synthase activity in plasma using LC-MS/MS. Clin Chim Acta 2015;438:261–5.
[23] Krijt J, Kopecka J, Hnizda A, Moat S, Kluijtmans LA, Mayne P, Kozich V. Determination of cystathionine beta-synthase activity in human plasma by LC-MS/MS: potential use in diagnosis of CBS deficiency. J Inherit Metab Dis 2011;34:49–55.
[24] Pedre B, Dick TP. 3-Mercaptopyruvate sulfurtransferase: an enzyme at the crossroads of sulfane sulfur trafficking. Biol Chem 2021;402:223–37.
[25] Hipolito A, Nunes SC, Vicente JB, Serpa J. Cysteine aminotransferase (CAT): a pivotal sponsor in metabolic remodeling and an ally of 3-mercaptopyruvate sulfurtransferase (MST) in cancer. Molecules 2020;25:3984.
[26] Shibuya N, Koike S, Tanaka M, Ishigami-Yuasa M, Kimura Y, Ogasawara Y, et al. A novel pathway for the production of hydrogen sulfide from D-cysteine in mammalian cells. Nat Commun 2013;4:1366.
[27] Frasdorf B, Radon C, Leimkuhler S. Characterization and interaction studies of two isoforms of the dual localized 3-mercaptopyruvate sulfurtransferase TUM1 from humans. J Biol Chem 2014;289:34543–56.
[28] Modis K, Coletta C, Erdelyi K, Papapetropoulos A, Szabo C. Intramitochondrial hydrogen sulfide production by 3-mercaptopyruvate sulfurtransferase maintains mitochondrial electron flow and supports cellular bioenergetics. FASEB J 2013;27:601–11.
[29] Nagahara N, Ito T, Kitamura H, Nishino T. Tissue and subcellular distribution of mercaptopyruvate sulfurtransferase in the rat: confocal laser fluorescence and immunoelectron microscopic studies combined with biochemical analysis. Histochem Cell Biol 1998;110:243–50.
[30] Tomita M, Nagahara N, Ito T. Expression of 3-mercaptopyruvate sulfurtransferase in the mouse. Molecules 2016;21:1707.
[31] Philipp TM, Will A, Richter H, Winterhalter PR, Pohnert G, Steinbrenner H, Klotz LO. A coupled enzyme assay for detection of selenium-binding protein 1 (SELENBP1) methanethiol oxidase (MTO) activity in mature enterocytes. Redox Biol 2021;43:101972.
[32] Pol A, Renkema GH, Tangerman A, Winkel EG, Engelke UF, de Brouwer APM, et al. Mutations in SELENBP1, encoding a novel human methanethiol oxidase, cause extraoral halitosis. Nat Genet 2018;50:120–9.
[33] Raucci R, Colonna G, Guerriero E, Capone F, Accardo M, Castello G, Costantini S. Structural and functional studies of the human selenium binding protein-1 and its involvement in hepatocellular carcinoma. Biochim Biophys Acta 2011;1814:513–22.
[34] Steinbrenner H, Micoogullari M, Hoang NA, Bergheim I, Klotz LO, Sies H. Selenium-binding protein 1 (SELENBP1) is a marker of mature adipocytes. Redox Biol 2019;20:489–95.
[35] Libiad M, Vitvitsky V, Bostelaar T, Bak DW, Lee HJ, Sakamoto N, et al. Hydrogen sulfide perturbs mitochondrial bioenergetics and triggers metabolic reprogramming in colon cells. J Biol Chem 2019;294:12077–90.
[36] Libiad M, Yadav PK, Vitvitsky V, Martinov M, Banerjee R. Organization of the human mitochondrial hydrogen sulfide oxidation pathway. J Biol Chem 2014;289:30901–10.
[37] Zuhra K, Tome CS, Forte E, Vicente JB, Giuffre A. The multifaceted roles of sulfane sulfur species in cancer-associated processes. Biochim Biophys Acta Bioenerg 2021;1862:148338.
[38] Hildebrandt TM, Grieshaber MK. Three enzymatic activities catalyze the oxidation of sulfide to thiosulfate in mammalian and invertebrate mitochondria. FEBS J 2008;275:3352–61.
[39] Malagrino F, Zuhra K, Mascolo L, Mastronicola D, Vicente JB, Forte E, Giuffre A. Hydrogen sulfide oxidation: adaptive changes in mitochondria of SW480 colorectal cancer cells upon exposure to hypoxia. Oxid Med Cell Longev 2019;2019:8102936.
[40] Landry AP, Moon S, Bonanata J, Cho US, Coitino EL, Banerjee R. Dismantling and rebuilding the trisulfide cofactor demonstrates its essential role in human sulfide quinone oxidoreductase. J Am Chem Soc 2020;142:14295–306.
[41] Landry AP, Moon S, Kim H, Yadav PK, Guha A, Cho US, Banerjee R. A catalytic trisulfide in human sulfide quinone oxidoreductase catalyzes coenzyme A persulfide synthesis and inhibits butyrate oxidation. Cell Chem Biol 2019;26:1515–1525.e1514.
[42] Jackson MR, Melideo SL, Jorns MS. Human sulfide:quinone oxidoreductase catalyzes the first step in hydrogen sulfide metabolism and produces a sulfane sulfur metabolite. Biochemistry 2012;51:6804–15.
[43] Landry AP, Ballou DP, Banerjee R. H_2S oxidation by nanodisc-embedded human sulfide quinone oxidoreductase. J Biol Chem 2017;292:11641–9.
[44] Pettinati I, Brem J, McDonough MA, Schofield CJ. Crystal structure of human persulfide dioxygenase: structural basis of ethylmalonic encephalopathy. Hum Mol Genet 2015;24:2458–69.
[45] Johnson-Winters K, Tollin G, Enemark JH. Elucidating the catalytic mechanism of sulfite oxidizing enzymes using structural, spectroscopic, and kinetic analyses. Biochemistry 2010;49:7242–54.
[46] Goubern M, Andriamihaja M, Nubel T, Blachier F, Bouillaud F. Sulfide, the first inorganic substrate for human cells. FASEB J 2007;21:1699–706.
[47] Abou-Hamdan A, Guedouari-Bounihi H, Lenoir V, Andriamihaja M, Blachier F, Bouillaud F. Oxidation of H_2S in mammalian cells and mitochondria. Methods Enzymol 2015;554:201–28.
[48] Modis K, Ju Y, Ahmad A, Untereiner AA, Altaany Z, Wu L, et al. S-Sulfhydration of ATP synthase by hydrogen sulfide stimulates mitochondrial bioenergetics. Pharmacol Res 2016;113:116–24.
[49] Olson KR, Gao Y, Arif F, Arora K, Patel S, DeLeon ER, et al. Metabolism of hydrogen sulfide (H_2S) and production of reactive sulfur species (RSS) by superoxide dismutase. Redox Biol 2018;15:74–85.
[50] Olson KR, Clear KJ, Derry PJ, Gao Y, Ma Z, Wu G, et al. Coenzyme Q10 and related quinones oxidize H_2S to polysulfides and thiosulfate. Free Radic Biol Med 2022;182:119–31.
[51] Scheller AS, Philipp TM, Klotz LO, Steinbrenner H. Altered capacity for H_2S production during the spontaneous differentiation of Caco-2 cells to colonocytes due to reciprocal regulation of CBS and SELENBP1. Antioxidants (Basel) 2022;11:1957.
[52] Bonifacio VDB, Pereira SA, Serpa J, Vicente JB. Cysteine metabolic circuitries: druggable targets in cancer. Br J Cancer 2021;124:862–79.
[53] Kimura H. Hydrogen polysulfide (H_2S_n) signaling along with hydrogen sulfide (H_2S) and nitric oxide (NO). J Neural Transm (Vienna) 2016;123:1235–45.
[54] Paul BD, Snyder SH. H_2S: a novel gasotransmitter that signals by sulfhydration. Trends Biochem Sci 2015;40:687–700.

[55] Paul BD, Snyder SH. Protein sulfhydration. Methods Enzymol 2015;555:79–90.

[56] Millikin R, Bianco CL, White C, Saund SS, Henriquez S, Sosa V, et al. The chemical biology of protein hydropersulfides: studies of a possible protective function of biological hydropersulfide generation. Free Radic Biol Med 2016;97:136–47.

[57] Cuevasanta E, Moller MN, Alvarez B. Biological chemistry of hydrogen sulfide and persulfides. Arch Biochem Biophys 2017;617:9–25.

[58] Das TN, Huie RE, Neta P, Padmaja S. Reduction potential of the sulfhydryl radical: pulse radiolysis and laser flash photolysis studies of the formation and reactions of center dot SH and $HSSH^{\bullet -}$ in aqueous solutions. J Phys Chem A 1999;103:5221–6.

[59] Cuevasanta E, Lange M, Bonanata J, Coitino EL, Ferrer-Sueta G, Filipovic MR, Alvarez B. Reaction of hydrogen sulfide with disulfide and sulfenic acid to form the strongly nucleophilic persulfide. J Biol Chem 2015;290:26866–80.

[60] Akaike T, Ida T, Wei FY, Nishida M, Kumagai Y, Alam MM, et al. Cysteinyl-tRNA synthetase governs cysteine polysulfidation and mitochondrial bioenergetics. Nat Commun 2017;8:1177.

[61] Paul BD, Snyder SH. H_2S signalling through protein sulfhydration and beyond. Nat Rev Mol Cell Biol 2012;13:499–507.

[62] Filipovic MR, Zivanovic J, Alvarez B, Banerjee R. Chemical biology of H_2S signaling through persulfidation. Chem Rev 2018;118:1253–337.

[63] Mustafa AK, Gadalla MM, Sen N, Kim S, Mu W, Gazi SK, et al. H_2S signals through protein S-sulfhydration. Sci Signal 2009;2:ra72.

[64] Krishnan N, Fu C, Pappin DJ, Tonks NK. H_2S-induced sulfhydration of the phosphatase PTP1B and its role in the endoplasmic reticulum stress response. Sci Signal 2011;4:ra86.

[65] Sen N, Paul BD, Gadalla MM, Mustafa AK, Sen T, Xu R, et al. Hydrogen sulfide-linked sulfhydration of NF-kappaB mediates its antiapoptotic actions. Mol Cell 2012;45:13–24.

[66] Mustafa AK, Sikka G, Gazi SK, Steppan J, Jung SM, Bhunia AK, et al. Hydrogen sulfide as endothelium-derived hyperpolarizing factor sulfhydrates potassium channels. Circ Res 2011;109:1259–68.

[67] Bianco CL, Toscano JP, Fukuto JM. Chapter 2—an integrated view of the chemical biology of NO, CO, H_2S, and O_2 A2—Ignarro, Louis J. In: Freeman BA, editor. Nitric oxide. 3rd ed. Academic Press; 2017. p. 9–21.

[68] Vitvitsky V, Yadav PK, An S, Seravalli J, Cho US, Banerjee R. Structural and mechanistic insights into hemoglobin-catalyzed hydrogen sulfide oxidation and the fate of polysulfide products. J Biol Chem 2017;292:5584–92.

[69] Vitvitsky V, Yadav PK, Kurthen A, Banerjee R. Sulfide oxidation by a noncanonical pathway in red blood cells generates thiosulfate and polysulfides. J Biol Chem 2015;290:8310–20.

[70] Nicholls P, Marshall DC, Cooper CE, Wilson MT. Sulfide inhibition of and metabolism by cytochrome c oxidase. Biochem Soc Trans 2013;41:1312–6.

[71] Petersen LC. The effect of inhibitors on the oxygen kinetics of cytochrome c oxidase. Biochim Biophys Acta 1977;460:299–307.

[72] Borisov VB, Siletsky SA, Paiardini A, Hoogewijs D, Forte E, Giuffre A, Poole RK. Bacterial oxidases of the cytochrome bd family: redox enzymes of unique structure, function, and utility as drug targets. Antioxid Redox Signal 2021;34:1280–318.

[73] Forte E, Borisov VB, Falabella M, Colaco HG, Tinajero-Trejo M, Poole RK, et al. The terminal oxidase cytochrome bd promotes sulfide-resistant bacterial respiration and growth. Sci Rep 2016;6:23788.

[74] Rahman MA, Cumming BM, Addicott KW, Pacl HT, Russell SL, Nargan K, et al. Hydrogen sulfide dysregulates the immune response by suppressing central carbon metabolism to promote tuberculosis. Proc Natl Acad Sci USA 2020;117:6663–74.

[75] Rahman MA, Glasgow JN, Nadeem S, Reddy VP, Sevalkar RR, Lancaster Jr JR, Steyn AJC. The role of host-generated H_2S in microbial pathogenesis: new perspectives on tuberculosis. Front Cell Infect Microbiol 2020;10:586923.

[76] Cirino G, Szabo C, Papapetropoulos A. Physiological roles of hydrogen sulfide in mammalian cells, tissues and organs. Physiol Rev 2022 (online ahead of print).

[77] Szabo C. Hydrogen sulphide and its therapeutic potential. Nat Rev Drug Discov 2007;6:917–35.

[78] Wallace JL, Wang R. Hydrogen sulfide-based therapeutics: exploiting a unique but ubiquitous gasotransmitter. Nat Rev Drug Discov 2015;14:329–45.

[79] Nagy P, Palinkas Z, Nagy A, Budai B, Toth I, Vasas A. Chemical aspects of hydrogen sulfide measurements in physiological samples. Biochim Biophys Acta 2014;1840:876–91.

[80] Carballal S, Trujillo M, Cuevasanta E, Bartesaghi S, Moller MN, Folkes LK, et al. Reactivity of hydrogen sulfide with peroxynitrite and other oxidants of biological interest. Free Radic Biol Med 2011;50:196–205.

[81] Benchoam D, Cuevasanta E, Moller MN, Alvarez B. Persulfides, at the crossroads between hydrogen sulfide and thiols. Essays Biochem 2020;64:155–68.

[82] Ono K, Akaike T, Sawa T, Kumagai Y, Wink DA, Tantillo DJ, et al. Redox chemistry and chemical biology of H_2S, hydropersulfides, and derived species: implications of their possible biological activity and utility. Free Radic Biol Med 2014;77:82–94.

[83] Petrovic D, Kouroussis E, Vignane T, Filipovic MR. The role of protein persulfidation in brain aging and neurodegeneration. Front Aging Neurosci 2021;13:674135.

[84] Zivanovic J, Kouroussis E, Kohl JB, Adhikari B, Bursac B, Schott-Roux S, et al. Selective persulfide detection reveals evolutionarily conserved antiaging effects of S-sulfhydration. Cell Metab 2020;31:207.

[85] Paulsen CE, Carroll KS. Cysteine-mediated redox signaling: chemistry, biology, and tools for discovery. Chem Rev 2013;113:4633–79.

[86] Doka E, Pader I, Biro A, Johansson K, Cheng Q, Ballago K, et al. A novel persulfide detection method reveals protein persulfide- and polysulfide-reducing functions of thioredoxin and glutathione systems. Sci Adv 2016;2. e1500968.

[87] Cuadrado A, Rojo AI, Wells G, Hayes JD, Cousin SP, Rumsey WL, et al. Therapeutic targeting of the NRF2 and KEAP1 partnership in chronic diseases. Nat Rev Drug Discov 2019;18:295–317.

[88] Kolluru GK, Shackelford RE, Shen X, Dominic P, Kevil CG. Sulfide regulation of cardiovascular function in health and disease. Nat Rev Cardiol 2022.

[89] Giovinazzo D, Bursac B, Sbodio JI, Nalluru S, Vignane T, Snowman AM, et al. Hydrogen sulfide is neuroprotective in

Alzheimer's disease by sulfhydrating GSK3beta and inhibiting Tau hyperphosphorylation. Proc Natl Acad Sci USA 2021;118. e2017225118.

[90] Paul BD, Sbodio JI, Xu R, Vandiver MS, Cha JY, Snowman AM, Snyder SH. Cystathionine gamma-lyase deficiency mediates neurodegeneration in Huntington's disease. Nature 2014;509:96–100.

[91] Bibli SI, Hu J, Looso M, Weigert A, Ratiu C, Wittig J, et al. Mapping the endothelial cell S-sulfhydrome highlights the crucial role of integrin sulfhydration in vascular function. Circulation 2021;143:935–48.

[92] Katsouda A, Valakos D, Dionellis VS, Bibli SI, Akoumianakis I, Karaliota S, et al. MPST sulfurtransferase maintains mitochondrial protein import and cellular bioenergetics to attenuate obesity. J Exp Med 2022;219. e20211894.

[93] Ascencao K, Szabo C. Emerging roles of cystathionine beta-synthase in various forms of cancer. Redox Biol 2022;53:102331.

[94] Szabo C. The re-emerging pathophysiological role of the cystathionine-beta-synthase—hydrogen sulfide system in Down syndrome. FEBS J 2020;287:3150–60.

[95] Panagaki T, Randi EB, Augsburger F, Szabo C. Overproduction of H2S, generated by CBS, inhibits mitochondrial Complex IV and suppresses oxidative phosphorylation in Down syndrome. Proc Natl Acad Sci USA 2019;116:18769–71.

[96] Marechal D, Brault V, Leon A, Martin D, Lopes Pereira P, Loaec N, et al. Cbs overdosage is necessary and sufficient to induce cognitive phenotypes in mouse models of Down syndrome and interacts genetically with Dyrk1a. Hum Mol Genet 2019;28:1561–77.

[97] Zhang S, Li F, Younes M, Liu H, Chen C, Yao Q. Reduced selenium-binding protein 1 in breast cancer correlates with poor survival and resistance to the anti-proliferative effects of selenium. PLoS One 2013;8:e63702.

[98] Szabo C. Roles of hydrogen sulfide in the pathogenesis of diabetes mellitus and its complications. Antioxid Redox Signal 2012;17:68–80.

[99] Zuhra K, Augsburger F, Majtan T, Szabo C. Cystathionine-beta-Synthase: molecular regulation and pharmacological inhibition. Biomolecules 2020;10:697.

[100] Janosik M, Kery V, Gaustadnes M, Maclean KN, Kraus JP. Regulation of human cystathionine beta-synthase by S-adenosyl-L-methionine: evidence for two catalytically active conformations involving an autoinhibitory domain in the C-terminal region. Biochemistry 2001;40:10625–33.

[101] Mendes MI, Colaco HG, Smith DE, Ramos RJ, Pop A, van Dooren SJ, et al. Reduced response of cystathionine beta-synthase (CBS) to S-adenosylmethionine (SAM): identification and functional analysis of CBS gene mutations in homocystinuria patients. J Inherit Metab Dis 2014;37:245–54.

[102] Agrawal N, Banerjee R. Human polycomb 2 protein is a SUMO E3 ligase and alleviates substrate-induced inhibition of cystathionine beta-synthase sumoylation. PLoS One 2008;3:e4032.

[103] d'Emmanuele di Villa Bianca R, Mitidieri E, Fusco F, Russo A, Pagliara V, Tramontano T, et al. Urothelium muscarinic activation phosphorylates CBS(Ser227) via cGMP/PKG pathway causing human bladder relaxation through H_2S production. Sci Rep 2016;6:31491.

[104] Mosharov E, Cranford MR, Banerjee R. The quantitatively important relationship between homocysteine metabolism and glutathione synthesis by the transsulfuration pathway and its regulation by redox changes. Biochemistry 2000;39:13005–11.

[105] Niu WN, Yadav PK, Adamec J, Banerjee R. S-glutathionylation enhances human cystathionine beta-synthase activity under oxidative stress conditions. Antioxid Redox Signal 2015;22:350–61.

[106] Eto K, Kimura H. A novel enhancing mechanism for hydrogen sulfide-producing activity of cystathionine beta-synthase. J Biol Chem 2002;277:42680–5.

[107] Celano L, Gil M, Carballal S, Duran R, Denicola A, Banerjee R, Alvarez B. Inactivation of cystathionine beta-synthase with peroxynitrite. Arch Biochem Biophys 2009;491:96–105.

[108] Taoka S, Ohja S, Shan X, Kruger WD, Banerjee R. Evidence for heme-mediated redox regulation of human cystathionine beta-synthase activity. J Biol Chem 1998;273:25179–84.

[109] Taoka S, West M, Banerjee R. Characterization of the heme and pyridoxal phosphate cofactors of human cystathionine beta-synthase reveals nonequivalent active sites. Biochemistry 1999;38:7406.

[110] Cherney MM, Pazicni S, Frank N, Marvin KA, Kraus JP, Burstyn JN. Ferrous human cystathionine beta-synthase loses activity during enzyme assay due to a ligand switch process. Biochemistry 2007;46:13199–210.

[111] Pazicni S, Cherney MM, Lukat-Rodgers GS, Oliveriusova J, Rodgers KR, Kraus JP, Burstyn JN. The heme of cystathionine beta-synthase likely undergoes a thermally induced redox-mediated ligand switch. Biochemistry 2005;44:16785–95.

[112] Singh S, Madzelan P, Stasser J, Weeks CL, Becker D, Spiro TG, et al. Modulation of the heme electronic structure and cystathionine beta-synthase activity by second coordination sphere ligands: the role of heme ligand switching in redox regulation. J Inorg Biochem 2009;103:689–97.

[113] Kabil O, Weeks CL, Carballal S, Gherasim C, Alvarez B, Spiro TG, Banerjee R. Reversible heme-dependent regulation of human cystathionine beta-synthase by a flavoprotein oxidoreductase. Biochemistry 2011;50:8261–3.

[114] Carballal S, Cuevasanta E, Marmisolle I, Kabil O, Gherasim C, Ballou DP, et al. Kinetics of reversible reductive carbonylation of heme in human cystathionine beta-synthase. Biochemistry 2013;52:4553–62.

[115] Carballal S, Madzelan P, Zinola CF, Grana M, Radi R, Banerjee R, Alvarez B. Dioxygen reactivity and heme redox potential of truncated human cystathionine beta-synthase. Biochemistry 2008;47:3194–201.

[116] Vicente JB, Colaco HG, Mendes MI, Sarti P, Leandro P, Giuffre A. NO* binds human cystathionine beta-synthase quickly and tightly. J Biol Chem 2014;289:8579–87.

[117] Vicente JB, Colaco HG, Sarti P, Leandro P, Giuffre A. S-Adenosyl-l-methionine modulates CO and NO* binding to the human H_2S-generating enzyme cystathionine beta-synthase. J Biol Chem 2016;291:572–81.

[118] Weeks CL, Singh S, Madzelan P, Banerjee R, Spiro TG. Heme regulation of human cystathionine beta-synthase activity: insights from fluorescence and Raman spectroscopy. J Am Chem Soc 2009;131:12809–16.

[119] Singh S, Banerjee R. PLP-dependent H_2S biogenesis. Biochim Biophys Acta 2011;1814:1518–27.

[120] Taoka S, Banerjee R. Characterization of NO binding to human cystathionine beta-synthase: possible implications of the effects of

CO and NO binding to the human enzyme. J Inorg Biochem 2001;87:245–51.

[121] Vicente JB, Malagrino F, Arese M, Forte E, Sarti P, Giuffre A. Bioenergetic relevance of hydrogen sulfide and the interplay between gasotransmitters at human cystathionine beta-synthase. Biochim Biophys Acta 2016;1857:1127–38.

[122] Sun Q, Collins R, Huang S, Holmberg-Schiavone L, Anand GS, Tan CH, et al. Structural basis for the inhibition mechanism of human cystathionine gamma-lyase, an enzyme responsible for the production of H_2S. J Biol Chem 2009;284:3076–85.

[123] Yadav PK, Vitvitsky V, Kim H, White A, Cho US, Banerjee R. S-3-carboxypropyl-l-cysteine specifically inhibits cystathionine gamma-lyase-dependent hydrogen sulfide synthesis. J Biol Chem 2019;294:11011–22.

[124] Luo C, Ji D, Li Y, Cao Y, Zhang S, Yan W, et al. Abnormal nitration and S-sulfhydration modification of Sp1-CSE-H_2S pathway trap the progress of hyperhomocysteinemia into a vicious cycle. Free Radic Biol Med 2021;164:20–33.

[125] Fernandes DGF, Nunes J, Tome CS, Zuhra K, Costa JMF, Antunes AMM, et al. Human cystathionine gamma-lyase is inhibited by s-nitrosation: a new crosstalk mechanism between NO and H_2S. Antioxidants (Basel) 2021;10:1391.

[126] Wang J, Jia G, Li H, Yan S, Qian J, Guo X, et al. H_2O_2-mediated oxidative stress enhances cystathionine gamma-lyase-derived H_2S synthesis via a sulfenic acid intermediate. Antioxidants (Basel) 2021;10:1488.

[127] Bibli SI, Hu J, Sigala F, Wittig I, Heidler J, Zukunft S, et al. Cystathionine gamma lyase sulfhydrates the RNA binding protein human antigen R to preserve endothelial cell function and delay atherogenesis. Circulation 2019;139:101–14.

[128] Bian Y, Song C, Cheng K, Dong M, Wang F, Huang J, et al. An enzyme assisted RP-RPLC approach for in-depth analysis of human liver phosphoproteome. J Proteom 2014;96:253–62.

[129] Nagahara N, Katayama A. Post-translational regulation of mercaptopyruvate sulfurtransferase via a low redox potential cysteine-sulfenate in the maintenance of redox homeostasis. J Biol Chem 2005;280:34569–76.

[130] Modis K, Asimakopoulou A, Coletta C, Papapetropoulos A, Szabo C. Oxidative stress suppresses the cellular bioenergetic effect of the 3-mercaptopyruvate sulfurtransferase/hydrogen sulfide pathway. Biochem Biophys Res Commun 2013;433:401–7.

[131] Ishida YI, Kayama T, Kibune Y, Nishimoto S, Koike S, Suzuki T, et al. Identification of an argpyrimidine-modified protein in human red blood cells from schizophrenic patients: a possible biomarker for diseases involving carbonyl stress. Biochem Biophys Res Commun 2017;493:573–7.

[132] Ying Q, Ansong E, Diamond AM, Yang W. A critical role for cysteine 57 in the biological functions of selenium binding protein-1. Int J Mol Sci 2015;16:27599–608.

[133] Jung M, Kasamatsu S, Matsunaga T, Akashi S, Ono K, Nishimura A, et al. Protein polysulfidation-dependent persulfide dioxygenase activity of ethylmalonic encephalopathy protein 1. Biochem Biophys Res Commun 2016;480:180–6.

[134] Choudhary C, Kumar C, Gnad F, Nielsen ML, Rehman M, Walther TC, et al. Lysine acetylation targets protein complexes and co-regulates major cellular functions. Science 2009;325:834–40.

[135] Rardin MJ, Newman JC, Held JM, Cusack MP, Sorensen DJ, Li B, et al. Label-free quantitative proteomics of the lysine acetylome in mitochondria identifies substrates of SIRT3 in metabolic pathways. Proc Natl Acad Sci USA 2013;110:6601–6.

[136] Park J, Chen Y, Tishkoff DX, Peng C, Tan M, Dai L, et al. SIRT5-mediated lysine desuccinylation impacts diverse metabolic pathways. Mol Cell 2013;50:919–30.

[137] Lundby A, Secher A, Lage K, Nordsborg NB, Dmytriyev A, Lundby C, Olsen JV. Quantitative maps of protein phosphorylation sites across 14 different rat organs and tissues. Nat Commun 2012;3:876.

[138] Pacher P. Cyanide emerges as an endogenous mammalian gasotransmitter. Proc Natl Acad Sci USA 2021;118. e2108040118.

[139] Zuhra K, Szabo C. The two faces of cyanide: an environmental toxin and a potential novel mammalian gasotransmitter. FEBS J 2022;289:2481–515.

[140] Randi EB, Zuhra K, Pecze L, Panagaki T, Szabo C. Physiological concentrations of cyanide stimulate mitochondrial Complex IV and enhance cellular bioenergetics. Proc Natl Acad Sci USA 2021;118. e2026245118.

[141] Cortese-Krott MM, Kuhnle GG, Dyson A, Fernandez BO, Grman M, DuMond JF, et al. Key bioactive reaction products of the NO/H_2S interaction are S/N-hybrid species, polysulfides, and nitroxyl. Proc Natl Acad Sci USA 2015;112:E4651–60.

[142] Cortese-Krott MM, Koning A, Kuhnle GGC, Nagy P, Bianco CL, Pasch A, et al. The reactive species interactome: evolutionary emergence, biological significance, and opportunities for redox metabolomics and personalized medicine. Antioxid Redox Signal 2017;27:684–712.

Chapter 12

Intestinal redox regulation and inflammatory bowel disease

Hideya Iwaki[1,2] and Hozumi Motohashi[2]

[1]*Department of Gastroenterology, Tohoku University Graduate School of Medicine, Sendai, Japan;* [2]*Department of Gene Expression Regulation, Institute of Development, Aging and Cancer, Tohoku University, Sendai, Japan*

Key takeaway

Inflammatory bowel disease (IBD), intestine, redox regulation, Keap1, Nrf2, ferroptosis.

Introduction

Intestinal epithelial cells (IECs) reside in a unique environment in terms of redox status. Due to the suboxic and anoxic conditions of the intestinal lumen and the supply of oxygenated blood from submucosal vessels, IECs are regarded as being located at the anoxic−oxic interface. Under this unique condition, IECs are likely to be subjected to redox fluctuations (Fig. 12.1). In the normal intestine, optimal levels of reactive oxygen species (ROS) perform beneficial functions such as signal transduction for cell proliferation and differentiation and as a defense against intestinal pathogens.

Inflammatory bowel disease (IBD) refers to chronic relapsing autoimmune disorders of the gastrointestinal tract. Because its age of onset is relatively young, lifelong medical support is required for IBD patients. Although numerous studies have been conducted to try to cure IBD, many questions remain regarding the pathophysiological mechanisms causing IBD. The redox environment in the intestine is closely linked to the causes and prognoses of chronic inflammation in IBD. Considering that the efficacy

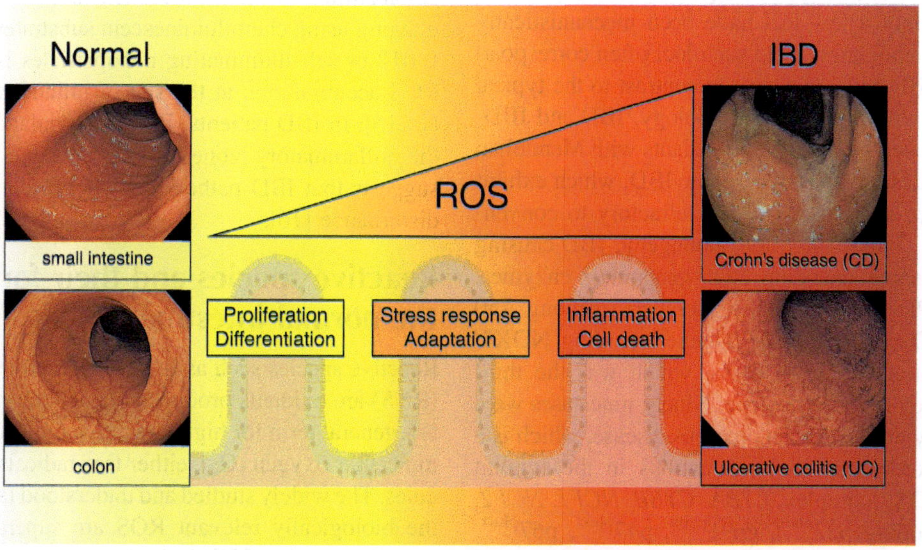

FIGURE 12.1 Different responses of the intestine to various levels of reactive oxygen species (ROS). IECs have their own optimal ROS levels under physiological conditions. Under normal unstressed conditions, IECs, including intestinal stem cells, are in a state of proliferation and differentiation. An appropriate level of ROS is needed for activation of the Wnt and Notch signaling pathways. In the chronic inflammatory milieu, increased ROS causes cell death, and in turn, intracellular molecules released from injured tissues (damage-associated molecular patterns (DAMPs)) further exacerbate inflammation. The four images are endoscopic images of the small intestine and colon: the left images show the small intestine and colon in the healthy status, whereas the right images are from CD patients with longitudinal ulcers and UC patients showing spontaneous bleeding and ulceration.

Modulation of Oxidative Stress. https://doi.org/10.1016/B978-0-443-19247-0.00015-1

of currently available therapeutic drugs for IBD is not entirely satisfactory, the development of new therapeutics is awaited, for which pharmaceutical intervention with redox regulators may be a promising approach.

Pathophysiology of IBD and its relation to redox disturbance

IBD refers to chronic relapsing autoimmune disorders of the gastrointestinal tract and is categorized into two major classes, ulcerative colitis (UC) and Crohn's disease (CD). In UC patients, ulcerations occur mainly on the mucosal surface of the colon, whereas in CD patients, longitudinal ulcerations occur mainly in the small intestine and occasionally in the colon. The peak age for UC onset is 30–40 years and for CD onset, is 20–30 years [1]. Furthermore, after the onset of the disease, patients require lifelong medical support, regular check-ups (blood tests, imaging, endoscopies, etc.) and treatment according to their current inflammatory status [2,3]. IBD is a disease of increasing global concern as the IBD incidence is on the rise worldwide [4]. In Europe, the United States, and Australia, the incidence has risen and currently reached a plateau as high as 0.3%. In Africa, Asia, and South America, the morbidity and prevalence are still lower than those in Western countries, but a rapid rise in IBD incidence is continuing.

IBD is considered a multifactorial disease caused by a complex interaction of genetic factors, the immune system, intestinal bacterial flora, and environmental factors. Genetic polymorphisms in more than 250 genetic loci have been found to be associated with a high risk of IBD [5,6]. Among them, only a few loci have been mechanistically linked to IBD pathogenesis, and such loci often correspond to monogenic IBD-causing genes. In contrast to the typical idiopathic IBD with multifactorial etiology, IBD and IBD-like diseases caused by monogenic variants with Mendelian inheritance are described as monogenic IBD, which exhibit especially severe symptoms and are refractory to conventional therapies. Importantly, the monogenic IBD-causing genes include some encoding ROS-generating enzymes, namely, NADPH oxidase family members. Among 750 monogenic IBD cases, the *CYBB* gene encoding NOX2/gp91^{phox} was mutated in 68 cases, which was the third highest frequency for a single gene. Ninety-nine cases were accompanied by chronic granulomatous disease, which is a monogenic disorder caused by mutations in the subunit genes of the NOX2 complex, *CYBA, CYBB, NCF1, NCF2*, and *NCF4* encoding p22^{phox}, gp91^{phox}, p47^{phox}, p67^{phox}, and p40^{phox}, respectively, and is the second most common background disorder of monogenic IBD [7]. NOX1 and dual oxidase 2 (DUOX2) missense mutations are reported in patients with VEO-IBD (very-early-onset IBD), which is a distinct subset of pediatric CD characterized by disease onset under 6 years of age [8]. All of these mutations attenuate their enzymatic activities, leading to a reduction in ROS production, which causes the functional impairment of the protective function by neutrophils and IECs (Fig. 12.2).

Environmental factors also have profound influences on IBD pathology, especially idiopathic IBD with multifactorial etiology. A wide variety of environmental factors have been proposed as causes and prerequisites of IBD, including smoking, dietary habits, lifestyle, and air pollution [9]. A retrospective cohort study showed a positive correlation between exposure to oxidants in childhood and the development of IBD [10]. Redox disturbance caused by environmental factors is likely to play significant roles in the pathogenesis of IBD.

Several mouse models could help in understanding the pathogenesis of IBD and assist in the design of novel therapeutic concepts. The dextran sulfate sodium (DSS) colitis model is a simple and convenient chemical colitis model in which 1%–5% DSS is dissolved in the mouse's drinking water [11]. DSS is a water-soluble, negatively charged sulfated polysaccharide with a highly variable molecular weight ranging from 5 to 1400 kDa. DSS destroys the intestinal barrier function and induces an immune response and cytokine production, which results in mucosal erosion and crypt abscesses similar to UC [12].

The 2,4,6-trinitrobenzene sulfonic acid (TNBS) colitis model induces colitis by intrarectal injection of TNBS and ethanol, which act as a hapten to disrupt the intestinal barrier [13]. Administration of TNBS colitis results in the appearance of cobblestone-like ulcerations in the distal colon similar to CD. In these chemical colitis models, ROS imaging using chemiluminescent substrates such as luminol L-012 or self-illuminating nanoparticles is performed, and ROS accumulation at the site of inflammation is observed [14,15]. In IBD patients, ROS accumulation is observed in the inflammatory zone of the intestine, which strongly suggests that IBD pathogenesis is closely related to redox disturbance [16].

Reactive species and their formation in the normal intestine

Reactive species such as ROS and reactive nitrogen species (RNS) are oxidants produced via cellular metabolism. ROS is a general term for highly reactive molecules derived from molecular oxygen (O_2), either free radicals or neutral molecules. The widely studied and understood family members of the biologically relevant ROS are superoxide ($O_2^{\bullet-}$), hydroxyl radicals ($OH^{\bullet-}$), hydrogen peroxide (H_2O_2), and hypochlorous acid (HOCl) [17]. RNS includes nitric oxide (NO) and its derivatives, such as nitrosonium cation (NO^+), nitroxyl anion (NO^-), and peroxynitrite ($ONOO^-$) [18]. The intestinal levels of ROS and RNS are influenced by various

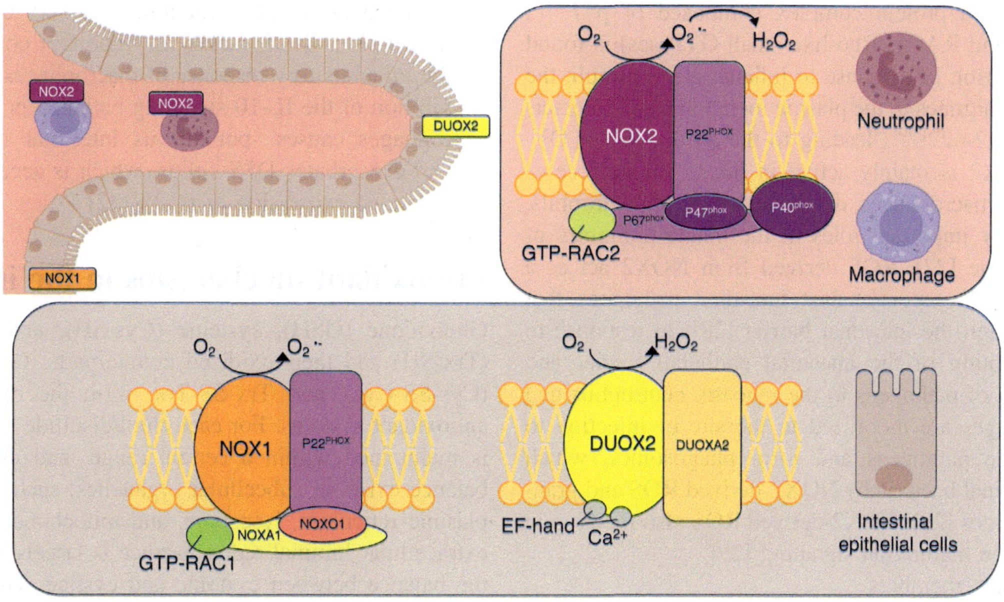

FIGURE 12.2 NADPH oxidase (NOX) family members strongly contribute to reactive oxygen species (ROS) generation in intestinal tissue. Innate immune cells express NOX2, which binds to $p22^{phox}$ and forms the NOX2 complex. The cytosolic subunits $p47^{phox}$, $p67^{phox}$, $p40^{phox}$ and RAC2, GTP-binding proteins, activate the NOX2 complex. Similarly, the NOX1-$p22^{phox}$ complex is activated by the subunits NOXO1, NOXA1 and RAC1 in IECs. DUOX2 forms a heterodimer with DUOXA2 and has two EF-hand motifs, which bind Ca^{2+} and activate this heterodimer.

factors and they regulate the proliferation, differentiation, and apoptosis of IECs. Under normal physiological conditions, ROS produced in the intestine activate the Wnt and Notch signaling pathways and prevent opportunistic infection by inducing innate immunity.

Intriguingly, sleep deprivation causes ROS accumulation in the intestine, leading to pathological consequences [19]. Sleep loss causes an increase in DNA damage and apoptosis in IECs in mice and flies and shortens the lifespan of flies. These detrimental effects of sleep loss are all rescued by overexpression of antioxidant enzymes in flies. The major sources of ROS and RNS in the intestine are NOX family members, nitric oxide synthase (NOS), and the mitochondrial electron transport chain [20]. In this review article, we focus on the former two.

1) NOX family members (Fig. 12.2)
NOX is a membrane protein with six transmembrane α-helices, consisting of the seven-member NOX family of NOX1-5 and DUOX1-2 [21]. NOX1-3 and NOX5 use NADPH as an electron donor for the extracellular generation of $O_2^{\cdot-}$ by one-electron reduction of O_2. $O_2^{\cdot-}$ is spontaneously converted to H_2O_2, and superoxide dismutase (SOD) promotes this conversion. NOX4 and DUOX1-2 directly extracellularly produce H_2O_2 by two-electron reduction of O_2. The produced H_2O_2 is taken up into the cell via aquaporin channels [22]. The major NOX family members contributing to intestinal physiology are NOX1 and DUOX2, which are mainly expressed in IECs, and NOX2, which is mainly expressed in innate immune cells.
NOX1 forms a heterodimer with $p22^{PHOX}$, which requires a regulatory protein complex composed of NOXO1, NOXA1, and RAC1 for enzymatic activation [21]. In situ hybridization analysis in mice shows that NOX1 is expressed in the lower two-thirds of crypts in the colon and that a similar expression pattern is observed in the small intestine but with less abundance [23]. In human tissues by in situ hybridization [24], NOX1 expression is low in the small intestine and high in the colon. Within the colon, NOX1 expression is higher in the left colon than in the right colon. The highest expression is observed in the colonic crypts, and its expression decreases incrementally from the crypts to the apex of the villus. NOX1 contributes to ROS accumulation during inflammation because the expression of intestinal epithelium NOX1 is increased by TNFα and IFN-γ [25,26].
DUOX2 forms a functionally stable heterodimer with DUOXA2, and the EF-hand of the N-terminal cytoplasmic region of DUOX2 is a Ca^{2+} binding motif that activates DUOX2 to produce H_2O_2 in a cellular Ca^{2+} concentration-dependent manner [21]. In the human intestine, the expression of DUOX2/DUOXA2 is detected in the whole intestine, especially in the cecum and colon epithelium.
NOX2 forms a heterodimer with $p22^{phox}$, which is located in the plasma membrane. Under unstressed

conditions, a protein complex composed of p47^{phox}, p67^{phox}, and RAC1 (Rho-like small GTPases) is found in the cytosol. In response to inflammatory stimuli, the complex migrates to the plasma membrane and interacts with NOX2-p22^{phox}, leading to the production of $O_2^{\bullet-}$ [21]. NOX2 is mainly active in innate immune cells, including macrophages, dendritic cells, and neutrophils, which play important roles in the innate immunity of the intestine [27]. ROS derived from NOX2 act as a bactericidal weapon against intestinal pathogens that pass through the intestinal barrier [28]. In response to the disruption of the intestinal epithelial barrier and migration of pathogens to the mucosa, neutrophils and macrophages are mobilized to the site of infection to engulf the pathogens and form phagosomes, which kill intestinal bacteria by NOX2-derived ROS and granular enzymes [28]. NOX2-derived ROS also function in phagosome maturation signaling [29]

2) NOS family members

NOS is a family of enzymes that catalyze the production of nitric oxide (NO) from L-arginine. The NOS family consists of NOS1 (neuronal NOS, nNOS), NOS2 (inducible NOS, iNOS), and eNOS (endothelial NOS, eNOS). NO and O_2 cause nitrosation stress and oxidative stress, both of which are mainly caused by iNOS induction in the inflammatory milieu [30]. Elevated expression of iNOS was detected by immunohistochemistry and semiquantification of mRNA expression in the inflamed intestinal epithelium of a DSS colitis mouse model [31]. iNOS makes an important contribution to the inflammatory response of macrophages. Genetic inhibition of the IL-10 signaling pathway in mouse macrophages causes spontaneous intestinal inflammation and exacerbates DSS colitis, which is accompanied by increased expression of iNOS [32]

Antioxidant mechanisms in the intestine

Glutathione (GSH), cysteine (Cys-SH), and thioredoxin (Trx-SH) and their oxidized counterparts, GSSG, cystine (Cys-SS-Cys), and Trx-SS-Trx, form the major cellular antioxidant systems. For each thiol/disulfide pair, the ratio is maintained within a certain range, and distinct redox balance exists in subcellular organelles, such as the endoplasmic reticulum, lysosome, and mitochondria [33]. The extracellular luminal redox balance is largely governed by the balance between cysteine and cystine. These thiol/disulfide balances are likely to reflect distinctive redox control nodes of metabolic processes and networks of enzymatic reactions. In IBD patients, the GSH/GSSG ratio of the intestinal mucosa decreases with increasing inflammation [34].

GSH is present abundantly in cells, as high as a millimolar order of concentration, as a biologically active reduced thiol, and it is synthesized through two ATP-requiring enzymatic steps in the cytosol (Fig. 12.3) [35].

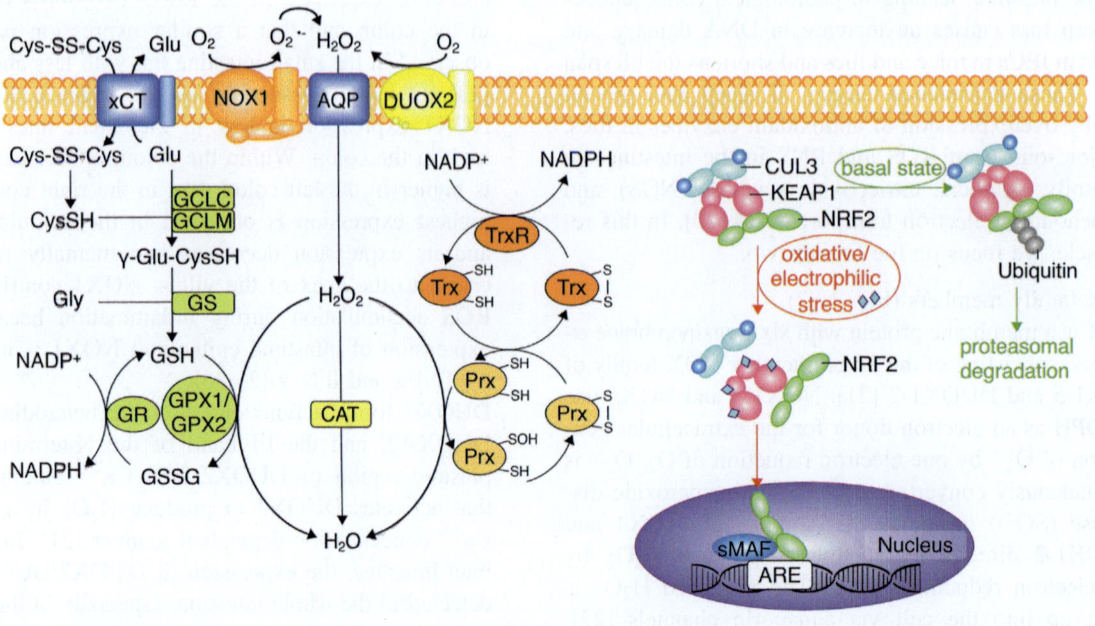

FIGURE 12.3 Glutathione and thioredoxin antioxidant system and KEAP1-NRF2 system. Glutathione and thioredoxin form two major antioxidant systems in cells. NRF2 directly regulates genes encoding xCT, GCLC, GCLM, GS, GPX2, GR, CAT, PRX1, TRX and TRXR. When cells are exposed to oxidative/electrophilic stress, NRF2 is stabilized and induces all of these genes, resulting in activation of the glutathione and thioredoxin antioxidant systems. AQP: aquaporin.

γ-Glutamylcysteine (γ-Glu-CysSH) is synthesized from glutamate and cysteine via glutamate cysteine ligase (GCL), which is the first step serving as a rate-limiting reaction of glutathione synthesis. The second step is the conjugation of γ-Glu-CysSH and glycine catalyzed by glutathione synthetase [36]. GCL consists of two subunits, a catalytic subunit encoded by the *GCLC* gene and a regulatory subunit encoded by the *GCLM* gene. GSH peroxidases (GPX) utilize GSH to quench reactive oxygen species, including hydrogen peroxide and lipid peroxides. The oxidized glutathione GSSG is reduced back to GSH by glutathione reductase (GR), which consumes NADPH. The major contributions of GPX1 and GPX2 were shown in an experiment using mouse genetics. Although disruption of *Gpx1* or *Gpx2* in mice does not result in apparent abnormalities, simultaneous disruption of Gpx1 and Gpx2 causes spontaneous colitis [37]. The intestinal mucosa of *Gpx1*:*Gpx2* double-deficient mice loses virtually all GSH-dependent ability to reduce hydrogen peroxide, resulting in ileocolitis [38].

For sufficient production of GSH, a sufficient supply of glutamate, cysteine, and glycine is needed. Among them, cysteine availability is rate-limiting because cysteine is less abundant than glutamate and glycine in plasma and cells. Major cysteine sources are cystine from the food, cysteine synthesis via transsulfuration from methionine, and cysteine recycling from GSH by γ-glutamyltranspeptidase (GGT), called the γ-glutamyl cycle [35]. In the γ-glutamyl cycle, extracellular GSH is degraded by GGT into γ-glutamyl amino acid and cysteinyl-glycine, and cysteinyl-glycine is further degraded into glycine and cysteine by dipeptidase. The released cysteine is taken up by cells via neutral amino acid transport systems, such as ASCT1, which is encoded by the *SLC1A4* gene, and ASCT2, which is encoded by *SLC1A5*. If the released cysteine is oxidized to cystine, cystine is taken up via a cystine-glutamate antiporter, which consists of xCT encoded by *SLC7A11* and CD98 encoded by *SLC3A2*, and it is reduced again to cysteine in the cytoplasm [39].

A glutamate supply is also necessary because it is an essential building block of GSH and because cystine is taken up in exchange for glutamate via xCT. Two major pathways for glutamate supply to IECs are glutamine deamination by glutaminase and uptake via glutamate transporters. Glutamate transporters are mostly expressed in neural tissues, but EAAT3 encoded by SLC1A1 is also found in the brush borders of the intestine [40].

The thioredoxin system is another important antioxidant system (Fig. 12.3) [41]. Thioredoxin reduces disulfide-bonded molecules, and the oxidized thioredoxin is converted back to the reduced form by thioredoxin reductase (TrxR), consuming NADPH. Peroxiredoxin (Prx) is one of the main targets of the Trx system. Prx quenches ROS and is recycled by the reduced form of Trx. In IECs, Trx, TrxR, and Prx are expressed in both the small intestine and colon [42]. Of note, transgenic mice overexpressing human Trx are resistant to DSS colitis, and administration of recombinant human Trx alleviates intestinal inflammation in mice. The effect of recombinant Trx was tested in DSS colitis model mice and IL-10-deficient mice with spontaneous colitis [43]. Based on these results, an elevation of serum Trx levels in IBD patients with active inflammation can be interpreted as an anti-inflammatory response.

In addition to these antioxidant systems, catalase and superoxide dismutases also contribute to reducing ROS levels. Catalase decomposes hydrogen peroxide to oxygen and water in intracellular peroxisomes. Catalase activity in peripheral leukocytes of CD patients is lower than that of healthy controls regardless of the inflammatory status of the patients [44]. In UC patients, genetic polymorphisms in the promoter region of the catalase gene have been reported [45]. In addition, microarray analysis showed that catalase expression is significantly decreased in the inflammatory mucosa of UC patients [46].

Gene regulation of antioxidant systems

The Kelch-like ECH-associated protein 1 (KEAP1)-NF-E2-related factor 2 (NFE2L2/NRF2)-system plays a central role in the defense mechanisms against redox disturbances (Fig. 12.3) [47]. NRF2 is a potent transcriptional activator, and it regulates a battery of genes whose products are involved in antioxidant and detoxification functions. KEAP1 is a negative regulator of NRF2 by enhancing its ubiquitination and subsequent degradation in the proteasome. More precisely, KEAP1 is an adaptor subunit of a Cullin 3 (CUL3)-based ubiquitin E3 ligase. Under unstressed conditions, NRF2 binds to the KEAP1-CUL3 complex in the cytoplasm, which mediates ubiquitination and subsequent degradation of NRF2 by the proteasome, suppressing NRF2 pathway activity [48]. Upon exposure to oxidative/electrophilic stress, cysteine residues of KEAP1 are directly modified by oxidation and alkylation, resulting in a decline in the ubiquitin E3 ligase activity of the KEAP1-CUL3 complex. NRF2 is then stabilized and activates its target genes. In the nucleus, NRF2 heterodimerizes with small musculoaponeurotic fibrosarcoma (sMAF) proteins and activates transcription by binding to antioxidant responsive elements (AREs), which reside in regulatory regions of NRF2 target genes, including those encoding antioxidant proteins and detoxification enzymes [49].

Nrf2 exhibits potent anti-inflammatory effects, for which two mechanisms have been proposed: one is a direct effect by inhibition of the transcriptional expression of proinflammatory cytokine genes, and the other is an indirect effect by induction of antioxidant genes [50]. In the

DSS colitis model, Nrf2-deficient mice show exacerbation of colitis and a significant increase in the expression of proinflammatory mediators/cytokines such as COX-2, iNOS, IL-1β, IL-6, and TNFα [51]. Examination of bone marrow-derived macrophages implies direct involvement of NRF2 in the inhibition of proinflammatory genes, such as IL6 and IL1b [52]. NRF2 target genes involved in antioxidant function and detoxification are also induced in the inflamed intestine of IBD patients. *SLC7A11*, which encodes a cystine transporter xCT, is one such NRF2 target gene, and it regulates the uptake of cystine, which is utilized for GSH production [53]. Microarray analysis of mRNA shows increased expression of *SLC7A11* in inflammatory mucosa compared with noninflammatory mucosa in IBD patients [46]. *ABCC1* is another NRF2 target gene encoding the multidrug resistance-associated protein MRP1 [54]. MRP1 expression is induced in the inflamed intestine of IBD patients, and increased MRP1 expression is detected at the basolateral membrane of IECs [55]. Because MRP1 is responsible for the export of cysteinyl-leukotriene C4 (LTC_4), a lipid mediator inducing apoptosis, enhanced expression of MRP1 is likely to protect IECs. Consistently, Mrp1-deficient mice show aggravation of DSS colitis, although increased severity in the TNBS intestinal inflammation model is not apparent [56].

Redox balance impacts the differentiation and proliferation of IECs

IECs are composed of different cell populations in crypts and villi: intestinal stem cells and panate cells in crypts, intestinal cells differentiated from stem cells and tuft cells in villi, and apical intestinal cells at the tips of villi. Intestinal stem cells in crypts proliferate into progenitor cells, which differentiate into various cell types, including panate cells, goblet cells, and intestinal cells (enterocytes and colonocytes). The panate cells remain in the crypts, whereas other intestinal cells migrate to the tip of the villi and differentiate into apical enterocytes [56]. The villus tip enterocytes undergo spontaneous apoptosis at 4−5 days after the onset of differentiation from stem cells and are shed into the lumen, completing the regeneration cycle [57].

The redox state of IECs is important for cell growth regulation. Evaluation of the redox potential of the Caco-2 cell line shows that the intracellular GSH/GSSG redox state (Eh) changes according to the cell growth state; the Eh varies between −260 and −230 mV during proliferation, −220 and −190 mV during differentiation, and −170 and −150 mV during apoptosis [58,59]. Disturbance of these optimal redox balances causes aberrant behaviors of IECs. For example, insufficient ROS production induces aberrant differentiation of intestinal stem cells. NOX1-deficient mice reveal a massive conversion of progenitor cells into post-mitotic goblet cells at the cost of colonocytes due to the concerted repression of the phosphatidylinositol 3-kinase (PI3K)/AKT/Wnt/β-catenin and Notch1 signaling pathways, which strictly control intestinal stem cell self-renewal, cell proliferation, migration, and differentiation [60]. Excessive ROS production suppresses cell proliferation in crypts [61]. Especially after genotoxic damage, disruption of TP53-induced glycolysis regulatory phosphatase (TIGAR) increases intracellular ROS levels, leading to the impairment of crypt proliferation [61], as TIGAR exerts an antioxidant function by enhancing NADPH production by diverting the metabolic flux from the main glycolytic pathway toward the pentose phosphate pathway [62]. Too much reduction in ROS is also unfavorable for crypt proliferation. The crypt cell proliferation induced by Wnt signaling in a mouse model of APC deletion requires RAC1, a component of the NOX1 complex, for ROS generation [63], implying that certain levels of ROS enhance cell proliferation. Notably, simultaneous loss of TIGAR and RAC1, which should increase and decrease ROS, respectively, cooperatively suppresses crypt proliferation [61]. With these results, context-dependent optimal ROS levels and redox balances for the physiological turnover of intestinal epithelium appear to be determined by multiple independent and intertwined signaling pathways.

The KEAP1-NRF2 system makes an important contribution to intestinal epithelial cell growth through the intricate regulation of ROS [64]. In Drosophila, NRF2 induces the expression of antioxidant genes and provides a reducing environment for intestinal stem cells, which is cytoprotective and prevents excessive proliferation by limiting S-phase entry. Regulation of intestinal stem cell proliferation by the Keap1-Nrf2 system balances tissue regeneration and growth and maintains homeostasis of intestinal barrier function.

Ferroptosis of IECs in IBD

The intestinal epithelium forms an interface between the internal milieu of the body and the intestinal lumen bacteria. One of the important functions of the intestinal epithelium is serving as a barrier to keep bacteria inside the intestine. The intestinal epithelial barrier is composed of mucus and tight junctions produced by epithelial cells, and they are modulated by interactions with the gut microbiota and the immune system [65]. Due to chronic inflammation in IBD, the intestinal epithelium, which plays important roles in intestinal barrier function, undergoes several cell death pathways, including apoptosis, necrosis, necroptosis, pyroptosis, and ferroptosis [66]. Among these cell death pathways, ferroptosis is directly associated with IBD and ROS [67].

Ferroptosis is characterized by iron accumulation, excessive ROS production, and overwhelming lipid peroxidation. Iron-dependent peroxidation of polyunsaturated

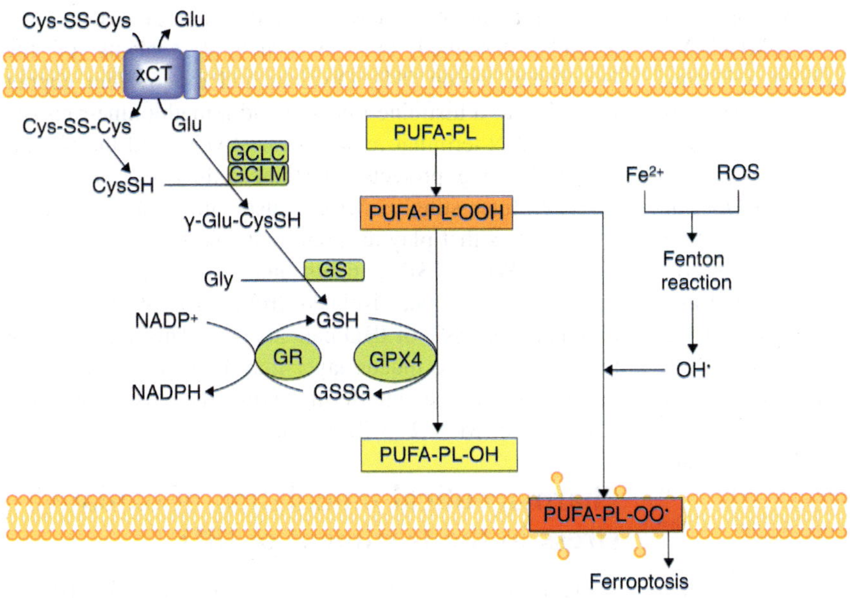

FIGURE 12.4 Ferroptosis and its regulation. Ferroptosis is a cell death triggered by the generation of lipid peroxides and related radicals (PUFA-PL-OO•), which damage cellular membrane integrity. GPX4 converts PUFA-PL-OOH to nontoxic PUFA-PL-OH with the help of GSH. GSH depletion and/or GPX4 inhibition triggers ferroptosis through the accumulation of intracellular ROS and overwhelming lipid peroxidation. By the Fenton reaction, ROS and Fe^{2+} generate OH•, which converts PUFA-PL-OOH to PUFA-PL-OO•.

fatty acids (PUFAs) causes the disruption of cell membranes and cell death (Fig. 12.4) [68,69]. Hydrogen peroxide (H_2O_2) produces $OH^{\bullet-}$ via a Fenton reaction catalyzed by Fe^{2+}. The Fe^{3+} produced from this reaction is reduced back to Fe^{2+} by H_2O_2, hydroperoxyl radicals ($HO_2^{\bullet}$) and/or organic radical intermediates, enabling the catalytic behavior of the Fe^{2+}/Fe^{3+} system to generate ROS [70]. $OH^{\cdot}$ peroxidizes PUFA of phospholipids (PUFA-PL) to generate PUFA-PL-hydroperoxides (PUFA-PL-OOH), and PUFA-PL-OOH undergoes reduction by GSH via GPX4 to nonlethal PUFA-PL alcohols (PUFA-PL-OH) [69]. When this GPX4-mediated reducing reaction is impaired by GPX4 inhibition or GSH depletion, PUFA-PL-OOH accumulates intracellularly, leading to ferroptotic cell death [71].

IBD and ferroptosis are thought to be closely related. Microarray analysis using colonic biopsy samples from UC patients and controls showed significantly altered expression of ferroptosis-related genes. In the DSS colitis mouse model, ferroptosis is induced in IECs, and the ferroptosis inhibitors ferrostatin-1 and deferoxamine alleviate colitis [71]. In CD patients, GPX4 activity is decreased in the small intestinal mucosa in the inflammatory state, which may be closely related to ferroptosis [72]. In addition, administration of arachidonic acid, one of the PUFAs, to *Gpx4*-deficient IECs induces an inflammatory response. In heterozygotes of intestinal epithelium-specific *Gpx4* knockout mice, severe intestinal inflammation is induced on a PUFA-enriched Western diet. These results suggest that a PUFA-enriched Western diet poses a risk for developing IBD by conferring susceptibility to ferroptosis on IECs.

Mucus as an important component of the intestinal barrier

A vast number of bacterial species reside in the intestinal lumen in a symbiotic relationship with their host: an estimated 10 million to 10 billion bacteria in the small intestine and an estimated 100 trillion cells in the colon [73]. Mucus serves as an important component of the intestinal barrier that protects the body by keeping an enormous number of intestinal bacteria as well as dangerous substances, including food antigens and toxins, inside the intestine. The mucus layer of the intestine differs from site to site [74]. In the small intestine, there is a single layer of mucus that can be easily removed. In the colon, the mucus consists of two layers, a sterile inner layer firmly attached to the epithelium and a loose outer layer.

Mucins are the major components of mucus and are secreted by goblet cells. Mucins are glycosylated proteins, and their core structures are mucin domains that are extensively decorated by *O*-linked glycans, which bind water and give mucus its gel-like properties [75]. Mucin family proteins are composed of transmembrane mucins and gel-forming mucins [76]. The former contains MUC3, MUC4, MUC12, MUC13, and MUC17, and the latter contains MUC2, MUC5AC, MUC5B, and MUC6. Transmembrane mucins are involved in intracellular signal transduction, whereas gel-forming mucins are secreted from goblet cells and serve as the skeleton of the mucin layer.

Their expression is influenced by the redox status of the intestinal tissue environment. In Caco-2, an enterocytederived cell line, DUOX2 regulates the expression of MUC3, one of the transmembrane mucins, and MUC5AC, one of the gel-forming mucins [77]. In addition, epidermal growth factor (EGF) stimulation induces the expression of DUOX2, MUC2, MUC3, and MUC5AC, and DUOX2 knockdown reduces MUC3 and MUC5AC expression but not MUC2, suggesting that DUOX2-dependent ROS generation plays a role in the regulation of mucin production. Notably, the NOD-like receptor family pyrin domain containing 6 (NLRP6) inflammasome has been reported as a link between ROS and mucin, specifically MUC2 in this case [74]. Evaluation of MUC2 secretion in mouse colonic explants or cell suspensions shows a positive correlation between MUC2 secretion and ROS levels. The NLRP6 inflammasome is activated by ROS from NOX/DUOX and triggers calcium ion–dependent compound exocytosis of MUC2 mucin. Thus, the tissue ROS level is one of the important regulators of mucus formation.

MUC2, one of the gel-forming mucins, is the main mucus layer component secreted from goblet cells, and it is associated with IBD. A critical function of MUC2 has been shown in the analysis of *Muc2*-deficient mice, which develop spontaneous intestinal inflammation, severe colitis in the DSS colitis model, and colon cancer [78,79]. MUC2 packing in goblet cells and its release from goblet cells are regulated by the intracellular pH and Ca^{2+} concentration [80]. After being released from goblet cells, MUC2 undergoes crosslinking by transglutaminase 3, resulting in the formation of a stable mucus layer [81]. A structural feature of gel-forming mucins, including MUC2, is the presence of cysteine-rich domains at the N-terminal and C-terminal regions and those interspersing the central mucin domains, which play an important role in mucin multimerization by forming a disulfide bridge [75]. The cysteine-rich nature of the gel-forming mucins is likely to confer susceptibility to redox disturbance on the mucus layer. Indeed, sulfide produced by gut sulfate-reducing bacteria (SRB) was shown to reduce disulfide bonds of the MUC2 multimer, drive its denaturation, and allow microbial access to the mucus layer [82]. Under anaerobic conditions in the intestinal lumen, SRB, which are obligate anaerobes, use sulfate as a terminal electron acceptor and produce sulfide, thereby obtaining energy for growth [83]. Sulfides and trisulfides are found in the feces of normal mice, and both are significantly reduced when SRB is reduced by antibiotics [82]. Hydrogen sulfide is suggested to cleave intra- and intermolecular disulfide bonds in the MUC2 multimer, which should result in the dissociation of mucin monomers and the breakdown of the network structure of mucus layers. The MUC2 protein in the fecal mucus from mice treated with antibiotics to eliminate intestinal SRB was observed as a high molecular weight band, whereas MUC2 was observed as a low molecular weight band after treatment with reducing agents such as dithiothreitol and Na_2S [82]. In addition, a new protective role of MUC2 was recently described by the structural analysis of the N-terminal region [84]. Divalent and monovalent copper ions bind to a histidine-rich site and a methionine-rich site of MUC2 N-terminal region, respectively, and the mucin-copper binding protects intestinal cells from the copper toxicity. Interestingly, MUC2 also allows an uptake of copper irons that play an important role in cells as a trace element. When IBD patients and healthy controls were compared, SRB was isolated from 24% of healthy individuals and 68% of IBD patients [85]. This suggests that the quality of the mucus layer may be changed by SRB-generating sulfide interfering with the disulfide bond structures of MUC2 in IBD patients.

Pharmaceutical modulation of oxidative stress in the treatment of IBD

There are only a few types of therapeutic agents for IBD: 5-aminosalicylic acid (5-ASA), steroids, immunosuppressive drugs, and monoclonal antibody drugs [2,3]. Clinically relevant side effects of these treatments are 5-ASA intolerance and immunosuppression. Long-term administration of steroids occasionally causes osteoporosis and steroid psychosis. Effective therapeutics with fewer side effects are eagerly awaited. Modulation and normalization of the redox balance in intestinal tissues are desirable goals for developing new therapeutics for IBD.

In fact, 5-ASA possesses antioxidant activity. The beneficial effects of 5-ASA are exerted as a potent antioxidant that reduces ROS levels in the inflamed colonic tissues of UC patients [86]. 5-ASA together with flavonoids suppresses ROS levels, resulting in the inhibition of neutrophil extracellular trap formation in activated neutrophils [87]. In UC patients, clinical studies with 5-ASA in combination with an additional antioxidant, N-acetylcysteine, show a higher clinical remission rate and lower serum proinflammatory cytokine levels than 5-ASA alone [88].

A unique approach that takes advantage of elevated ROS levels in inflammatory tissues has been proposed, which is a gene editing technology combined with a specific delivery system in response to ROS [89]. Thioketal linkers have been reported to be ROS-cleavable structures due to their susceptibility to oxidative degradation [90], and they can be utilized for drug delivery specifically to tissues with high ROS levels, such as inflammatory tissues. Utilizing this technique, a Cas9-encoding plasmid was delivered to the mouse inflammatory colon lesion for inflammation-specific genome editing, enabling the induction of genome editing according to the local pathological condition [89]. Alternatively, a combination of gene editing and organoid transplantation is a promising approach for the effective treatment of IBD. While intestinal organoids are very useful in vitro experimental tools allowing various genetic manipulations by genome editing for stem cell studies, organoids can also be transplanted in vivo, serving as a preclinical tool for regenerative medicine [91]. A DSS-induced colitis model was used for organoid transplantation, in which organoids were infused into the luminal space of the colon. The organoids were successfully integrated into areas with epithelial damage, as donor-derived cells were detected in the injured areas but not in the healthy areas. Inflamed regions with epithelial damage are likely to have open stem cell niches that can accommodate the integration of donor stem cells within the organoids.

Inhibition of ferroptosis is another approach for IBD treatment in terms of correcting redox imbalance. Mucosal ROS production is increased in UC in proportion to disease activity, and iron chelators are known to reduce ROS production and ameliorate colonic symptoms in IBD [92]. In a DSS colitis mouse model, ferroptosis inhibitors (ferrostatin-1, liproxstatin-1, deferprone, and butylated hydroxyanisole) suppressed inflammation [93]. Curcurigoside (CUR) is a phytoconstituent with antioxidant and anti-inflammatory properties that protects against UC ferroptosis through the promotion of GPX4 [94]. CUR increases selenium sensitivity and enhances GPX4 expression levels in the IEC-6 rat intestinal epithelial cell line, while GPX4 silencing inhibits the protective effect of CUR on cell death and oxidative stress accumulation in ferroptotic IECs.

Elimination of ROS from the inflammatory site of IBD intestine using probiotics is another unique approach [95]. One of the orally administered probiotics, *Escherichia coli* Nissle 1917 (ECN), was genetically engineered to overexpress catalase and superoxide dismutase and applied for IBD treatment, allowing for the effective removal of ROS from inflamed tissues. The genome-edited ECN was coated with chitosan/sodium alginate and administered to mouse colitis models induced by various chemicals (DSS, TNBS, and oxazolone), and it successfully alleviated intestinal inflammation.

In human studies, probiotics are considered safe food additives conferring a health benefit on the host. For example, *Lactobacilli* have beneficial effects in maintaining intestinal homeostasis and suppressing intestinal bacteria that are harmful to IBD [96]. Probiotic therapy using *Lactobacilli* has beneficial effects in the adjuvant therapy of IBD. Probiotic strains produce growth factors supporting the healthy turnover of IECs and antimicrobial substances that kill harmful microorganisms. Intriguingly, when ROS production by NOX family members is inhibited in mouse IECs, ROS-generating bacteria are enriched in the microbiota and they suppress virulent factors generated by pathogenic *Citrobacter* [96]. Thus, the redox balance in the intestine is maintained in a cooperative interaction between commensal bacteria and epithelial cells, and how to maintain and reconstruct the integrity of the redox balance control system is an important viewpoint for the development of IBD treatment.

Concluding remarks

The intestinal epithelium is an interface between the internal milieu of the body, which provides oxic conditions, and the external intestinal lumen, which provides anoxic conditions. Regulation of the redox balance fluctuation within the permissible range is necessary to maintain the healthy status of the intestinal epithelium. NOX family members that generate ROS play protective roles at a physiological level and detrimental roles at a pathological level. Pathways regulated by ROS, especially the Wnt and Notch signaling pathways, have large impacts on intestinal epithelial differentiation and proliferation. The KEAP1-NRF2 system provides another ROS-responding pathway, directly ROS sensing by KEAP1 and transcriptional activation of a battery of genes by NRF2, to induce cytoprotective and antioxidative effects, contributing to the facilitation of the resolution of inflammation. Pharmaceutical intervention with these redox regulators will provide new therapeutics. In addition, reactive species that induce ferroptosis of IECs would be effective therapeutic targets. Maintaining a healthy state of the mucus layer, for which the redox balance in the intestinal lumen appears to be a critical regulator, would be another therapeutic target. Further clarification of the molecular mechanisms regulating the intestinal redox balance will add new layers of therapeutic approaches.

References

[1] Cosnes J, Gowerrousseau C, Seksik P, Cortot A. Epidemiology and natural history of inflammatory bowel diseases. Gastroenterology 2011;140:1785–1794.e4.

[2] Lamb CA, Kennedy NA, Raine T, Hendy PA, Smith PJ, Limdi JK, et al. British Society of Gastroenterology consensus guidelines on the management of inflammatory bowel disease in adults. Gut 2019;68:s1–106.

[3] Matsuoka K, Kobayashi T, Ueno F, Matsui T, Hirai F, Inoue N, et al. Evidence-based clinical practice guidelines for inflammatory bowel disease. J Gastroenterol 2018;53:305–53.

[4] Ng SC, Shi HY, Hamidi N, Underwood FE, Tang W, Benchimol EI, et al. Worldwide incidence and prevalence of inflammatory bowel disease in the 21st century: a systematic review of population-based studies. Lancet 2017;390:2769–78.

[5] Graham DB, Xavier RJ. Pathway paradigms revealed from the genetics of inflammatory bowel disease. Nature 2020;578:527–39.

[6] Agrawal M, Allin KH, Petralia F, Colombel J-F, Jess T. Multiomics to elucidate inflammatory bowel disease risk factors and pathways. Nat Rev Gastroenterol Hepatol 2022;19:399–409.

[7] Nambu R, Warner N, Mulder DJ, Kotlarz D, McGovern DPB, Cho J, et al. A systematic review of monogenic inflammatory bowel disease. Clin Gastroenterol Hepatol 2022;20:e653–63.

[8] Hayes P, Dhillon S, O'Neill K, Thoeni C, Hui KY, Elkadri A, et al. Defects in nicotinamide-adenine dinucleotide phosphate oxidase genes NOX1 and DUOX2 in very early onset inflammatory bowel disease. CMGH 2015;1:489–502.
[9] Ananthakrishnan AN, Bernstein CN, Iliopoulos D, Macpherson A, Neurath MF, Raja Ali RA, et al. Environmental triggers in IBD: a review of progress and evidence. Nat Rev Gastroenterol Hepatol 2018;15:39–49.
[10] Elten M, Benchimol EI, Fell DB, Kuenzig ME, Smith G, Chen H, et al. Ambient air pollution and the risk of pediatric-onset inflammatory bowel disease: a population-based cohort study. Environ Int 2020;138.
[11] Okayasu I, Hatakeyama S, Yamada M, Ohkusa T, Inagaki Y, Nakaya R. A novel method in the induction of reliable experimental acute and chronic ulcerative colitis in mice. Gastroenterology 1990;98:694–702.
[12] Eichele DD, Kharbanda KK. Dextran sodium sulfate colitis murine model: an indispensable tool for advancing our understanding of inflammatory bowel diseases pathogenesis. World J Gastroenterol 2017;23:6016–29.
[13] Elson CO, Beagley KW, Sharmanov AT, Fujihashi K, Kiyono H, Tennyson GS, et al. Hapten-induced model of murine inflammatory bowel disease: mucosa immune responses and protection by tolerance. J Immunol 1996;157:2174–85.
[14] Wirtz S, Popp V, Kindermann M, Gerlach K, Weigmann B, Fichtner-Feigl S, et al. Chemically induced mouse models of acute and chronic intestinal inflammation. Nat Protoc 2017;12:1295–309.
[15] Xu X, An H, Zhang D, Tao H, Dou Y, Li X, et al. A self-illuminating nanoparticle for inflammation imaging and cancer therapy. Sci Adv 2019;5:eaat2953.
[16] McKenzie S, Baker M, Buffinton G, Doe W. Evidence of oxidant-induced injury to epithelial cells during inflammatory bowel disease. J Clin Invest 1996;1:136–41.
[17] Mittal M, Siddiqui MR, Tran K, Reddy SP, Malik AB. Reactive oxygen species in inflammation and tissue injury. Antioxid Redox Signal 2014;20:1126–67.
[18] Dröge W. Free radicals in the physiological control of cell function. Physiol Rev 2002;82:47–95.
[19] Vaccaro A, Kaplan Dor Y, Nambara K, Pollina EA, Lin C, Greenberg ME, et al. Sleep loss can cause death through accumulation of reactive oxygen species in the gut. Cell 2020;181:1307–1328.e15.
[20] Aviello G, Knaus UG. ROS in gastrointestinal inflammation: rescue or sabotage? Br J Pharmacol 2017;174:1704–18.
[21] Sumimoto H. Structure, regulation and evolution of Nox-family NADPH oxidases that produce reactive oxygen species. FEBS J 2008;275:3249–77.
[22] Bienert GP, Chaumont F. Aquaporin-facilitated transmembrane diffusion of hydrogen peroxide. Biochim Biophys Acta Gen Subj 2014;1840:1596–604.
[23] Geiszt M, Lekstrom K, Brenner S, Hewitt SM, Dana R, Malech HL, et al. NAD(P)H oxidase 1, a product of differentiated colon epithelial cells, can partially replace glycoprotein 91 phox in the regulated production of superoxide by phagocytes. J Immunol 2003;171:299–306.
[24] Szanto I, Rubbia-Brandt L, Kiss P, Steger K, Banfi B, Kovari E, et al. Expression of NOXI, a superoxide-generating NADPH oxidase, in colon cancer and inflammatory bowel disease. J Pathol 2005;207:164–76.
[25] Mouzaoui S, Djerdjouri B, Makhezer N, Kroviarski Y, El-Benna J, Dang PM-C. Tumor necrosis factor-α-induced colitis increases NADPH oxidase 1 expression, oxidative stress, and neutrophil recruitment in the colon: preventive effect of apocynin. Mediators Inflamm 2014;2014:312484.
[26] Kuwano Y, Kawahara T, Yamamoto H, Teshima-Kondo S, Tominaga K, Masuda K, et al. Interferon-activates transcription of NADPH oxidase 1 gene and upregulates production of superoxide anion by human large intestinal epithelial cells. Am J Physiol Cell Physiol 2006;290:433–43.
[27] Babior BM, Lambeth JD, Nauseef W. The neutrophil NADPH oxidase. Arch Biochem Biophys 2002;397:342–4.
[28] Fournier BM, Parkos CA. The role of neutrophils during intestinal inflammation. Mucosal Immunol 2012;5:354–66.
[29] Micheau O, Ichim G, Jacquin E, Hodge S, Asare PF, Roscioli E, et al. LC3-associated phagocytosis (LAP): a potentially influential mediator of efferocytosis-related tumor progression and aggressiveness. Front Oncol 2020;1:1298.
[30] Kolios G, Valatas V, Ward SG. Nitric oxide in inflammatory bowel disease: a universal messenger in an unsolved puzzle. Immunology 2004;113:427–37.
[31] Tuin A, Poelstra K, de Jager-Krikken A, Bok L, Raaben W, Velders MP, et al. Role of alkaline phosphatase in colitis in man and rats. Gut 2009;58:379–87.
[32] Li B, Alli R, Vogel P, Geiger TL. IL-10 modulates DSS-induced colitis through a macrophage-ROS-NO axis. Mucosal Immunol 2014;7:869–78.
[33] Circu ML, Aw TY. Intestinal redox biology and oxidative stress. Semin Cell Dev Biol 2012;23:729–37.
[34] Sido B, Hack V, Hochlehnert A, Lipps H, Herfarth C, Dröge W. Impairment of intestinal glutathione synthesis in patients with inflammatory bowel disease. Gut 1998;42:485–92.
[35] Lu SC. Regulation of glutathione synthesis. Mol Aspects Med 2009;30:42–59.
[36] Dalton TP, Chen Y, Schneider SN, Nebert DW, Shertzer HG. Genetically altered mice to evaluate glutathione homeostasis in health and disease. Free Radic Biol Med 2004;37:1511–26.
[37] Steven Esworthy R, Aranda R, Marti NG, Doroshow JH, Binder SW, Chu F, et al. Mice with combined disruption of Gpx1 and Gpx2 genes have colitis. Am J Physiol Gastrointest Liver Physiol 2001;281:G848–55.
[38] Chu FF, Esworthy RS, Doroshow JH. Role of Se-dependent glutathione peroxidases in gastrointestinal inflammation and cancer. Free Radic Biol Med 2004;36:1481–95.
[39] Gauthier-Coles G, Vennitti J, Zhang Z, Comb WC, Xing S, Javed K, et al. Quantitative modelling of amino acid transport and homeostasis in mammalian cells. Nat Commun 2021;12:5282.
[40] Ping Jin X, bin Peng J, Huang F, Zhu YN, Fei J, Guo LH. A mRNA molecule encoding truncated excitatory amino acid car-rier 1 (EAAC1) protein (EAAC2) is transcribed from an indepen-dent promoter but not an alternative splicing event. Cell Res 2002;12:257–62.
[41] Lu J, Holmgren A. The thioredoxin antioxidant system. Free Radic Biol Med 2014;66:75–87.
[42] Godoy JR, Funke M, Ackermann W, Haunhorst P, Oesteritz S, Capani F, et al. Redox atlas of the mouse. Immunohistochemical detection of glutaredoxin-, peroxiredoxin-, and thioredoxin-family proteins in various tissues of the laboratory mouse. Biochim Biophys Acta Gen Subj 2011;1810:2–92.

[43] Tamaki H, Nakamura H, Nishio A, Nakase H, Ueno S, Uza N, et al. Human thioredoxin-1 ameliorates experimental murine colitis in association with suppressed macrophage inhibitory factor production. Gastroenterology 2006;131:1110–21.
[44] Beltŕan B, Nos P, Dasí F, Iborra M, Bastida G, Martínez M, et al. Mitochondrial dysfunction, persistent oxidative damage, and catalase inhibition in immune cells of naïve and treated Crohn's disease. Inflamm Bowel Dis 2010;16:76–86.
[45] Khodayari S, Salehi Z, Asl SF, Aminian K, Gisomi NM, Dalivandan ST. Catalase gene C-262T polymorphism: importance in ulcerative colitis. J Gastroenterol Hepatol 2013;28:819–22.
[46] Palmieri O, Creanza TM, Bossa F, Palumbo O, Maglietta R, Ancona N, et al. Genome-wide pathway analysis using gene expression data of colonic mucosa in patients with inflammatory bowel disease. Inflamm Bowel Dis 2015;21:1260–8.
[47] Motohashi H, Yamamoto M. Nrf2-Keap1 defines a physiologically important stress response mechanism. Trends Mol Med 2004;10:549–57.
[48] Suzuki T, Yamamoto M. Molecular basis of the Keap1-Nrf2 system. Free Radic Biol Med 2015;88:93–100.
[49] Motohashi H, O'connor T, Katsuoka F, Douglas Engel J, Yamamoto M. Integration and diversity of the regulatory network composed of Maf and CNC families of transcription factors. Gene 2002;294:1–12.
[50] Yamamoto XM, Kensler TW, Motohashi H. The KEAP1-NRF2 system: a thiol-based sensor-effector apparatus for maintaining redox homeostasis. Physiol Rev 2018;98:1169–203.
[51] Khor TO, Huang MT, Kwon KH, Chan JY, Reddy BS, Kong AN. Nrf2-deficient mice have an increased susceptibility to dextran sulfate sodium-induced colitis. Cancer Res 2006;66:11580–4.
[52] Kobayashi EH, Suzuki T, Funayama R, Nagashima T, Hayashi M, Sekine H, et al. Nrf2 suppresses macrophage inflammatory response by blocking proinflammatory cytokine transcription. Nat Commun 2016;7:11624.
[53] Sasaki H, Sato H, Kuriyama-Matsumura K, Sato K, Maebara K, Wang H, et al. Electrophile response element-mediated induction of the cystine/glutamate exchange transporter gene expression. J Biol Chem 2002;277:44765–71.
[54] Hayashi A, Suzuki H, Itoh K, Yamamoto M, Sugiyama Y. Transcription factor Nrf2 is required for the constitutive and inducible expression of multidrug resistance-associated protein 1 in mouse embryo fibroblasts. Biochem Biophys Res Commun 2003;310:824–9.
[55] Blokzijl H, van Steenpaal A, vander Borght S, Bok LIH, Libbrecht L, Tamminga M, et al. Up-regulation and cytoprotective role of epithelial multidrug resistance-associated protein 1 in inflammatory bowel disease. J Biol Chem 2008;283:35630–7.
[56] Tessa ten Hove T, Drillenburg P, Wijnholds J, te Velde AA, van Deventer SJH. Differential susceptibility of multidrug resistance protein-1 deficient mice to DSS and TNBS-induced colitis. Dig Dis Sci 2002;47:2056–63.
[57] Clevers H. The intestinal crypt, a prototype stem cell compartment. Cell 2013;154:274.
[58] Jones DP. Redox potential of GSH/GSSG couple: assay and biological significance. Methods Enzymol 2002;348:93–112.
[59] Nkabyo YS, Ziegler TR, Gu LH, Watson WH, Jones DP. Glutathione and thioredoxin redox during differentiation in human colon epithelial (Caco-2) cells. Am J Physiol Gastrointest Liver Physiol 2002;283:G1352–9.
[60] Coant N, ben Mkaddem S, Pedruzzi E, Guichard C, Tréton X, Ducroc R, et al. NADPH oxidase 1 modulates WNT and NOTCH1 signaling to control the fate of proliferative progenitor cells in the colon. Mol Cell Biol 2010;30:2636–50.
[61] Cheung EC, Lee P, Ceteci F, Nixon C, Blyth K, Sansom OJ, et al. Opposing effects of TIGAR-and RAC1-derived ROS on Wnt-driven proliferation in the mouse intestine. Genes Dev 2016;30:52–63.
[62] Zhang X, Qin Z, Wang J. The role of p53 in cell metabolism. Acta Pharmacol Sin 2010;31:1208–12.
[63] Myant KB, Cammareri P, McGhee EJ, Ridgway RA, Huels DJ, Cordero JB, et al. ROS production and NF-κB activation triggered by RAC1 facilitate WNT-driven intestinal stem cell proliferation and colorectal cancer initiation. Cell Stem Cell 2013;12:761–73.
[64] Hochmuth CE, Biteau B, Bohmann D, Jasper H. Redox regulation by keap1 and Nrf2 controls intestinal stem cell proliferation in drosophila. Cell Stem Cell 2011;8:188–99.
[65] Lu P, Xie M, Snelson M, Ménard S, Barbara G, Raffaella Barbaro M, et al. Inflammatory and microbiota-related regulation of the intestinal epithelial barrier. Front Nutr 2021;8:718356.
[66] Subramanian S, Geng H, Tan X-D, Li Xue Bao S. Cell death of intestinal epithelial cells in intestinal diseases. Sheng Li Xue Bao 2020;72:308–24.
[67] Xu S, He Y, Lin L, Chen P, Chen M, Zhang S. The emerging role of ferroptosis in intestinal disease. Cell Death Dis 2021;12:289.
[68] Dixon SJ, Lemberg KM, Lamprecht MR, Skouta R, Zaitsev EM, Gleason CE, et al. Ferroptosis: an iron-dependent form of non-apoptotic cell death. Cell 2012;149:1060–72.
[69] Stockwell BR. Ferroptosis turns 10: emerging mechanisms, physiological functions, and therapeutic applications. Cell 2022;185:2401–21.
[70] Sirés I, Garrido JA, Rodríguez RM, Brillas E, Oturan N, Oturan MA. Catalytic behavior of the Fe^{3+}/Fe^{2+} system in the electro-Fenton degradation of the antimicrobial chlorophene. Appl Catal B 2007;72:382–94.
[71] Xu M, Tao J, Yang Y, Tan S, Liu H, Jiang J, et al. Ferroptosis involves in intestinal epithelial cell death in ulcerative colitis. Cell Death Dis 2020;11:86.
[72] Mayr L, Grabherr F, Schwärzler J, Reitmeier I, Sommer F, Gehmacher T, et al. Dietary lipids fuel GPX4-restricted enteritis resembling Crohn's disease. Nat Commun 2020;11:1775.
[73] de Vos WM, Tilg H, Van Hul M, Cani PD. Gut microbiome and health: mechanistic insights. Gut 2022;71:1020–32.
[74] Birchenough GMH, Nyström EEL, Johansson MEV, Hansson GC. A sentinel goblet cell guards the colonic crypt by triggering Nlrp6-dependent Muc2 secretion. Science June 24, 2016;352(6293):1535–42.
[75] Johansson MEV, Hansson GC. Immunological aspects of intestinal mucus and mucins. Rev Immunol 2016;16:639–49.
[76] Paone P, Cani PD. Mucus barrier, mucins and gut microbiota: the expected slimy partners? Gut 2020;69:2232–43.
[77] Damiano S, Morano A, Ucci V, Accetta R, Mondola P, Paternò R, et al. Dual oxidase 2 generated reactive oxygen species selectively mediate the induction of mucins by epidermal growth factor in enterocytes. Int J Biochem Cell Biol 2015;60:889–93.
[78] Velcich A, Yang W, Heyer J, Fragale A, Nicholas C, Viani S, et al. Colorectal cancer in mice genetically deficient in the mucin Muc2. Science 2002;295:1726–9.

[79] Van der Sluis M, De Koning BA, De Bruijn AC, Velcich A, Meijerink JP, Van Goudoever JB, et al. Muc2-deficient mice spontaneously develop colitis, indicating that MUC2 is critical for colonic protection. Gastroenterology 2006;131:117–29.

[80] Ambort D, Johansson MEV, Gustafsson JK, Nilsson HE, Ermund A, Johansson BR, et al. Calcium and pH-dependent packing and release of the gel-forming MUC2 mucin. Proc Natl Acad Sci USA 2012;109:5645–50.

[81] Sharpen JDA, Dolan B, Nyström EEL, Birchenough GMH, Arike L, Martinez-Abad B, et al. Transglutaminase 3 crosslinks the secreted gel-forming mucus component Mucin-2 and stabilizes the colonic mucus layer. Nat Commun 2022;13:45.

[82] Ijssennagger N, Belzer C, Hooiveld GJ, Dekker J, van Mil SWC, Müller M, et al. Gut microbiota facilitates dietary heme-induced epithelial hyperproliferation by opening the mucus barrier in colon. Proc Natl Acad Sci USA 2015;112:10038–43.

[83] Muyzer G. The ecology and biotechnology of sulphate-reducing bacteria. Nat Rev Microbiol 2008;6:441–54.

[84] Reznik N, Gallo AD, Rush KW, Javitt G, Fridmann-Sirkis Y, Ilani T, et al. Intestinal mucin is a chaperone of multivalent copper. Cell September 29, 2022. S0092-8674(22)01193-X.

[85] Loubinoux J, Bronowicki J-P, Pereira IAC, Mougenel J-L, Faou AE. Sulfate-reducing bacteria in human feces and their association with inflammatory bowel diseases. FEMS Microbiol Ecol 2006;40:107–12.

[86] Managlia E, Katzman RB, Brown JB, Barrett TA. Antioxidant properties of mesalamine in colitis inhibit phosphoinositide 3-kinase signaling in progenitor cells. Inflamm Bowel Dis 2013;19:2051–60.

[87] Kirchner T, Hermann E, Möller S, Klinger M, Solbach W, Laskay T, et al. Flavonoids and 5-aminosalicylic acid inhibit the formation of neutrophil extracellular traps. Mediators Inflamm 2013;2013:710239.

[88] Guijarro LG, Mate J, Gisbert JP, Luis Perez-Calle J, Marín-Jimenez I, Arriaza E, et al. N-acetyl-L-cysteine combined with mesalamine in the treatment of ulcerative colitis: randomized, placebo-controlled pilot study. World J Gastroenterol 2008;14:2851–7.

[89] Yan X, Pan Q, Xin H, Chen Y, Ping Y. Genome-editing prodrug: targeted delivery and conditional stabilization of CRISPR-Cas9 for precision therapy of inflammatory disease. Sci Adv 2021;7:eabj0624.

[90] Liu B, Thayumanavan S. Mechanistic investigation on oxidative degradation of ROS-responsive thioacetal/thioketal moieties and their implications. Cell Rep Phys Sci 2020;1:100271.

[91] Watanabe S, Kobayashi S, Ogasawara N, Okamoto R, Nakamura T, Watanabe M, et al. Transplantation of intestinal organoids into a mouse model of colitis. Nat Protoc 2022;17:649–71.

[92] Millar AD, Rampton DS, Blake DR. Effects of iron and iron chelation in vitro on mucosal oxidant activity in ulcerative colitis. Aliment Pharmacol Ther 2000;14:1163–8.

[93] Chen Y, Zhang P, Chen W, Chen G. Ferroptosis mediated DSS-induced ulcerative colitis associated with Nrf2/HO-1 signaling pathway. Immunol Lett 2020;225:9–15.

[94] Wang S, Liu W, Wang J, Bai X. Curculigoside inhibits ferroptosis in ulcerative colitis through the induction of GPX4. Life Sci 2020;259:118356.

[95] Zhou J, Li M, Chen Q, Li X, Chen L, Dong Z, et al. Programmable probiotics modulate inflammation and gut microbiota for inflammatory bowel disease treatment after effective oral delivery. Nat Commun 2022;13:3432.

[96] Basso PJ, Câmara NOS, Sales-Campos H. Microbial-based therapies in the treatment of inflammatory bowel disease—an overview of human studies. Front Pharmacol 2019;9:1571.

Chapter 13

Applications of plant-derived products in photodynamic therapy

Francesco Cimino, Antonella Saija and Antonio Speciale
Department of Chemical, Biological, Pharmaceutical and Environmental Sciences, University of Messina, Messina, Italy

Introduction

Photodynamic therapy (PDT) is a promising noninvasive therapy useful in the treatment of different pathologies, including cancer and microbial infections [1–3]. The main components of PDT include a photosensitizer (PS), molecular oxygen, and light irradiation. These components are not toxic to cells individually, but when a PS is light irradiated in the presence of oxygen, these can initiate a photochemical reaction that generates highly reactive species and causes significant toxicity. Although the therapeutic properties of light for the treatment of various diseases in dermatology were known in ancient civilizations, PDT has significantly developed in the last 100 years. The interest in PDT started with the discovery of hematoporphyrin derivative (HpD) by Lipson and Schwartz in 1960 as PS [4,5]. Twenty years later, a HpD known as Photofrin (porfimer sodium; QLT, Vancouver, BC, Canada) was approved for treatment of various cancers in several countries representing the first PS commercially available drug. Although the main application of PDT is cancer treatment, due to its capability to destroy tumoral cells, also nononcologic applications have been explored in recent years, highlighting the potential to be effectively employed in pathogen-related conditions for fighting bacteria, fungi, viruses, and protozoa [6,7].

Although several first- and second-generation types of PS (porphyrin-based sensitizers and nonporphyrin derivatives, respectively) have been introduced for PDT application, their clinical usage is limited by various drawbacks, such as lack of chemical purity, long half-life, tissue accumulation, and poor capability to penetrate tissues. Thus, it is evident the necessity to find new PS with potent pharmaceutical properties and overcome the shortcomings of conventional PS. There are a number of research studies demonstrating that natural compounds with photosensitizing abilities can be isolated from plants and be potentially useful as alternatives to known PS to be employed to combat cancer and microbial infections. The main advantages of plant-derived PS for PDT are represented by their good pharmacological properties together with low systemic cytotoxicity to normal cells and negligible side effects.

Up today, the main plant-derived PS investigated for cancer PDT and antimicrobial PDT (aPDT) include chlorophylls (Chls) and Chl metabolites, curcumin (CUR), thiophenes, alkaloids, and anthraquinones (Fig. 13.1). Chls are natural pigments, widely present in terrestrial plants, and able to absorb a lot of the light. They showed a strong absorption at the range of 600–700 nm with a high singlet oxygen ($^1O_2$) quantum yield, so being an attractive alternative PS in PDT. Chls obtained from a wide variety of sources is a mixture of two compounds, mainly Chl a and b. The latter differs from Chl a by the presence of an aldehyde group in place of the methyl one. Also, several Chl metabolites are known for their activity and selectivity as PS. In fact, enzymatic degradation of Chl produces a lot of metabolites such as pheophorbide upon the loss of the phytol chain and Mg dechelation, and purpurin 18 (Pu-18) obtained by oxidative cleavage of pheophorbide and its esters. Thanks to their chemico-physical properties, these compounds were studies as potential alternatives for PDT. Pu-18 occurs, for example, in spinach leaves, seaweed, and cyanobacterium *Spirulina maxima*. Pheophorbide a [(3S,4S)-9-ethenyl-14-ethyl-21(methoxycarbonyl)-4,8,13,18-tetramethyl-20-oxo-3-phorbinepropanoic acid] (Fig. 13.1) is formed in algae and higher plants and was isolated for the first time from *Scutellaria barbata* D. Don.

The food colorant CUR, found in the rhizome of *Curcuma longa* of the Zingiberaceae family, consists of two symmetrical feruloyl moieties connected through a methylene group; orally consumed for centuries in several countries, it has been proven safe for humans and thus useful for prevention and treatment of a variety of diseases (Fig. 13.1).

Modulation of Oxidative Stress. https://doi.org/10.1016/B978-0-443-19247-0.00008-4

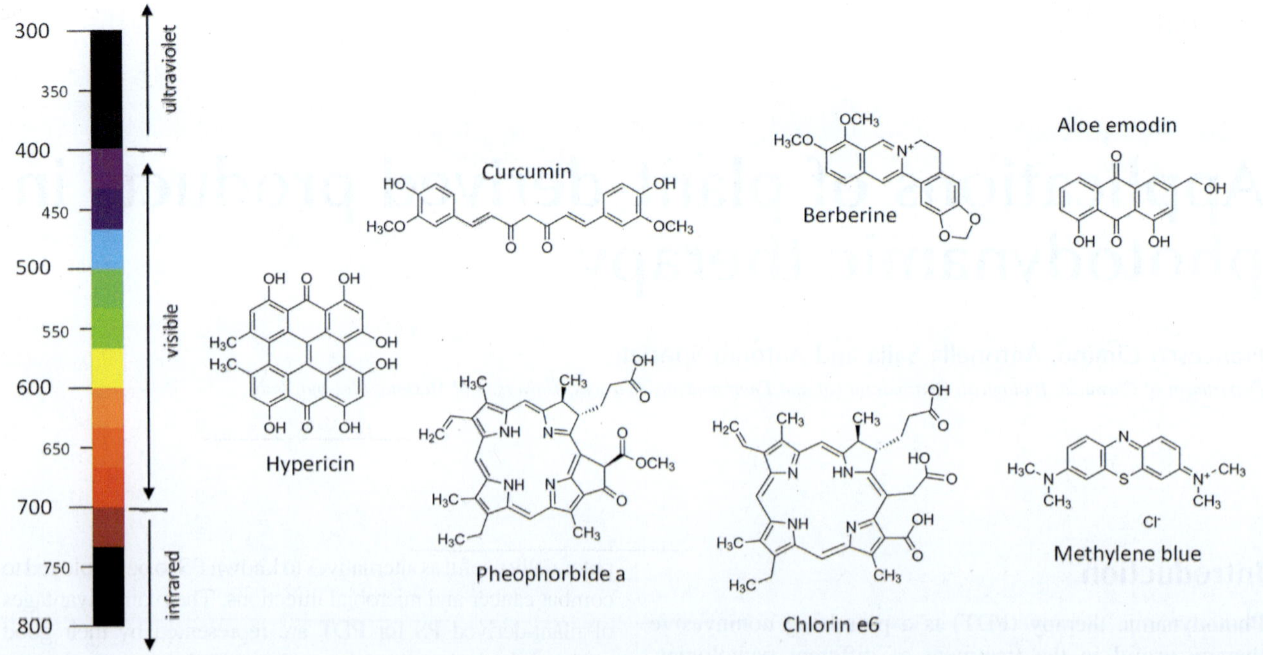

FIGURE 13.1 Chemical structures of the main plant-derived PSs investigated for cancer PDT and aPDT with ranges of irradiation wavelengths used for their activation. Aloe-emodin, 380–500 nm; berberine, 405–447 nm; chlorin e6, 690 nm; curcumin, 405–485 nm; hypericin, 530–620 nm; methylene blue, 660 nm; pheophorbide a, 610–690 nm.

Thiophenes (compounds formed by heterocyclic aromatic rings made up of one sulfur and four carbon atoms) are secondary metabolites derived from plants belonging to the *Asteraceae* family. Alkaloids, a diverse secondary metabolites group from higher plants, contain a heterocyclic structure with a nitrogen atom in the ring. Nitrogen-containing alkaloids are normally photoactive in nature; in particular, berberine (BBR) is a significant isoquinoline alkaloid found in several plant families such as *Annonaceae, Papaveraceae, Berberidaceae, Juglandaceae, Magnoliaceae, Ranunculaceae* and *Rutaceae*. Anthraquinones are the largest group among natural quinones from higher plants and include several hundred compounds, such as purpurin, aloe emodin, and hypericin (HY) (Fig. 13.1). Purpurin (1,2,4-trihydroxyanthraquinone) is a polyketide derivative of the 9,10-anthracenedione ring, mostly isolated from the roots of the perennial herb *Rubia cordifolia*. Aloe emodin (AEm) (1,8-dihydroxy-3-hydroxyl-methylanthraquinone) is the main bioactive component of *Rheum palmatum* (rhubarb) and *Aloe vera*, while emodin (1,3,8-trihydroxy-6-methylanthraquinone) is present in a wide range of higher plant taxa, including those from the *Rhamnaceae*, *Polygonaceae*, *Fabaceae* and *Asteraceae* families. The naphthodianthrone HY (4,5,7,4′,5′,7′-hexahydroxy-2,2-dimethylnaphtodi anthrone) is a well-known natural PS found in some plant species of the genus *Hypericum,* especially *Hypericum perforatum* L. (Fig. 13.1).

The purpose of this chapter was to provide an updated review of the state-of-the-art research conducted in the last decade on the potential applications of plant-derived products in PDT both for the treatment of neoplastic pathologies and for the inactivation of infectious disease-related pathogens.

Photodynamic therapy

As said before, the main components of PDT include a PS, molecular oxygen, and light irradiation. More exactly, PDT consists of the administration of a PS combined with light irradiation with proper wavelength in the presence of oxygen [8–11] generating singlet oxygen ($^1O_2$), and cytotoxic reactive species accumulation that in turn causes damage to biomolecules. Generally, the efficacy of PDT depends on PS type, dosage, light source and fluence rate, and time exposure. The choice of light source is commonly based on PS nature and absorption spectra, as well as on the characteristics of the targets [1]. The success of clinical practice of PDT relies also on the appropriate light delivery and sufficient PS and oxygen concentration in the target tissue [12,13], as well as the light sources (usually lasers or light emitting diodes [LEDs]) and delivery devices (optical fibers) [14].

A photopharmacological effect is always triggered by energy decay. Fluorescence and phosphorescence are common examples of decay, but these do not produce biological effects. Besides the formation of a PS conformational isomer and the initiation of a photochemical reaction of the PS, there are two more relevant forms of photopharmaceutical decay, which are the formation of PS-radical, and the formation of singlet oxygen.

The photophysical processes involved in PDT are illustrated in the Jablonski-diagram reported in Fig. 13.2. Starting with a PS in its energetically lowest state (the ground state, GS), the absorption of light yields an excited form of the PS. Several excited states occur higher up the PS's GS, and the change in energetic level differs on the light energy absorbed.

Irradiating PS with appropriate wavelengths of light produces changes from its singlet GS (S0) to the short-lived first excited singlet-state (S1), and the transferred energy can be released as fluorescence or by internal conversion returning to S0 state. Otherwise, the S1 PS can also be switched to the relatively long-lived first excited triplet state (T1) by intersystem crossing and coming back to S0 by emitting phosphorescence. However, during this step, the energy can be transferred to biological molecules or molecular oxygen producing reactive oxygen species (ROS) and then biomolecules damages [15].

Two types of photochemical pathways are proposed. In the type I reaction, the triplet-state PS can react directly with an organic molecule or substrate that can donate an electron to PS producing a radical anion or cation. Even if this process occurs under hypoxic conditions (typical in the inner center of tumor tissues), in presence of oxygen, a radical cascade involves ROS so producing reactive hydroxyl ($HO^{\cdot}$) and the superoxide anion radicals ($O_2^{\cdot}$) [11,16]. Conversely, in the type II reactions, energy is transferred from T1 PS to molecular oxygen producing singlet oxygen as the main cytotoxic agent in PDT (Fig. 13.2). Since singlet oxygen lifetime is short (4 μs in water) [17], its generation site is important for PDT outcome. Additionally, a modified type I (MTO) mechanism has been suggested, paralleled to type I and II, where T1 PS interacts directly with available free radicals [18]. The effects of PDT are circumscribed to the site of free radical production since their short half-life (10–300 ns) and a small diffusion distance (around 10–55 nm) [19]. However, among the three mechanisms discussed, the type II is proposed as the main and clinically most important pathway involved in PDT [20] also because PS works as catalyst and generally is not rapidly degenerated.

Blue, red, and infrared are the most common light sources in PDT. UV or blue light can excite the molecule into higher energetic states than any red light can, since the shorter the wave, the higher the energy. Furthermore, the wavelengths below 800 nm are mostly used in PDT than higher wavelengths (above 800 nm), which are lacking photodynamic reactions. Conversely, blue light penetrates the tissue less than red and infrared lights. In fact,

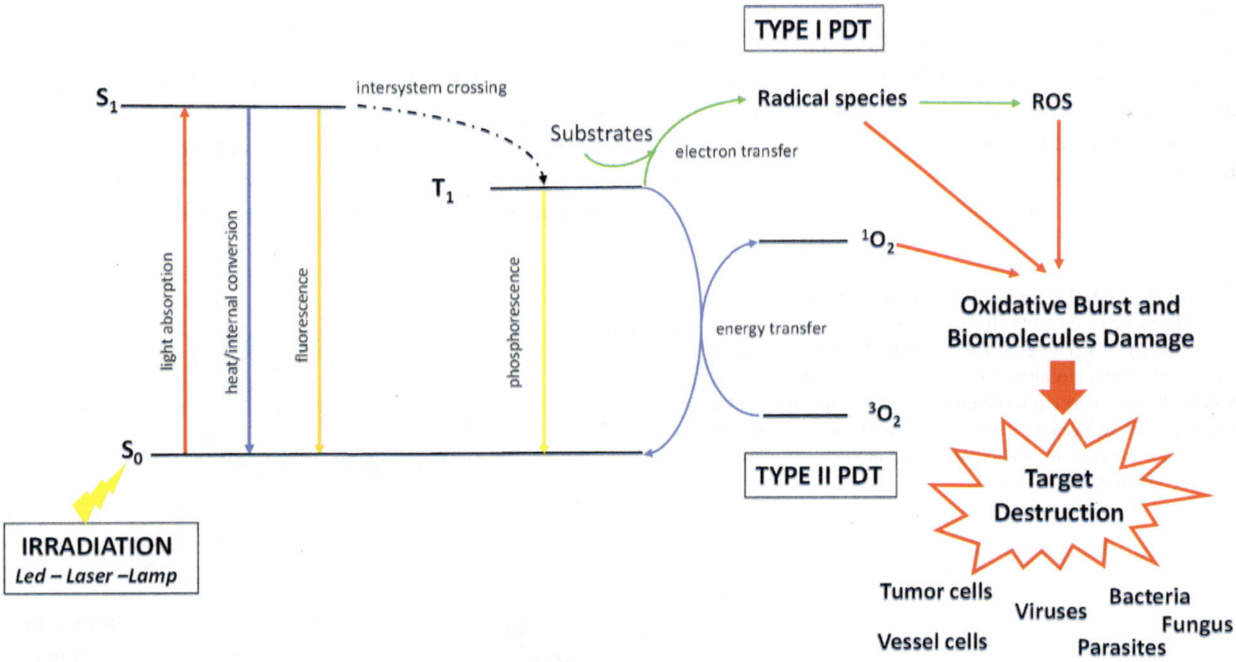

FIGURE 13.2 Jablonski-diagram reporting the photophysical processes involved in PDT. Exposure to light with appropriate wavelength activates the PS from its singlet ground state (S0) to the short-lived first excited singlet-state (S1). Then, it can return to the S0-state by emitting the absorbed energy as fluorescence or by internal conversion. Alternatively, it can convert to the relatively long-lived first excited triplet state (T1) by intersystem crossing, and then return to the S0-state by emitting phosphorescence. However, energy transfer from T1 to biological substrates (type I reactions) or molecular oxygen (type II reactions) generates ROS, which produce biomolecules damages.

penetration of light through tissue is highly complex since light is either dispersed or absorbed when it enters tissue, depending on tissue type and light wavelength. The "phototherapeutic window" wavelength range (600–850 nm) is the one most used in conventional PDT, due to the absorption of lower wavelength light by the important endogenous chromophores (adenine and dihydronicotinamide in the reduced form of nicotinamide adenine dinucleotide [NADH], collagen, lipopigments, deoxyhemoglobin, flavins, and melanin), the reduced light scattering at longer wavelengths, and the absorption of wavelengths greater than 1300 nm [11,21,22].

Main criteria for ideal PS should include some important aspects [11,23–27]. Firstly, PS should possess a high extinction coefficient at the selected absorption wavelength. In particular, longer wavelengths are useful when higher tissue penetration, and minimum light scattering is required; inversely, the range of 400–420 nm is suitable for superficial treatment disorders. Additionally, PS should be stable in solution, and in serum or plasma, it should possess good photochemical reactivity with high yields and long lifetime of triplet state, free radical production efficiency, reduced dark toxicity, organism or cell type specificity, and last but not least, it should have a good bioavailability.

Cancer and PDT

Cancer is a leading cause of death worldwide [28,29] characterized by uncontrolled growth and proliferation of cells due to an accumulation of genetic alterations. Actual therapy includes surgery, radiotherapy, and chemotherapy that can also be combined to improve efficacy and resistance. However, chemotherapy is often limited due to a lower selectivity of available drugs toward cancer cells. For this reason, new strategies need to be developed to improve target selectivity of anticancer drugs.

PDT's cancer cell death mechanism is started after the activation of administrated PS using a specific light wavelength and may occur in three main pathways: apoptosis, necrosis, and autophagy [30,31] (Fig. 13.3). Along with the direct cellular toxicity, other mechanisms such as vascular shutdown and local inflammatory reactions contribute to the effects of PDT [32–35] (Fig. 13.3). In fact, after PS administration, it can favorably accumulate in tumor tissues during the drug-to-light interval (DLI) [36]. High DLI allows optimal redistribution of the PS in cellular compartments (cellular-PDT), while lower DLI mainly targets tumor vasculature (vascular-PDT) [37,38].

PS is transported bound to circulating cells in the blood and reaches organ or tumor by diffusion throughout the parenchyma [10]. However, PS accumulates mainly in cancer tissue, not affecting healthy tissues [39], through mechanisms that are not fully understood. One potential mechanism involves low-density lipoproteins (LDL) [2] since PS combines mainly with these transporters. In fact, LDL supply cholesterol for membrane production especially in rapidly dividing cancer cells so improving PS uptake. Additionally, cells with augmented mitotic activity showed increased expression of LDL receptor on their surface playing an important role in PS delivery to cancer tissue [11,40,41].

Additional hypothesis involves the lipophilic nature of some anionic PS that become neutrally charged in tumor environment characterized by low pH producing a trapping effect [10].

Ultimately, PDT selective illumination of the target tissue with light allows a definite site of action reducing the undesired effects in the healthy tissues.

The efficacy of PDT-induced cell death is affected by different conditions such as subcellular localization and bioavailability. In particular, lipophilic PS accumulate

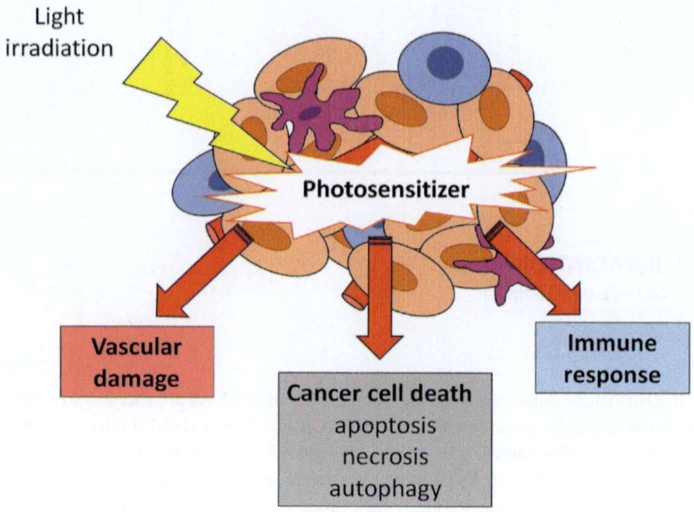

FIGURE 13.3 Mechanisms of PDT-induced anticancer activity. The PDT-induced modes of cell death include apoptosis, necrosis, and autophagy, depending on the cell type, PS type or concentration, intracellular localization, light dose, and oxygen partial pressure. PS can induce immunogenic cell death mediated by the antigenicity of dying/dead cancer cells. Additionally, PDT can damage blood vessels in tumors inducing morphological changes of vessel and hypoxia.

mainly in the membranes of the cellular organelles, such as the endoplasmic reticulum, Golgi apparatus, and mitochondria; inversely, hydrophilic PS accumulation involves the endocytic pathway [35].

However, one important limit of PDT is represented by the low concentration of molecular oxygen in tumor tissues [42]. Many solid cancers showed hypoxic conditions due to altered microcirculation and aberrant tumor propagation [43,44]. Furthermore, tumor hypoxia promotes metastasis and increases resistance to the ROS-generated PDT [45].

Antimicrobial photodynamic therapy

Antibiotics have the potential to combat infectious diseases; however, their efficacy in therapy of infectious diseases is challenged by the emergence of multidrug-resistant (MDR) pathogens. Antimicrobial resistance (AMR) occurring in bacteria, viruses, fungi, and parasites is considered a global health problem and announced by the World Health Organization (WHO) as one of the top 10 worldwide health threats facing human beings. The misuse of antimicrobials makes almost all disease-causing microorganisms resistant to drugs used to treat them [46].

aPTD is suggested as a good alternative due to the broad-spectrum action affecting a broad range of microorganisms such as bacteria, yeasts, fungi, and parasitic protozoa, as well as viruses. Interestingly, independently of their drug-resistance profiles, many MDR bacteria are sensitive to aPDT [3,47] (Fig. 13.4).

The efficacy of aPDT usually is related to the type and concentration of PS and the microorganism targeted [48–50]. In particular, the Gram-positive bacteria present a layer of only peptidoglycan and lipoteichoic acid that is relatively permeable; on the contrary, Gram-negative bacteria possess a more complex cell wall structure, comparatively nonporous, with an inner cytoplasmic membrane and an outer membrane separated by the peptidoglycan-containing periplasm. Fungi have an intermediate permeability between these two classes of bacteria. Besides this, cysts formed by protozoa also represent challenging targets.

Although the broad spectrum of action, aPTD is selective for microbial cells, causing low toxicity to host cells, thanks to the faster binding of PS to the microbial membranes compared to host cells due to the greater affinity of PS to the microorganism [51].

aPDT produces ROS that in turn impairs microbial biomolecules inducing microbe growth inhibition and death [52,53]; the antimicrobial activity of aPDT can be obtained against planktonic cells and/or biofilms growing microorganisms. The proposed antimicrobial mechanisms of aPDT involve interaction with the external structures, i.e., cell wall, cell membrane, or virus capsid and envelope, leakage of cellular components or inactivation of membrane transport systems and enzymes and/or damage to DNA [3]. Additionally, internalized PS can also induce intracellular oxidative damage [3].

Assumed the multitargeted properties of aPDT, it is supposed that the resistance development is extremely limited [54]. However, although rarely and still contained, it has been reported that microbes can adapt and escape to this therapy [52,53,55].

Furthermore, the time required to aPDT to kill the microorganism is very short, about a few seconds, while antimicrobial drugs need few hours up to days to induce their effects [56]. Additionally, the selective illumination of the target site reduces the undesired effects on host tissues [57].

Plant-derived products in anticancer PDT

Plant drugs used as PS in anticancer PDT

Many phototoxic constituents were reported in various plant species that have been shown to be equally effective as of conventional PS. For these reasons, natural

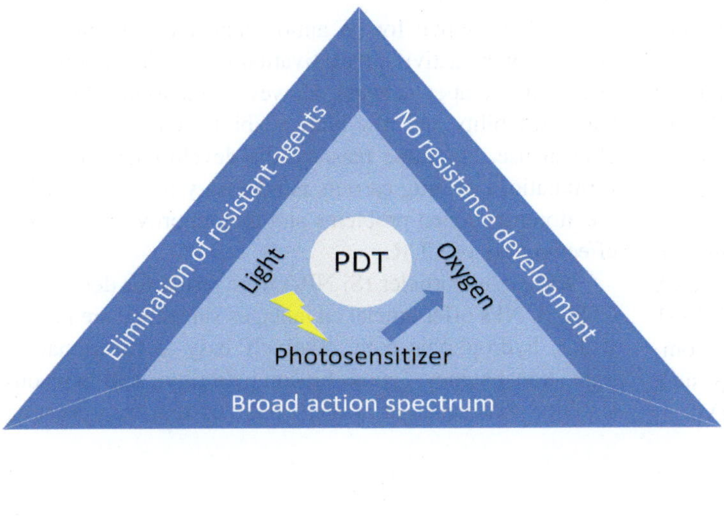

FIGURE 13.4 Advantages of antimicrobial photodynamic therapy (aPDT). aPTD has a broad spectrum of action and can kill a wide range of microbes such as bacteria, fungi and protozoa, as well as inactivate viruses. Interestingly, major multidrug-resistant bacteria are sensitive to aPDT, irrespective of their drug resistance profiles. Furthermore, given the multi-target nature of aPDT, it is assumed that the possibility for microorganisms to develop resistance is very limited.

compounds with photosensitizing abilities can be isolated from plants and used as alternatives for conventional PS in PDT. Furthermore, combinations of PDT with other approaches, such as chemotherapy, radiotherapy, immunotherapy, or even phytotherapy, could represent a useful strategy against various types of cancer. In fact, compared to the single one, combination therapies can reduce side effects and can efficiently reduce cancer cell proliferation. Additionally, combination therapies can improve the drug uptake into the cancer cells and tumors, improving anticancer therapy response. For all these reasons, PDT combination therapy can be a promising and useful approach to overcome drug-resistant tumors while reducing adverse effect [58].

However, problems due to lack of selectivity, poor water-solubility, photosensitivity, and potential toxic effects on healthy tissues reduce clinical utility of PDT approaches. Recently, new emerging drug delivery targeted approaches have been developed able to overcome these issues improving the delivery of PSs to tumor tissues, the specificity, and the efficiency.

HY is a promising plant-based PS, thanks to its photosensitizing properties, tumoritropic migratory characteristics, and low cytotoxicity [59,60]. HY can diffuse into tumor cells via endocytosis, and it localizes in various cellular or subcellular regions. However, the PDT efficacy of HY may be compromised due to lower HY intracellular concentration, irradiation conditions, cell type, and the oxygen pressure in it. Additionally, PDT with HY is also able to induce molecular responses that support tumor survival and regrowth with development of resistance, or activation of repair mechanisms or drug efflux transporters in different in vitro models (Caco-2 and HT-29) [61]. Additionally, studies demonstrated that low-dose HY-PDT induces drug resistance as demonstrated in a fractionated light regime with a longer dark period [62]. For all these reasons, ideal conditions need to be established in order to make HY-PDT safe and effective.

Šemeláková et al. tested **HY** effects using HT-29 and HCT-116 human colorectal carcinoma cells irradiated with suboptimal low-dose PDT (530−620 nm) at 50 and 30 nM, respectively [63]. Low dose of HY-PDT showed no significant proapoptotic effects in HT-29 cells, while altered cellular morphology and caspase-3 activation in HCT-116 cells were observed confirming different sensitivity of cell lines to PDT. Additionally, HY-PDT induced accumulation of cells in the S-phase, mostly at the expense of the G1/G0. However, low-dose HY-PDT reduced clonogenic survival and increased ROS in HT-29 cells although induced mRNA level of MMP-2 and -9. Interestingly, low-dose HY-PDT induced apoptosis in combination with bioactive compounds naturally occurring in plants of *Hypericum* spp. such as hyperforin or its stable derivative aristoforin at 5 μM.

Another requirement of a successful HY-PDT is a sufficient intracellular concentration that can be affected by drug efflux transporters. Jendželovský and coworkers tested the modulations of HY intracellular content by some of the well-known membrane drug efflux proteins in the effectiveness of HY-PDT using human leukemia cell lines with different levels of MDR and resistance-associated proteins (MRP) and breast cancer resistance protein (BCRP) [64]. The authors demonstrated that the efflux of HY from cancer cells exerted by BCRP is the first key step in affecting HY cellular accumulation and HY-PDT efficacy. HY (10−100 nM) treatment and light activation (530−620 nm) induced cells death and caspase-3 in MDR1 and MRP1 overexpressed cells starting from 50 nM. Inversely, BCRP overexpression protected human leukemia cells from HY-PDT-induced cytotoxicity and proapoptotic effects confirming that HY is a substrate of BCRP so contributing to cancer drug resistance.

The nanotechnology use in PDT has flagged new opportunities for cancer treatment and has developed great potential in recent era [65]. Nanoparticles (NPs) drug delivery systems have attracted great attention, thanks to their biocompatibility, low toxicity, ability to overcome biological barriers, and versatility in delivering different drugs. The incorporation of NPs with PS can increase PS water solubility, protect them from undesirable degradation, and finally enhance tissue targeting improving pharmacokinetic parameters of PDT.

Magnetic drug targeting (MDT) is one of the most promising approaches in cancer therapy since the selective accumulation of the particles is manipulated by external magnetic fields to reach the target area. Superparamagnetic iron oxide nanoparticles (SPIONs) with an HY-linked functionalized dextran coating were prepared and tested in human T-cell leukemia Jurkat cells following irradiation with LED white light [66]. Drug-loaded particles induced cell death in a concentration and exposure time-dependent manner, and this effect was associated to ROS production supporting the potential role of combined MDT and PDT for cancer therapy.

CUR is known for its antioxidant, anti-inflammatory, and anticancer activity. Its activation with light empowers it as a phototherapeutic agent. However, due to the very poor water solubility and low bioavailability, CUR has limited clinical use. For these reasons, the development of stable formulations of drug carriers is necessary in order to solve the aforementioned problems and then improve therapeutic effectiveness of CUR.

Silica nanoparticles (Si NPs) were tested for delivery of CUR. Si NPs offer crucial advantages since they are porous with a hydrophobic core, relatively easy to functionalize, light transparency, good biocompatibility, and aqueous stability. Ghazaelan et al. demonstrated that incorporating

CUR with Si NPs increased CUR solubility. CUR-Si NPs induced cytotoxicity in human melanoma cancer A375 cells after PDT with blue light irradiation (465 nm) [67]. CUR-Si NPs associated to PDT were effective in a dose-dependent way in cancer cells (but not in normal fibroblasts), producing growth inhibition and apoptosis through ROS generation.

Similarly, Sing and coworkers tested phototoxicity (blue light 420 nm) of CUR-Si NPs in tumor spheroids of Nt-8e oral cancer cells which mimic avascular tumors [68]. These CUR-Si NPs showed higher uptake in spheroids compared to free CUR, thanks to their negative surface potential and probably via endocytosis cellular internalization. Spheroids treated with CUR-Si NPs complex and light showed larger inhibition in growth and migration of cells and enhanced ROS generation as compared to spheroids treated with free CUR under similar conditions. However, big spheroids showed lower CUR uptake compared to the small ones; this was consistent with lower dark toxicity and higher resistance to photodynamic damage exhibited by big spheroids as compared to the small spheroids. Additionally, since the phototoxicity of CUR requires oxygen for ROS generation, the different effects were associated also to hypoxic region generated by big spheroids. Involvement of ROS was also confirmed by the authors since exposing spheroids to glutathione (GSH) reduced CUR-Si NPs phototoxicity. Compared to free CUR that induced apoptosis following PDT, CUR-Si NPs induced cell necrosis probably through the release of lytic enzymes from lysosomes where they mainly accumulate.

Lipid formulations are proposed as an alternative strategy to improve the effect of PS in PDT. For example, pegylated liposomes (Plip) exhibit longer circulation time among all drug delivery systems. CUR encapsulated in liposomes composed from hydrogenated soy phosphatidylcholine (HSPC) exhibited higher stability and cellular uptake [69]. CUR showed significant phototoxicity after blue light low irradiation (380–500 nm) compared to the free compound in melanoma MUG-Mel2 and squamous cell carcinoma SCC-25. This is mainly due to different cellular uptake since free CUR interacts with outer cellular membrane, while liposomes enter the cell through an endosomal route with improved CUR bioavailability. CUR Plip PDT induced early and late apoptosis via increased proapoptotic Bax protein expression and reduced cancer cell migration contributing to malignant cell metastasis inhibition. Interestingly, these effects were not observed in normal HaCaT human epidermal keratinocytes.

Another system able to overcome CUR limitations is represented by polymeric NPs. Poly(lactic-co-glycolic acid) (PLGA) is a biocompatible and biodegradable polymer widely used for production of NPs able to offer continuous in vitro release of encapsulated drug for long periods of time. PLGA CUR NPs were prepared and tested for PDT (457 nm) in human ovarian adenocarcinoma cell line SK-OV-3 [70]. PLGA CUR NPs showed improved physicochemical properties compared to free CUR. PLGA CUR NPs following PDT induced nuclear damage probably via ROS production, while free CUR was unable to exert toxic effects. As previously discussed, irradiation affects membrane integrity, and this improved free CUR uptake by diffusion without showing PDT effects.

However, although many studies reported the involvement of ROS in the phototoxicity of CUR and other PS, Paunovic et al. demonstrated a different mechanism for CUR involving specific molecular proapoptotic pathways [71]. CUR NPs, prepared by tetrahydrofuran/water solvent exchange, exposed to blue light (470 nm) exerted phototoxicity in B16 mouse melanoma, H460 human lung cancer, and U251 human glioma cell lines. In the latter cell line, the most sensitive to CUR phototoxicity, the involvement of JNK in mitochondria-dependent apoptosis was demonstrated inducing a significant loss of mitochondrial membrane potential after 15 min of treatment. The activated JNK, in fact, translocates to mitochondria and modulates the activity of Bcl2 proapoptotic protein. Interestingly, neither oxidative stress nor ROS production was observed, and the effects of CUR NPs PDT were not reverted by reference antioxidant compounds in U251 cells. Furthermore, the authors suggest that blue light irradiation improves the cellular uptake of CUR NPs since CUR NPs alone were not found in treated U251 cells not exposed to blue light.

Other systems have been studied to overcome solubility and bioavailability problems of CUR. Among these, metal-based complexes have been proposed as a new emerging class of PDT agents. These metal complexes are useful not only for ligating the metal to various chromophores but also for their intrinsic PS properties since can offer many more excited-state electronic configurations depending on metal used. These complexes are stable in human plasma, photostable upon continuous LED irradiation, and absorb in the red region of the spectrum that has greater tissue penetration. Hosseinzadeh et al. tested CUR complexes with cerium ions, to improve the solubility and stability of CUR. These authors demonstrated that CUR alone was not able to induce cytotoxicity after blue light irradiation (465 nm) in A375 human malignant melanoma and MDA-MB-231 breast cancer cell lines up to 200 μg/mL [72]. Conversely CUR–cerium complexes following PDT improved efficacy starting from 10 to 25 μg/mL in both cancer cells. Additionally, cells treatment with CUR–cerium complexes before PDT induced marked nuclear condensation and fragmentation like also apoptotic bodies compared to free CUR. Although Hosseinzadeh and coworkers further confirmed the role of drug delivery systems, they proved also that preexposure (before cerium-CUR complexes) to red light (660 nm) induced cell death, suggesting that light affects membrane potential of cells and mitochondria and then CUR uptake. Interestingly, pretreatment by red light did not show any effect on free CUR treatment.

Banerjee et al. tested a new transition metal complex based on oxovanadium(IV) with CUR in order to improve its bioavailability [73]. In addition, to increase the aqueous solubility and cellular uptake of the complexes, the authors derivatized the OH groups of CUR by glucose before complexing with oxovanadium(IV). The carbohydrate attached complexes were better internalized compared to the noncarbohydrate analogues, probably due to higher rate of glucose uptake of cancer cells. Furthermore, the complexes showed significant photocytotoxicity in visible light (400–700 nm) showing DNA cleavage activity by generating ROS in HaCaT, HeLa, and MCF-7 cells.

Recently, layered double hydroxides (LDH), also called anionic nanoclays, have been developed as nano-drug delivery systems; they are based on a network of divalent and trivalent metal cations crosslinked with hydroxide anions and contain charge balancing interlayer anions. Thanks to its biocompatibility and biodegradability, distinctive anionic exchange property and pH-dependent drug release property in acidic environments, typical of cancer tissues, CUR intercalation with LDH has been tested following PDT (blue LED, 465 nm) in MDA-MB-231 human breast cancer cell line [74]. CUR-LDH following PDT induced cells death in a dose-dependent way confirming photodynamic activities compared to free CUR. In another paper, the same authors characterized the mechanisms of in vitro phototoxicity of this nanosystem [75]. CUR-LDH (25 and 100 μg/mL) followed by PDT induced autophagy, apoptosis, and G0/G1 cell cycle arrest, and these effects were associated to ROS production in MDA-MB-231 cancer cells.

Chls have appeared as attractive alternative PDT sensitizers although they are rapidly degraded when exposed to light outside of their native and protective environment. For this reason, the use of proper drug delivery systems has been implemented in order to overcome Chls clinical limitations.

Plasmonic Au NPs have been proposed as nanocarriers able to deliver drugs to the target area. These systems can be easily functionalized with therapeutic agents through covalent, noncovalent, and intermolecular interactions. Additionally, the use of noble metal NPs as photothermal agents has received much attention since they showed antitumor capability via photothermal effect. Combining PDT with other phototherapies such as photothermal therapy (PTT) demonstrates great potential to overcome the limitations of each method improving the treatment efficacy. PTT was reported to increase blood flow which would carry oxygen to the hypoxic tumor and improve permeability that in turn increase penetration of PS into the tumor.

Chl b-Au Nanocomplexes (NCs) were tested for the PDT following diode-pumped solid-state (DPSS) laser (650 nm) in HepG2 and MCF7 cells [76]. Chl b-Au NCs PDT reduced cell growth in both cell lines although an improved inhibitory effect was observed in MCF-7. On the contrary, testing PTT using a green laser (532 nm), falling in the plasmon band of Au NPs, induced some inhibition only at higher concentrations confirming high efficiency of PDT versus PTT.

Effective sources of Chls from vegetable extracts have been investigated in order to obtain formulations able to overcome stability and pharmacokinetic problems.

Pan et al. prepared a polymer hydrogel shell in situ on tumor Hela cells by the photopolymerization of poly (ethylene glycol) double acrylates (PEGDA) and a *Spinacia oleracea* L. extract (SOLE), which is a mixture containing Chls, under near infrared (NIR) irradiation [77]. PEGDA hydrogel is a highly biocompatible hydrogel since its hydrophilic ethylene oxide segments are nontoxic to cells; besides to be a photoinitiator, SOLE is a natural PS for cancer PDT. SOLE within the hydrogel affected Hela cells viability following irradiation (660 nm), while no significant difference in Chinese Hamster Ovary (CHO) control cells was observed. This effect was associated to ROS production since, under laser irradiation, SOLE induced the generation of $^1O_2$ probably by excitation energy transfer from triplet chlorophylls to molecular oxygen. However, $^1O_2$ production was reduced by ~12% and ~68% when the light was blocked by pig skin tissues with thicknesses of 2 and 6 mm, respectively. Interestingly, this thin and semitransparent shell formed on the Hela cells has the double advantage to retain the PS around the tumor cell producing a higher $^1O_2$ concentration and to prevent its rapid diffusion to normal tissue.

Similarly, an amaranth extract (AE) rich in chlorophyll derivatives was tested for PDT using a new composite hydrogel containing reduced graphene oxide (rGO) and gold NPs (AuNPs) [78]; this hydrogel is projected to form a shell on in situ cancer cells and to combine the efficacy of PTT and PDT. rGO represents a good support for self-assembly of supramolecular hydrogels, while AuNPs were homodispersed in the hydrogel giving an improved photothermal property. AE worked as both a reductant and cross-linking agent as well as PS. Following NIR irradiation (808 nm NIR laser) AE improved photothermal efficiency of rGO and AuNPs. At the same extent, data demonstrated that AuNPs and rGO have a synergistic effect on accelerating the generation of $^1O_2$ from AE following NIR irradiation at 660 nm. GO/AE/AuNPs showed extremely higher anticancer efficiency following NIR irradiation in HeLa cells than single precursors rGO/AE or AE at each concentration.

Cluster-structured NPs (CNPs) were prepared from Fe_3O_4 nanocrystals along with a chlorophyll-Fe(II)

(Fe_3O_4@Chl/Fe) and functionalized with 4-carboxyphenylboronic acid (CPBA) to improve cellular internalization targeting glycoproteins on cancer cells. These CNPs were tested for PDT and chemodynamic therapy (CDT) adjuvant [79]. Fe-based CNP induced ROS by CDT mediated Fenton like reactions improving PDT effects. In particular, Fe_3O_4@Chl/Fe CNPs induced phototoxicity following PDT (660 nm LED light), and this effect was improved by CPBA functionalization in human bladder carcinoma cells (T24). Additionally, CDT−PDT combination therapy significantly reduced tumor growth and increased the survival rate of orthotopic MB49-bearing mice inducing an immunostimulatory microenvironment downregulating Programmed Cell Death Ligand 1 (PD-L1) pathway.

There are many chlorophyll metabolites known for their activity and selectivity as PS. Pyropheophorbide a (PPa), a degradation product of chlorophyll widely present in nature, is considered a highly potent PS [80]. PPa was reported as endowed with anticancer activity. PPa PDT (quartz-halogen lamp filter cut-on 610 nm) induced cytotoxicity on human breast tumor MCF-7 cells in a dose-dependent way. However, these effects were also observed in normal human mammary epithelial cells so limiting its potential use in PDT without protecting other normal tissue from illumination [81]. PPa PDT induced apoptosis in MCF-7 cells was confirmed by mitochondrial membrane permeabilization, cytochrome *c* release, caspase 9 activation, and then DNA fragmentation, and these effects were associated to dose-dependent ROS production. Additionally, an accumulation of cells in the G2/M phase versus G1 was observed through the dose-dependent increase in p53 level and decrease in p21. In vivo single dose of PPa i.v. following irradiation (laser light 675 nm) reduced MCF-7 cell growth in a xenograft nude mice model, although a slight tumor regrowth was observed after 9 days.

In order to improve its solubility, PPa was loaded in liposomes based on dipalmitoylphosphatidylcholine (DPPC), cholesterol, and 1,2-distearoyl-sn-glycero-3-phosphoethanolamine-N-PEG_{5k} [DSPE-$mPEG_{5k}$] [80]. PPa liposomes were efficiently internalized, probably via endocytosis, in 4T1 murine breast cancer cells. Under laser irradiation (690 nm), PPa liposomes induced significant phototoxicity on 4T1 murine breast cancer cells. Additionally, they induced ROS generation and destroyed lysosomal membrane structure inducing apoptosis. In vivo data confirmed previous observation since intravenous PPa liposomes plus laser irradiation remarkably inhibited tumor growth in Balb/c mice bearing 4T1 tumors without affecting normal organs.

Pu-18, another degradation product of chlorophyll, induced high cytotoxic effects on 2D 4T1 breast cancer cells following PDT (630 nm), while a reduced efficiency was observed in 3D 4T1 spheroids (irradiated at 630 nm light) probably due to limited penetration depth [82]. Pu-18 was distributed mainly in lysosomes and produced ROS following irradiation that in turn induced apoptosis via lysosomal and mitochondrial damage. Using an in vivo 4T1 breast cancer xenograft female Balb/c mice model, after intratumoral administration, Pu-18 retains into cancer cells for 4 days and following PDT (660-nm laser light) a reduction of tumor growth and weight was observed.

However, due to Pu-18 hydrophobicity, aggregation and preferential localization in lipid vesicles and lysosomes were observed. Additionally, PDT quickly induces Pu-18 degradation into less active compounds. For all these reasons, drug delivery systems can overcome Pu-18 limitations improving pharmacokinetic profile and effectiveness.

So, in order to increase Pu-18 bioavailability, solid lipid NPs (SLNs) were tested as lipid-based drug delivery system providing better absorption through biological barriers, extended blood half-life and decreased liver first-pass metabolism [83]. Pu-18 was entrapped in a lipid matrix via the preparation of an oil-in-water phase, using lauric acid (LA), palmitic acid (PA), or glycerol monostearate (GMS). GMS provided the smallest, most homogeneous, and most stable NPs, suggesting that longer-carbon-chain lipids had a higher affinity for Pu-18. All the formulations of Pu-18-loaded SLNs following PDT (LED light 418 nm) induced phototoxicity in HeLa cells, better for GMS NPs, and this effect was improved compared to pure Pu-18. On the contrary, in A549 cells, no differences were observed between lipid NP formulations and pure Pu-18 providing support for cell type-dependent of these formulations.

Another important natural PS for PDT is represented by BBR, which possesses a range of pharmacological properties including anticancer activities. Its advantages are represented by easy production and low cost even if BBR showed toxicity and poor water solubility that limit its clinical use. BBR mechanisms involved in PDT include electron transfers producing free radicals and energy transfer generating $^1O_2$.

An alkaloidal protoberberine fraction (BBR-F) from *Chelidonium majus* L., consisting of BBR, coptisine, and in minimal amount stylopine, dihydroberberine, and N-methylstylopine, was tested for PDT on cervical carcinoma cells (HeLa and C33A) that are respectively positive and negative for integrated human papilloma virus (HPV) DNA [84]. Following irradiation (LED 405 nm), BBR-F did not affect cell viability of normal human fibroblast control cells while induced cellular toxicity in both cancer cell lines, through ROS generation and then loss of mitochondrial membrane integrity and caspase activation. However, HPV-negative C33A cells were more susceptible to BBR-F PDT.

Protoberberine alkaloids such as BBR, jatrorrhizine and coralyne confirmed phototoxicity following ultraviolet A

(UVA) exposure (wavelength >360 nm) in human lung carcinoma (A549), skin carcinoma (A431), and human osteosarcoma (U2-OS) cell lines while the compounds alone were practically ineffective [85]. Interestingly, while BBR PDT-induced apoptosis was associated to ROS generation and mitochondrial membrane permeabilization, coralyne revealed an O_2-independent mechanism. Since N-acetyl-L-cysteine, a known antioxidant, was able to revert the effects of BBR only. Data showed that coralyne following UVA induced DNA damage generating double strand breaks in A549 cells with an apoptosis-independent mechanism and the effect was mediated by replication machinery.

Liu et al. demonstrated also the in vitro antiproliferative and proapoptotic effects of BBR-PDT (laser light 405 nm) on HeLa cells like also in glioma U-118 MG, U-251 MG cells and immortalized HaCaT keratinocytes [86]. The nude mouse HeLa xenograft female BALB/c mice model confirmed the in vitro effects with a tumor size reduction in BBR-PDT group compared to control one. At molecular level, BBR-PDT inhibited activation of the phosphoinositide 3-kinases (PI3K)-protein kinase B (PKB)-mammalian target of rapamycin (mTOR) pathway, and the phosphorylation of p70s6K and rps6 in HeLa cells, and this effect was stronger compared to BBR treatment. Since the PI3K-PKB-mTOR pathway, vital for growth and survival of cancer cells, is inhibited by ROS, the involvement of $^1O_2$ was supposed.

At the same extent, BBR following light irradiation (447 nm) reduced cell viability in human renal carcinoma cells (ACHN, 786-O) and human immortalized renal tubular epithelial cells (HK-2) inducing ROS generation, autophagy, and apoptosis, and these effects were not observed in the dark [87]. Additionally, BBR associated with PDT triggered metabolites changes, such as lysine, formate and lactate levels, related to inhibition of cell proliferation, migration, and angiogenesis respectively. Similarly, Carriero et al. demonstrated BBR-PDT cytotoxic and proapoptotic effects (blue LED source, 447 nm) in high-grade astrocytoma (T98G, U87-MG, U373-MG, and U138-MG) and low-grade pediatric astrocytoma (Res186) cell lines compared to rat normal astrocytes [88].

In order to improve BBR bioavailability, new formulations have been proposed as drug delivery systems. BBR nanoemulsion showed phototoxic effects following laser irradiation (447 nm) in cervical carcinoma cell line (Caski) and, at a lower degree, in immortalized nontumorigenic human skin keratinocytes (HaCaT) [89]. At the same extent, BBR nanoemulsion induced ROS generation better in Caski than in HaCaT cells. Compared to other studies, Floriano et al. were not able to detect caspase-3 activation following BBR-PDT; this effect was instead revealed by other authors using free BBR in the same cell lines and experimental conditions (LED irradiation at 447 nm) [90].

The research by Nowak-Perlak et al. evidenced the phototoxic and anticancerous effects of emodin and AEm on SCC-25 cells (cutaneous squamous cell carcinoma), MUG-Mel2 cells (melanoma) and HaCaT cells (normal skin cells) irradiated with blue light (380–500 nm) [91]. Although emodin and AEm are isomers and differ only in the position of one hydroxyl group, the findings show that both substances affect skin cancer cells and normal keratinocytes in different ways, appearing AEm a more potent growth inhibitor than emodin. Similarly, Liu et al. reported a study on inhibition of human oral squamous cell carcinoma in vitro and in vivo, using AEm mediated PDT [92]. Following irradiation with 405 nm laser light, distinct morphology changes of oral mucosa carcinoma KB cells and inhibition of cell migration were found; cell proliferation block in G1 phase and apoptosis increase were related to massive ROS generation, upregulation of caspase-3 and Bax protein levels, and downregulation of Bcl-2. When tested in vivo in SPF BALB/c-nu nude mice bearing KB tumor, good therapeutic effect, and safety were shown.

Ferroptosis is an iron-dependent programmed cell death modality, that is closely associated with accumulation of intracellular ROS, and thus can effectively enhance the antitumor effects of PDT strongly contributing to disrupt intracellular redox homeostasis. The study from Wu et al. attempted to explore if AEm acts as a PS and activate ferroptosis pathway, due to a specific inhibiting activity to glutathione S-transferase P1 (GSTP1, a key protein for ferroptosis) [93]. AEm@RBC/Fe nanocrystals (NCrs) were prepared to obtain an AEm NCrs (made using poloxamer-407) cores and further modification of red blood cells (RBC) membranes and ferritin (a major intracellular iron storage protein, which can be recognized by tumor cells overexpressing transferrin receptor protein 1 [TfR1]). The presence of ferritin was fundamental to provide both sufficient oxygen for oxygen-dependent and Fe^{3+} for iron-dependent ferroptosis in tumor cells. The efficacy was in vitro demonstrated on human oral squamous carcinoma HSC-3 cells (with over-expressed TfR1 and also transfected to overexpress GSTP1) following irradiation with 405 nm laser. Furthermore, the biomimetization of AEm NCrs with ferritin-decorated RBC membranes facilitated the prolonged circulation and cancer targeting of this nanosystem in vivo in mice bearing HSC-3 tumor. So, the employment of AEm may be useful to achieve a successful combined PDT/ferroptosis synergistic therapy.

AEm-induced PDT was explored also in human gastric cancer cells (SGC-7901) [94]. The AEm and AEm-PDT (with LED light 430 nm) demonstrated a significant inhibition of proliferation of human gastric cancer cells in dose-dependent and energy-dependent manners. Upregulation of caspase-9 and caspase-3 protein levels was also observed, indicating that the mitochondrial pathway may be involved. Another interesting study from Li et al. explored the combined effect of r-caspase-3 gene transfection with PDT on gastric cancer cells using AEm-encapsulated nanoliposomes (based on L-α-phosphatidylcholine/cholesterol), which acted as gene carrier as well as a PS carrier [95]. Nano-AEm-mediated r-caspase-3 gene transfection coupled with PDT (with LED light 430 nm) appeared useful to significantly inhibit the proliferation rate and to increase the apoptotic rate in human gastric cancer cells.

Angiogenesis plays an important role in tumor growth and metastasis. An essential step in angiogenesis involves the formation of tube-like structures during matrix degradation, rearrangement, and apoptosis of endothelial cells. Chen et al. investigated the mechanisms of photocytotoxicity induced by AEm in human umbilical vein endothelial cells (HUVECs) [96]. PDT was performed using blue LED irradiation (430 nm). Mitochondrial mechanisms of apoptotic cell death were observed in AEm PDT-treated cells; the capacity of migration and invasion of HUVECs were inhibited by AEm PDT. AEm PDT-induced cellular apoptotic cell death via the mitochondria pathways as well as inhibited cell migration invasion and angiogenesis via p38, extracellular signal-regulated kinase (ERK) and mitogen-activated protein kinase (MAPK) signal pathways.

The anthraquinone parietin is known for its capability to act as a PS against bacteria and cancer cells [97]. To overcome its hydrophobicity, it was loaded in liposomes based on tetraether lipid (TEL) and DPPC; the incorporation of thc bipolar TEL molecules (consisting of two biphytanyl chains attached to hydrophilic headgroups by ether linkages at both ends) is used to allow the production of liposomes with increased membrane rigidity, so avoiding premature PS release into the bloodstream. The phototoxicity of this system under irradiation at 457 nm was demonstrated on triple-negative breast cancer cell line MDA-MB-231 [98]. Furthermore, the chorioallantoic membrane (CAM) assay was used to demonstrate the PDT-induced vascular damage induced by parietin liposomes in combination with exposure to blue laser (440 nm). The same assay was used to verify the photodestructive effect on the microvasculature of CUR loaded in DSPG:DSPC [1,2-distearoyl-sn-glycero-3-phospho-(1′-rac-glycerol)/2-distearoyl-sn-glycero-3-phosphocholine] or DSPC:TEL liposomes under irradiation with led blue light (405 nm) [99], as well as that of HY loaded in liposomes consisting of DSPC or DPPC/TEL together with laser irradiation at 633 nm [100].

Other plant-derived drugs as PS in anticancer PDT

Embelin, a natural compound isolated from *Embelia ribes* (a medicinal plant used in the Indian system of medicine), has been tested for its photodynamic activity in Ehrlich's ascites carcinoma (EAC) cells [101]. These cells were maintained in the peritoneal cavity of male Swiss albino mice for 3 weeks for maturation before being aspirated and used in in vivo and in vitro assays. Embelin showed phototoxicity (600 nm) in EAC cells. Additionally, mature EAC were subcutaneously injected for solid tumor development for PDT testing of Embelin. Intraperitoneal Embelin following tumor irradiation with visible light for 2 weeks or 90 days showed significant reduction of tumor volume and incidence, and these effects were more pronounced at 90 days. Embelin mechanism involved apoptosis, as demonstrated by reduced Bcl-2/Bax ratio, probably via oxidative stress. Additionally, pattern of tumor markers like myeloperoxidase (MPO), beta-D-glucuronidase, and rhodanese were normalized after embelin PDT treatment.

Anthraquinones isolated from leaves and stem of *Heterophyllaea pustulata* have been demonstrated for their phototoxic effects. Rubiadin and soranjidiol are the most interesting compounds of this group. The photosensitizing properties of soranjidiol were better than rubiadin exposing breast cancer MCF-7c3 cells (MCF-7 transfected with procaspase-3 cDNA) to light energy (420 nm) [102]. These drugs were localized mainly in cytoplasmic region and apoptosis was confirmed by nuclear condensation and DNA fragmentation. However, a different mechanism was proposed since rubiadin-induced caspase-3 canonical pro-apoptotic pathway while soranjidiol induced calpain non-canonical programmed cell death. The combination of rubiadin and soranjidiol PDT demonstrated a synergistic effect of these two molecules. Interestingly, 1-methyl ether derivates showed distinctive activity profile due to different cellular uptake [103]. Rubiadin derivate showed no activity in MCF-7c3 cells following irradiation due to very low uptake. Inversely, soranjidiol derivate improved the photodynamic activity compared to parent compound.

Acanthopanacis cortex (AC) extract was tested as potential PS in human laryngeal epithelial cancer cells (KB and Hep-2 cells) [104]. Following irradiation (LED 625 nm), AC extract induced cell toxicity with an increased ROS generation, and this effect was not observed in dark exposed cells. Additionally, AC extract induced apoptosis via B-cell lymphoma protein 2 (Bcl-2)-associated X (Bax) and poly-(ADP)-ribose polymerase (PARP) activation. Unfortunately, no data were reported regarding compounds contained so that these effects cannot be attributed to a specific PS.

Oil extracted from the fruit of acai, *Euterpe oleracea* Martius (Arecaceae), a palm tree native to the Amazon estuary, has been tested for its photodynamic activity thanks to the contained phytochemicals such as phenolics, flavonoids, and anthocyanins [105]. Even if these compounds have been reported for their anticancer activity, their role as PS has been evaluated in vitro using B16F10 murine melanoma cells and confirmed in vivo in xenograft of B16F10 in C57BL/6 female mice. Due to the hydrophobic nature of acai oil, it was nanoemulsified, producing small sized and monodisperse nanodroplet, in order to improve the bioavailability. Acai oil nanoemulsion (NanoA) following PDT (660 nm) showed significant phototoxicity in B16F10, inducing late apoptosis/necrosis. Data were also confirmed in vivo since NanoA reduced tumor volume, and this effect was further and significantly improved with a higher ratio value of necrotic area to tumor area. However, no information was reported to identify the components responsible for its PS effect.

Plant-derived drugs in combination to PDT and chemotherapy

There is large evidence that an interesting approach for treatment of cancer might be the combination of PDT and/or chemotherapy with plant-derived drugs used not as PS but due to other therapeutic properties. For example, the flavonoid rutoside (quercetin-3-O-rutinoside) has been tested in combination with methylene blue (MB) as PS on A375 melanoma cells [106]. MB is a well-known dye effective in PDT due to its ability to produce singlet oxygen. Rutoside pretreatment made the A375 cells sensitive to G1 arrest after MB-PDT (red light at 660 nm) increasing the cells in early and late apoptosis phases compared to control probably via ROS induction. Interestingly, post treatment of the A375 melanoma cells with rutoside after MB-PDT reduced the phototoxic effects of MB.

An acetone extract from *Rubus fairholmianus* root (RFSA) in combination with sulfonated zinc-phthalocyanines (ZnPcSmix), known for their PS properties, was assayed in MCF-7 cells [107]. RFSA combination with ZnPcSmix-PDT (laser at 680 nm) improved phototoxicity compared to RFSA-PDT alone. An increase in late apoptotic cells was observed in combination therapy, compared to RFSA-PDT, inducing caspase3/7 activities and cytochrome C release, and these effects were associated to significant ROS production so demonstrating the additive or synergistic effects of this combination treatment.

Similarly, catechin (CA), a flavonoid well known for its antioxidant but also anticancer activities, was tested in combination with the ZnPcSmix in PDT in A549 lung cancer cells [108]. CA followed ZnPcSmix-PDT (laser at 680 nm) improved phototoxicity compared to ZnPcSmix-PDT alone inducing apoptosis thus confirming the usefulness of combination therapy.

Ficus carica ethanolic leaf extract (FC), containing coumarins such as bergapten and psoralen and flavonoids such as rutin, luteolin, and quercetin, was tested for combination with Aluminum(Al)-PcSmix-PDT (laser at 630 nm) and the chemotherapics doxorubicin (Dox) or dacarbazine (DTIC) in rhabdomyosarcoma (RD) cells [109]. Data confirmed that the cytotoxicity was enhanced in the FC combination with chemotherapeutic agents (FC + Dox and FC + DTIC) and further improved following AlPcSmix mediated PDT. The combination index values confirmed synergistic properties of di- and tri-combinations with FC.

Additionally, phytotherapy may be useful to overcome PDT-induced drug resistance. Han and coworkers demonstrated that chlorin e6 (Ce6) PDT induced expression of ataxia telangiectasia mutated protein (ATM), p53 and γ-H2A.X, markers of self-repair response, and enhanced expression of glutathione peroxidase 4 (GPX4) in Lewis cells (LLC) lung cancer cell model, inducing drug resistance [110]. GPX4, typically overexpressed after DNA damage response (DDR), mitigates the intracellular ROS production so reducing PDT mechanisms. Dihydroartemisinin (DHA), a natural compound from *Artemisia annua*, is able to stimulate ferroptosis. DHA was evaluated as pretreatment followed by Ce6 PDT (690 nm laser) in LLC. DHA pretreatment of LLC following Ce6 PDT was able to significantly augment the intracellular ROS content by blocking GPX4 expression induced by PDT and so improving apoptosis induction.

Similarly, oleanolic acid (OA) Ce6 self-assembled NPs were projected for synergistic chemo/sono-photodynamic cancer therapy under laser irradiation at 680 nm and ultrasound irradiation in PC9 and 4T1 cells [111]. This was associated with synergic effects of OA able to induce mitochondrial depolarization, apoptosis, and cell cycle arrest in cancer cells. Additionally, compared to dark exposed, OACe6 following PDT (680 nm) reduced tumor weight and growth in an in vivo 4T1 mammary tumor xenograft model.

Plant-derived products in aPDT

Plant-derived drugs as PS against bacterial infections

aPDT has some characteristics that make it interesting and possibly useful to complement conventional antibiotic therapy. In particular, it shows no cross-resistance with antibiotics and low dark toxicity, meaning that toxicity is largely absent outside the irradiated zone [55].

Many researchers evaluated the applicability of various plant-derived natural products as PS in aPDT for the treatment of dental caries, chronic and inflammatory dental infections, and bacterial skin infections. Two issues need to be taken into particular consideration. Microbial biofilm describes a sessile community in which microbial cells are firmly attached to the substratum and embedded in extracellular polymeric matrix. Microbial biofilms account for up to 80% of all bacterial and fungal infections in humans.

Since biofilm-associated pathogens are particularly resistant to antibiotic treatment, new approaches such as aPDT are needed to be developed to combat clinically relevant biofilms such as oral and dental biofilms and wound infections [112]. Furthermore, infections caused by AMR bacteria are serious global health concerns. The high prevalence of methicillin-resistant *Staphylococcus aureus* (MRSA) causing skin and soft tissue infections in both the community and healthcare settings challenges the limited options of effective antibiotics and motivates the search for alternative therapeutic solutions, such as aPDT [113].

aPDT have been reported to be effective in dentistry against periodontal bacteria, caries-related strains, and peri-implantitis-related bacteria (*Porphyromonas gingivalis*, *Streptococcus mutans* and *Lactobacillus* spp., streptococci, *Actinomyces* spp., lactobacilli, *Bifidobacterium* spp., *Prevotella intermedia*, *Fusobacterium* spp., etc). However, most dental diseases such as dental caries and periodontitis are caused by biofilms attached to the tissue surface. In these conditions, the better choice is to use short-wavelength visible light, for maximizing the light energy for effectively killing the bacteria although with a lower penetration depth.

CUR is one of the most studied PS for aPDT [114], especially in the field of oral infections [115]. Lee et al. [116] investigated the effects of CUR and *Curcuma xanthorrhiza* extract (CXE) containing xanthorrhizol or of a mixture of these products as PS against *S. mutans* using a colony-forming-unit assay. The Gram-positive sucrose-dependent bacteria *S. mutans* participates in dental biofilm formation when conditions related to sucrose fermentation by-products decrease the normal oral pH and alter the balance of the demineralization/remineralization process, leading to demineralization process and promoting the formation of cavities. Xanthorrhizol is expected to easily penetrate the surface of a biofilm since in comparison with CUR its molecular weight is lower (218.33 and 368.38 g/mol, respectively) and its solubility is about tenfold higher (28.90 and 2.68 μg/mL, respectively). Irradiation was performed using LED light at 405 nm; interestingly, medical devices equipped with a 405 nm LED light source are marketed and used for caries and/or plaque detection. CUR alone did not show any antimicrobial activity in the dark, as opposed to the extract alone and in combination with CUR. Conversely, the viability of *S. mutans* in the presence of CUR, CXE, and a mixture of these two components was substantially reduced during irradiation. However, the phototoxicity varied with PS solubility and concentration; in fact, the antimicrobial photodynamic activity of CUR was decreased at higher concentrations while that of CXE increased with increasing concentration. These observations could be due to CUR not being dissolved sufficiently at concentrations over 10^4 ng/mL. Thus, combining CUR and CXE with a 405 nm LED may be a novel method of applying aPDT.

Similarly, Hwang et al. [117] evaluated in vitro the aPDT activity of two extracts of *Curcuma* and *Chlorella* on biofilms of *S. mutans,* irradiated with LED light (405 nm) for 5 min. aPDT significantly decreased the number of viable cells and the live/dead cell ratio.

S. aureus is commonly found in the healthy oral cavities, especially in the presence of prosthetic devices, and some oral infections such as endodontic infection and mucositis are associated with *S. aureus*, but a fundamental obstacle to eliminate the *S. aureus* strains is the development of antibiotic resistant microorganisms, such as MRSA. Ribeiro et al. [118] evaluated the activity of CUR (0.1−20 μM) as PS against *S. aureus*, both MRSA and methicillin-susceptible (MSSA), exposed to LED light (455 nm). PDT with CUR 5 to 20 μM resulted in photo-killing of MSSA and (although at the highest dose of 20 μM) MRSA.

Saitawee et al. [119] evaluated the antibacterial activity of a *C. longa* extract as PS against *Aggregatibacter actinomycetemcomitans,* a pathogenic bacteria associated with aggressive periodontitis and poorly responding to conventional treatment. Irradiation (blue LED light, 420−480 nm) considerably increased the antibacterial activity of the extract, with 0.78 μg/mL extract solution and light showing complete absence of *A. actinomycetemcomitans*.

Mendez et al. [120] evaluated the aPDT activity of CUR, at different preirradiation times (PIT), against bacterial biofilms prepared from infected dentin obtained from donors and grown for 3 or 5 days. The biofilms were treated with 600 μM CUR and irradiated with blue LED light (455 ± 30 nm). CUR alone (PIT = 5 min) and all combinations of CUR and LED light, significantly reduced the vitality of 3-day biofilms, whereas only CUR plus LED using PIT of 2 or 5 min were effective in reducing the vitality of 5-day biofilms.

Rocha et al. [121] reported CUR-aPDT efficacy on biofilms of *Enterococcus faecalis* (one of the bacterial species most commonly involved in failure of endodontic treatment and post-treatment of apical periodontitis) incubated in bovine bone cavities. In particular, they confirmed the higher activity of CUR when irradiated with blue LED light (450 nm) compared to the not irradiated. In another study [121], the same research group prepared a mouthwash based on a microemulsion with CUR for disinfecting the oral cavity. CUR microemulsion (30 or 60 μg/mL) combined with irradiation (blue LED light at 430 nm for 10 or 30 min) were effective, in terms of CFU/mL reduction, against biofilms of *E. coli*, MRSA, and *Candida albicans*. The PS activity of a commercially available extract of *C. longa,* as well as that of *Citrus lemon*, *Hamamelis virginiana,* and *H. perforatum* extracts, has been confirmed by Nardini et al. [122] on *E. faecalis* culture in planktonic form and on biofilm upon irradiation at 460, 405 and 660 nm (depending on features of the investigated PS materials). Significant microbial reduction was observed both the planktonic and biofilm forms with all the extracts.

Due to the limitations associated with CUR for its poor water solubility, instability at physiological pH, and low bioavailability, many researchers have developed micro- and nanoformulations to improve its therapeutic effects [123]. Similar formulations have been prepared and evaluated also in the field of aPDT. In particular, the natural cationic and biodegradable polymer chitosan may be used to modify the surface features of NPs and to improve their adherence to the bacteria. Agel et al. prepared CUR encapsulated cationic NPs using PLGA, poly(vinyl alcohol), and chitosan [124]. Their aPDT activity was tested in vitro against the Gram-positive *Staphylococcus saprophyticus* subsp. bovis and the Gram-negative *E. coli* DH5 alpha, using irradiation with blue light (457 nm). Surface charge modification with chitosan increased adherence to the bacteria and structural damage upon photodynamic treatment, finally increasing the antibacterial phototoxicity of CUR-loaded NPs. Zhang et al. [125], instead, developed CUR-loaded chitosan-coated AuNPs, as a pH stimulus-responsive drug delivery system able to anchor to the cell membrane. These NPs were able to release CUR in a pH-dependent manner, facilitating the drug delivery to the acidic bacterial infection environment; furthermore, AuNPs acted not only as a nano-carrier but also as photothermal material effectively absorbing near-infrared light. Moreover, compared with free CUR, these NPs improved photoinactivation of *S. aureus* and *E. coli* under dual wavelength irradiation of 405 + 808 nm. Santezi et al. investigated the aPDT efficacy of CUR in dimethylsulfoxide solution (CUR-S) and in three different bioadhesive formulations: a CUR-loaded chitosan hydrogel with a poloxamer (CUR-CHIH), a CUR-loaded liquid crystal precursor system (CUR-LCP), a CUR-loaded microemulsion (CUR-ME) [126]. In vitro experiments showed that, under blue light irradiation (440−460 nm), CUR-S was the only formulation able to significantly reduce biofilm viability of *C. albicans* and *Lactobacillus casei*. There was a significant reduction in the viability of *S. mutans* biofilms when CUR-S and CUR-LCP were applied. Furthermore, in situ experiments showed antimicrobial efficacy against *S. mutans*. These findings confirm that the phototoxic effects of CUR have a high relation with the type of formulation in which it is loaded.

Silva et al. investigated two distinct CUR-based formulations based on either complexation with methyl-β-cyclodextrin (MβCD), MβCDC-CUR, or dissolution in a choline chloride (ChCl): glycerol (Gly) deep eutectic solvent (DES), DES-CUR, to be used as phototherapeutic agents for blue-light (irradiation 400−550 nm) aPDT approaches [127]. Unlike MβCD-CUR, DES-CUR showed good biological properties and high photoresponsivity, displaying relevant phototoxicity against bacterial pathogens (*Escherichia coli* ATCC 25922 and *Staphylococcus aureus* ATCC 25923). Finally, graphene quantum dots (GQDs) may be used as a carrier for PS delivery, due to small size, wide surface area, and good biocompatibility but also possess PS activity. So, Mushtaq et al. prepared CUR-loaded GQDs and demonstrated their enhancement of aPDT activity of CUR against *Pseudomonas aeruginosa*, MRSA, *E. coli*, and *C. albicans* under irradiation with blue light (405 nm) [128].

The use of HY, as well as that of *H. perforatum* extracts, as PS in aPDT has been evaluated in various studies, such as the one by Nardini et al. [122] cited above. Vollmer et al. studied the aPDT activity of an *H. perforatum* extract on in situ oral biofilms, prepared using intraoral devices in healthy volunteers. Irradiation was performed ex situ with visible light (with an accessory orange filter in the range of 570−780 nm) combined with water-filtered infrared-A (to accentuate the amount of infrared-A radiation in the range of 780−1400 nm) [129]. *H. perforatum* extract showed significant photoactivation at 32 mg/mL, and completely eradicated all biofilms. Delcanale et al. reported the aPDT concentration and irradiation time-dependent activity of an extract obtained from flowering stems of *H. perforatum* against planktonic *S. aureus* [130]. Irradiation was performed with green LED light for 5 or 10 min (515 nm). Fagopyrins, belonging to naphthodianthrones and structurally similar to HY, are known to act as PS. Buckwheat plants contain protofagopyrins, which are converted to fagopyrins when the plant extract is exposed to light. Kim et al. studied the aPDT activity of fagopyrin F-rich fraction obtained from Tartary buckwheat (*Fagopyrum tataricum*) flower extract exposed to lights against both planktonic and biofilms form of *S. mutans* [131]. Irradiation with blue light (450 nm) significantly increased the phototoxicity of the extract, with inhibition of *S. mutans* viability and biofilm formation.

The aPDT activity of HY against both planktonic and biofilm-forming MRSA and MSSA has been reported by Garcia et al. [132]. After a preincubation with HY, irradiation was performed with LED light (602 ± 10 nm). The 5 min preincubation combined with 10 min irradiation showed bactericidal effects against the planktonic forms, whereas longer preincubation (24 h) and 30 min irradiation were needed to obtain a photoactivity against biofilms.

Propionibacterium acnes is one of the species of the genus *Propionibacterium* that can colonize pilosebaceous ducts, as observed in acne, a chronic disease affecting the pilosebaceous units. Barroso et al. reported the in vitro photodynamic activity of different concentrations of HY against *Propionibacterium acnes* biofilms under irradiation with different energies of low-level laser (660 nm) [133]. An in vivo study on HY-aPDT was performed by Chan et al. on a wound infection model in mice using a panel of clinically relevant MRSA [134]. The activity of HY was compared with that of pheophorbide a as well as that of MB. The irradiation was performed at 610 nm for MB and pheophorbide a or 590 nm for HY for 20 min. HY showed lower minimum bactericidal concentration values compared to pheophorbide a and MB, as well as better wound healing via re-epithelization. Also, HY dark toxicity on neutrophils (the first line of defense recruited to the site of infection) was significantly lower than that of the other two compounds. Also, BBR-based aPDT was shown to be potentially useful in treatment of skin infectious disease. In fact, the combined effect of blue LED irradiation and BBR on *Pseudomonas aeruginosa* and *S. aureus* was reported [135]; this effect prevented the formation of biofilms and destroy the microbial biofilms.

As to plant-derived extracts rich in chlorophylls as PS, Alam et al. studied the aPDT activity of an ethanolic extract and a PS-enriched fraction, containing six pheophorbide compounds, obtained from *Tripterygium wilfordii* [136]. Their strong aPDT activity was demonstrated under irradiation with LED red light (660 nm) both in vitro against MSSA, MRSA, *Staphylococcus epidermidis*, *Streptococcus pyogenes*, and *C. albicans*, as well as in an in vivo model using *Caenorhabditis elegans*. Also da Silva Souza Campanholi et al. reported the aPDT activity of an extract of *Tetragonia tetragonoides*, rich in chlorophylls, against *S. aureus* irradiated for 20 min with red LED light (665 nm) [137]. Treatment induced a dose-dependent damage of the cell wall of the pathogen, without significant toxicity in healthy cells. Plant extracts containing chlorophyll can be used as PS for aPDT against bacterial dental infections. For example, the extract obtained from the aerial organs of *Dioscorea altissima*, containing chlorophyll, and incorporated into glass ionomer cement (GIC, whose antimicrobial activity is due to the sealing property based on calcium chelation and fluoride release) was tested as a PS in aPDT against biofilm formation by *S. mutans*, using laser light at 660 nm [138]. The extract potentiated the antimicrobial action of GIC against *S. mutans* and laser irradiation increased this activity. Conversely, Mamone et al. demonstrated the aPDT activity of extracts from three Argentinean plants (*Solanum verbascifolium* flower, *Tecoma stans* flower, and *Cissus verticillata* root) against *S. epidermidis*; in these studies, plant leaves and stems were discarded to avoid possible chlorophyll interference [139]. Bacterial suspensions of *S. epidermidis* were preincubated for 60 min and irradiated with artificial visible light for 40 min.

Finally, aPDT may be successfully employed for treatment of halitosis. A randomized, controlled clinical trial on 44 individuals was performed to evaluate the ability of a *Bixa orellana* extract as PS to reduce halitosis, a condition in which bacteria in the coating of the tongue dorsum are believed to be the main cause since they produce volatile sulfur compounds [140]. For aPDT, the *Bixa orellana* extract was irradiated with a blue-violet LED (395–480 nm). Results showed an immediate reduction of halitosis, although the reduction was not maintained after 7 days.

Of course, plant-based products may be used for aPDT as PS also in fields different from bacteria-sustained oral or skin diseases. For example, CUR might be used as a protective agent in the control of bacteria and bacterial biofilms in food products. *Listeria monocytogenes* may be mostly transmitted through contaminated food (such as cold meats, cheese, and smoked products) and can cause listeriosis, a not very frequent infection but potentially lethal among adults and neonates. *L. monocytogenes* is relatively frequent on surfaces of working spaces of the food industry and adheres to surfaces, forming dense biofilms highly resistant to common disinfectants. Since CUR is approved by EU as a food additive (E100), the activity of a CUR-rich extract of *Curcuma longa* and commercial CUR as PS on *Listeria innocua* biofilm and planktonic forms has been investigated [141]; *L. innocua* is a good surrogate of *L. monocytogenes* being genetically, ecologically, and phenotypically close to this pathogen. In this study, following irradiation with blue light (400–500 nm) for 30 min, CUR resulted more effective than the extract, and planktonic cells were much more susceptible to CUR-aPDT than biofilms. Furthermore, the efficacy of CUR-aPDT following irradiation with blue LED light (462 ± 3 nm) against *Escherichia coli* and *S. aureus*, two foodborne pathogens, was investigated [142] in freshly squeezed orange juice. Le et al. compared the antimicrobial activity of CUR with that of AEm against *S. aureus* and *E. coli* under PDT [143]. The aPDT efficacy was shown to be based on the number of absorbed photons, since the degree of bacterial inactivation was correlated to the absorbed photons and the concentration of PS [143]. In particular, AEm was more effective than CUR against both *S. aureus* and *E. coli*, while *E. coli* was more resistant to PDT than *S. aureus*.

Finally, Sarker and Ahn [144] examined the application of two extracts from *Chamaecyparis obtusa* and *Moringa oleifera*, as natural PS for water disinfection of MDR bacteria and total coliforms from secondary effluent in full-scale municipal wastewater treatment plants. Irradiation with white LED increased the intrinsic antibacterial effect of the extracts. *E. coli* was more resistant than *S. aureus*, requiring a longer irradiation time for complete inactivation.

Plant-derived drugs as PS against fungal infections

Photodynamic therapy represents a new promising alternative treatment strategy against superficial fungal infections. In this context, one of the most studied natural compounds is CUR [115]. Dovigo et al. evaluated CUR

(20–40 μM) as PS against planktonic and biofilm forms of clinical isolates of *C. albicans*, *Candida tropicalis*, and *Candida glabrata*, exposed to LED light 440–460 nm, showing significant antifungal effects [145]. The same research group later evaluated CUR-PDT against biofilms of three isolates of *Candida dubliniensis* from HIV-positive patients [146]. *C. dubliniensis*, phenotypically similar to *C. albicans*, has been isolated from different groups of patients, including immunocompromised patients, and so may be more difficult to eradicate. Biofilms were treated with CUR (20–40 μM), incubated in the dark for 20 min, and then irradiated with LED light (455 nm). CUR-PDT significantly reduced the metabolism of the *C. dubliniensis* biofilms, and biofilms required a longer preirradiation time to allow CUR penetration than planktonic forms. The need of longer preirradiation time for CUR penetration into biofilms compared to planktonic cultures was previously reported also in cultures of *C. albicans* and *C. glabrata* [147]. The activity of CUR-PDT was also evidenced on multispecies biofilms of *C. albicans*, *C. glabrata*, and *S. mutans* [148] using CUR (80–120 μM) and irradiation with LED blue light (440–460 nm).

Casu et al. examined how an MDR oral clinical isolate of *C. albicans* responded to aPDT that used a CUR/H_2O_2 3% formulation as a PS and was exposed to various light sources (traditional irradiation at 460 nm or polarized light source at 380–3400 nm) [149]. One has to note that polarized light has a major ability to enter the yeast cell wall. Both light sources were able to activate the PS formulation. An interesting difference was observed in the cell-generation-time (CGTOD) after PDT treatment, since the polarized light was more active compared to the source of 460 nm (16 and 8 h, respectively). These data evidence the existence of an inhibition window time, in which the majority of cells are in metabolic shock, a phenomenon caused by PT-induced radicals under PDT.

As to the mechanisms involved in the PDT effects of CUR, in the study by Carmello et al. [150], the effects of sublethal CUR-PDT with blue light (455 nm) on DNA damage was investigated in *C. albicans*. CUR-PDT, but also light alone, induced DNA damage, although the presence of CUR significantly slowed DNA repair. More recently, the effects of PDT with CUR or with the chlorin derivative photodithazine as PS in combination with LED light (blue or red light, respectively) on the expression of genes associated with adhesion and biofilm formation (agglutinin-like sequence [ALS]-1 and hyphal wall protein 1 [HPW1]) and with oxidative stress response (adenylate cyclase-associated protein [CAP1], catalase 1 [CAT1], and superoxide dismutase 1 [SOD1]) were investigated in *C. albicans* [151]. PDT with both the PS reduced the expression of all the five genes, with a decrease of *C. albicans* virulence and adaptability to oxidative stress. Similarly, Ma et al. observed a downregulation of hypha-specific and biofilm-related genes (enhanced filamentous growth protein 1 [EFG1], Unscheduled meiotic 6 [UME6], Hypha-specific G1 cyclin-related protein 1 [HGC1], and Extent of cell elongation protein 1 [ECE1]) in three *C. albicans* strains (ATCC 90028 and two clinical isolates from HIV and oral lichen planus patients' oral cavities) treated with CUR irradiated with LED light (455 nm), together with inhibition of hyphal growth, cell separation, and defective biofilm formation [152].

Hsieh et al. evaluated CUR-PDT alone and in combination with the antifungal fluconazole against *C. albicans*, following irradiation with blue light [153]. CUR-PDT effectively eradicated *C. albicans* biofilms and enhanced the activity of fluconazole when used in combination.

A study on CUR-PDT antifungal activity in an in vivo model of oral candidiasis was conducted [154]. In this study, mice, immunosuppressed with two subcutaneous injections of prednisolone, were orally inoculated with *C. albicans* and, after 5 days, received topical CUR (up to 80 μM) and were irradiated with LED light (455 nm). CUR-PDT induced a significant reduction in *C. albicans* viability without any harm to the host tissue. Sakima et al. encapsulated CUR in anionic and cationic NPs synthesized using polylactic acid and dextran sulfate and evaluated its photodynamic effects following blue light irradiation for 5 consecutive days on a model of oral candidiasis in immunosuppressed mice [155]. No antifungal effect for anionic CUR-NPs was observed, very likely due to the negative charge of the formulation that promotes repulsion against the negative charge of biofilm matrix and the *C. albicans* cell wall. Conversely, cationic CUR-NPs reduces *C. albicans* even in the absence of light.

AEm has been investigated in vitro as a PS on azole-sensitive and azole-resistant *C. albicans*. Irradiation was performed with white light (400–780 nm) [156]. AEm, not showing toxicity in the dark, effectively inactivated *C. albicans* cells in a concentration-dependent manner when irradiated. Moreover, irradiation increased the entry of AEm into *C. albicans* cells and induced damage to the fungal cell wall, cytoplasm, nucleus, and the surface. The combination with irradiation was effective in *C. albicans* strains regardless of whether resistant or not to azole. Thus, the authors suggested AEm could represent a potential PS antifungal PDT against drug-resistant *C. albicans* strains.

Trichophyton rubrum is responsible for the majority of dermatophytosis [156]. The efficacy of AEm-mediated aPDT was investigated against *T. rubrum* microconidia in vitro, as well as against *T. rubrum*-caused tinea corporis in vivo in a guinea pig model and against *T. unguium* ex vivo. AEm-mediated aPDT (irradiation with blue light 435 nm) effectively inactivated *T. rubrum* microconidia, through generation of abundant intracellular ROS, exhibited strong inhibitory effect on growth of *T. rubrum*.

The results were confirmed also in the in vivo and ex vivo experiments, suggesting that AEm is a potential PS for the photodynamic treatment of dermatophytosis caused by *T. rubrum*, although its permeability in skin and nails needs to be improved.

Giacone et al. investigated the PDT activity against *C. albicans* of two root organic extracts obtained from *Tagetes minuta*, a source of thiophenes, compounds whose antifungal activity is enhanced by irradiation with UVA [157]. These extracts inhibited virulence factors of *Candida*, such as adherence to epithelial surfaces and germ tube formation. The same research group also evaluated the PDT activity against *C. albicans* of various organic extracts obtained from different parts of *Thymophylla pentachaeta* var. belenidium, another plant containing photoactive thiophenes [158]. Hexane and dichloromethane extracts from roots exhibited high photodynamic antifungal activity against *C. albicans* under UVA light irradiation and decreased the adherence of *C. albicans* to buccal epithelial cells. Finally, the in vitro photodynamic antifungal activity of hexane and ethanol extracts from aerial parts of *Alternanthera maritima* (containing steroids, triterpenes, and flavonoids) was demonstrated against two *C. dubliniensis* strains, under irradiation with a 685 nm diode laser [159].

Plant-derived drugs as PS against viral infections

The first trials on antiviral PDT date back to the early 1970s, when Felber et al. [160], after rupturing early vesicular lesions caused by herpes simplex virus (HSV), applied Neutral Red with subsequent exposure to fluorescent light, with 18 out of 20 patients with symptomatic improvements, superior to those obtained in 12 control patients. However, after all this time still photodynamic antiviral therapy had not reached the expected clinical significance.

At the molecular level, the antiviral activity of PDT is based on the ability of the different types of PS, after irradiation with light and the subsequent generation of ROS, to hit and damage capsid proteins and envelope lipids, and to destroy the integrity of viral genetic material [161]. In particular, the multitarget mechanism of PDT differentiates it from other antiviral drugs and makes the development of resistance unlikely. Moreover, antioxidant enzymes, such as superoxide dismutase, catalase, and peroxidase, do not protect against singlet oxygen, the main ROS on which the antiviral activity of PDT is based [162].

Antiviral activity of several PS belonging to different classes has been investigated over the years. Their potential activity is usually assessed against viral suspensions as well as in cell cultures infected with a virus to estimate the effective doses not toxic to the host cells and to evaluate their ability to inactivate not only free virus particles but also intracellular viruses [163,164].

Randazzo et al. assessed the in vitro antiviral activity of CUR, as PS, and LED blue light (464–476 nm) on feline calicivirus (FCV) and murine norovirus (MNV-1), as surrogates of norovirus (NoV), one of the most important seafood- and water-borne viruses and the cause of many acute gastroenteritis outbreaks [165]. Photoactivated CUR resulted more active against FCV than MNV-1. The findings showed a positive correlation between temperature and inactivation, and the antiviral activity was concentration-dependent up to 50 μg/mL. Instead, photoactivated CUR showed only slight activity against MNV-1, even when CUR and light doses were increased (50 μg/mL of CUR and 120 min of light irradiation). Wu et al. investigated the activity of CUR and LED blue light (470 nm) against MNV-1 both cultured in buffer and bio-accumulated in oysters [166]. Results showed that the infectivity of MNV-1 was significantly inhibited both if cultivated in buffer and extracted from the gut of oysters at CUR 20 μM, and that virus inactivation was dose-dependent. The authors also reported significant damage to viral nucleic acids and alteration of virus morphology due to changes in viral capsid protein structures. Thus, treatment of oysters with photodynamically activated CUR might be an efficacious method to inactivate food-borne NoV.

More recently, Pourhajibagher et al. evaluated the ability of CUR-PLGA NPs irradiated with blue laser (450 ± 10 nm) to inactivate severe acute respiratory syndrome coronavirus 2 (SARS-CoV-2) in plasma samples of infected patients, by evaluating the effects of treated plasma on Vero cells [167]. Irradiated Cur@PLGA-NPs exhibited in vitro anti-SARS-CoV-2 activity in plasma, without cytotoxic effects in Vero cells exposed to treated plasma and without any adverse effect on plasma quality.

McCormick et al. evaluated the antiviral photodynamic activity of PhytoQuin (previously known as Orthoquin), a PS with antimicrobial properties obtained from an ethanolic extract of *Polygonum cuspidatum* [168,169]. The main components of these extract were polydatin, resveratrol, anthraglycoside B, rhein, emodin, and physcion. Under irradiation with visible light, PhytoQuin inhibited *herpes simplex virus* (HSV-1 and HSV-2, two enveloped DNA viruses) infection of target cells, with a reduction of plaque formation that was light-dependent. Inhibition of vesicular stomatitis virus (an enveloped RNA virus) resulted instead light-independent [168]. The activity of PhytoQuin-PDT was later evaluated on two human coronaviruses, the alphacoronavirus HCoV-229E and the betacoronavirus HCoV-OC43, in cultured cells. The observed antiviral effect was light-dependent and caused disruption of HCoV particle integrity allowing for the digestion of viral RNA by exogenous ribonucleases. Using lentiviruses pseudotyped with the SARS-CoV-2 Spike protein (S), the authors confirmed again a strong, light-dependent antiviral effect of PhytoQuin, which prevented Spike protein-mediated entry into human cells. The authors also found that the PhytoQuin constituent emodin had a light-dependent antiviral activity similar to that of PhytoQuin, demonstrating its importance in this extract antiviral activity [169].

Mugas et al. investigated the in vitro antiviral activity of purified anthraquinones obtained from *Heterophyllaea pustulata* as PS in PDT against HSV-1, using Vero cells as host cells [170]. Irradiation was performed with an actinic lamp emitting in the range between 380 and 480 nm with a maximum at 420 nm. Soranjidiol and 5,5′-bisoranjidiol, showing poor antiherpetic activity at their maximum noncytotoxic concentration when nonirradiated, exhibited instead significant photo-induced effects.

The antiviral activity of HY as PS in PDT has been reported against various types of viruses, such as Sindbis virus and Murine cytomegalovirus, hepatitis B, and HIV-1, acting by binding to the viral envelope and inhibiting viral fusion with target cells [164,171–175]. In these studies, it was found that the antiviral activity of HY and derivatives is strongly enhanced by light [176] and that they are effective against enveloped viruses but not against nonenveloped viruses [177].

Plant-derived drugs potentially effective for photolarvicidal activity

Mosquito-borne diseases represent a critical health problem worldwide, especially in tropical and subtropical countries. In fact, mosquitoes are the most common vectors known for transmitting deadly diseases, such as dengue, malaria, West Nile fever, and Zika [178,179]. In cases where vaccines or effective drugs are lacking, the prevention and control of these infections are fundamentally dependent on efficient control of the spread of the vector.

Bagnato and coworkers research group [180–182] focused its research on CUR as photolarvicide against *Aedes aegypti*, the main vector of the arboviruses causing dengue, chikungunya, Zika, and yellow fever [178]. The authors investigated at first two different formulations of CUR, one with sucrose and the other with D-mannitol (both with a w/w CUR:vehicle ratio of 1:99), sugars added to improve solubility and palatability of CUR [180]. Photolarvicidal activity was evaluated in cups containing tap water in external environment with 8 h exposure to direct or indirect sunlight, since CUR absorbs photons in the blue region of sunlight spectra (range of 300–500 nm, with maximum at 420 nm). For both formulations, the photolarvicidal activity was significantly lower under direct sunlight exposure, although relevant also under indirect exposure. The formulation with D-mannitol resulted more efficient due to the higher permeability in the peritrophic membrane of the larvae, causing irreversible damage to their digestive tube epithelium. The environmental safety of these formulations has been supported by the studies on morphological changes in the nontarget species *Danio rerio* (Zebrafish) gills. In a following study, they observed a delay in development time, changes in sex ratio and reduction in longevity, when larvae were exposed to sublethal concentrations of CUR/D-mannitol under a 12:12 h light:dark photoperiod [181]. In a third study, the same research group evaluated four CUR/D-mannitol formulations with different w/w proportions under light irradiation. The 50:50 w/w formulation resulted as the most effective, causing an extrusion into the intestine and peritrophic membrane, as well as the one with the shortest internalization and longest elimination time [182].

Conclusion

Current PDT is based on the mutual action of PS, light and oxygen to induce toxic effects on animal cells as well as on bacteria, fungi, viruses, and protozoa. The conventional phototoxic mechanism comprises light absorption by the PS and the consequent generation of an excited triplet state that can contribute to electron transfer processes typically leading to the formation of ROS or singlet oxygen through different mechanisms [11]. Thanks to the high reactivities and short lifetimes of activated PS, it produces local cytotoxic effects so reducing adverse effects on healthy tissues. Recently several plant-based PS have been reported for their photoactivity, with the advantages of low or no adverse effects compared to synthetic products and comparable efficiency with conventional PS. Cancer treatment is surely the main application of PDT, however also potential nononcologic applications have been evidenced in particular concerning infectious conditions at the level of the skin or the oral cavity.

Despite the continuous progress in drug discovery, cancer is considered one of the most common death causes. Tumors have developed many mechanisms at molecular level able to protect cancer cells from chemotherapy. In this scenario, PDT for cancer treatment evidenced a feasible, safe and reliable therapy, also taking into consideration the different action mechanisms through which PDT can avoid cancer cell replication and tumor growth [183]. The principal plant-derived PS investigated for cancer PDT include CUR, HY, BBR and chlorophyll derivatives, as well as several other thiophenes, alkaloids, and anthraquinones compounds. These drugs, following PDT, reduce the cancer cells number by inhibiting cellular proliferation and inducing necrosis or apoptosis depending on the employed concentration. Synergism between plant-based PS has been reported as also combination with other physical approaches (e.g., hyperthermia), which are able to improve the phototoxic effects.

At the same extent, various plant-derived natural products have been evaluated as PS in aPDT for the treatment of dental caries, chronic and inflammatory dental infections, and skin infections, representing an emerging field in the era of antibiotic resistance. Potentially, aPDT offers an important advantage over established antibiotic therapy, such as its ability to kill bacteria, irrespective of the MDR status, and rapid inactivation of pathogens. However, the most important aspect is the lack of development of resistance to plant-based aPDT, which has not yet been reported. Also in the light of the tragic events related to the COVID-19 pandemic, the data evidencing the antiviral activity of PDT based on plant-derived drugs as PS appear to be of particular interest.

Since some factors limit the application of plant-derived PS, the future development of PDT involves the use of nanotechnology able to overcome bioavailability problems of these compounds and to promote their selective accumulation in the target tissue or cells. Additionally, nanosystems could provide multi-functionality properties with multitarget or multitherapy approaches.

With the collection of chemically diverse plant-based PS, PDT might ultimately extend its clinical breakthrough as a promising alternative approach against cancer and multiresistant pathogens.

References

[1] Correia JH, et al. Photodynamic therapy review: principles, photosensitizers, applications, and future directions. Pharmaceutics 2021;13(9).

[2] Kwiatkowski S, et al. Photodynamic therapy—mechanisms, photosensitizers and combinations. Biomed Pharmacother 2018;106:1098−107.

[3] Youf R, et al. Antimicrobial photodynamic therapy: latest developments with a focus on combinatory strategies. Pharmaceutics 2021;13(12).

[4] Dougherty TJ, et al. Photoradiation therapy. II. Cure of animal tumors with hematoporphyrin and light. J Natl Cancer Inst 1975;55(1):115−21.

[5] Dougherty TJ HB, Schwartz S, Winkelman JW, Lipson RL. Historical perspective. In: Henderson BW, editor. Photodynamic therapy: basic principles and clinical applications. 1st ed. New York: CRC Press; 1992. p. 1−15.

[6] Yoo SW, et al. Non-oncologic applications of nanomedicine-based phototherapy. Biomedicines 2021;9(2).

[7] Niculescu A-G, Grumezescu AM. Photodynamic therapy—an up-to-date review. Appl Sci 2021;11(8):3626.

[8] Allison RR, Moghissi K. Photodynamic therapy (PDT): PDT mechanisms. Clin Endosc 2013;46(1):24−9.

[9] Robertson CA, Evans DH, Abrahamse H. Photodynamic therapy (PDT): a short review on cellular mechanisms and cancer research applications for PDT. J Photochem Photobiol B 2009;96(1):1−8.

[10] Castano AP, Demidova TN, Hamblin MR. Mechanisms in photodynamic therapy: part two-cellular signaling, cell metabolism and modes of cell death. Photodiagnosis Photodyn Ther 2005;2(1):1−23.

[11] Castano AP, Demidova TN, Hamblin MR. Mechanisms in photodynamic therapy: part one-photosensitizers, photochemistry and cellular localization. Photodiagnosis Photodyn Ther 2004;1(4):279−93.

[12] Passos SK, Tedesco AC, Eid DR, Lacava ZG. Bowen disease treated with PDT using ALA in nanostructured vehicle and two light deliveries: a case report. J Am Acad Dermatol 2011;64(2 Suppl. 1):AB141.

[13] Kruijt B, et al. A dedicated applicator for light delivery and monitoring of PDT of intra-anal intraepithelial neoplasia. Photodiagnosis Photodyn Ther 2010;7(1):3−9.

[14] Siewert B, Stuppner H. The photoactivity of natural products—an overlooked potential of phytomedicines? Phytomedicine 2019;60:152985.

[15] Foote CS. Definition of type I and type II photosensitized oxidation. Photochem Photobiol 1991;54(5):659.

[16] Najafi M, et al. Hypoxia in solid tumors: a key promoter of cancer stem cell (CSC) resistance. J Cancer Res Clin Oncol 2020;146(1):19−31.

[17] Hamblin MR, Mróz P. Advances in photodynamic therapy: basic, translational, and clinical. In: Artech House engineering in medicine & biology series. Boston, Mass: Artech House; 2008. p. 559. 20 p. of plates.

[18] Gal D. Effect of photosensitizers in chemical and biological processes: the MTO mechanism in photodynamic therapy. Biochem Biophys Res Commun 1992;186(2):1032−6.

[19] Muniyandi K, et al. Role of photoactive phytocompounds in photodynamic therapy of cancer. Molecules 2020;25(18).

[20] Zuluaga MF, Lange N. Combination of photodynamic therapy with anti-cancer agents. Curr Med Chem 2008;15(17):1655−73.

[21] Wilson BC, Jeeves WP, Lowe DM. In vivo and post mortem measurements of the attenuation spectra of light in mammalian tissues. Photochem Photobiol 1985;42(2):153−62.

[22] Szacilowski K, et al. Bioinorganic photochemistry: frontiers and mechanisms. Chem Rev 2005;105(6):2647−94.

[23] O'Connor AE, Gallagher WM, Byrne AT. Porphyrin and non-porphyrin photosensitizers in oncology: preclinical and clinical advances in photodynamic therapy. Photochem Photobiol 2009;85(5):1053−74.

[24] Allison RR, Sibata CH. Oncologic photodynamic therapy photosensitizers: a clinical review. Photodiagnosis Photodyn Ther 2010;7(2):61−75.

[25] Brandis AS, Salomon Y, Scherz A. Chlorophyll sensitizers in photodynamic therapy. In: Grimm B, et al., editors. Chlorophylls and bacteriochlorophylls: biochemistry, biophysics, functions and applications. Dordrecht: Springer Netherlands; 2006. p. 461−83.

[26] Yoon I, Li JZ, Shim YK. Advance in photosensitizers and light delivery for photodynamic therapy. Clin Endosc 2013;46(1):7−23.

[27] Sharma SK, et al. Drug discovery of antimicrobial photosensitizers using animal models. Curr Pharm Des 2011;17(13):1303−19.

[28] Senapati S, et al. Controlled drug delivery vehicles for cancer treatment and their performance. Signal Transduct Target Ther 2018;3:7.

[29] Boyle P, Levin B, editors. World cancer report 2008. International Agency for Research on Cancer (IARC); 2008.

[30] Mishchenko T, et al. Which cell death modality wins the contest for photodynamic therapy of cancer? Cell Death Dis 2022;13(5):455.

[31] Mroz P, et al. Cell death pathways in photodynamic therapy of cancer. Cancers (Basel) 2011;3(2):2516−39.

[32] Castano AP, et al. Photodynamic therapy plus low-dose cyclophosphamide generates antitumor immunity in a mouse model. Proc Natl Acad Sci USA 2008;105(14):5495−500.

[33] Garg AD, et al. Photodynamic therapy: illuminating the road from cell death towards anti-tumour immunity. Apoptosis 2010;15(9):1050–71.

[34] Firczuk M, et al. Approaches to improve photodynamic therapy of cancer. Front Biosci (Landmark Ed) 2011;16(1):208–24.

[35] George BP, Abrahamse H. A review on novel breast cancer therapies: photodynamic therapy and plant derived agent induced cell death mechanisms. Anticancer Agents Med Chem 2016;16(7): 793–801.

[36] Rajendran M. Quinones as photosensitizer for photodynamic therapy: ROS generation, mechanism and detection methods. Photodiagnosis Photodyn Ther 2016;13:175–87.

[37] Donohoe C, et al. Cell death in photodynamic therapy: from oxidative stress to anti-tumor immunity. Biochim Biophys Acta Rev Cancer 2019;1872(2):188308.

[38] Chen B, et al. Vascular and cellular targeting for photodynamic therapy. Crit Rev Eukaryot Gene Expr 2006;16(4):279–305.

[39] Kurokawa H, Ito H, Matsui H. Porphylipoprotein accumulation and porphylipoprotein photodynamic therapy effects involving cancer cell-specific cytotoxicity. Int J Mol Sci 2021;22(14).

[40] Cruz PM, et al. The role of cholesterol metabolism and cholesterol transport in carcinogenesis: a review of scientific findings, relevant to future cancer therapeutics. Front Pharmacol 2013;4:119.

[41] Hamblin MR, Newman EL. Photosensitizer targeting in photodynamic therapy. II. Conjugates of haematoporphyrin with serum lipoproteins. J Photochem Photobiol B 1994;26(2):147–57.

[42] Wen J, et al. Mitochondria-targeted nanoplatforms for enhanced photodynamic therapy against hypoxia tumor. J Nanobiotechnol 2021;19(1):440.

[43] Li X, et al. Innovative strategies for hypoxic-tumor photodynamic therapy. Angew Chem Int Ed Engl 2018;57(36):11522–31.

[44] Liu JN, Bu W, Shi J. Chemical design and synthesis of functionalized probes for imaging and treating tumor hypoxia. Chem Rev 2017;117(9):6160–224.

[45] Ruan C, et al. Nanomaterials for tumor hypoxia relief to improve the efficacy of ROS-generated cancer therapy. Front Chem 2021;9:649158.

[46] Laxminarayan R, et al. Access to effective antimicrobials: a worldwide challenge. Lancet 2016;387(10014):168–75.

[47] Sabino CP, et al. Global priority multidrug-resistant pathogens do not resist photodynamic therapy. J Photochem Photobiol B 2020;208:111893.

[48] Ribeiro M, et al. Photodynamic therapy and combinatory treatments for the control of biofilm-associated infections. Lett Appl Microbiol 2022;75(3):548–64.

[49] Tavares A, et al. Antimicrobial photodynamic therapy: study of bacterial recovery viability and potential development of resistance after treatment. Mar Drugs 2010;8(1):91–105.

[50] de Freitas LM, et al. Antimicrobial photodynamic therapy enhanced by the peptide aurein 1.2. Sci Rep 2018;8(1):4212.

[51] Pereira Rosa L. Antimicrobial photodynamic therapy: a new therapeutic option to combat infections. J Med Microbiol Diagn 2014;03(04):1000158.

[52] Hanakova A, et al. The application of antimicrobial photodynamic therapy on *S. aureus* and *E. coli* using porphyrin photosensitizers bound to cyclodextrin. Microbiol Res 2014;169(2–3):163–70.

[53] Kashef N, Hamblin MR. Can microbial cells develop resistance to oxidative stress in antimicrobial photodynamic inactivation? Drug Resist Updat 2017;31:31–42.

[54] Marasini S, Leanse LG, Dai T. Can microorganisms develop resistance against light based anti-infective agents? Adv Drug Deliv Rev 2021;175:113822.

[55] Liu Y, et al. Antibacterial photodynamic therapy: overview of a promising approach to fight antibiotic-resistant bacterial infections. J Clin Transl Res 2015;1(3):140–67.

[56] Hamblin MR. Antimicrobial photodynamic inactivation: a bright new technique to kill resistant microbes. Curr Opin Microbiol 2016;33:67–73.

[57] Hamblin MR, Hasan T. Photodynamic therapy: a new antimicrobial approach to infectious disease? Photochem Photobiol Sci 2004;3(5):436–50.

[58] Khdair A, et al. Nanoparticle-mediated combination chemotherapy and photodynamic therapy overcomes tumor drug resistance. J Control Release 2010;141(2):137–44.

[59] Jendželovská Z, et al. Hypericin in the light and in the dark: two sides of the same coin. Front Plant Sci 2016;7:560.

[60] Xu L, et al. Hypericin-photodynamic therapy inhibits the growth of adult T-cell leukemia cells through induction of apoptosis and suppression of viral transcription. Retrovirology 2019;16(1):5.

[61] Kōlōç Süloğlu A, et al. Evaluation of apoptotic cell death mechanisms induced by hypericin-mediated photodynamic therapy in colon cancer cells. Turk J Biol 2016;40:539–46.

[62] Sackova V, et al. Hypericin-mediated photocytotoxic effect on HT-29 adenocarcinoma cells is reduced by light fractionation with longer dark pause between two unequal light doses. Photochem Photobiol 2005;81(6):1411–6.

[63] Semelakova M, et al. The pro-apoptotic and anti-invasive effects of hypericin-mediated photodynamic therapy are enhanced by hyperforin or aristoforin in HT-29 colon adenocarcinoma cells. J Photochem Photobiol B 2012;117:115–25.

[64] Jendzelovsky R, et al. Breast cancer resistance protein is the enemy of hypericin accumulation and toxicity of hypericin-mediated photodynamic therapy. Biomed Pharmacother 2019;109:2173–81.

[65] Nkune NW, Abrahamse H. Nanoparticle-based drug delivery systems for photodynamic therapy of metastatic melanoma: a review. Int J Mol Sci 2021;22(22).

[66] Unterweger H, et al. Hypericin-bearing magnetic iron oxide nanoparticles for selective drug delivery in photodynamic therapy. Int J Nanomed 2015;10:6985–96.

[67] Ghazaeian M, et al. Curcumin-silica nanocomplex preparation, hemoglobin and DNA interaction and photocytotoxicity against melanoma cancer cells. J Biomol Struct Dyn 2021;39(17):6606–16.

[68] Singh SP, Sharma M, Gupta PK. Evaluation of phototoxic effects of curcumin loaded in organically modified silica nanoparticles in tumor spheroids of oral cancer cells. BioNanoScience 2015;5(1):10–21.

[69] Wozniak M, et al. The comparison of in vitro photosensitizing efficacy of curcumin-loaded liposomes following photodynamic therapy on melanoma MUG-Mel2, squamous cell carcinoma SCC-25, and normal keratinocyte HaCaT cells. Pharmaceuticals (Basel) 2021;14(4).

[70] Duse L, et al. Photodynamic therapy of ovarian carcinoma cells with curcumin-loaded biodegradable polymeric nanoparticles. Pharmaceutics 2019;11(6).

[71] Paunovic V, et al. c-Jun N-terminal kinase-dependent apoptotic photocytotoxicity of solvent exchange-prepared curcumin nanoparticles. Biomed Microdevices 2016;18(2):37.

[72] Hosseinzadeh R, et al. Preparation of cerium-curcumin and cerium-quercetin complexes and their LEDs irradiation assisted anticancer effects on MDA-MB-231 and A375 cancer cell lines. Photodiagnosis Photodyn Ther 2021;34:102326.

[73] Banerjee S, et al. Remarkable enhancement in photocytotoxicity and hydrolytic stability of curcumin on binding to an oxovanadium(IV) moiety. Dalton Trans 2015;44(9):4108–22.

[74] Khorsandi K, Hosseinzadeh R, Fateh M. Curcumin intercalated layered double hydroxide nanohybrid as a potential drug delivery system for effective photodynamic therapy in human breast cancer cells. RSC Adv 2015;5(114):93987–94.

[75] Khorsandi K, Hosseinzadeh R, Shahidi FK. Photodynamic treatment with anionic nanoclays containing curcumin on human triple-negative breast cancer cells: cellular and biochemical studies. J Cell Biochem 2019;120(4):4998–5009.

[76] Alexeree S, et al. A novel synthesis of a chlorophyll b-gold nanoconjugate used for enhancing photodynamic therapy: in vitro study. Photodiagnosis Photodyn Ther 2021;35:102444.

[77] Pan L, et al. A novel composite hydrogel initiated by *Spinacia oleracea* L. extract on Hela cells for localized photodynamic therapy. Mater Sci Eng C Mater Biol Appl 2017;75:1448–55.

[78] Chang G, et al. Reduced graphene oxide/amaranth extract/AuNPs composite hydrogel on tumor cells as integrated platform for localized and multiple synergistic therapy. ACS Appl Mater Interfaces 2015;7(21):11246–56.

[79] Chin YC, et al. Iron oxide@chlorophyll clustered nanoparticles eliminate bladder cancer by photodynamic immunotherapy-initiated ferroptosis and immunostimulation. J Nanobiotechnology 2022;20(1):373.

[80] Zhou H, et al. Plant-derived chlorophyll derivative loaded liposomes for tri-model imaging guided photodynamic therapy. Nanoscale 2019;11(42):19823–31.

[81] Hoi SW, et al. Photodynamic therapy of pheophorbide a inhibits the proliferation of human breast tumour via both caspase-dependent and -independent apoptotic pathways in in vitro and in vivo models. Phytother Res 2012;26(5):734–42.

[82] Huang P, et al. Photodynamic treatment with purpurin 18 effectively inhibits triple negative breast cancer by inducing cell apoptosis. Lasers Med Sci 2021;36(2):339–47.

[83] Yeo S, et al. Synthesis and design of purpurin-18-loaded solid lipid nanoparticles for improved anticancer efficiency of photodynamic therapy. Pharmaceutics 2022;14(5).

[84] Warowicka A, et al. Protoberberine compounds extracted from *Chelidonium majus* L. as novel natural photosensitizers for cancer therapy. Phytomedicine 2019;64:152919.

[85] Bhattacharyya R, et al. Differential modes of photosensitisation in cancer cells by berberine and coralyne. Free Radic Res 2017;51(7–8):723–38.

[86] Liu H-Q, et al. Photodynamic therapy enhanced the antitumor effects of berberine on HeLa cells. Open Chem 2019;17(1):413–21.

[87] Lopes TZ, et al. Berberine associated photodynamic therapy promotes autophagy and apoptosis via ROS generation in renal carcinoma cells. Biomed Pharmacother 2020;123:109794.

[88] Carriero F, et al. Berberine photo-activation potentiates cytotoxicity in human astrocytoma cells through apoptosis induction. J Pers Med 2021;11(10).

[89] Floriano BF, et al. Effect of berberine nanoemulsion photodynamic therapy on cervical carcinoma cell line. Photodiagnosis Photodyn Ther 2021;33:102174.

[90] Oliveira PM, et al. Effect of berberine associated with photodynamic therapy in cell lines. Photodiagnosis Photodyn Ther 2020;32:102045.

[91] Nowak-Perlak M, et al. The comparison of the efficiency of emodin and aloe-emodin in photodynamic therapy. Int J Mol Sci 2022;23(11).

[92] Liu YQ, et al. Inhibitory effect of aloe emodin mediated photodynamic therapy on human oral mucosa carcinoma in vitro and in vivo. Biomed Pharmacother 2018;97:697–707.

[93] Wu M, et al. Biomimetic photosensitizer nanocrystals trigger enhanced ferroptosis for improving cancer treatment. J Control Release 2022;352:1116–33.

[94] Lin HD, et al. The effect of aloe-emodin-induced photodynamic activity on the apoptosis of human gastric cancer cells: a pilot study. Oncol Lett 2017;13(5):3431–6.

[95] Li KT, et al. The effect of aloe emodin-encapsulated nanoliposome-mediated r-caspase-3 gene transfection and photodynamic therapy on human gastric cancer cells. Cancer Med 2016;5(2):361–9.

[96] Chen Q, et al. Photodynamic therapy mediated by aloe-emodin inhibited angiogenesis and cell metastasis through activating MAPK signaling pathway on HUVECs. Technol Cancer Res Treat 2018;17. 1533033818785512.

[97] Mugas ML, et al. Photodynamic therapy of tumour cells mediated by the natural anthraquinone parietin and blue light. J Photochem Photobiol B 2021;214:112089.

[98] Ayoub AM, et al. Photodynamic and antiangiogenic activities of parietin liposomes in triple negative breast cancer. Biomater Adv 2022;134:112543.

[99] Duse L, et al. Low level LED photodynamic therapy using curcumin loaded tetraether liposomes. Eur J Pharm Biopharm 2018;126:233–41.

[100] Plenagl N, et al. Photodynamic therapy—hypericin tetraether liposome conjugates and their antitumor and antiangiogenic activity. Drug Deliv 2019;26(1):23–33.

[101] Joy B, et al. Embelin (2,5-dihydroxy-3-undecyl-p-benzoquinone): a bioactive molecule isolated from *Embelia ribes* as an effective photodynamic therapeutic candidate against tumor in vivo. Phytomedicine 2014;21(11):1292–7.

[102] Rumie Vittar NB, et al. Photochemotherapy using natural anthraquinones: rubiadin and soranjidiol sensitize human cancer cell to die by apoptosis. Photodiagnosis Photodyn Ther 2014;11(2):182–92.

[103] Comini LR, et al. Photodynamic activity of anthraquinones isolated from *Heterophyllaea pustulata* Hook f. (Rubiaceae) on MCF-7c3 breast cancer cells. Phytomedicine 2011;18(12):1093–5.

[104] Shi S, et al. Acanthopanacis Cortex extract: a novel photosensitizer for head and neck squamous cell carcinoma therapy. Photodiagnosis Photodyn Ther 2019;26:142–9.

[105] Monge-Fuentes V, et al. Photodynamic therapy mediated by acai oil (*Euterpe oleracea* Martius) in nanoemulsion: a potential treatment for melanoma. J Photochem Photobiol B 2017;166:301–10.

[106] Khorsandi K, Hosseinzadeh R, Chamani E. Molecular interaction and cellular studies on combination photodynamic therapy with rutoside for melanoma A375 cancer cells: an in vitro study. Cancer Cell Int 2020;20:525.

[107] George BP, Abrahamse H, Hemmaragala NM. Anticancer effects elicited by combination of Rubus extract with phthalocyanine photosensitiser on MCF-7 human breast cancer cells. Photodiagnosis Photodyn Ther 2017;19:266–73.

[108] Senapathy GJ, George BP, Abrahamse H. Enhancement of phthalocyanine mediated photodynamic therapy by catechin on lung cancer cells. Molecules 2020;25(21).

[109] Aziz B, et al. Study of synergistic effects of *Ficus carica* leaves extract mediated chemo-photodynamic therapy on rhabdomyosarcoma cells. Photodiagnosis Photodyn Ther 2021;36:102565.

[110] Han N, et al. Ferroptosis triggered by dihydroartemisinin facilitates chlorin e6 induced photodynamic therapy against lung cancerthrough inhibiting GPX4 and enhancing ROS. Eur J Pharmacol 2022;919:174797.

[111] Zheng Y, et al. A nanosensitizer self-assembled from oleanolic acid and chlorin e6 for synergistic chemo/sono-photodynamic cancer therapy. Phytomedicine 2021;93:153788.

[112] de Melo WC, et al. Photodynamic inactivation of biofilm: taking a lightly colored approach to stubborn infection. Expert Rev Anti Infect Ther 2013;11(7):669–93.

[113] Dharmaratne P, et al. Contemporary approaches and future perspectives of antibacterial photodynamic therapy (aPDT) against methicillin-resistant *Staphylococcus aureus* (MRSA): a systematic review. Eur J Med Chem 2020;200:112341.

[114] Singh L, et al. Curcumin as a natural remedy for atherosclerosis: a pharmacological review. Molecules 2021;26(13).

[115] Santezi C, Reina BD, Dovigo LN. Curcumin-mediated photodynamic therapy for the treatment of oral infections-a review. Photodiagnosis Photodyn Ther 2018;21:409–15.

[116] Lee HJ, et al. Antibacterial photodynamic therapy with curcumin and *Curcuma xanthorrhiza* extract against *Streptococcus mutans*. Photodiagnosis Photodyn Ther 2017;20:116–9.

[117] Hwang HR, et al. Effect of antimicrobial photodynamic therapy with Chlorella and Curcuma extract on *Streptococcus mutans* biofilms. Photodiagnosis Photodyn Ther 2021;35:102411.

[118] Ribeiro AP, et al. Phototoxic effect of curcumin on methicillin-resistant *Staphylococcus aureus* and L929 fibroblasts. Lasers Med Sci 2013;28(2):391–8.

[119] Saitawee D, et al. Photodynamic therapy of *Curcuma longa* extract stimulated with blue light against *Aggregatibacter actinomycetemcomitans*. Photodiagnosis Photodyn Ther 2018;22:101–5.

[120] Cusicanqui Méndez DA, et al. The effectiveness of curcumin-mediated antimicrobial photodynamic therapy depends on pre-irradiation and biofilm growth times. Photodiagnosis Photodyn Ther 2019;27:474–80.

[121] Rocha MP, et al. Photodynamic therapry with curcumin in the reduction of enterococcus faecalis biofilm in bone cavity: rMicrobiological and spectral fluorescense analysis. Photodiagnosis Photodyn Ther 2021;33:102084.

[122] Nardini EF, et al. The potential of commercially available phytotherapeutic compounds as new photosensitizers for dental antimicrobial PDT: a photochemical and photobiological in vitro study. Photodiagnosis Photodyn Ther 2019;27:248–54.

[123] Chopra H, et al. Curcumin nanoparticles as promising therapeutic agents for drug targets. Molecules 2021;26(16).

[124] Agel MR, et al. Curcumin loaded nanoparticles as efficient photoactive formulations against gram-positive and gram-negative bacteria. Colloids Surf B Biointerfaces 2019;178:460–8.

[125] Zhang Y, et al. Curcumin-loaded multifunctional chitosan gold nanoparticles: an enhanced PDT/PTT dual-modal phototherapeutic and pH-responsive antimicrobial agent. Photodiagnosis Photodyn Ther 2022;39:103011.

[126] Santezi C, et al. Photodynamic potential of curcumin in bioadhesive formulations: optical characteristics and antimicrobial effect against biofilms. Photodiagnosis Photodyn Ther 2021;35:102416.

[127] Silva E, et al. Comparing deep eutectic solvents and cyclodextrin complexes as curcumin vehicles for blue-light antimicrobial photodynamic therapy approaches. Photochem Photobiol Sci 2022;21(7):1159–73.

[128] Mushtaq S, et al. Potentiation of antimicrobial photodynamic therapy by curcumin-loaded graphene quantum dots. Photochem Photobiol 2022;98(1):202–10.

[129] Vollmer A, et al. Antimicrobial photoinactivation using visible light plus water-filtered infrared-A (VIS + wIRA) and *Hypericum perforatum* modifies in situ oral biofilms. Sci Rep 2019;9(1):20325.

[130] Delcanale P, et al. Photodynamic action of *Hypericum perforatum* hydrophilic extract against *Staphylococcus aureus*. Photochem Photobiol Sci 2020;19(3):324–31.

[131] Kim J, et al. Antibacterial photodynamic inactivation of fagopyrin F from Tartary buckwheat (*Fagopyrum tataricum*) flower against *Streptococcus mutans* and its biofilm. Int J Mol Sci 2021;22(12).

[132] García I, et al. Antimicrobial photodynamic activity of hypericin against methicillin-susceptible and resistant *Staphylococcus aureus* biofilms. Future Microbiol 2015;10(3):347–56.

[133] Barroso RA, et al. Antimicrobial photodynamic therapy against propionibacterium acnes biofilms using hypericin (*Hypericum perforatum*) photosensitizer: in vitro study. Lasers Med Sci 2021;36(6):1235–40.

[134] Chan BCL, et al. Hypericin and pheophorbide a mediated photodynamic therapy fighting MRSA wound infections: a translational study from in vitro to in vivo. Pharmaceutics 2021;13(9).

[135] Safai SM, Khorsandi K, Falsafi S. Effect of berberine and blue LED irradiation on combating biofilm of *Pseudomonas aeruginosa* and *Staphylococcus aureus*. Curr Microbiol 2022;79(12):366.

[136] Alam ST, et al. Natural photosensitizers from *Tripterygium wilfordii* and their antimicrobial photodynamic therapeutic effects in a *Caenorhabditis elegans* model. J Photochem Photobiol B 2021;218:112184.

[137] da Silva Souza Campanholi K, et al. Photodamage on *Staphylococcus aureus* by natural extract from *Tetragonia tetragonoides* (Pall.) Kuntze: clean method of extraction, characterization and photophysical studies. J Photochem Photobiol B 2020;203:111763.

[138] Chiode MMM, et al. Plant extract incorporated into glass ionomer cement as a photosensitizing agent for antimicrobial photodynamic therapy on *Streptococcus mutans*. Photodiagnosis Photodyn Ther 2022;38:102788.

[139] Mamone L, et al. Photodynamic inactivation of Gram-positive bacteria employing natural resources. J Photochem Photobiol B 2014;133:80–9.

[140] Gonçalves MLL, et al. Antimicrobial photodynamic therapy with *Bixa orellana* extract and blue LED in the reduction of halitosis-A randomized, controlled clinical trial. Photodiagnosis Photodyn Ther 2020;30:101751.

[141] Bonifácio D, et al. Photodynamic inactivation of Listeria innocua biofilms with food-grade photosensitizers: a curcumin-rich extract of *Curcuma longa* vs commercial curcumin. J Appl Microbiol 2018;125(1):282–94.

[142] Bhavya ML, Umesh Hebbar H. Efficacy of blue LED in microbial inactivation: effect of photosensitization and process parameters. Int J Food Microbiol 2019;290:296–304.

[143] Le TD, Phasupan P, Nguyen LT. Antimicrobial photodynamic efficacy of selected natural photosensitizers against food pathogens: impacts and interrelationship of process parameters. Photodiagnosis Photodyn Ther 2020;32:102024.

[144] Sarker MAR, Ahn YH. Green phytoextracts as natural photosensitizers in LED-based photodynamic disinfection of multidrug-resistant bacteria in wastewater effluent. Chemosphere 2022;297:134157.

[145] Dovigo LN, et al. Susceptibility of clinical isolates of Candida to photodynamic effects of curcumin. Lasers Surg Med 2011;43(9):927–34.

[146] Sanitá PV, et al. Curcumin-mediated anti-microbial photodynamic therapy against *Candida dubliniensis* biofilms. Lasers Med Sci 2018;33(4):709–17.

[147] Andrade MC, et al. Effect of different pre-irradiation times on curcumin-mediated photodynamic therapy against planktonic cultures and biofilms of *Candida* spp. Arch Oral Biol 2013;58(2):200–10.

[148] Quishida CC, et al. Photodynamic inactivation of a multispecies biofilm using curcumin and LED light. Lasers Med Sci 2016;31(5):997–1009.

[149] Casu C, Orrù G, Scano A. Curcumin/H_2O_2 photodynamically activated: an antimicrobial time-response assessment against an MDR strain of *Candida albicans*. Eur Rev Med Pharmacol Sci 2022;26(23):8841–51.

[150] Carmello JC, et al. Genotoxic effect of photodynamic therapy mediated by curcumin on *Candida albicans*. FEMS Yeast Res 2015;15(4):fov018.

[151] Jordão CC, et al. Antimicrobial photodynamic therapy reduces gene expression of *Candida albicans* in biofilms. Photodiagnosis Photodyn Ther 2020;31:101825.

[152] Ma J, et al. Antifungal effect of photodynamic therapy mediated by curcumin on *Candida albicans* biofilms in vitro. Photodiagnosis Photodyn Ther 2019;27:280–7.

[153] Hsieh YH, et al. An in vitro study on the effect of combined treatment with photodynamic and chemical therapies on *Candida albicans*. Int J Mol Sci 2018;19(2).

[154] Dovigo LN, et al. Curcumin-mediated photodynamic inactivation of *Candida albicans* in a murine model of oral candidiasis. Med Mycol 2013;51(3):243–51.

[155] Sakima VT, et al. Antimicrobial photodynamic therapy mediated by curcumin-loaded polymeric nanoparticles in a murine model of oral candidiasis. Molecules 2018;23(8).

[156] Ma W, et al. The effects of aloe emodin-mediated antimicrobial photodynamic therapy on drug-sensitive and resistant *Candida albicans*. Photochem Photobiol Sci 2020;19(4):485–94.

[157] Giacone L, et al. Photodynamic activity of *Tagetes minuta* extracts against superficial fungal infections. Med Mycol 2020;58(6):797–809.

[158] Cordisco E, et al. Evaluation of the antifungal photodynamic activity of *Thymophylla pentachaeta* extracts against *Candida albicans* and its virulence factors. Phytomedicine 2021;90:153608.

[159] Gasparetto A, et al. Extracts from *Alternanthera maritima* as natural photosensitizers in photodynamic antimicrobial chemotherapy (PACT). J Photochem Photobiol B 2010;99(1):15–20.

[160] Felber TD, et al. Photodynamic inactivation of herpes simplex: report of a clinical trial. JAMA 1973;223(3):289–92.

[161] Wiehe A, O'Brien JM, Senge MO. Trends and targets in antiviral phototherapy. Photochem Photobiol Sci 2019;18(11):2565–612.

[162] Wainwright M, Crossley KB. Photosensitising agents—circumventing resistance and breaking down biofilms: a review. Int Biodeterior Biodegrad 2004;53(2):119–26.

[163] Conrado PCV, et al. A systematic review of photodynamic therapy as an antiviral treatment: potential guidance for dealing with SARS-CoV-2. Photodiagnosis Photodyn Ther 2021;34:102221.

[164] Sobotta L, et al. Photosensitizers mediated photodynamic inactivation against virus particles. Mini Rev Med Chem 2015;15(6):503–21.

[165] Randazzo W, Aznar R, Sánchez G. Curcumin-mediated photodynamic inactivation of norovirus surrogates. Food Environ Virol 2016;8(4):244–50.

[166] Wu J, et al. Virucidal efficacy of treatment with photodynamically activated curcumin on murine norovirus bio-accumulated in oysters. Photodiagnosis Photodyn Ther 2015;12(3):385–92.

[167] Pourhajibagher M, et al. Robust antimicrobial photodynamic therapy with curcumin-poly (lactic-co-glycolic acid) nanoparticles against COVID-19: a preliminary in vitro study in Vero cell line as a model. Photodiagnosis Photodyn Ther 2021;34:102286.

[168] Monjo AL, et al. Photodynamic inactivation of herpes simplex viruses. Viruses 2018;10(10).

[169] Duguay BA, et al. Photodynamic inactivation of human coronaviruses. Viruses 2022;14(1).

[170] Mugas ML, et al. Inactivation of herpes simplex virus by photosensitizing anthraquinones isolated from Heterophyllaea pustulata. Planta Med 2021;87(9):716–23.

[171] Lopez-Bazzocchi I, Hudson JB, Towers GH. Antiviral activity of the photoactive plant pigment hypericin. Photochem Photobiol 1991;54(1):95–8.

[172] Hudson JB, Lopez-Bazzocchi I, Towers GHN. Antiviral activities of hypericin. Antivir Res 1991;15(2):101–12.

[173] Lenard J, Rabson A, Vanderoef R. Photodynamic inactivation of infectivity of human immunodeficiency virus and other enveloped viruses using hypericin and rose bengal: inhibition of fusion and syncytia formation. Proc Natl Acad Sci USA 1993;90(1):158–62.

[174] Yip L, et al. Antiviral activity of a derivative of the photosensitive compound hypericin. Phytomedicine 1996;3(2):185–90.

[175] Moraleda G, et al. Inhibition of duck hepatitis B virus replication by hypericin. Antivir Res 1993;20(3):235–47.

[176] Hudson JB, Harris L, Towers GHN. The importance of light in the anti-HIV effect of hypericin. Antivir Res 1993;20(2):173–8.

[177] Miskovsky P. Hypericin-a new antiviral and antitumor photosensitizer: mechanism of action and interaction with biological macromolecules. Curr Drug Targets 2002;3(1):55–84.

[178] Girard M, et al. Arboviruses: a global public health threat. Vaccine 2020;38(24):3989–94.

[179] Sharma M, Kumar V. Mosquito-larvicidal Binary (BinA/B) proteins for mosquito control programs-advancements, challenges, and possibilities. Curr Res Insect Sci 2022;2:100028.

[180] de Souza LM, et al. Curcumin in formulations against *Aedes aegypti*: mode of action, photolarvicidal and ovicidal activity. Photodiagnosis Photodyn Ther 2020;31:101840.

[181] Mezzacappo NF, et al. Curcumin/d-mannitol as photolarvicide: induced delay in larval development time, changes in sex ratio and reduced longevity of *Aedes aegypti*. Pest Manag Sci 2021;77(5):2530–8.

[182] Garbuio M, et al. Formulations of curcumin and d-mannitol as a photolarvicide against *Aedes aegypti* larvae: sublethal photolarvicidal action, toxicity, residual evaluation, and small-scale field trial. Photodiagnosis Photodyn Ther 2022;38:102740.

[183] Oniszczuk A, et al. The potential of photodynamic therapy (PDT)-experimental investigations and clinical use. Biomed Pharmacother 2016;83:912–29.

Chapter 14

Hopes and disappointments related to the use of flavonoids in therapeutical approaches

Lidia Gaffke[a], Karolina Pierzynowska[a], Zuzanna Cyske, Estera Rintz, Magdalena Podlacha, Grzegorz Mincewicz and Grzegorz Węgrzyn

Department of Molecular Biology, Faculty of Biology, University of Gdansk, Gdansk, Poland

Introduction—Antioxidant activities of flavonoids and beyond

Among various metabolites produced by plants, flavonoids reveal high chemical variability and tremendous biological activities [1]. This group of compounds is classified as molecules containing a phenylchromene backbone (a skeleton with 15 carbon atoms forming two phenyl rings and an additional heterocyclic ring with the embedded oxygen atom) with specific side moieties (Fig. 14.1). These specific moieties determine classification of flavonoids, with the major groups of these compounds identified as flavones, isoflavones, flavanols, flavonols, flavanones, anthocyanidins, and chalcones, all of them represented by different molecules (Fig. 14.1) [2]. In plants, flavonoids play different roles, including regulation of growth and ripening, control of development, contribution to creation of colors of flowers, protection against microorganisms, repulsion of herbivores, resistance to various environmental stresses, and others [1]. However, in this chapter, we will focus on their effects on animal and human organisms rather than on benefits they provide to plants.

In fact, biological activities of flavonoids discovered in cells, tissues and organs of humans and animals are numerous and differential, indicating the influence of these plant metabolites on various processes and functions. The most pronounced biologically relevant features of flavonoids are their antioxidative properties. As reviewed recently [2], they are expressed according to several different mechanisms. First, flavonoids can be scavengers of reactive oxygen species (ROS) which directly decreases levels of these deleterious molecules. Second, flavonoids can activate antioxidant enzymes, thus decreasing ROS levels through such a secondary mechanism. However, other indirect actions of flavonoids enhance their antioxidant effects. These include inhibition of NAPDH oxidases and stimulation of chelating properties of some metal ions. In addition, actions of flavonoids may lead to elevation of levels of α-tocopheryl radicals and enhancement of mitigation of the oxidative stress by these compounds, as well as by nitric oxide, low-molecular-weight antioxidants, and increased concentrations of uric acid [2]. Since it is commonly accepted that the oxidative stress has deleterious effects in many diseases, the antioxidative properties of flavonoids are recognized as general health profits of these plant metabolites. Nevertheless, other activities of flavonoids may potentially provide perhaps even more important benefits for human health, especially in preventing or treatment of various diseases. Anti-inflammatory effects of administration of different flavonoids were broadly described in the literature and summarized recently [3]. Such effects may reflect abilities of these plant metabolites to interact with and influence activities of many proteins operating as mediators in the signal transduction cascades (like various kinases) and more direct regulators of gene expression processes [1,2,4–6]. Moreover, various other processes occurring in cells and tissues can be regulated in a profitable way due to such activities of flavonoids, making them candidates for therapeutics in a broad spectrum of diseases. In fact, these compounds have been proposed as potential drugs in as diverse disorders as cancer, microbial infections, neurodegenerative diseases, diabetes, cardiovascular manifestations, metabolic diseases, allergies, and others [5–11]. Unfortunately, despite very

[a]Equal contributions

Modulation of Oxidative Stress. https://doi.org/10.1016/B978-0-443-19247-0.00013-8

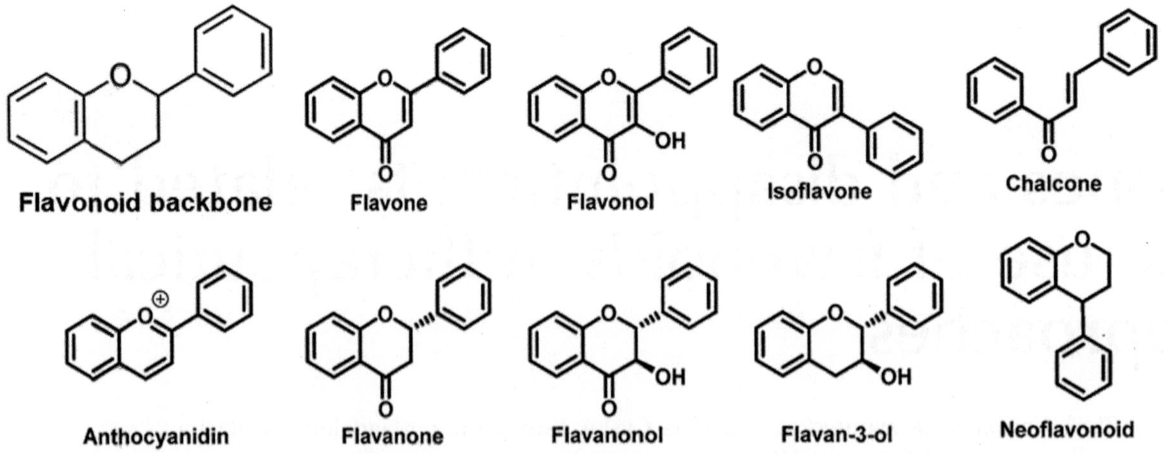

Flavonoid class	Examples
Flavones	Apigenin, Luteolin
Flavonols	Kaempferol, Quercetin
Isoflavones	Daidzein, Genistein, Glycitein
Chalcones	Chalcone, Naringenin chalcone
Anthocyanidins	Cyanidin, Pelargonidin, Petunidin
Flavanones	Hesperetin, Naringenin
Flavanonols	Dihydrokaempferol, Taxifolin
Flavan-3-ols	Catechin, Gallocatechin 3-gallate
Neoflavonoids	Calophyllolide, Dalbergichromene

FIGURE 14.1 Flavonoids and their major classes (*upper panel*) and examples of specific compounds from these groups (*lower panel*).

encouraging results of experiments on cellular and animals models of various diseases, clinical trials indicated that efficacy of flavonoids was often either doubtful or minor. On the other hand, epidemiological data strongly suggest health benefits and decreased risks for many diseases when flavonoids are consumed in relatively large amounts as elements of diet [1–11]. This makes the global picture of therapeutical effects of flavonoids very unclear. Despite a large body of literature in the field of the medical use of these compounds (the search of the PubMed database for the combination of terms "flavonoids" and "therapy" gave 47,985 records at 24th September 2022), there are still huge controversies regarding the therapeutical potential of flavonoids, resulting in great hopes and serious disappointments in this field.

Considering the presence of almost 50 thousand research papers published in the area of the use of flavonoids for therapeutical applications, in this chapter, we did not aim to review such a huge body of data. In fact, many excellent review papers have been published recently in this field, considering specific use of flavonoids for treatment of various diseases (see for example Refs. [1–11]), and a general scheme of a variability of therapeutical applications of these compounds is demonstrated in Fig. 14.2. Instead, we aimed to present a few overviews on attempts to develop specific medical applications of these plant metabolites, and one more detailed description of the works on the use of particular flavonoid in a specific disease. Thus, we have chosen to present three general stories about studies on the use of flavonoids in cancer, infectious diseases, neurodegenerative diseases, and one very specific case of research on development of a potential therapy for an inherited metabolic disorder. Then, we attempted to answer the questions why did clinical trials not necessaryily confirm results of preclinical studies with flavonoids and what should be done further to explore the undoubted therapeutic potential of these compounds?

Flavonoids as anticancer compounds

Anticancer properties of flavonoids are perhaps the most widely studied features of these compounds in the light of their potential medical use. The search of the PubMed database for the combination of terms "flavonoids" and

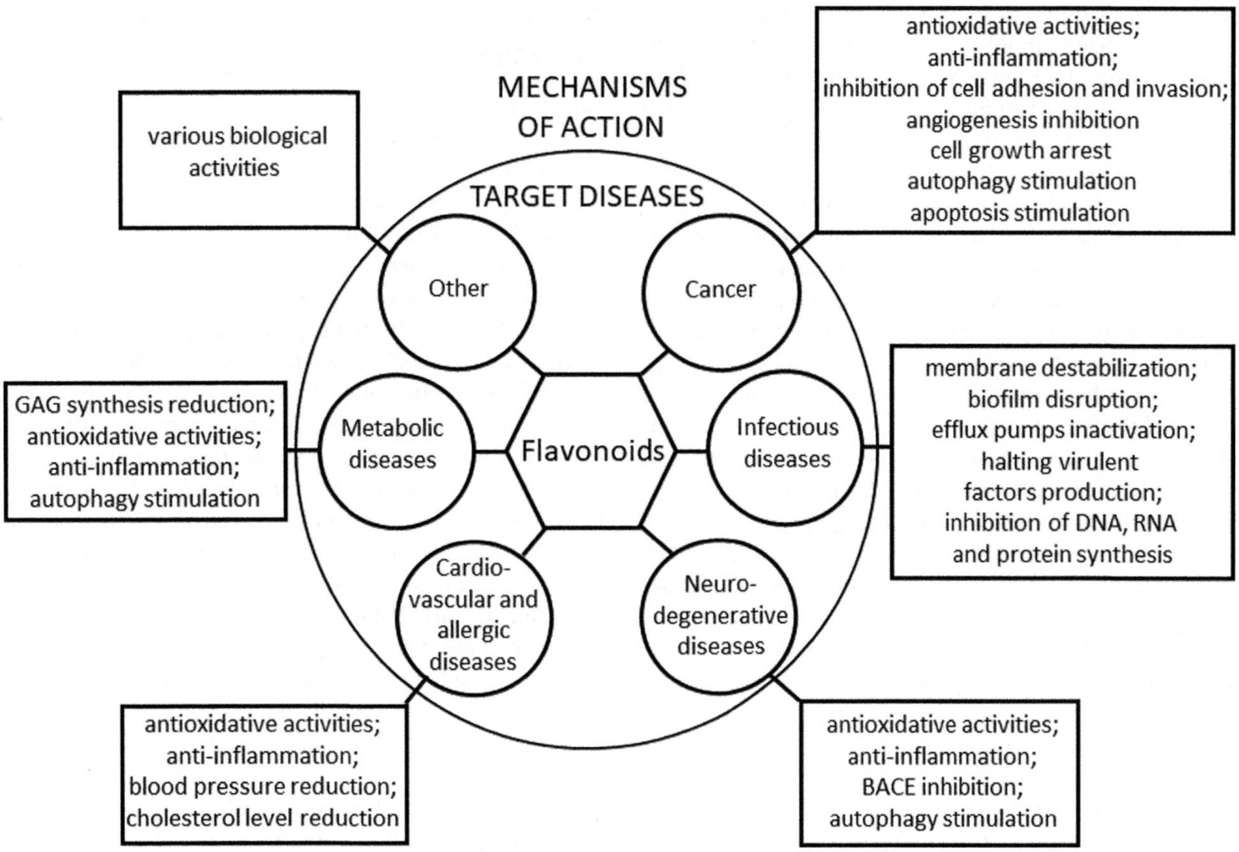

FIGURE 14.2 A simplified overview of the possible therapeutic applications of flavonoids. Targeted groups of diseases are indicated, together with major mechanisms of actions of flavonoids.

"cancer" gave 26,288 records at 24th September 2022; this indicates that more than 50% of published reports in the field of potential therapeutical use of flavonoids concerned their anticancer activities. Therefore, considering the number of great review articles in this field recently published in the literature (1459 records in the last 5 years, as for the PubMed database on 24th September 2022), here we will provide an overview and comments rather than a detailed review of the subject.

As summarized recently [12], numerous studies demonstrated anticancer actions of flavonoids. Conclusions of such experimental works were corroborated by epidemiological analyses which strongly suggested that consumption of foods rich in flavonoids decreases the risk of development of cancer [12]. It was proposed that actions of flavonoids against cancer cells are based on various biological activities of these compounds, among which scavenging of ROS, anti-inflammatory properties, inhibition of activities of protein kinases, halting metastasis by interfering with cell adhesion and invasion, angiogenesis inhibition, downregulation of cell growth efficiency, and stimulation of autophagy and apoptosis are crucial [12]. Literature analyses led to the conclusion that the most promising compounds from the discussed group are following molecules (presented here in alphabetical order): apigenin, casticin, epigallocatechin, galangin, genistein, kaempferol, luteolin, naringenin, pelargonidin, quercetin, vitexin, and wogonin [12]. Moreover, these compounds may act against cancer cells both alone or in combination with other anticancer drugs, enhancing their efficiency.

Many studies were focused on understanding molecular mechanisms of anticancer actions of flavonoids. From results of these research studies, it appears clear that there is no single or predominant mechanism of such biological effects, but rather a combination of various activities leads to the final effects. Moreover, different types of cancers may be sensitive to different actions of flavonoids. For example, breast cancer cells may be sensitive to flavonoid-mediated actions because of the interference with the mTOR signaling pathway, resulting in changes in the control of autophagy, cell growth, proliferation, and apoptosis [13,14]. In addition, modulation of the Bcl-2 activity in the p53-mediated signaling pathway may be especially important in the stimulation of apoptosis in cancer cells of different types [15]. Moreover, the crucial role of autophagy stimulation in flavonoid-mediated anticancer activities has been confirmed recently on the basis of extensive analysis of published research reports [16]. On the other hand, it was suggested that in the treatment of melanoma cells with different flavonoids (apigenin, epigallocatechin-3-gallate, kaempferol, naringenin, and silybin), the modulation of functions of the receptor tyrosine kinase and the Wnt protein, causing changes in efficiencies of signal transduction pathways dependent on these factors may be the major mechanisms [17]. The variability of mechanisms of anticancer properties of flavonoids is supported by results of other analyses which indicated crucial roles of ROS-mediated processes by apigenin, epigallocatechin gallate, hesperetin, luteolin, naringenin, and quercetin [18]. Another analysis indicated that flavonoids are involved in various epigenetic regulations that may affect the development of cancer cells; these include DNA methylation, histone modifications, and modulation of activities of miRNA and other noncoding regulatory RNAs [19]. One should also note that gut microbiota dysbiosis can indirectly stimulate carcinogenesis, thus, any compounds that are beneficial for keeping proper microbiome may prevent cancer development. In this light, it was indicated that through reshaping gut microbiota, flavonoids can exert anticarcinogenic properties [20]. Furthermore, some flavonoids can be converted by bacteria into bioactive metabolites which enhance their anticancer activities [20]. This concerns both the colorectal cancer and other cancer types [21]. Finally, it is important to remember that mechanisms of actions of various flavonoids differ in details. For example, quercetin stimulates apoptotic pathways in cancer cells through modulating activities of p53, NF-κB, MAPK, JAK/STAT, PI3K/AKT, and Wnt/β-catenin. In addition to regulating these pathways, quercetin controls the levels of noncoding RNAs (ncRNAs), including miRNAs, which are involved in carcinogenesis and tumor suppression [22]. On the other hand, kaempferol acts mainly through both activation of JAK/STAT3, PI3K/AKT, and NF-κB, and interference with TNF-induced activation of MAPK [23].

In summary, various flavonoids revealed effective anticancer activities against different types of cancers in in vitro and preclinical studies. On the other hand, authors of recent comprehensive review articles indicated that published clinical trials with flavonoids as potential anticancer drugs are scarce, and their results are often inconclusive [12–23]. The difficulties in studies on efficacy of these compounds in clinical trials include problems with choosing appropriate dose and duration of the treatment, as well as interpretation of the data due to high variability of mechanisms of their actions. Therefore, at the current stage of our knowledge, we are unsure about actual potential of flavonoids in treatment of cancers.

Antibacterial and antiviral effects of flavonoids

Due to the antibiotic crisis, expressed as appearance of many strains of pathogenic bacteria resistant to many, if not all, known antibiotics, it is an urgent need to discover previously unknown antibiotics and/or to develop alternative antibacterial therapies [24]. The use of flavonoids can be considered as one of options, as these compounds were reported to possess various activities to combat pathogenic bacteria. Such antibacterial properties of flavonoids have been reviewed and discussed recently [25]. The first point is that different compounds from this group were demonstrated as antimicrobials against various pathogenic bacteria. Examples are pathogenic *Escherichia coli*, *Helicobacter pylori*, *Klebsiella pneumoniae*, *Mycobacterium tuberculosis*, *Porphyromonas gingivalis*, *Pseudomonas aeruginosa*, *Staphylococcus aureus*, and others. Then, flavonoids either inhibit bacterial growth or kill bacterial cells according to different mechanisms, including both direct and indirect mechanisms. For direct actions, flavonoids can affect the stability of the bacterial cell membrane, inhibit formation of bacterial biofilm, make efflux pumps ineffective, and interfere with production of virulence factors [25].

Interestingly, when sensitivity of various bacteria (both Gram-positive (*Bacillus subtilis*, *Micrococcus luteus*, *Sarcina* sp., and *Staphylococcus aureus*) and Gram-negative (*Citrobacter freundii*, *Escherichia coli*, *Klebsiella pneumoniae*, *Proteus vulgaris*, *Pseudomonas aeruginosa*, *Salmonella enterica*, *Serratia marcescens*, and *Vibrio harveyi*)) to various flavonoids (apigenin, daidzein, genistein, kaempferol, and naringenin) was tested, differential patterns of antimicrobial activities of each investigated compound have been demonstrated [26]. Molecular studies indicated that growth of sensitive bacteria was inhibited due to global inhibition of synthesis of DNA, RNA, and proteins [27]. Moreover, bacteriostatic rather than bactericidal effects were detected [27]. Importantly, analyses of activities of several plant extracts rich in flavonoids indicated different, significantly less effective, antimicrobial effects than purified compounds [28]. Moreover, contrary to purified flavonoids which were demonstrated to be generally safe to animals and humans, treatment of cultures of human cells with such extracts caused their decreased viability [28].

Since multidrug resistance of bacteria is often dependent on actions of efflux pumps which remove antibiotics from the cells, inhibition of these molecular machines may be crucial to resurrect the potential of previously discovered antibacterial compounds. Indeed, flavonoids were demonstrated to be able to inhibit bacterial efflux pumps [29]. Interestingly, some flavonoids, like genistein, can both halt DNA and RNA syntheses and inactivate efflux pumps [27,29].

Therefore, one might consider to use combinations of flavonoids and classical antibiotics in treatment of patients infected with pathogenic bacteria, otherwise resistant to many antibiotics. Recent discussions indicated the importance of modeling of biologically active molecules to optimize their desired functions. Such modeling was performed for flavonoids as antimicrobial compounds, and some important suggestions on how to plan development of molecules with higher antibacterial potential could be provided [30]. This type of studies is especially important in development of drugs against bacteria that are particularly difficult to combat, like *Mycobacterium tuberculosis*. Indeed, extensive studies on searching for antituberculosis agents led to identification of over 100 flavonoids expressing such activities [31].

When considering infectious diseases, it is necessary to mention antiviral activities of flavonoids. In fact, many studies, summarized recently [32,33], indicated that these compounds can be active against various viruses, including influenza viruses, coronaviruses, herpes simplex viruses, enteroviruses, arboviruses, Dengue virus, Zika virus, and others. Mechanisms of these inhibitions of viral development are different, from inhibition of replication of viral genetic material, through direct binding to virions and interactions of essential viral proteins, to modulation of the host immune response and increasing viability of cells [32]. Stimulation of the host defense processes, like autophagy, and protection against other stresses, like oxidative stress, can also be especially helpful in managing viral infections of human or mammalian cells and organisms [33]. Interestingly, the use of flavonoids has been suggested as a potential treatment to alleviate and shorten the deleterious period associated with the post-COVID-19 syndrome [34].

Despite all the beneficial effects of antibacterial and antiviral activities of flavonoids, one should note that vast majority of studies performed to date in this subject were conducted either in vitro or with the use of animal models. Therefore, the serious limitation is a lack of solid studies with patients, especially clinical trials. This might be, however, especially difficult to organize as still antibiotic therapy is the first choice treatment of patients infected with pathogenic bacteria, and there are still other methods of treatment of viral infections. Similarly, any potential trials with combination of already approved drugs with flavonoids might not be easy.

The potential use of flavonoids in neurodegenerative diseases

Neurodegenerative diseases are especially difficult to treat due to their complicated pathomechanisms and problems with efficient delivery of putative drugs to the central nervous system (CNS). On the other hand, this group of diseases is characterized by very severe symptoms and exclusion of patients from normal life. Therefore, development of effective therapies for diseases in which functions of the brain are affected is an urgent medical need.

It was suggested by various authors (and summarized recently) that flavonoids may have beneficial effects in treatment of various neurodegenerative disease, including the most frequent one (and at the same time one of the most devastating disorders)—the Alzheimer's diseases [35]. The neuroprotective activities of flavonoids may arise from already mentioned (in previous sections of this chapter) antioxidative and anti-inflammatory properties [35]. Acting as ROS scavengers and stimulators of NRF2-ARE and PPAR-γ, they can effectively reduce the oxidative stress, while by downregulation of pathways dependent on NF-κB, MAPK, and ERK, they cause a decrease in the efficiency of inflammation, especially neuroinflammation [35]. In addition, negative regulation of AchE and BchE may lead to flavonoid-mediated modulation of neurotransmitters, whereas positive regulation of CREB can facilitate proneuronotrophic processes [35].

Apart from the above-mentioned general activities of flavonoids, there are also indications that one of isoflavones, genistein, has an especially strong potential in development of therapies for neurodegenerative diseases, including Alzheimer's disease. By acting more specifically, it can inhibit production of beta-amyloid (one of the major pathogenic factors in the latter disease) by blocking the activity of BACE (also called the β-site APP cleaving enzyme 1 or β-secretase) [36,37]. A huge advantage of the use of genistein in disorders caused by accumulation of various aggregates (which is common in many neurodegenerative diseases) is the ability of this isoflavone to simulate autophagy, while giving little or no adverse effects. In fact, autophagy activation has been proposed recently as an especially promising way to treat neurodegenerative diseases through degradation of insoluble aggregates which are otherwise toxic for cells, with neurons being particularly sensitive to them [38]. In fact, studies on cellular and animal models of Huntington's disease (another neurodegenerative disorder) and Alzheimer's disease indicated that genistein was able not only to stimulate autophagy and lead to disappearance of aggregates of mutant huntingtin [39,40] and beta-amyloid and hyperphosphorylated tau protein [41] but also to correct behavior of rats being an animal model of Alzheimer's disease, including memory and cognitive functions [41]. Such a multimodal action of genistein might be especially important in developing treatment strategies for various neurodegenerative diseases where action on a single target may be highly insufficient in attempts to find a really effective therapy [42]. This strategy is also compatible with the idea of the use of one drug for treatment of many diseases that opens a way for introducing a therapy that could be available for patients suffering from a battery of both common and rare diseases (note that commercialization of any drug for a rare disease is extremely difficult due to various economic barriers) [43]. Interestingly, genistein has been proposed also a compound which might be effective in treatment of memory impairment [44] and in age-related diseases, including senile dementia and others [45]. Therefore, one might even speculate that genistein might be efficient in protecting the brains against senescence and age-related neurodegeneration in the brain.

Despite all the above overviewed promising activities of flavonoids, their use against neurodegenerative diseases is restricted mainly to preclinical studies. Some primary clinical trials did not indicate sufficient benefits when using flavonoids in Alzheimer's patients [46]. On the other hand, very low doses of these compounds were used relative to those employed in experiments with cellular or animal models, and bioavailability issues were not sufficiently addressed. Therefore, flavonoids still remain only a hope for effective drugs against neurodegenerative diseases.

The case of the use of genistein in mucopolysaccharidoses

Mucopolysaccharidoses (MPS) are a group of lysosomal storage diseases (LSD) caused by mutations in genes encoding enzymes involved in degradation of glycosaminoglycans (GAGs), complex sugars playing various roles in tissue structures and functions and cell signaling [47]. Due to the absence or severe deficiency in one of such enzymes, GAGs cannot be degraded and accumulate(s) in lysosomes and outside of these organelles. This causes a cascade of changes in cell physiology, functions of tissues and organs, and finally the disorders in whole organism. The symptoms of MPS are very severe and occur in virtually all organs; however, they appear usually at the age of several years, thus, proper diagnosis is difficult and takes sometimes a relatively long time [48]. Nevertheless, once the symptoms appear, they progress considerably, causing severe disabilities of patients whose expected life span is about 2 decades on average [47,48]. Depending on dysfunction of a specific enzyme (appearing as a result of genetic mutations), 13 types of MPS are distinguished [49]. Despite the fact that some treatments are currently used for a few MPS types, like enzyme replacement therapy (ERT) or hematopoietic stem cells transplantation, no therapy for neuronopathic types is available, mainly because the therapeutic, intravenously administered, recombinant enzyme cannot cross the blood–brain barrier efficiently [50–52].

In the light of severity of neuronopathic MPS and a lack of effective treatment, various potential therapies have been considered [53–59]. Among them, the use of genistein, a flavonoid from the group of isoflavones, was proposed. The idea was that genistein might impair synthesis of GAGs, as early studies indicated that epidermal growth factor (EGF) is required for maximal synthesis of these sugars, and this isoflavone can bind to the receptor of this protein, called EGFR (reviewed previously in detail, see Ref. [60]). Such impairment of synthesis of GAGs could restore the balance between production and degradation of these compounds, especially in the presence of residual activity of the deficient enzyme, thus resulting in a decrease in the storage [61]. Indeed, experiments with cultures of fibroblast derived from MPS patients indicated that GAG synthesis is significantly less effective in the presence of genistein [62]. Moreover, pathogenic structures in MPS cells disappeared after incubation of cultures with this compound [62]. Such effects have been confirmed by different research groups [63,64]. Moreover, it was confirmed that the down-regulation of GAG synthesis is due to genistein-mediated inhibition of protein kinase activity of EGFR [65].

The encouraging results of experiments with cell cultures led to studies on animal models of MPS. Treatment of MPS II [66] and MPS IIIB [67] mouse models with genistein led to a significant decrease in GAG storage in these animals. When the orally administered genistein dose was increased up to 160 mg/kg/day, the storage reduction was also evident in the brain which was accompanied by correction of behavior of MPS IIIB mice, without any significant adverse effects [68]. Positive effects of genistein alone or in combination with another flavonoid, kaempferol, have also been reported in the MPS I model [69]. Other in vitro studies suggested that apart from genistein, some other natural and synthetic flavonoids could cause a decrease in the GAG storage and reduction of the oxidative stress in MPS cells [70–77].

In the light of a high efficacy of genistein in the experiments with cellular and animal models of MPS mentioned above, medical experiments and clinical trials with patients have been conducted. The first studies were performed using soy isoflavone extracts, rather than purified genistein. However, a significant limitation of studies based on the extracts is a huge variability between the commercial products marked as isoflavone-rich mixtures, as it was demonstrated that the actual content of flavonoids in different products can vary significantly from those indicated in the labels [78]. Nevertheless, results of preliminary clinical studies with MPS patients and a standardized isoflavone-rich soy extract (confirmed to contain the declared amounts of isoflavones) revealed a statistically significant decrease in urinary GAG levels, improvement in hair morphology and some cognitive benefits [79]. A 2-year follow-up study confirmed the beneficial effects of genistein in MPS III patients [80]. On the other hand, another similar study with MPS III patients treated with low doses of genistein (provided as a soy isoflavone extract) showed no correction of disability [81]. In contrast, the range of joint motion has been evidently improved in MPS II patients treated in a similar way [82]. Positive effects of genistein were more pronounced if 2–3-times higher doses (relative to previously used 5 mg/kg/day) were applied to treat MPS III patients [83].

The first randomized clinical trial with placebo control has been performed also with MPS III patients. Administration of genistein caused a significant decrease in urinary and plasma GAGs, however, no effects on total behavior scores could be observed [84]. It was suggested that the doses of genistein, administered orally as soy isoflavone extracts, might be too low, because high efficacy of genistein in studies with MPS IIIB mice were evident at 160 mg/kg/day [68]. Therefore, safety of a similar dose (150 mg/kg/day) of synthetic genistein provided to MPS patients was tested, to indicate that this isoflavone is safe for as long treatment as 2 years [85,86]. This opened the possibility to conduct a clinical trial with a high dose of genistein. Results of such a single center, double-blinded, randomized, placebo-controlled study with open-label extension phase has been published recently [87]. Although the study group of MPS III patients was quite small (21 participants), statistical analyses of the obtained results could be performed and indicated a significant reduction in urinary GAG levels after treatment with genistein; however, no evidence of clinical efficacy could be measured [87]. Therefore, efficacy of genistein in treatment of MPS patients had been questioned.

Along with differential results in clinical studies with patients treated with genistein, results of some investigations of cellular and animal models became also controversial. Namely, it was reported that genistein could cause an increase in levels of GAGs in MPS I cells [88]. This was in contrast to previous studies demonstrating an opposite effect, that is, a disease in GAG concentrations in cells treated with genistein [62–65]. Subsequent analyses suggested that these discrepancies in results might appear due to cell line–specific differences in responses to genistein treatment [89]. Another contradictory feature of genistein reported in different articles is the safety of this compound. Although in most in vitro studies this isoflavone was assessed as safe to human cells [62–65,71,75], one work indicated a genistein-related damage od DNA in MPS IVA cells [90]. No explanation of this discrepancy in results was provided to date. Similarly, adverse effects of genistein at the dose of 160 mg/kg/day were reported for MPS I mice, which included a decreased length of both femur and the whole body and frequent scrotal hernia and scrotal hydrocele [91]. In contrast, neither such adverse effects of genistein nor other negative changes after administration of this isoflavone were observed previously in MPS II and MPS IIIB mice, as well as in control wild-type mice [66,68]. One might suggest that different animal models might respond differently to genistein, but at the moment, this can be only a speculation.

The presented case of studies on the use of genistein in MPS is an example of difficulties in medical applications of flavonoids and indication of possible controversies between hopes and disappointments in this field. Most primary reports describing effects of genistein in reducing synthesis rate and levels of GAGs were very encouraging for development of potential drugs for treatment of MPS patients [62–65]. Such a hope was strengthened by results of experiments with two MPS mice models [66–68]. Even preliminary clinical studies were encouraging [79,80,82,83]. Despite some reports indicating an increase in GAG concentrations in cells [88,90] and appearance of adverse effects in animals treated with genistein [91], majority of reports did not mention such problems [62–77,92]. The discrepancy between results of in vitro studies might arise from potential cell line-specific effects of genistein [89]. However, it is more difficult to explain different efficacies observed in clinical trials. Although in all clinical studies performed to date, decreases in GAG levels were reported, some reports showed positive clinical effects [79,80,82,83] while others could not demonstrate clinical improvement [81,84,87]. It is not clear what are the reasons for these differences. One problem is a rarity of the MPS disease and thus, a low number of patients participating in clinical studies. Along with this, both age of patients and their clinical state varied significantly from person to person, making the analyses of results especially difficult. In addition, some crucial parameters which should be tested in MPS patients arc cxtremely difficult to investigate. They are exemplified by assessment of cognitive skills, mental development, and behavioral characteristics which are almost impossible to quantify in a precise manner in severely affected children suffering from MPS [93]. Thus, solid conclusions on efficacy of flavonoids, like genistein, in treatment of MPS are very hard to reach, and the advice for further researchers might be to take into consideration a battery of different aspects and factors which can influence the results of studies. A summary of hopes and disappointments in the use of genistein for treatment of MPS is presented in Fig. 14.3, along with some comments that might explain the discrepancies in the reported results.

Concluding remarks

The description of selected features of flavonoids and their potential applications in treatment of patients suffering from various diseases (like cancer, infectious diseases, neurodegenerative diseases) and presentation of the history of the use of genistein, an isoflavone, as a potential drug for mucopolysaccharidosis, shown here as a case study, indicate hopes and disappointments related to the employment of these compounds as therapeutic agents. Generally, many in vitro studies (especially those performed with

The use of genistein in mucopolysaccharidoses

Hopes	Disappointments	Comments
	In vitro studies	
Inhibition of GAG synthesis	Stimulation of GAG synthesis	Possible cell line-specific effects
	Experiments with animal models	
Safety (no adverse effects) Reduction of GAG levels Correction of behavior	Adverse effects	Possible differences between animal models
	Clinical experiments and trials	
Safety (no adverse effects) Reduction of GAG levels Improvement in some symptoms	Little or no clinical improvement	Bioavailability issues

FIGURE 14.3 A summary of hopes of disappointments in the use of genistein (an isoflavone) in treatment of mucopolysaccharidoses (MPS).

cell cultures) and experiments with animal models of diseases indicated high efficiency of flavonoids is either diminishing of primary biochemical causes of the diseases or improving processes which are otherwise impaired due to the disease progress. On the other hand, clinical trials with flavonoids as drugs for specific diseases are either lacking or demonstrated little or no clinical improvements of patients. In the light of such discrepancies, one should ask about the reasons of them.

A general problem is the use of very different concentrations of flavonoids by different researchers. This makes a reliable comparison of results difficult, if not impossible at all. Another serious drawback is often treatment of cells, animals, or humans with extracts which should contain certain amounts of flavonoids, instead of purified or synthetic compounds. As it was demonstrated experimentally, various extracts contain very different amounts of flavonoids, sometimes dozens of times lower than those declared by manufacturers [78], and even different lots of the same product might differ considerably in this parameter. Therefore, such experiments are hardly reproducible. Moreover, the presence of other compounds in such extracts (beside flavonoids) might modulate actions of biologically active molecules. This can lead to discrepancies between results obtained with pure compounds and extracts [28]. Another problem which is sometimes overlooked is bioavailability of flavonoids which is generally not high [94]. Ignoring this problem might lead to negative results of clinical studies even if preclinical experiments indicated high efficiency in reducing specific disorders. Finally, it is necessary to take into consideration the multimodal action of flavonoids. The multiple biological activities of these compounds, from antioxidative and anti-inflammatory properties, through interactions with different proteins and changing biochemical pathways, to indirect influencing the physiological processes, are rarely considered together; most often only one function of the studied molecule is investigated which may easily lead to misinterpretation of the results and to serious confusions. On the other hand, such multiple activities of flavonoids can be profitable for potential drugs in the case of many diseases, especially those of complex pathomechanisms. The use of multiple-function compounds might be effective in therapeutical approaches which are based on combination therapies. In fact, flavonoids have been proposed to be used in such strategies of drug development [95–97]. Despite these profits of multiple biological activities of flavonoids, the same features may be considered as their drawbacks. Namely, many pharmaceutical companies focus their research on development of new drugs which have a single, well-defined molecular target [43]. Obviously, this strategy can lead to detailed characterization of the mode of action of the putative drug; however, a great potential of flavonoids may be lost. Moreover, natural compounds are not attractive molecules for development of therapies for rare diseases, purely due to economic barriers [43].

In summary, it appears that flavonoids have a great potential as putative drugs for many diseases (which is a hope) but to avoid hardly interpretable or false-negative results (which are disappointing and may cause a loss of interest in further experiments), more careful studies are necessary which should take into consideration various activities of these plant metabolites, the range of concentrations in which they are active, and their bioavailability.

Acknowledgments

The work of authors on flavonoids was supported by National Science Center, Poland (grant no. 2018/29/N/NZ2/00802 to L.G., and grant no. 2019/35/N/NZ2/00505 to E.R.), and by Fundacja Sanfilippo, Poland (grant 21.01.2019 to G.W.).

References

[1] Dias MC, Pinto DCGA, Silva AMS. Plant flavonoids: chemical characteristics and biological activity. Molecules 2021;26(17):5377. https://doi.org/10.3390/molecules26175377.

[2] Shen N, Wang T, Gan Q, Liu S, Wang L, Jin B. Plant flavonoids: classification, distribution, biosynthesis, and antioxidant activity. Food Chem 2022;383:132531. https://doi.org/10.1016/j.foodchem.2022.132531.

[3] Al-Khayri JM, Sahana GR, Nagella P, Joseph BV, Alessa FM, Al-Mssallem MQ. Flavonoids as potential anti-inflammatory molecules: a review. Molecules 2022;27(9):2901. https://doi.org/10.3390/molecules27092901.

[4] Gouveia HJCB, Urquiza-Martínez MV, Manhães-de-Castro R, et al. Effects of the treatment with flavonoids on metabolic syndrome components in humans: a systematic review focusing on mechanisms of action. Int J Mol Sci 2022;23(15):8344. https://doi.org/10.3390/ijms23158344.

[5] Sharifi-Rad J, Quispe C, Imran M, et al. Genistein: an integrative overview of its mode of action, pharmacological properties, and health benefits. Oxid Med Cell Longev 2021;2021:3268136. https://doi.org/10.1155/2021/3268136.

[6] Fan X, Fan Z, Yang Z, et al. Flavonoids-natural gifts to promote health and longevity. Int J Mol Sci 2022;23(4):2176. https://doi.org/10.3390/ijms23042176.

[7] Azeem M, Hanif M, Mahmood K, Ameer N, Chughtai FRS, Abid U. An insight into anticancer, antioxidant, antimicrobial, antidiabetic and anti-inflammatory effects of quercetin: a review. Polym Bull (Berl) 2022:1−22. https://doi.org/10.1007/s00289-022-04091-8 (published online ahead of print, January 30, 2022).

[8] Roy A, Khan A, Ahmad I, et al. Flavonoids a bioactive compound from medicinal plants and its therapeutic applications. BioMed Res Int 2022;2022:5445291. https://doi.org/10.1155/2022/5445291.

[9] Sok Yen F, Shu Qin C, Tan Shi Xuan S, et al. Hypoglycemic effects of plant flavonoids: a review. Evid Based Complement Altern Med 2021;2021:2057333. https://doi.org/10.1155/2021/2057333.

[10] de Almeida Brasiel PG, Guimarães FV, Rodrigues PM, Bou-Habib DC, Carvalho VF. Therapeutic efficacy of flavonoids in allergies: a systematic review of randomized controlled trials. J Immunol Res 2022;2022:8191253. https://doi.org/10.1155/2022/8191253.

[11] Popiolek-Kalisz J, Fornal E. The impact of flavonols on cardiovascular risk. Nutrients 2022;14(9):1973. https://doi.org/10.3390/nu14091973.

[12] Forni C, Rossi M, Borromeo I, et al. Flavonoids: a myth or a reality for cancer therapy? Molecules (Basel, Switzerland) 2021;26(12):3583. https://doi.org/10.3390/molecules26123583.

[13] Hussain Y, Khan H, Alam W, et al. Flavonoids targeting the mTOR signaling cascades in cancer: a potential crosstalk in anti-breast cancer therapy. Oxid Med Cell Longev 2022;2022:4831833. https://doi.org/10.1155/2022/4831833.

[14] Park MY, Kim Y, Ha SE, et al. Function and application of flavonoids in the breast cancer. Int J Mol Sci 2022;23(14):7732. https://doi.org/10.3390/ijms23147732.

[15] Rahman N, Khan H, Zia A, et al. Bcl-2 modulation in p53 signaling pathway by flavonoids: a potential strategy towards the treatment of cancer. Int J Mol Sci 2021;22(21):11315. https://doi.org/10.3390/ijms222111315.

[16] Silva GVS, Lopes ALVFG, Viali IC, et al. Therapeutic properties of flavonoids in treatment of cancer through autophagic modulation: a systematic review. Chin J Integr Med 2022. https://doi.org/10.1007/s11655-022-3674-9 (in press).

[17] Coutinho TE, Souto EB, Silva AM. Selected flavonoids to target melanoma: a perspective in nanoengineering delivery systems. Bioengineering (Basel) 2022;9(7):290. https://doi.org/10.3390/bioengineering9070290.

[18] Slika H, Mansour H, Wehbe N, et al. Therapeutic potential of flavonoids in cancer: ROS-mediated mechanisms. Biomed Pharmacother 2022;146:112442. https://doi.org/10.1016/j.biopha.2021.112442.

[19] Fatima N, Baqri SSR, Bhattacharya A, et al. Role of flavonoids as epigenetic modulators in cancer prevention and therapy. Front Genet 2021;12:758733. https://doi.org/10.3389/fgene.2021.758733.

[20] Wang M, Yu F, Zhang Y, Chang W, Zhou M. The effects and mechanisms of flavonoids on cancer prevention and therapy: focus on gut microbiota. Int J Biol Sci 2022;18(4):1451−75. https://doi.org/10.7150/ijbs.68170.

[21] Pereira-Wilson C. Can dietary flavonoids be useful in the personalized treatment of colorectal cancer? World J Gastrointest Oncol 2022;14(6):1115−23. https://doi.org/10.4251/wjgo.v14.i6.1115.

[22] Asgharian P, Tazekand AP, Hosseini K, et al. Potential mechanisms of quercetin in cancer prevention: focus on cellular and molecular targets. Cancer Cell Int 2022;22(1):257. https://doi.org/10.1186/s12935-022-02677-w.

[23] Amjad E, Sokouti B, Asnaashari S. A systematic review of anti-cancer roles and mechanisms of kaempferol as a natural compound. Cancer Cell Int 2022;22(1):260. https://doi.org/10.1186/s12935-022-02673-0.

[24] Cook MA, Wright GD. The past, present, and future of antibiotics. Sci Transl Med 2022;14(657):eabo7793. https://doi.org/10.1126/scitranslmed.abo7793.

[25] Song L, Hu X, Ren X, Liu J, Liu X. Antibacterial modes of herbal flavonoids combat resistant bacteria. Front Pharmacol 2022;13:873374. https://doi.org/10.3389/fphar.2022.873374.

[26] Ulanowska K, Majchrzyk A, Moskot M, Jakóbkiewicz-Banecka J, Węgrzyn G. Assessment of antibacterial effects of flavonoids by estimation of generation times in liquid bacterial cultures. Biologia 2007;62:132−5. https://doi.org/10.2478/s11756-007-0042-3.

[27] Ulanowska K, Tkaczyk A, Konopa G, Wegrzyn G. Differential antibacterial activity of genistein arising from global inhibition of DNA, RNA and protein synthesis in some bacterial strains. Arch Microbiol 2006;184(5):271–8. https://doi.org/10.1007/s00203-005-0063-7.

[28] Pierzynowska K, Rzeszótko A, Blendowska A, et al. Differential effects of various soy isoflavone dietary supplements (nutraceuticals) on bacterial growth and human fibroblast viability. Acta Biochim Pol 2018;65(2):325–32. https://doi.org/10.18388/abp.2018_2596.

[29] Waditzer M, Bucar F. Flavonoids as inhibitors of bacterial efflux pumps. Molecules 2021;26(22):6904. https://doi.org/10.3390/molecules26226904.

[30] Shamsudin NF, Ahmed QU, Mahmood S, et al. Antibacterial effects of flavonoids and their structure-activity relationship study: a comparative interpretation. Molecules 2022;27(4):1149. https://doi.org/10.3390/molecules27041149.

[31] Rabaan AA, Alhumaid S, Albayat H, et al. Promising anti-mycobacterial activities of flavonoids against *Mycobacterium* sp. drug targets: a comprehensive review. Molecules 2022;27(16):5335. https://doi.org/10.3390/molecules27165335.

[32] Castro E Silva JH, Souza JT, Schitine C, Júnior AFS, Bastos EMS, Costa SL. Pharmacological potential of flavonoids against neurotropic viruses. Pharmaceuticals (Basel) 2022;15(9):1149. https://doi.org/10.3390/ph15091149.

[33] Zhang X, Chen S, Li X, Zhang L, Ren L. Flavonoids as potential antiviral agents for porcine viruses. Pharmaceutics 2022;14(9):1793. https://doi.org/10.3390/pharmaceutics14091793.

[34] Bardelčíková A, Miroššay A, Šoltýs J, Mojžiš J. Therapeutic and prophylactic effect of flavonoids in post-COVID-19 therapy. Phytother Res 2022;36(5):2042–60. https://doi.org/10.1002/ptr.7436.

[35] Minocha T, Birla H, Obaid AA, et al. Flavonoids as promising neuroprotectants and their therapeutic potential against Alzheimer's disease. Oxid Med Cell Longev 2022;2022:6038996. https://doi.org/10.1155/2022/6038996.

[36] Liao W, Jin G, Zhao M, Yang H. The effect of genistein on the content and activity of α- and β-secretase and protein kinase C in Aβ-injured hippocampal neurons. Basic Clin Pharmacol Toxicol 2013;112(3):182–5. https://doi.org/10.1111/bcpt.12009.

[37] Youn K, Park JH, Lee S, et al. BACE1 inhibition by genistein: biological evaluation, kinetic analysis, and molecular docking simulation. J Med Food 2018;21(4):416–20. https://doi.org/10.1089/jmf.2017.4068.

[38] Pierzynowska K, Gaffke L, Cyske Z, et al. Autophagy stimulation as a promising approach in treatment of neurodegenerative diseases. Metab Brain Dis 2018;33(4):989–1008. https://doi.org/10.1007/s11011-018-0214-6.

[39] Pierzynowska K, Gaffke L, Hać A, et al. Correction of Huntington's disease phenotype by genistein-induced autophagy in the cellular model. Neuromol Med 2018;20(1):112–23. https://doi.org/10.1007/s12017-018-8482-1.

[40] Pierzynowska K, Gaffke L, Cyske Z, Węgrzyn G. Genistein induces degradation of mutant huntingtin in fibroblasts from Huntington's disease patients. Metab Brain Dis 2019;34(3):715–20. https://doi.org/10.1007/s11011-019-00405-4.

[41] Pierzynowska K, Podlacha M, Gaffke L, et al. Autophagy-dependent mechanism of genistein-mediated elimination of behavioral and biochemical defects in the rat model of sporadic Alzheimer's disease. Neuropharmacology 2019;148:332–46. https://doi.org/10.1016/j.neuropharm.2019.01.030.

[42] Mas-Bargues C, Borrás C, Viña J. The multimodal action of genistein in Alzheimer's and other age-related diseases. Free Radic Biol Med 2022;183:127–37. https://doi.org/10.1016/j.freeradbiomed.2022.03.021.

[43] Pierzynowska K, Kamińska T, Węgrzyn G. One drug to treat many diseases: unlocking the economic trap of rare diseases. Metab Brain Dis 2020;35(8):1237–40. https://doi.org/10.1007/s11011-020-00617-z.

[44] Fuloria S, Yusri MAA, Sekar M, et al. Genistein: a potential natural lead molecule for new drug design and development for treating memory impairment. Molecules 2022;27(1):265. https://doi.org/10.3390/molecules27010265.

[45] Mas-Bargues C, Borrás C, Viña J. Genistein, a tool for geroscience. Mech Ageing Dev 2022;204:111665. https://doi.org/10.1016/j.mad.2022.111665.

[46] Gleason CE, Fischer BL, Dowling NM, et al. Cognitive effects of soy isoflavones in patients with Alzheimer's disease. J Alzheimers Dis 2015;47(4):1009–19. https://doi.org/10.3233/JAD-142958.

[47] Nagpal R, Goyal RB, Priyadarshini K, et al. Mucopolysaccharidosis: a broad review. Indian J Ophthalmol 2022;70(7):2249–61. https://doi.org/10.4103/ijo.IJO_425_22.

[48] Wiśniewska K, Wolski J, Gaffke L, Cyske Z, Pierzynowska K, Węgrzyn G. Misdiagnosis in mucopolysaccharidoses. J Appl Genet 2022;63(3):475–95. https://doi.org/10.1007/s13353-022-00703-1.

[49] Węgrzyn G, Pierzynowska K, Pavone LM. Editorial: molecular aspects of mucopolysaccharidoses. Front Mol Biosci 2022;9:874267. https://doi.org/10.3389/fmolb.2022.874267.

[50] Sahin O, Thompson HP, Goodman GW, Li J, Urayama A. Mucopolysaccharidoses and the blood-brain barrier. Fluids Barriers CNS 2022;19(1):76. https://doi.org/10.1186/s12987-022-00373-5.

[51] McBride KL, Flanigan KM. Update in the mucopolysaccharidoses. Semin Pediatr Neurol 2021;37:100874. https://doi.org/10.1016/j.spen.2021.100874.

[52] Khan SA, Tomatsu SC. Mucolipidoses overview: past, present, and future. Int J Mol Sci 2020;21(18):6812. https://doi.org/10.3390/ijms21186812.

[53] Pierzynowska K, Gaffke L, Cyske Z, et al. Oxidative stress in mucopolysaccharidoses: pharmacological implications. Molecules 2021;26(18):5616. https://doi.org/10.3390/molecules26185616.

[54] Rintz E, Pierzynowska K, Podlacha M, Węgrzyn G. Has resveratrol a potential for mucopolysaccharidosis treatment? Eur J Pharmacol 2020;888:173534. https://doi.org/10.1016/j.ejphar.2020.173534.

[55] Parini R, Deodato F. Intravenous enzyme replacement therapy in mucopolysaccharidoses: clinical effectiveness and limitations. Int J Mol Sci 2020;21(8):2975. https://doi.org/10.3390/ijms21082975.

[56] Losada Díaz JC, Cepeda Del Castillo J, Rodriguez-López EA, Alméciga-Díaz CJ. Advances in the development of pharmacological chaperones for the mucopolysaccharidoses. Int J Mol Sci 2019;21(1):232. https://doi.org/10.3390/ijms21010232.

[57] Pierzynowska K, Gaffke L, Podlacha M, Brokowska J, Węgrzyn G. Mucopolysaccharidosis and autophagy: controversies on the contribution of the process to the pathogenesis and possible therapeutic applications. Neuromol Med 2020;22(1):25–30.

[58] Christensen CL, Ashmead RE, Choy FYM. Cell and gene therapies for mucopolysaccharidoses: base editing and therapeutic delivery to

the CNS. Diseases 2019;7(3):47. https://doi.org/10.3390/diseases7030047.

[59] Sawamoto K, Stapleton M, Alméciga-Díaz CJ, et al. Therapeutic options for mucopolysaccharidoses: current and emerging treatments. Drugs 2019;79(10):1103–34. https://doi.org/10.1007/s40265-019-01147-4.

[60] Węgrzyn A. Gene expression-targeted isoflavone therapy. IUBMB Life 2012;64(4):307–15. https://doi.org/10.1002/iub.1007.

[61] Jakóbkiewicz-Banecka J, Wegrzyn A, Wegrzyn G. Substrate deprivation therapy: a new hope for patients suffering from neuronopathic forms of inherited lysosomal storage diseases. J Appl Genet 2007;48(4):383–8. https://doi.org/10.1007/BF03195237.

[62] Piotrowska E, Jakóbkiewicz-Banecka J, Barańska S, et al. Genistein-mediated inhibition of glycosaminoglycan synthesis as a basis for gene expression-targeted isoflavone therapy for mucopolysaccharidoses. Eur J Hum Genet 2006;14(7):846–52. https://doi.org/10.1038/sj.ejhg.5201623.

[63] Arfi A, Richard M, Gandolphe C, Scherman D. Storage correction in cells of patients suffering from mucopolysaccharidoses types IIIA and VII after treatment with genistein and other isoflavones. J Inherit Metab Dis 2010;33(1):61–7. https://doi.org/10.1007/s10545-009-9029-2.

[64] Otomo T, Hossain MA, Ozono K, Sakai N. Genistein reduces heparan sulfate accumulation in human mucolipidosis II skin fibroblasts. Mol Genet Metab 2012;105(2):266–9. https://doi.org/10.1016/j.ymgme.2011.10.015.

[65] Jakóbkiewicz-Banecka J, Piotrowska E, Narajczyk M, Barańska S, Wegrzyn G. Genistein-mediated inhibition of glycosaminoglycan synthesis, which corrects storage in cells of patients suffering from mucopolysaccharidoses, acts by influencing an epidermal growth factor-dependent pathway. J Biomed Sci 2009;16(1):26. https://doi.org/10.1186/1423-0127-16-26.

[66] Friso A, Tomanin R, Salvalaio M, Scarpa M. Genistein reduces glycosaminoglycan levels in a mouse model of mucopolysaccharidosis type II. Br J Pharmacol 2010;159(5):1082–91. https://doi.org/10.1111/j.1476-5381.2009.00565.x.

[67] Malinowska M, Wilkinson FL, Bennett W, et al. Genistein reduces lysosomal storage in peripheral tissues of mucopolysaccharide IIIB mice. Mol Genet Metab 2009;98(3):235–42. https://doi.org/10.1016/j.ymgme.2009.06.013.

[68] Malinowska M, Wilkinson FL, Langford-Smith KJ, et al. Genistein improves neuropathology and corrects behaviour in a mouse model of neurodegenerative metabolic disease. PLoS One 2010;5(12):e14192. https://doi.org/10.1371/journal.pone.0014192.

[69] Węsierska M, Kloska A, Medina DL, et al. Cellular and gene expression response to the combination of genistein and kaempferol in the treatment of mucopolysaccharidosis type I. Int J Mol Sci 2022;23(3):1058. https://doi.org/10.3390/ijms23031058.

[70] Kloska A, Jakóbkiewicz-Banecka J, Narajczyk M, Banecka-Majkutewicz Z, Węgrzyn G. Effects of flavonoids on glycosaminoglycan synthesis: implications for substrate reduction therapy in Sanfilippo disease and other mucopolysaccharidoses. Metab Brain Dis 2011;26(1):1–8. https://doi.org/10.1007/s11011-011-9233-2.

[71] Kloska A, Narajczyk M, Jakóbkiewicz-Banecka J, et al. Synthetic genistein derivatives as modulators of glycosaminoglycan storage. J Transl Med 2012;10:153. https://doi.org/10.1186/1479-5876-10-153.

[72] Moskot M, Montefusco S, Jakóbkiewicz-Banecka J, et al. The phytoestrogen genistein modulates lysosomal metabolism and transcription factor EB (TFEB) activation. J Biol Chem 2014;289(24):17054–69. https://doi.org/10.1074/jbc.M114.555300.

[73] Moskot M, Jakóbkiewicz-Banecka J, Kloska A, et al. Modulation of expression of genes involved in glycosaminoglycan metabolism and lysosome biogenesis by flavonoids. Sci Rep 2015;5:9378. https://doi.org/10.1038/srep09378.

[74] Moskot M, Gabig-Cimińska M, Jakóbkiewicz-Banecka J, Węsierska M, Bocheńska K, Węgrzyn G. Cell cycle is disturbed in mucopolysaccharidosis type II fibroblasts, and can be improved by genistein. Gene 2016;585(1):100–3. https://doi.org/10.1016/j.gene.2016.03.029.

[75] Fumić B, Jablan J, Cinčić D, Zovko Končić M, Jug M. Cyclodextrin encapsulation of daidzein and genistein by grinding: implication on the glycosaminoglycan accumulation in mucopolysaccharidosis type II and III fibroblasts. J Microencapsul 2018;35(1):1–12. https://doi.org/10.1080/02652048.2017.1409819.

[76] Pierzynowska K, Gaffke L, Jankowska E, et al. Proteasome composition and activity changes in cultured fibroblasts derived from mucopolysaccharidoses patients and their modulation by genistein. Front Cell Dev Biol 2020;8:540726. https://doi.org/10.3389/fcell.2020.540726.

[77] Jacques CED, Lopes FF, Poletto E, et al. Evaluation of oxidative stress and mitochondrial function in a type II mucopolysaccharidosis cellular model: in vitro effects of genistein and coenzyme Q10. Metab Brain Dis 2022. https://doi.org/10.1007/s11011-022-01062-w (in press).

[78] Piotrowska E, Jakóbkiewicz-Banecka J, Wegrzyn G. Different amounts of isoflavones in various commercially available soy extracts in the light of gene expression-targeted isoflavone therapy. Phytother Res 2010;24(Suppl. 1):S109–13. https://doi.org/10.1002/ptr.2944 (published correction appears in Phytother Res April 2010;24(4):632).

[79] Piotrowska E, Jakóbkiewicz-Banecka J, Tylki-Szymanska A, et al. Genistin-rich soy isoflavone extract in substrate reduction therapy for Sanfilippo syndrome: an open-label, pilot study in 10 pediatric patients. Curr Ther Res Clin Exp 2008;69(2):166–79. https://doi.org/10.1016/j.curtheres.2008.04.002.

[80] Piotrowska E, Jakobkiewicz-Banecka J, Maryniak A, et al. Two-year follow-up of Sanfilippo disease patients treated with a genistein-rich isoflavone extract: assessment of effects on cognitive functions and general status of patients. Med Sci Monit 2011;17(4):CR196–202. https://doi.org/10.12659/msm.881715.

[81] Delgadillo V, O'Callaghan Mdel M, Artuch R, Montero R, Pineda M. Genistein supplementation in patients affected by Sanfilippo disease. J Inherit Metab Dis 2011;34(5):1039–44. https://doi.org/10.1007/s10545-011-9342-4.

[82] Marucha J, Tylki-Szymańska A, Jakóbkiewicz-Banecka J, et al. Improvement in the range of joint motion in seven patients with mucopolysaccharidosis type II during experimental gene expression-targeted isoflavone therapy (GET IT). Am J Med Genet A 2011;155A(9):2257–62. https://doi.org/10.1002/ajmg.a.34146.

[83] Malinová V, Węgrzyn G, Narajczyk M. The use of elevated doses of genistein-rich soy extract in the gene expression-targeted isoflavone therapy for Sanfilippo disease patients. JIMD Rep 2012;5:21–5. https://doi.org/10.1007/8904_2011_87.

[84] de Ruijter J, Valstar MJ, Narajczyk M, et al. Genistein in Sanfilippo disease: a randomized controlled crossover trial. Ann Neurol 2012;71(1):110–20. https://doi.org/10.1002/ana.22643.

[85] Kim KH, Dodsworth C, Paras A, Burton BK. High dose genistein aglycone therapy is safe in patients with mucopolysaccharidoses involving the central nervous system. Mol Genet Metab 2013;109(4):382–5. https://doi.org/10.1016/j.ymgme.2013.06.012.

[86] Jurecka A, Tylki-Szymańska A. Gynecomastia in MPS IIIA boys: related to treatment or precocious puberty? Mol Genet Metab 2014;111(2):61–2. https://doi.org/10.1016/j.ymgme.2013.10.008.

[87] Ghosh A, Rust S, Langford-Smith K, et al. High dose genistein in Sanfilippo syndrome: a randomised controlled trial. J Inherit Metab Dis 2021;44(5):1248–62. https://doi.org/10.1002/jimd.12407.

[88] Kingma SD, Wagemans T, IJlst L, Wijburg FA, van Vlies N. Genistein increases glycosaminoglycan levels in mucopolysaccharidosis type I cell models. J Inherit Metab Dis 2014;37(5):813–21. https://doi.org/10.1007/s10545-014-9703-x.

[89] Lan Y, Li X, Liu X, et al. Genistein enhances or reduces glycosaminoglycan quantity in a cell type-specific manner. Cell Physiol Biochem 2018;47(4):1667–81. https://doi.org/10.1159/000490985.

[90] Negretto GW, Deon M, Burin M, et al. In vitro effect of genistein on DNA damage in leukocytes from mucopolysaccharidosis IVA patients. Mol Genet Metab 2014;111(2):205–8. https://doi.org/10.1016/j.ymgme.2013.11.011.

[91] Kingma SD, Wagemans T, IJlst L, et al. Adverse effects of genistein in a mucopolysaccharidosis type I mouse model. JIMD Rep 2015;23:77–83. https://doi.org/10.1007/8904_2015_432.

[92] Brokowska J, Gaffke L, Pierzynowska K, Cyske Z, Węgrzyn G. Cell cycle disturbances in mucopolysaccharidoses: transcriptomic and experimental studies on cellular models. Exp Biol Med 2022. https://doi.org/10.1177/15353702221114872. 15353702221114872.

[93] Cyske Z, Anikiej-Wiczenbach P, Wisniewska K, et al. Sanfilippo syndrome: optimizing care with a multidisciplinary approach. J Multidiscip Healthc 2022;15:2097–110. https://doi.org/10.2147/JMDH.S362994.

[94] Billowria K, Ali R, Rangra NK, Kumar R, Chawla PA. Bioactive flavonoids: a comprehensive review on pharmacokinetics and analytical aspects. Crit Rev Anal Chem 2022:1–15. https://doi.org/10.1080/10408347.2022.2105641 (published online ahead of print, August 5, 2022).

[95] Vladu AF, Ficai D, Ene AG, Ficai A. Combination therapy using polyphenols: an efficient way to improve antitumoral activity and reduce resistance. Int J Mol Sci 2022;23(18):10244. https://doi.org/10.3390/ijms231810244.

[96] Chen Z, Zhang SL. The role of flavonoids in the prevention and management of cardiovascular complications: a narrative review. Ann Palliat Med 2021;10(7):8254–63. https://doi.org/10.21037/apm-21-1343.

[97] Szczechowiak K, Diniz BS, Leszek J. Diet and Alzheimer's dementia—nutritional approach to modulate inflammation. Pharmacol Biochem Behav 2019;184:172743. https://doi.org/10.1016/j.pbb.2019.172743.

Chapter 15

Omega-3 nutritional intervention as therapeutic co-adjuvant approach to improve Rett syndrome clinical and biochemical features

Valeria Cordone[1], **Alessandra Pecorelli**[1,2] **and Giuseppe Valacchi**[1,2,3]

[1]*Department of Environmental Sciences and Prevention, University of Ferrara, Ferrara, Italy;* [2]*Animal Science Department, Plants for Human Health Institute, North Carolina State University, Kannapolis Research Campus, Kannapolis, NC, United States;* [3]*Department of Food and Nutrition, Kyung Hee University, Seoul, South Korea*

Key takeaways

- This chapter focuses on the role of omega-3 polyunsaturated fatty acids (PUFAs) as possible nutritional intervention in Rett syndrome, a rare genetic neurodevelopmental disorder with metabolic and multisystem disturbances.
- To date, there is no cure for Rett syndrome. Researchers are investigating different approaches including gene therapy, although this option seems to be still a big challenge before translation in clinical practice. Thus, therapies/co-adjuvants aimed at ameliorating the symptomatic picture of the pathology represent a more concrete goal.
- Supplementation with omega-3 PUFAs has beneficial effects in various diseases, even though attention should be paid to doses/concentrations and oxidation of these molecules.
- Omega-3 PUFAs supplementation in Rett syndrome patients exhibited beneficial effects on inflammatory state, redox homeostasis, myocardial function, fatty acid composition of erythrocyte membranes, and the overall clinical features.

Introduction

Omega-3 polyunsaturated fatty acids (PUFAs) have well-demonstrated beneficial effects as anti-inflammatory/immune-modulatory molecules and regulate multiple biological functions (i.e., blood pressure, maternal/child health, correct neurological development) [1].

Rett syndrome (RTT), although classified as a rare disease, is the second most prevalent cause of severe mental retardation in girls [2]. Even if the neurologic signs are prominent, an oxInflammatory condition, characterized by a combination of oxidative stress together with a subclinical inflammatory state, may contribute to the onset and progression of RTT multisystem co-morbidities [3,4]. To date, RTT has no definitive cure. However, a multitude of in vitro and in vivo studies investigated molecules able to ameliorate both neurologic and nonneurologic RTT manifestations.

The present chapter has the aim to describe the role of omega-3 PUFAs as possible partial therapeutic agents in controlling inflammation, in restoring homeostasis to multiple disrupted cellular pathways, and in improving symptoms of a complex pathology, like RTT.

Rett syndrome: A multisystem pathology with genetic cause

Rett syndrome (OMIM # 312750) is a devastating neurodevelopmental disorder, with a prevalence rate of approximately 1:10,000 female live births [2,5]. In the classic form of RTT, the onset of the pathology typically occurs postnatally, after a phase of apparently normal development and growth, with a stagnation and rapid developmental regression of acquired psychomotor skills (e.g., loss of purposeful hand skills and appearance of stereotypic movements), followed by severe mental retardation, seizures, motor impairment, ataxia, and autistic features [6]. In the 95% of cases, RTT is caused by mutations in the X-linked *MECP2* gene, encoding for methyl-CpG binding protein 2 (MeCP2), an ubiquitous epigenetic modulator responsible for modifying chromatin shaping, repressing/activating gene transcription, and controlling RNA/micro

Modulation of Oxidative Stress. https://doi.org/10.1016/B978-0-443-19247-0.00011-4

RNA processing [7,8]. *MECP2* mutations usually occur de novo (to date more than 800 RTT-causing mutations were confirmed), and some evidence suggest that most of mutations arise on the paternal inherited X chromosome [9,10]. Among all the different *MECP2* mutations, eight missense and nonsense mutations (R106W, R133C, T158M, R168X, R255X, R270X, R294X, and R306C, where X is an STOP codon) account for approximately 78% of all mutations in the disease [11]. C-terminal deletions account for another 8%, and large deletions constitute approximately 5% [12].

Anatomically, reduced brain volume in RTT patients is associated with abnormally small neuronal body size and densely packed neurons, presenting decreased dendritic complexity and spine density, particularly in layers III and V of the cerebral cortex, thalamus, substantia nigra, basal ganglia, amygdala, cerebellum, and hippocampus [13]. In addition, the dendrites of pyramidal neurons in the motor and frontal cortices are considerably shorter than in non-RTT brains [13]. MRI data even demonstrate selective reductions in the volume of the parietal and temporal lobes in female RTT patients, with relative preservation of the occipital lobe [14]. Hence, the aforementioned pre- and postsynaptic abnormalities in RTT brains (i.e., abnormal axonal number, reduced dendritic branching, and spine density) result in an overall decrease of synapse number and an abnormal excitatory/inhibitory balance [15].

Although neurological conditions are prominent, RTT even affects a wide array of nonneurological organs [16]. Multisystem disturbances, like respiratory (hyperventilation and apneas), gastrointestinal (feeding problems, dysphagia, gastroesophageal reflux, altered microbiota and constipation), orthopedic (scoliosis, high prevalence of fractures, and low bone mineral content), and cardiac (prolonged QT interval and arrhythmias) issues, are the most prevalent [17]. Urological dysfunctions (urinary tract infections, kidney stones, and urine retention), metabolic alterations (severe dyslipidemia, insulin resistance, and augmented levels of total cholesterol), and skeletal muscle troubles (hypotonia, muscle atrophy, and motor deterioration) are also nonneurological co-morbidities associated with RTT [18].

While most research studies are focused on the role of *MECP2* in the central nervous system, given its crucial involvement in the earliest stages of neurogenesis and neuronal migration, as well as in the later stages of synaptic and circuit development/plasticity [19–21], distinct clinical aspects found in *Mecp2* mutant animal models and RTT patients highlight the importance of MeCP2 in peripheral tissues (as recently reviewed by Ref. [18]). Indeed, findings on a *Mecp2* peripheral knockout mouse model exclusively expressing MeCP2 in neuronal and glial cells revealed that some symptoms of RTT arise independently of nervous system defects [22].

In addition, RTT patients show compromised signaling pathways and metabolic processes including alterations of cholesterol metabolism [23], in parallel with unbalanced redox homeostasis [24,25], dysfunctional mitochondrial bioenergetics [26–28], and chronic subclinical inflammatory condition [29,30], which act in a vicious circle defined as "OxInflammation" [4].

The first reports of an oxidative impairment and its potential role in RTT occurred about 2 decades ago, showing low serum vitamin E levels in RTT patients [31] and enhanced peroxidation-damage to membranes as well as reduced cytosolic superoxide-dismutase (SOD1) levels in red blood cells deriving from RTT patients [32]. Other papers then revealed that also 4-hydroxynonenal protein adducts (4-HNE-PAs) and non-protein-bound iron (NPBI) levels are increased in the systemic compartment of RTT subjects [33]. Since Fe(II) may contribute to oxidative stress via Fenton reaction [34], high NPBI levels are considered a pro-oxidant element.

Primary fibroblasts and peripheral blood mononuclear cells (PBMCs) isolated from Rett patients also showed enhanced levels of mitochondrial reactive oxygen species (ROS), hydrogen peroxide, and 4-HNE-PAs [24,35], together with altered activities of the main antioxidant enzymes (i.e., glutathione peroxidase, glutathione reductase, and thioredoxin reductase) and higher levels of oxidized glutathione [24,36]. Interestingly, oxidative stress and related damages are present in the brains of RTT presymptomatic mouse models (*Mecp2* knock-out and *Mecp2*^{308}) [37,38]. Whereas a marked improvement of mouse phenotypes, in parallel with decreased levels of brain oxidative markers, was found upon the re-expression of *Mecp2* [38], suggesting a crucial pathogenic role of redox imbalance in the disease.

Besides the altered redox homeostasis, RTT patients show a deregulation of acute phase response proteins [29], in parallel with a perturbed cytokine/chemokine profile, characterized by high serum levels of interleukin (IL)-3, IL-8, IL-9, IL-13, and IL-15 and corroborated by a Th2-shifted balance [39,40]. RTT PBMCs even present an upregulation of arachidonate 15-lipoxygenase (ALOX15) mRNA, an enzyme involved in the oxidation of PUFAs including linoleic acid and generation of bioactive lipid metabolites such as hydroxyoctadecadienoic acids (HODEs). ALOX15 transcript levels are correlated to augmented serum levels of 13-HODE in RTT patients [41]. In addition, studies on both fibroblasts and PBMCs derived from RTT patients evidenced a deregulated inflammasome response, a group of intracellular multiprotein complexes assembled in response to different stimuli (both pathogens and sterile stressors) and characterized by the activation of inflammatory caspase 1, able to activate the proinflammatory cytokines IL-1β and IL-18 [35,42]. Even macrophage populations, including microglia, are dysregulated in *Mecp2*-null mice [43,44], indeed pre-phenotypic and phenotypic RTT mice exhibited an impaired expression of genes associated with innate immunity and cellular stress responses in microglial population, suggesting an early potential role of these cells in the later onset of neurological symptoms [45].

Lastly, plasma levels of F_2-dihomo-isoprostanes (the main oxidation byproduct of adrenic acid, a specific element of myelin) and IL-18 were increased mostly in the early phases of classic RTT [35,46], suggesting that OxInflammatory markers may arise at the same time of the neuro-regression onset in RTT. Therefore, the vicious circle of redox-imbalance and chronic inflammatory state can be considered driving factors for the pathogenesis and progression of RTT [47].

Rett syndrome: From gene therapy challenges to co-adjuvants of current therapeutic strategies

Over the last 15 years, the proved reversibility of RTT-like neurological phenotype in *Mecp2*-knockout mice, by delayed restoration of *Mecp2* gene [48], inspired numerous groups to explore new therapeutic approaches designed to reverse RTT defects, to delay or prevent their onset or to ameliorate some phenotypic manifestations.

One of the most attractive possible interventions is targeting the primary underlying cause (i.e., the loss-of-function mutations in *MECP2*). The main gene therapy approach is *MECP2* gene augmentation that involves delivering a construct containing a wild type copy of *MECP2* coding region to affected cells, in order to restore gene function and, in turn, verify improved functions at molecular, cellular, network and whole body level. To date, just one approach of gene therapy for RTT (TSHA-102 from Taysha GTx) is currently pending approval by the U.S. Food and Drug Administration to start the clinical trials testing, while another one AVXS-201 from Novartis was recently terminated.

In this regard, several challenges make difficult the translation of gene therapy approaches from bench to clinics: 1, finding an appropriate way to control the expression of the exogenously derived gene; 2, the transduction of a sufficient number of cells; 3, the avoidance of off-target effect; 4, the X-chromosome inactivation; 5, finding a nontoxic and efficient vector system for patients; 6, choosing an optimal time for gene therapy intervention.

Regulation of MeCP2 levels within transduced cells is crucial, since MeCP2 is dosage-sensitive, its expression levels is dependent on the phenomena of gene dosage compensation, known as X-chromosome inactivation (XCI), and its overexpression is known to cause another condition called "*MECP2* duplication syndrome" [49,50]. Cells of male individuals affected by this pathology present two copies of *MECP2* gene on their single X-chromosome, thus leading to the production of too much protein. The disease is characterized by mental disability, delayed or absent speech development, autistic features, seizures, ataxia, and recurrent respiratory infections [49,51,52]. While females carrying *MECP2* duplication, in which most cells (about 80%) inactivate the X-chromosome with the duplication, however show anxiety and depression [53,54]. This picture suggests that to cure RTT subjects, correct levels of *MECP2* need to be provided, in particular, delivering additional copies of the gene to cells that already express the healthy copy has to be avoided.

About vectors currently in use for gene therapies, adeno-associated viruses (AAVs) are the most utilized [55]. AAV9 can cross the blood−brain barrier, infect neurons quite efficiently, and mediate long-term transgene expression [56,57]; however, the transduction efficiency showed in mouse models was not sufficient to completely rescue RTT-like phenotypes to the wild-type levels [58,59], and this vector induced severe, sometimes lethal, liver damages [60].

Moreover, since MeCP2 has been shown to play important roles in both neuronal development and adulthood processes [61], another issue is deciding the optimal time for gene therapy. It has been demonstrated that delivery of *MECP2* either in neonate or in adult mice can yield survival and phenotypic benefits, indicating that therapeutic interventions can be helpful across a wide range of ages [48,62]. However, it is not yet clarified whether a critical time window for *Mecp2* delivery would produce the most robust improvement of RTT symptoms. Furthermore, the re-expression of *MECP2* in RTT patients could likely induce an increase of brain volume, whereas RTT individuals have smaller head circumference than neurotypical people. Thus, curing young and adult RTT patients might require cranial surgery to prevent brain damages or fatalities [63].

Other gene-targeted strategies for RTT have been currently investigated: 1—the pharmacological overcome of *MECP2* early truncation mutation to produce full-length protein; 2—the recent development of the genomic editing system CRISPR/Cas9 to correct mainly *MECP2* point mutations; 3—the re-activation of the inactive X-chromosome. This latter seems an attractive treatment option as cells would use their own regulatory functions to produce just the right amount of MeCP2 protein, although the overdosage of other X-linked genes and in vivo efficiency have still to be investigated [63].

Thus, even though very promising, gene therapy strategies are still far to become a gold-standard treatment for this complex pathology.

Until now, 45 interventional trials for RTT have been listed in ClinicalTrials.gov [64], a registry of publicly and privately supported clinical studies conducted all over the world. The amelioration of quality of life is the main outcome measure for the pathology, which derives from clinical severity scores, communication assessments, breathing pattern analysis, and studying stereotypic hand movements [65]. Most of clinical trials involves the direct or indirect modulation of neurotransmission, primary aimed at mitigating neurological symptoms of the disease (i.e., gene/epigenetic modifiers; growth factor therapies, such as Trofinetide, a synthetic analog of the amino-terminal tripeptide of IGF-1, able to reduce neuroinflammation and support synaptic functions; brain-derived neurotrophic factor (BDNF) boosters, like Fingolimod; antidepressant; NMDA receptor antagonist, like Ketamine, able to ameliorate neurological dysfunction in RTT mouse models; serotonergic drugs; anticonvulsant drugs).

To date, treatment of RTT is purely symptomatic and supportive. In many cases, the physical symptoms of RTT can be managed with a robust regimen of therapies: occupational therapy, speech/language therapy, feeding assistance, physical therapy, and medications to reduce breathing and cardiac problems, to relieve indigestion and constipation, to control seizures, muscle stiffness, anxiety, or sleep difficulties [66]. Alternate therapies such as massage therapy, hippotherapy, and music therapy can also be part of the management program of RTT patients [3].

As reviewed by Katz and colleagues [66], a wide variety of nonclinical studies have been conducted especially in RTT mouse models (heterozygous *Mecp2*-deficient female and *Mecp2*-null male mice) to investigate molecules able to ameliorate neurologic and nonneurologic RTT manifestations. Among the latter, several natural-derived compounds showed promising effects in rescuing the redox imbalance (i.e., Trolox, a vitamin-E derivative and free radical scavenger; curcumin, a natural polyphenol acting as antioxidant and neuroprotective agent; coenzyme Q10, an antioxidant molecule influencing the energy state as well as the reduced glutathione (GSH)/oxidized glutathione (GSSG) ratio; EPI-743, an α-tocotrienol quinone) and as booster of mitochondrial metabolism (i.e., acetyl L-carnitine and L-carnitine, essential for mitochondrial energy production) [67–71]. Some of these molecules, such as EPI-743 and L-carnitine, demonstrated efficacy in restoring redox homeostasis, in increasing head circumference, oxygenation, and hand functions in clinical trials, although they did not meet all the primary endpoints of RTT severity score [66]. PUFAs have also been tested in clinical trials, with the purpose that oral supplementation of these compounds could potentially have therapeutic properties in RTT patients. Indeed, omega-3 PUFA treatment significantly improved the clinical severity score in parallel with a decreased levels of several oxidative stress markers in two pilot studies of patients with typical RTT [33,72] as discussed more in detail in the following sessions.

Omega-3 polyunsaturated fatty acids

Fatty acids (FAs) are hydrocarbons characterized by a methyl group on one end and a carboxyl group on the other. The carboxylic acid (−COOH) end of the chain is defined as "alpha," while the methyl ($-CH_3$) end is defined as the "tail" of the chain, thus as "omega" [73].

FAs modulate structure and functions of plasma membranes, regulate and mediate several immune responses, act as cellular messengers in signal transduction pathways, and take part into lipid transport elements, like chylomicrons and lipoproteins [74].

Saturated fatty acids, monounsaturated fatty acids (MUFAs), and PUFAs are the three major types of fatty acids. The acyl chain of saturated fatty acids contains no double bonds, whereas unsaturated fatty acids present one (MUFAs) or two or more double bonds (PUFAs). Depending on the location of the first double bond (C=C) from the terminal methyl end of the FA, PUFAs can be classified as omega-3 fatty acids (ω-3 or n-3 PUFAs) and omega-6 fatty acids (ω-6 or n-6 PUFAs). Since the enzymes desaturases, able to introduce double bonds in the n-3 and n-6 positions are not present in mammals, the human organism can synthesize all except two important fatty acids, termed as "linoleic acid" and "α-linolenic acid" [73].

Linoleic acid (LA, 18:2 n-6, where the first digit indicates the number of carbons, while the second one indicates the number of double bonds) is the precursor of the n-6 PUFAs, while α-linolenic acid (ALA, 18:3 n-3) is the precursor of the n-3 PUFAs. Omega-3 PUFAs include even stearidonic acid (SDA; 18:4 n-3), eicosapentaenoic acid (EPA; 20:5 n-3), docosapentaenoic acid (DPA; 22:5 n-3), and docosahexaenoic acid (DHA; 22:6 n-3) [1].

EPA and DHA can be synthesized in the human body using ALA as a precursor. However, bioconversion of ALA to EPA and DHA is limited; thus, an adequate dietary intake of long chain (LC) n-3 PUFAs is crucial. Phytoplankton and marine algae are important sources of omega-3 FAs. Good sources of plant oils containing ALA include walnut, edible seeds, clary sage seed oil, algal oil, flaxseed oil, chia seeds oil, Echium oil, and hemp oil, whereas safflower, sunflower, corn, and soybean oils are rich in linoleic acid (18:2 n-6) [75]. Common sources of animal EPA and DHA are represented by seafood, although fish do not actually produce these FAs, but they are produced by single-cell marine organisms that are consumed by fish. Other sources comprise squid oils, egg oil, and krill oil [75].

In recent years, a growing interest in n-3 PUFAs has risen due to their various roles in health promotion and disease risk reduction. Indeed, n-3 PUFAs regulate a wide variety of biological functions, which range from blood pressure, and maternal/child health to the correct neurological development and functioning of the brain and nervous system (e.g., learning ability, visual acuity, memory formation, and neuroprotection, being the precursors of neuroprotectin D1). They are even involved in counteracting pathologies, like cardiovascular disease, diabetes, and cancer [1]. In addition, lipid mediators produced from long-chain PUFAs, in particular, arachidonic acid (AA), the major end product in the n-6 series, and DHA and EPA in the n-3 series, play important roles in regulating inflammation and immune functions [76,77].

This topic and other n-3 PUFAs functions will be discussed more in detail in the next section ("The yin and yang of n-3 PUFAs").

The yin and yang of n-3 PUFAs

As already mentioned, the first part of this section will be focused to depict the role and molecular mechanisms of omega-3 fatty acids in helping to manage inflammatory conditions and other pathologies. Whereas the second part will highlight some side effects linked to an excessive consumption of n-3 PUFAs.

Omega-3 PUFAs exert their beneficial effects in regulating inflammatory processes through the following molecular mechanisms: 1, alteration of the physical properties of cell membrane; 2, substrate competition with n-6 AA; 3, conversion into anti-inflammatory, or better immune-modulating metabolites; and 4, influence on several cell signaling pathways.

n-3 PUFAs-induced alteration of the physical properties of cell membrane

n-3 PUFAs can be incorporated into membrane phospholipids of inflammatory cells, like $CD4^+$-T cells, macrophages, and B-cells, whose function is to help in maintaining membrane fluidity and in ensuring the appropriate environment for membrane proteins. n-3 PUFAs are even involved in influencing lipid raft formation [78,79]. In particular, on the basis of results obtained in B-cells, Kim and colleagues hypothesized that the increased raft size, upon EPA and DHA treatment, was accompanied by alterations in adaptive and innate functions [79].

Substrate competition with n-6 AA

PUFAs exert many of their biological actions through bioactive lipid mediators, generated by fatty acid oxygenases, like lipoxygenases (LOXs), cyclooxygenases (COXs), and cytochrome P450 monooxygenases (CYPs) [80]. Indeed, n-6 AA deriving from membrane phospholipids, after an inflammatory stimuli, is converted into eicosanoids, such as leukotrienes (LTs), prostaglandins (PGs), and lipoxins (LXs) via COX and LOX activities. Even n-3 PUFAs are present at the inflammation site, through their enzymatic transformation into bioactive mediators. The anti-inflammatory function of n-3 PUFAs occur by both competing with the formation of proinflammatory eicosanoids from n-6 AA, and generating metabolites with less potent activity than AA-derived molecules (Fig. 15.1) [81]. In particular, EPA and DHA are substrates of AA cascade enzymes (COX1/2, and 5-LOX), thus leading to reduced production of AA-derived eicosanoids, such as PGE_2, and increased production of n-3 PUFA-derived eicosanoids, like 5-series leukotrienes and 3-series prostanoids. These eicosanoids obtained from EPA, like PGE_3, exhibit decreased proinflammatory properties, as compared to eicosanoids generated from AA (Fig. 15.1) [82].

Conversion into anti-inflammatory or better immune-modulating metabolites

n-3 PUFAs' anti-inflammatory role is crucial in promoting the resolution of inflammation. The acute inflammatory response is normally beneficial and serves to protect the host from injuries and infections. Thus, the steps of acute inflammation are usually self-limited. Failure to resolve an acute inflammation may lead to the development of chronic inflammation, a hallmark of inflammatory diseases, like asthma, rheumatoid arthritis, and inflammatory bowel disease.

Resolution of inflammation is not only due to the passive end of proinflammatory stimuli, but also to an active process orchestrated by specialized proresolving mediators (SPMs). n-3 PUFAs are precursors of SPMs, like lipoxins, resolvins, protectins, and maresins (Fig. 15.1) [80]. DHA is the precursor of D-series resolvins (RvD1, RvD2, RvD3, RvD4), protectins (protectin D1), and maresins (MaR1), while EPA leads to the production of E-series resolvins (RvE1, RvE2, and RvE3) [80]. However, these SPMs act in combination with other mediators such as annexin A1 protein, microRNAs, cytokines, like TGF, and IL-10, and inhibitors of cyclin-dependent kinases [83].

SPMs are produced by macrophages and polymorphonuclear leukocytes (PMNs). SPMs biologic effects are specific for each molecule and comprise: suppression of cellular production of adhesion molecules, cytokines, ROS, and inflammatory transcription factors such as nuclear factor (NF)-κB. SPMs also induce an impairment of cellular functions, like neutrophil recruitment, infiltration, and transmigration, chemotaxis, and macrophage switching to anti-inflammatory phenotype M2 [80]. Moreover, SPMs action leads to increased uptake and removal of apoptotic bodies by phagocytic cells (a process known as "efferocytosis") and to augmented microbial killing. Hence, SPMs exhibit both immune suppressive properties upon inflammation and immune-stimulating effects (i.e., clearance of microbes and dead cells).

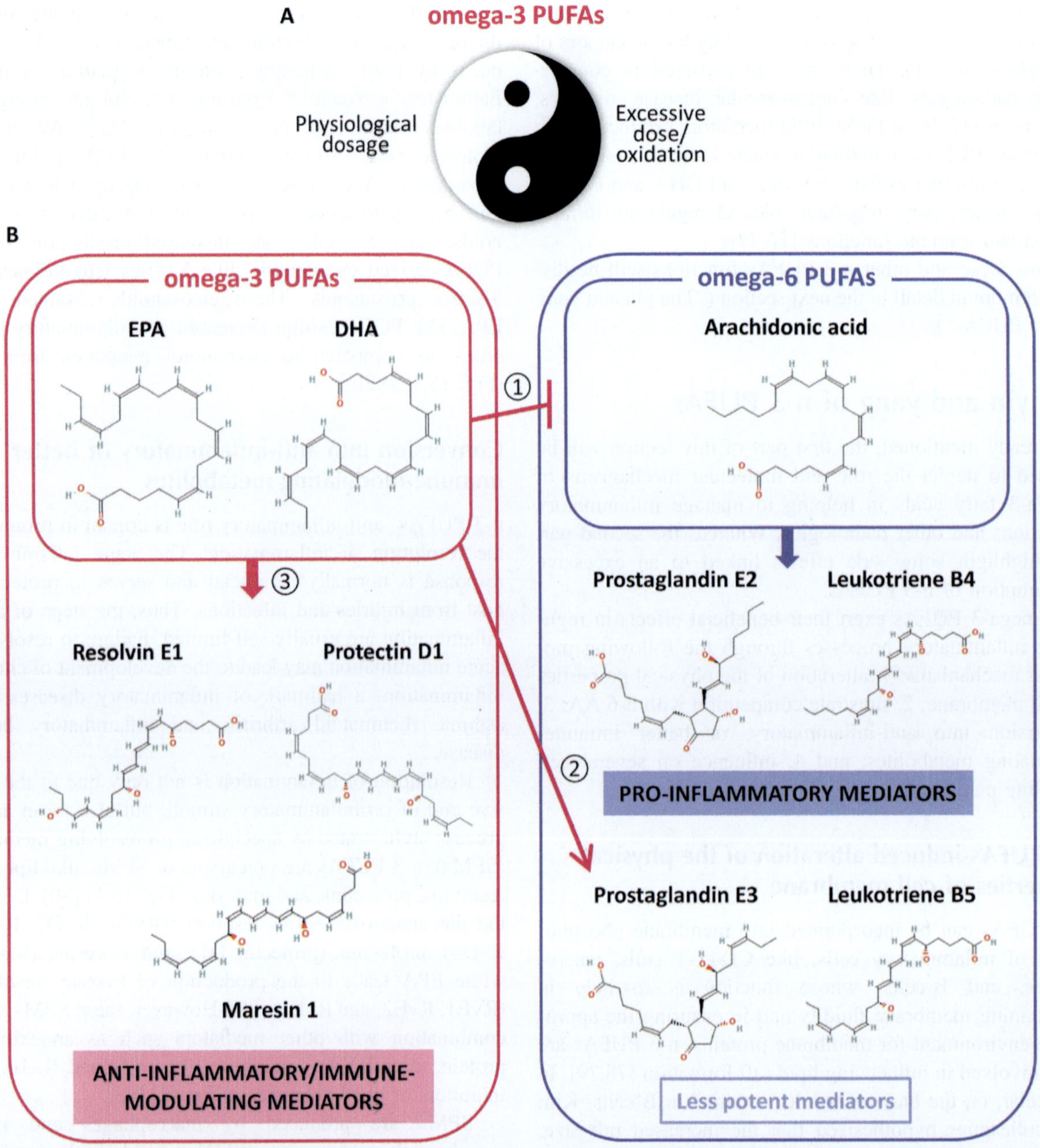

FIGURE 15.1 Main anti-inflammatory effects of omega-3 polyunsaturated fatty acids (PUFAs). (A) Despite the numerous beneficial properties of omega-3 PUFAs, attention should be given to the doses and oxidation state of these fatty acids, when used as co-treatment/therapeutic supplement to patients. (B) Omega-3 PUFAs, in particular eicosapentaenoic acid (EPA) and docosahexaenoic acid (DHA), exert their beneficial effects by the following mechanisms: (1) substrate competition with omega-6 arachidonic acid (AA) (2) generation of pro-inflammatory molecules (i.e., 3-series prostaglandins and 5-series leukotrienes); less potent than eicosanoids generated from AA; (3) conversion into anti-inflammatory/immune-modulating metabolites. *All the chemical structures were taken from Pubchem (https://pubchem.ncbi.nlm.nih.gov/).*

Influence on several cell signaling pathways

About the effects of n-3 PUFAs on cell signaling pathways, the direct modulation of G protein-coupled receptors (GPCRs) by EPA and DHA might contribute to their anti-inflammatory effects [84]. It has been demonstrated that GPR120 activation by DHA interacts with TGF-beta activated kinase 1 binding protein 1 (TAB1) via β-arrestin-2. This interaction could attenuate both toll-like receptor 4 (TLR4)- and tumor necrosis factor (TNF)-α-mediated inflammatory responses in macrophages and dendritic cells [85]. Moreover, enrichment of cellular phospholipid bilayer with n-3 PUFAs leads to an impaired dimerization and recruitment of TLR4, one of the main receptors upstream of

NF-κB activation [86,87]. EPA and DHA are also able to inhibit NF-κB signaling pathway and in turn reducing the expression of inflammation-related genes, by blocking IκB phosphorylation [88,89].

Then, n-3 PUFAs can directly affect inflammatory cells through intracellular fatty acid receptors, including transcription factors, like peroxisome proliferator-activated receptors (PPAR) α and γ [90].

As just described, omega-3 fatty acids have multiple anti-inflammatory properties. In addition, as recently reviewed by Zaloga [74], multiple scientific papers even showed the immune-suppressive properties of n-3 PUFAs and for these reasons fish oils are also used in the treatment of psoriasis, rheumatoid arthritis, inflammatory bowel disease, cachexia, dementia, and systemic lupus erythematosus [91]. Nevertheless, the anti-inflammatory and immune-suppressive effects of n-3 PUFAs can affect the response to microbial infection, whereas an intact immune response is required to eliminate the invading pathogen. Furthermore, the potential immune-suppressive functions of n-3 PUFAs may be harmful for patients with underlying immune-compromised states [74].

Recent papers even showed that DHA treatment, at certain doses, can trigger cell pyroptosis [92–94]. Pyroptosis is an inflammatory form of programmed cell death, which is triggered by inflammasome machinery responses and the activation of inflammatory caspases, like caspase-1 and caspase-4/5 (or caspase-11 in mice). The results are the cleavage of gasdermin D (GSDMD) to generate N-terminal fragments able to form pores in the plasma membrane, the release of proinflammatory cytokines, membrane swelling, and cell death [95]. Besides playing an important role in innate immune response, pyroptosis is also involved in sterile inflammatory processes [95]. Srikanth and colleagues [94] demonstrated that 30 μM DHA could promote anti-inflammatory effects in BV-2 microglial cell line challenged with lipopolysaccharides (LPS); while higher doses (>50 μM) of DHA induced pyroptosis without a proinflammatory stimulus, together with the increased activity of caspase-1 and the augmented gene expression of inflammatory cytokines (*Il1b*, *Il6*, *Tnf*, *Ifng*) and PUFA-metabolizing genes (*Alox5*, *Alox12*, *Alox15*, *Ptgs2*). Hence, this study showed that an excess of DHA is responsible for a proinflammatory process in microglial cells, with no pathogen infection.

Another concern about the use of n-3 PUFA treatments is linked to the safety of oxidized fish oil, one of the main omega-3-containing dietary supplements [96]. Indeed, due to multiple double bonds in the chemical structure, n-3 PUFAs are highly prone to spontaneous nonenzymatic oxidation, and oxidized fish oils could become ineffective or even harmful. n-3 PUFAs can be oxidized to primary lipid hydroperoxides and secondary oxidation products, like aldehydes and ketones [97], which are able to trigger the oxidation of other fatty acids (i.e., membrane lipids), producing further relatively stable lipid peroxides in a chain reaction, thus leading to cell damage and oxidative stress [98]. Indeed, the intake of marine omega-3-rich oils is able to induce augmented levels of plasma and urinary malondialdehyde both in mice and humans, as a consequence of peroxidized oil absorption and in vivo oxidation [99,100]. Then, several in vivo studies showed that lipid peroxidation takes part to the pathophysiological alterations of inflammation-related conditions, like neurodegenerative diseases [101,102].

In light of this, despite the numerous beneficial and anti-inflammatory properties of n-3 PUFAs, a special attention should be paid to the doses and oxidation state of these fatty acids, when used as co-treatment/therapeutic supplement to patients (Fig. 15.1).

n-3 PUFAs in Rett syndrome

Several evidence suggests that chronic inflammatory states may contribute to the progression of pathologic conditions, like cardiovascular diseases, fibrosis, autoimmune diseases, cancer, and neurologic disorders, including RTT [29,103].

n-3 PUFAs show anti-inflammatory activities, such as inducing the decrease of NF-κB activation, and repressing the gene expression of proinflammatory cytokines [88,89]. PUFAs exhibited beneficial effects in studies on attention-deficit hyperactivity disorder (ADHD), in treating depressive symptoms in major depression, and in counteracting symptoms of autism spectrum disorder (i.e., stereotypy, repetitive behavior, hyperactivity, and irritability) [104–106].

As showed in Fig. 15.2, in the last decade several studies demonstrated that n-3 PUFAs supplementation may affect the immune imbalance present in RTT patients, including the reversion of acute phase response (APR) protein expression directionality, and the downregulation of cytokine expression, like TNF-α and IL-37 [39,107]. Plasma samples proteome analysis showed that a 12-month n-3 PUFAs administration (DHA, 71.9 ± 13.9 mg/kg b.w./day and EPA, 115.5 ± 22.4 mg/kg b.w./day; the dose is 5–6 times higher than the standard one) in 24 RTT patients induced a decrease of proteins involved in APR (i.e., complement factor B, albumin, alpha-1-antitrypsin, and haptoglobin), and blood coagulation (i.e., fibrinogen alpha chain), and an increase of proteins associated to unfolded protein response (i.e., clusterin), transport pathways (i.e., retinol-binding protein 4, and vitamin D-binding protein), and lipid metabolism (i.e., apolipoprotein A-IV, and apolipoprotein A-I). In another study involving 16 RTT patients, who were administered with n-3 PUFAs oil for 12 months (DHA, 74.3 ± 6.8 mg/kg b.w./day and EPA, 119.7 ± 10.6 mg/kg b.w./day), the authors found a significant reduction of clinical severity score in fatty acids-

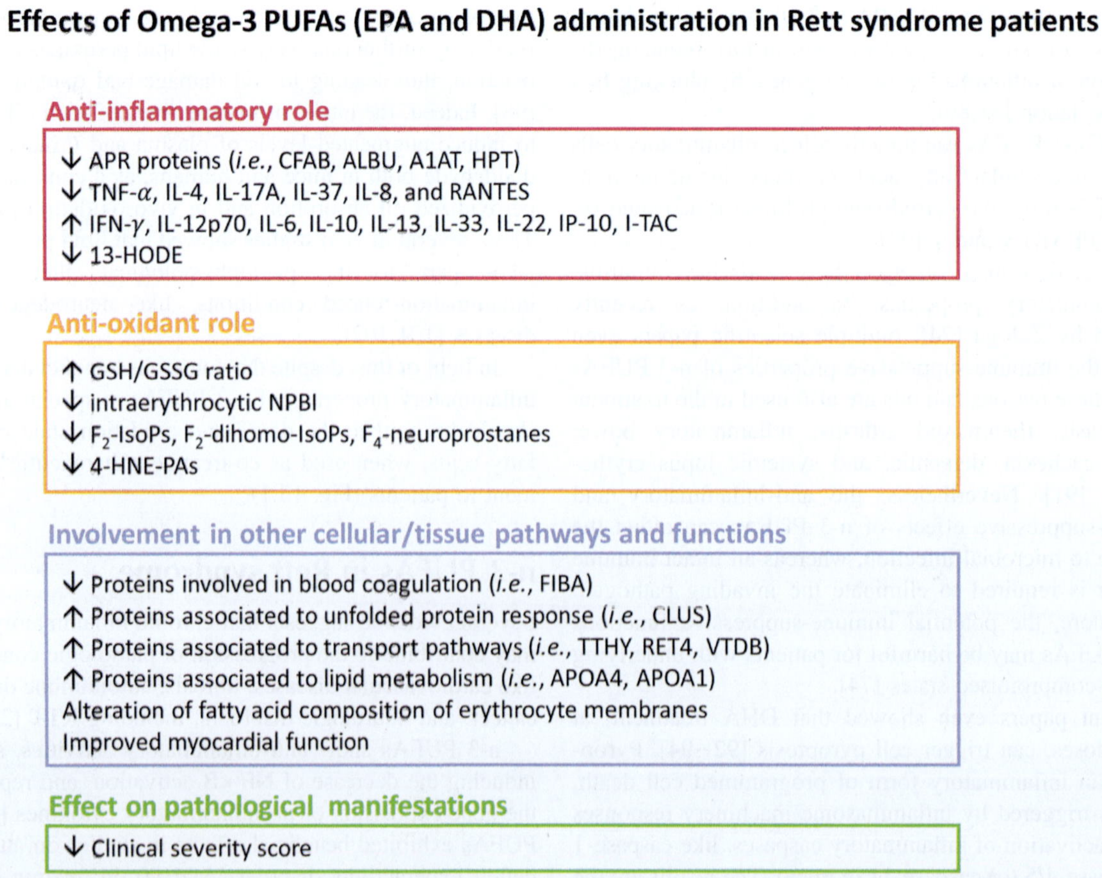

FIGURE 15.2 Main effects induced by omega-3 polyunsaturated fatty acids (PUFAs) administration on Rett syndrome subjects. *4-HNE-PAs*, 4-hydroxynonenal protein adducts; *A1AT*, alpha-1-antitrypsin; *APOA1*, apolipoprotein A-I; *APOA4*, apolipoprotein A-IV; *APR*, acute phase response; *CFAB*, complement factor B; *CLUS*, clusterin; *FIBA*, fibrinogen alpha chain; *GSH*, reduced glutathione; *GSSG*, oxidized glutathione; *HODE*, hydroxyoctadecadienoic acid; *HPT*, haptoglobin; *I-TAC*, INF–inducible T cell alpha chemoattractant; *IFN*, interferon; *IL*, interleukin; *IP-10*, IFN-γ-induced protein 10; *IsoPs*, isoprostanes; *NPBI*, non-protein-bound iron; *RANTES*, C–C motif chemokine 5; *RET4*, retinol-binding protein four; *TNF*, tumor necrosis factor; *TTHY*, transthyretin; *VTDB*, vitamin D-binding protein.

supplemented RTT subjects (as compared to untreated patients), in parallel with a significant reduction of TNF-α, IL-4, IL-17A, IL-37, IL-8, and RANTES plasma levels and an increase of interferon (IFN)-γ, IL-12p70, IL-6, IL-10, IL-13, IL-33, IL-22, IFN-γ-induced protein 10 (IP-10), and INF–inducible T cell alpha chemoattractant (I-TAC) levels [39]. Taken together, the prolonged PUFAs administration is able to strongly regulate the Th1-related cytokine pattern and T-reg lineage, as well as Th2-linked cytokines with the exception of IL-4, thus counteracting the proinflammatory status typical of the pathology [39]. In addition, it has been recently demonstrated that n-3 PUFAs could diminish serum HODEs levels in supplemented RTT patients [41]. The authors hypothesized that omega-3 fatty acids included into cell membranes after fish oil administration in RTT patients may diminish the metabolism of linoleic acid and, in turn, HODEs production, through a process of competitive inhibition (as described in the section "The yin and yang of n-3 PUFAs").

Beneficial effects of n-3 PUFAs on redox homeostasis [39,72,108–111], myocardial function [111], fatty acid composition of erythrocyte membranes [112], and clinical severity [72,108–110] of RTT patients were even reported (Fig. 15.2).

In particular, n-3 PUFAs-supplemented RTT patients for 6–12 months showed augmented systemic GSH/GSSG ratio and reduced levels of plasma and intraerythrocytic NPBI (two pro-oxidant factors), plasma F_2-isoprostanes (F_2-IsoPs, markers of systemic lipoperoxidation), F_2-dihomo-IsoPs (markers of glia membrane/brain white matter damage), F_4-neuroprostanes (F_4-NeuroPs, markers of neuronal membrane/brain gray matter damage), esterified F_2-IsoPs, and 4-HNE PAs of erythrocytic membranes [39,72,108–111]. Interestingly, the 6-month n-3 PUFAs fish oil supplementation in stage I RTT patients led to clear improvements in clinical features, such as motor/independent sitting, ambulation, hand use, language, nonverbal communication deficits, and breathing dysfunctions [109].

The authors hypothesized that these effects due to n-3 PUFAs treatment may be attributed to decreased oxidative stress, whose reduction might potentially affect different molecular targets (i.e., BDNF receptors, lipid peroxidation, or hemoglobin auto-oxidation), hence, possibly modifying the progression of the disorder [109].

Furthermore, a recent paper showed that DHA treatment on MeCP2 knockdown rat primary cortical astrocytes was able to increase MeCP2 protein expression, together with the levels of BDNF, ubiquinol cytochrome *c* reductase core protein (Uqcrc1) and NADH dehydrogenase (ubiquinone) flavoprotein 2 (Ndufv2), and the specific activities of mitochondrial respiratory complexes II and III, suggesting a potential role of DHA even in MeCP2-mediated mitochondrial dysfunctions [113].

Concluding remarks

To date, treatments for RTT patients are exclusively symptomatic and supportive. Although very promising and attractive, gene therapy approaches are still far to be translated from laboratory bench to clinical practice. Thus, nutritional interventions, especially those taking advantages of the anti-inflammatory properties of n-3 PUFAs (paying attention to the dose administered), represent potential therapeutic strategies, as they would modulate immune/inflammatory components and improve OxInflammation, thus alleviate multiple manifestations in RTT individuals.

Key terms

Rett syndrome. Rett syndrome is a neurodevelopmental disorder primarily affecting the female gender. In the majority of cases, it is caused by mutations in the X-linked *MECP2* gene.

Oxidative stress. Oxidative stress is the result of an imbalance between oxidant molecules and antioxidant defences, in favor of the former, leading to a disruption of redox signaling and biomolecular damages. While the maintenance of physiological levels of oxidants (termed "oxidative eustress") is essential for life functions through redox signaling.

Chronic subclinical inflammation. Chronic subclinical inflammation is defined as the persistence of unrecognized inflammatory processes, beyond their physiological functions, in which initiating trigger is often not well defined, and that results in impairment of tissue homeostasis and pathological conditions.

OxInflammation. OxInflammation is characterized by a permanent pro-oxidative milieu that interacts, in a feed-forward loop, to a not yet clinically detectable inflammatory process, leading to a chronic systemic/local damage, as a consequence of the interaction between oxidative stress and inflammatory mediators.

Omega-3 PUFAs. Omega-3 polyunsaturated fatty acids (PUFAs) are a class of fatty acids containing at least more than one double bond. Omega-3 fatty acids possess the first double bond (C=C) at the third carbon atom from the methyl end of the carbon chain. The human body is incapable of synthesizing omega-3 PUFAs.

References

[1] Shahidi F, Ambigaipalan P. Omega-3 polyunsaturated fatty acids and their health benefits. Annu Rev Food Sci Technol 2018;9:345–81. https://doi.org/10.1146/annurev-food-111317-095850.

[2] Neul JL, Kaufmann WE, Glaze DG, Christodoulou J, Clarke AJ, Bahi-Buisson N, et al. RettSearch Consortium, Rett syndrome: revised diagnostic criteria and nomenclature. Ann Neurol 2010;68:944–50. https://doi.org/10.1002/ana.22124.

[3] Gold WA, Krishnarajy R, Ellaway C, Christodoulou J. Rett syndrome: a genetic update and clinical review focusing on comorbidities. ACS Chem Neurosci 2018;9:167–76. https://doi.org/10.1021/acschemneuro.7b00346.

[4] Pecorelli A, Cervellati C, Hayek J, Valacchi G. OxInflammation in Rett syndrome. Int J Biochem Cell Biol 2016;81:246–53. https://doi.org/10.1016/j.biocel.2016.07.015.

[5] Fehr S, Bebbington A, Nassar N, Downs J, Ronen GM, de Klerk N, Leonard H. Trends in the diagnosis of Rett syndrome in Australia. Pediatr Res 2011;70:313–9. https://doi.org/10.1203/PDR.0b013e3182242461.

[6] Chahrour M, Zoghbi HY. The story of Rett syndrome: from clinic to neurobiology. Neuron 2007;56:422–37. https://doi.org/10.1016/j.neuron.2007.10.001.

[7] Amir RE, Van den Veyver IB, Wan M, Tran CQ, Francke U, Zoghbi HY. Rett syndrome is caused by mutations in X-linked MECP2, encoding methyl-CpG-binding protein 2. Nat Genet 1999;23:185–8. https://doi.org/10.1038/13810.

[8] Ip JPK, Mellios N, Sur M. Rett syndrome: insights into genetic, molecular and circuit mechanisms. Nat Rev Neurosci 2018;19:368–82. https://doi.org/10.1038/s41583-018-0006-3.

[9] Ehrhart F, Jacobsen A, Rigau M, Bosio M, Kaliyaperumal R, Laros JFJ, et al. A catalogue of 863 Rett-syndrome-causing MECP2 mutations and lessons learned from data integration. Sci Data 2021;8:10. https://doi.org/10.1038/s41597-020-00794-7.

[10] Girard M, Couvert P, Carrié A, Tardieu M, Chelly J, Beldjord C, Bienvenu T. Parental origin of de novo MECP2 mutations in Rett syndrome. Eur J Hum Genet 2001;9:231–6. https://doi.org/10.1038/sj.ejhg.5200618.

[11] Christodoulou J, Grimm A, Maher T, Bennetts B. RettBASE: the IRSA MECP2 variation database—a new mutation database in evolution. Hum Mutat 2003;21:466–72. https://doi.org/10.1002/humu.10194.

[12] Kyle SM, Vashi N, Justice MJ. Rett syndrome: a neurological disorder with metabolic components. Open Biol 2018;8:170216. https://doi.org/10.1098/rsob.170216.

[13] Armstrong D, Dunn JK, Antalffy B, Trivedi R. Selective dendritic alterations in the cortex of Rett syndrome. J Neuropathol Exp Neurol 1995;54:195–201. https://doi.org/10.1097/00005072-199503000-00006.

[14] Carter JC, Lanham DC, Pham D, Bibat G, Naidu S, Kaufmann WE. Selective cerebral volume reduction in Rett syndrome: a multiple-approach MR imaging study. AJNR Am J Neuroradiol 2008;29:436–41. https://doi.org/10.3174/ajnr.A0857.

[15] Banerjee A, Rikhye RV, Breton-Provencher V, Tang X, Li C, Li K, et al. Jointly reduced inhibition and excitation underlies circuit-wide changes in cortical processing in Rett syndrome. Proc Natl Acad Sci USA 2016;113:E7287–96. https://doi.org/10.1073/pnas.1615330113.

[16] Borloz E, Villard L, Roux J-C. Rett syndrome: think outside the (skull) box. Fac Rev 2021;10:59. https://doi.org/10.12703/r/10-59.

[17] Fu C, Armstrong D, Marsh E, Lieberman D, Motil K, Witt R, et al. Multisystem comorbidities in classic Rett syndrome: a scoping review. BMJ Paediatr Open 2020;4. https://doi.org/10.1136/bmjpo-2020-000731.

[18] Wang J, Xiao Y, Liu C, Huang Y, Petersen RB, Zheng L, Huang K. Emerging physiological and pathological roles of MeCP2 in non-neurological systems. Arch Biochem Biophys 2021;700:108768. https://doi.org/10.1016/j.abb.2021.108768.

[19] Bedogni F, Cobolli Gigli C, Pozzi D, Rossi RL, Scaramuzza L, Rossetti G, et al. Defects during Mecp2 null embryonic cortex development precede the onset of overt neurological symptoms. Cereb Cortex 2016;26:2517–29. https://doi.org/10.1093/cercor/bhv078.

[20] Kishi N, Macklis JD. MECP2 is progressively expressed in post-migratory neurons and is involved in neuronal maturation rather than cell fate decisions. Mol Cell Neurosci 2004;27:306–21. https://doi.org/10.1016/j.mcn.2004.07.006.

[21] Shahbazian MD, Antalffy B, Armstrong DL, Zoghbi HY. Insight into Rett syndrome: MeCP2 levels display tissue- and cell-specific differences and correlate with neuronal maturation. Hum Mol Genet 2002;11:115–24. https://doi.org/10.1093/hmg/11.2.115.

[22] Ross PD, Guy J, Selfridge J, Kamal B, Bahey N, Tanner KE, et al. Exclusive expression of MeCP2 in the nervous system distinguishes between brain and peripheral Rett syndrome-like phenotypes. Hum Mol Genet 2016;25:4389–404. https://doi.org/10.1093/hmg/ddw269.

[23] Segatto M, Trapani L, Di Tunno I, Sticozzi C, Valacchi G, Hayek J, Pallottini V. Cholesterol metabolism is altered in Rett syndrome: a study on plasma and primary cultured fibroblasts derived from patients. PLoS One 2014;9. https://doi.org/10.1371/journal.pone.0104834.

[24] Cervellati C, Sticozzi C, Romani A, Belmonte G, De Rasmo D, Signorile A, et al. Impaired enzymatic defensive activity, mitochondrial dysfunction and proteasome activation are involved in RTT cell oxidative damage. Biochim Biophys Acta 2015;1852:2066–74. https://doi.org/10.1016/j.bbadis.2015.07.014.

[25] Pecorelli A, Ciccoli L, Signorini C, Leoncini S, Giardini A, D'Esposito M, et al. Increased levels of 4HNE-protein plasma adducts in Rett syndrome. Clin Biochem 2011;44:368–71. https://doi.org/10.1016/j.clinbiochem.2011.01.007.

[26] Cicaloni V, Pecorelli A, Tinti L, Rossi M, Benedusi M, Cervellati C, et al. Proteomic profiling reveals mitochondrial alterations in Rett syndrome. Free Radic Biol Med 2020;155:37–48. https://doi.org/10.1016/j.freeradbiomed.2020.05.014.

[27] Crivellari I, Pecorelli A, Cordone V, Marchi S, Pinton P, Hayek J, et al. Impaired mitochondrial quality control in Rett Syndrome. Arch Biochem Biophys 2021;700:108790. https://doi.org/10.1016/j.abb.2021.108790.

[28] Shulyakova N, Andreazza AC, Mills LR, Eubanks JH. Mitochondrial dysfunction in the pathogenesis of Rett syndrome: implications for mitochondria-targeted therapies. Front Cell Neurosci 2017;11:58. https://doi.org/10.3389/fncel.2017.00058.

[29] Cortelazzo A, De Felice C, Guerranti R, Signorini C, Leoncini S, Pecorelli A, et al. Subclinical inflammatory status in Rett syndrome. Mediators Inflamm 2014;2014:480980. https://doi.org/10.1155/2014/480980.

[30] Pecorelli A, Cervellati C, Cordone V, Hayek J, Valacchi G. Compromised immune/inflammatory responses in Rett syndrome. Free Radic Biol Med 2020;152:100–6. https://doi.org/10.1016/j.freeradbiomed.2020.02.023.

[31] Formichi P, Battisti C, Dotti MT, Hayek G, Zappella M, Federico A. Vitamin E serum levels in Rett syndrome. J Neurol Sci 1998;156:227–30. https://doi.org/10.1016/s0022-510x(98)00035-5.

[32] Sierra C, Vilaseca MA, Brandi N, Artuch R, Mira A, Nieto M, Pineda M. Oxidative stress in Rett syndrome. Brain Dev 2001;23(Suppl. 1):S236–9. https://doi.org/10.1016/s0387-7604(01)00369-2.

[33] De Felice C, Ciccoli L, Leoncini S, Signorini C, Rossi M, Vannuccini L, et al. Systemic oxidative stress in classic Rett syndrome. Free Radic Biol Med 2009;47:440–8. https://doi.org/10.1016/j.freeradbiomed.2009.05.016.

[34] Dean RT, Fu S, Stocker R, Davies MJ. Biochemistry and pathology of radical-mediated protein oxidation. Biochem J 1997;324:1–18.

[35] Cordone V, Ferrara F, Pecorelli A, Guiotto A, Vitale A, Amicarelli F, et al. The constitutive activation of TLR4-IRAK1-NFκB axis is involved in the early NLRP3 inflammasome response in peripheral blood mononuclear cells of Rett syndrome patients. Free Radic Biol Med 2022;181:1–13. https://doi.org/10.1016/j.freeradbiomed.2022.01.017.

[36] Signorini C, Leoncini S, De Felice C, Pecorelli A, Meloni I, Ariani F, et al. Redox imbalance and morphological changes in skin fibroblasts in typical Rett syndrome. Oxid Med Cell Longev 2014;2014:1–10. https://doi.org/10.1155/2014/195935.

[37] Bebensee DF, Can K, Müller M. Increased mitochondrial mass and cytosolic redox imbalance in hippocampal astrocytes of a mouse model of Rett syndrome: subcellular changes revealed by ratiometric imaging of JC-1 and roGFP1 fluorescence. Oxid Med Cell Longev 2017;2017:3064016. https://doi.org/10.1155/2017/3064016.

[38] De Felice C, Della Ragione F, Signorini C, Leoncini S, Pecorelli A, Ciccoli L, et al. Oxidative brain damage in Mecp2-mutant murine models of Rett syndrome. Neurobiol Dis 2014;68:66–77. https://doi.org/10.1016/j.nbd.2014.04.006.

[39] Leoncini S, De Felice C, Signorini C, Zollo G, Cortelazzo A, Durand T, et al. Cytokine dysregulation in MECP2- and CDKL5-related Rett syndrome: relationships with aberrant redox homeostasis, inflammation, and ω-3 PUFAs. Oxid Med Cell Longev 2015;2015:421624. https://doi.org/10.1155/2015/421624.

[40] Pecorelli A, Cervellati F, Belmonte G, Montagner G, Waldon P, Hayek J, et al. Cytokines profile and peripheral blood mononuclear cells morphology in Rett and autistic patients. Cytokine 2016;77:180–8. https://doi.org/10.1016/j.cyto.2015.10.002.

[41] Pecorelli A, Cervellati C, Cordone V, Amicarelli F, Hayek J, Valacchi G. 13-HODE, 9-HODE and ALOX15 as potential players in Rett syndrome OxInflammation. Free Radic Biol Med 2019;134:598–603. https://doi.org/10.1016/j.freeradbiomed.2019.02.007.

[42] Pecorelli A, Cordone V, Messano N, Zhang C, Falone S, Amicarelli F, et al. Altered inflammasome machinery as a key player in the perpetuation of Rett syndrome oxinflammation. Redox Biol 2020;28:101334. https://doi.org/10.1016/j.redox.2019.101334.

[43] Cronk JC, Derecki NC, Ji E, Xu Y, Lampano AE, Smirnov I, et al. Methyl-CpG binding protein 2 regulates microglia and macrophage gene expression in response to inflammatory stimuli. Immunity 2015;42:679–91. https://doi.org/10.1016/j.immuni.2015.03.013.

[44] Schafer DP, Stevens B. Brains, blood, and guts: MeCP2 regulates microglia, monocytes, and peripheral macrophages. Immunity 2015;42:600–2. https://doi.org/10.1016/j.immuni.2015.04.002.

[45] Zhao D, Mokhtari R, Pedrosa E, Birnbaum R, Zheng D, Lachman HM. Transcriptome analysis of microglia in a mouse model of Rett syndrome: differential expression of genes associated with microglia/macrophage activation and cellular stress. Mol Autism 2017;8:17. https://doi.org/10.1186/s13229-017-0134-z.

[46] De Felice C, Signorini C, Durand T, Oger C, Guy A, Bultel-Poncé V, et al. F2-dihomo-isoprostanes as potential early biomarkers of lipid oxidative damage in Rett syndrome. J Lipid Res 2011;52:2287–97. https://doi.org/10.1194/jlr.P017798.

[47] Müller M. Disturbed redox homeostasis and oxidative stress: potential players in the developmental regression in Rett syndrome. Neurosci Biobehav Rev 2019;98:154–63. https://doi.org/10.1016/j.neubiorev.2018.12.009.

[48] Guy J, Gan J, Selfridge J, Cobb S, Bird A. Reversal of neurological defects in a mouse model of Rett syndrome. Science 2007;315:1143–7. https://doi.org/10.1126/science.1138389.

[49] D'Mello SR. MECP2 and the biology of MECP2 duplication syndrome. J Neurochem 2021;159:29–60. https://doi.org/10.1111/jnc.15331.

[50] Braunschweig D, Simcox T, Samaco RC, LaSalle JM. X-Chromosome inactivation ratios affect wild-type MeCP2 expression within mosaic Rett syndrome and Mecp2-/+ mouse brain. Hum Mol Genet 2004;13:1275–86. https://doi.org/10.1093/hmg/ddh142.

[51] Collins AL, Levenson JM, Vilaythong AP, Richman R, Armstrong DL, Noebels JL, et al. Mild overexpression of MeCP2 causes a progressive neurological disorder in mice. Hum Mol Genet 2004;13:2679–89. https://doi.org/10.1093/hmg/ddh282.

[52] Friez MJ, Jones JR, Clarkson K, Lubs H, Abuelo D, Bier J-AB, et al. Recurrent infections, hypotonia, and mental retardation caused by duplication of MECP2 and adjacent region in Xq28. Pediatrics 2006;118:e1687–95. https://doi.org/10.1542/peds.2006-0395.

[53] Chao H-T, Zoghbi HY. MeCP2: only 100% will do. Nat Neurosci 2012;15:176–7. https://doi.org/10.1038/nn.3027.

[54] Ramocki MB, Peters SU, Tavyev YJ, Zhang F, Carvalho CMB, Schaaf CP, et al. Autism and other neuropsychiatric symptoms are prevalent in individuals with MeCP2 duplication syndrome. Ann Neurol 2009;66:771–82. https://doi.org/10.1002/ana.21715.

[55] Chen YH, Keiser MS, Davidson BL. Viral vectors for gene transfer. Curr Protoc Mouse Biol 2018;8:e58. https://doi.org/10.1002/cpmo.58.

[56] Cappella M, Ciotti C, Cohen-Tannoudji M, Biferi MG. Gene therapy for ALS-A perspective. Int J Mol Sci 2019;20:E4388. https://doi.org/10.3390/ijms20184388.

[57] Liu D, Zhu M, Zhang Y, Diao Y. Crossing the blood-brain barrier with AAV vectors. Metab Brain Dis 2021;36:45–52. https://doi.org/10.1007/s11011-020-00630-2.

[58] Gadalla KKE, Bailey MES, Spike RC, Ross PD, Woodard KT, Kalburgi SN, et al. Improved survival and reduced phenotypic severity following AAV9/MECP2 gene transfer to neonatal and juvenile male Mecp2 knockout mice. Mol Ther 2013;21:18–30. https://doi.org/10.1038/mt.2012.200.

[59] Garg SK, Lioy DT, Cheval H, McGann JC, Bissonnette JM, Murtha MJ, et al. Systemic delivery of MeCP2 rescues behavioral and cellular deficits in female mouse models of Rett syndrome. J Neurosci 2013;33:13612–20. https://doi.org/10.1523/JNEUROSCI.1854-13.2013.

[60] Matagne V, Borloz E, Ehinger Y, Saidi L, Villard L, Roux J-C. Severe offtarget effects following intravenous delivery of AAV9-MECP2 in a female mouse model of Rett syndrome. Neurobiol Dis 2021;149:105235. https://doi.org/10.1016/j.nbd.2020.105235.

[61] Feldman D, Banerjee A, Sur M. Developmental dynamics of Rett syndrome. Neural Plast 2016;2016:6154080. https://doi.org/10.1155/2016/6154080.

[62] Giacometti E, Luikenhuis S, Beard C, Jaenisch R. Partial rescue of MeCP2 deficiency by postnatal activation of MeCP2. Proc Natl Acad Sci USA 2007;104:1931–6. https://doi.org/10.1073/pnas.0610593104.

[63] Clarke AJ, Abdala Sheikh AP. A perspective on "cure" for Rett syndrome. Orphanet J Rare Dis 2018;13:44. https://doi.org/10.1186/s13023-018-0786-6.

[64] ClinicalTrials.gov. Search of: interventional studies | Rett syndrome. 2022. https://clinicaltrials.gov/ct2/results?cond=Rett+Syndrome&age_v=&gndr=&type=Intr&rslt=&Search=Apply. [Accessed 2 September 2022].

[65] Katz DM, Berger-Sweeney JE, Eubanks JH, Justice MJ, Neul JL, Pozzo-Miller L, et al. Preclinical research in Rett syndrome: setting the foundation for translational success. Dis Models Mech 2012;5:733–45. https://doi.org/10.1242/dmm.011007.

[66] Katz DM, Bird A, Coenraads M, Gray SJ, Menon DU, Philpot BD, Tarquinio DC. Rett syndrome: crossing the threshold to clinical translation. Trends Neurosci 2016;39:100–13. https://doi.org/10.1016/j.tins.2015.12.008.

[67] Di Pierro D, Ciaccio C, Sbardella D, Tundo GR, Bernardini R, Curatolo P, et al. Effects of oral administration of common antioxidant supplements on the energy metabolism of red blood cells. Attenuation of oxidative stress-induced changes in Rett syndrome erythrocytes by CoQ10. Mol Cell Biochem 2020;463:101–13. https://doi.org/10.1007/s11010-019-03633-5.

[68] Ellaway CJ, Peat J, Williams K, Leonard H, Christodoulou J. Medium-term open label trial of L-carnitine in Rett syndrome. Brain Dev 2001;23(Suppl. 1):S85–9. https://doi.org/10.1016/s0387-7604(01)00346-1.

[69] Janc OA, Hüser MA, Dietrich K, Kempkes B, Menzfeld C, Hülsmann S, Müller M. Systemic radical scavenger treatment of a mouse model of Rett syndrome: merits and limitations of the vitamin E derivative Trolox. Front Cell Neurosci 2016;10:266. https://doi.org/10.3389/fncel.2016.00266.

[70] Panighini A, Duranti E, Santini F, Maffei M, Pizzorusso T, Funel N, et al. Vascular dysfunction in a mouse model of Rett syndrome and effects of curcumin treatment. PLoS One 2013;8:e64863. https://doi.org/10.1371/journal.pone.0064863.

[71] Schaevitz LR, Nicolai R, Lopez CM, D'Iddio S, Iannoni E, Berger-Sweeney JE. Acetyl-L-carnitine improves behavior and dendritic morphology in a mouse model of Rett syndrome. PLoS One 2012;7:e51586. https://doi.org/10.1371/journal.pone.0051586.

[72] Leoncini S, De Felice C, Signorini C, Pecorelli A, Durand T, Valacchi G, et al. Oxidative stress in Rett syndrome: natural history, genotype, and variants. Redox Rep 2011;16:145–53. https://doi.org/10.1179/1351000211Y.0000000004.

[73] Mir SM, Kanjilal S, Ahmed SU. Omega-3 fatty acids in inflammatory diseases. In: Hegde MV, Zanwar AA, Adekar SP, editors. Omega-3 fatty acids. Cham: Springer International Publishing; 2016. p. 141–55.

[74] Zaloga GP. Narrative review of n-3 polyunsaturated fatty acid supplementation upon immune functions, resolution molecules and lipid peroxidation. Nutrients 2021;13:662. https://doi.org/10.3390/nu13020662.

[75] Shahidi F, Miraliakbari H. Omega-3 (n-3) fatty acids in health and disease: part 1—cardiovascular disease and cancer. J Med Food 2004;7:387–401. https://doi.org/10.1089/jmf.2004.7.387.

[76] Molfino A, Amabile MI, Monti M, Muscaritoli M. Omega-3 polyunsaturated fatty acids in critical illness: anti-inflammatory, proresolving, or both? Oxid Med Cell Longev 2017;2017:5987082. https://doi.org/10.1155/2017/5987082.

[77] Simopoulos AP. Omega-3 fatty acids in inflammation and autoimmune diseases. J Am Coll Nutr 2002;21:495–505. https://doi.org/10.1080/07315724.2002.10719248.

[78] Rockett BD, Teague H, Harris M, Melton M, Williams J, Wassall SR, Shaikh SR. Fish oil increases raft size and membrane order of B cells accompanied by differential effects on function. J Lipid Res 2012;53:674–85. https://doi.org/10.1194/jlr.M021782.

[79] Kim W, Fan Y-Y, Barhoumi R, Smith R, McMurray DN, Chapkin RS. n-3 polyunsaturated fatty acids suppress the localization and activation of signaling proteins at the immunological synapse in murine CD4+ T cells by affecting lipid raft formation. J Immunol 2008;181:6236–43. https://doi.org/10.4049/jimmunol.181.9.6236.

[80] Serhan CN. Pro-resolving lipid mediators are leads for resolution physiology. Nature 2014;510:92–101. https://doi.org/10.1038/nature13479.

[81] Schmitz G, Ecker J. The opposing effects of n-3 and n-6 fatty acids. Prog Lipid Res 2008;47:147–55. https://doi.org/10.1016/j.plipres.2007.12.004.

[82] Simonetto M, Infante M, Sacco RL, Rundek T, Della-Morte D. A novel anti-inflammatory role of omega-3 PUFAs in prevention and treatment of atherosclerosis and vascular cognitive impairment and dementia. Nutrients 2019;11:2279. https://doi.org/10.3390/nu11102279.

[83] Basil MC, Levy BD. Specialized pro-resolving mediators: endogenous regulators of infection and inflammation. Nat Rev Immunol 2016;16:51–67. https://doi.org/10.1038/nri.2015.4.

[84] Im D-S. Omega-3 fatty acids in anti-inflammation (pro-resolution) and GPCRs. Prog Lipid Res 2012;51:232–7. https://doi.org/10.1016/j.plipres.2012.02.003.

[85] Oh DY, Talukdar S, Bae EJ, Imamura T, Morinaga H, Fan W, et al. GPR120 is an omega-3 fatty acid receptor mediating potent anti-inflammatory and insulin-sensitizing effects. Cell 2010;142:687–98. https://doi.org/10.1016/j.cell.2010.07.041.

[86] Chen X, Wu S, Chen C, Xie B, Fang Z, Hu W, et al. Omega-3 polyunsaturated fatty acid supplementation attenuates microglial-induced inflammation by inhibiting the HMGB1/TLR4/NF-κB pathway following experimental traumatic brain injury. J Neuroinflammation 2017;14:143. https://doi.org/10.1186/s12974-017-0917-3.

[87] Oppedisano F, Macrì R, Gliozzi M, Musolino V, Carresi C, Maiuolo J, et al. The anti-inflammatory and antioxidant properties of n-3 PUFAs: their role in cardiovascular protection. Biomedicines 2020;8:306. https://doi.org/10.3390/biomedicines8090306.

[88] Zhao Y, Joshi-Barve S, Barve S, Chen LH. Eicosapentaenoic acid prevents LPS-induced TNF-alpha expression by preventing NF-kappaB activation. J Am Coll Nutr 2004;23:71–8. https://doi.org/10.1080/07315724.2004.10719345.

[89] Zhao G, Etherton TD, Martin KR, Vanden Heuvel JP, Gillies PJ, West SG, Kris-Etherton PM. Anti-inflammatory effects of polyunsaturated fatty acids in THP-1 cells. Biochem Biophys Res Commun 2005;336:909–17. https://doi.org/10.1016/j.bbrc.2005.08.204.

[90] Gani OABSM, Sylte I. Molecular recognition of docosahexaenoic acid by peroxisome proliferator-activated receptors and retinoid-X receptor alpha. J Mol Graph Model 2008;27:217–24. https://doi.org/10.1016/j.jmgm.2008.04.008.

[91] Akbar U, Yang M, Kurian D, Mohan C. Omega-3 fatty acids in rheumatic diseases: a critical review. J Clin Rheumatol 2017;23:330–9. https://doi.org/10.1097/RHU.0000000000000563.

[92] Herr DR, Yam TYA, Tan WSD, Koh SS, Wong WSF, Ong W-Y, Chayaburakul K. Ultrastructural characteristics of DHA-induced pyroptosis. Neuromol Med 2020;22:293–303. https://doi.org/10.1007/s12017-019-08586-y.

[93] Pizato N, Luzete BC, Kiffer LFMV, Corrêa LH, de Oliveira Santos I, Assumpção JAF, et al. Omega-3 docosahexaenoic acid induces pyroptosis cell death in triple-negative breast cancer cells. Sci Rep 2018;8:1952. https://doi.org/10.1038/s41598-018-20422-0.

[94] Srikanth M, Chandrasaharan K, Zhao X, Chayaburakul K, Ong W-Y, Herr DR. Metabolism of docosahexaenoic acid (DHA) induces pyroptosis in BV-2 microglial cells. Neuromol Med 2018;20:504–14. https://doi.org/10.1007/s12017-018-8511-0.

[95] Broz P, Dixit VM. Inflammasomes: mechanism of assembly, regulation and signalling. Nat Rev Immunol 2016;16:407–20. https://doi.org/10.1038/nri.2016.58.

[96] Lange KW, Nakamura Y, Gosslau AM, Li S. Are there serious adverse effects of omega-3 polyunsaturated fatty acid supplements? J Food Bioact 2019;7. https://doi.org/10.31665/JFB.2019.7192.

[97] Arab-Tehrany E, Jacquot M, Gaiani C, Imran M, Desobry S, Linder M. Beneficial effects and oxidative stability of omega-3 long-chain polyunsaturated fatty acids. Trends Food Sci Technol 2012;25:24–33. https://doi.org/10.1016/j.tifs.2011.12.002.

[98] Albert BB, Cameron-Smith D, Hofman PL, Cutfield WS. Oxidation of marine omega-3 supplements and human health. BioMed Res Int 2013;2013:464921. https://doi.org/10.1155/2013/464921.

[99] Haglund O, Luostarinen R, Wallin R, Wibell L, Saldeen T. The effects of fish oil on triglycerides, cholesterol, fibrinogen and malondialdehyde in humans supplemented with vitamin E. J Nutr 1991;121:165–9. https://doi.org/10.1093/jn/121.2.165.

[100] Piché LA, Draper HH, Cole PD. Malondialdehyde excretion by subjects consuming cod liver oil vs a concentrate of n-3 fatty acids. Lipids 1988;23:370–1. https://doi.org/10.1007/BF02537352.

[101] Grimm MOW, Haupenthal VJ, Mett J, Stahlmann CP, Blümel T, Mylonas NT, et al. Oxidized docosahexaenoic acid species and lipid peroxidation products increase amyloidogenic amyloid precursor protein processing. Neurodegener Dis 2016;16:44–54. https://doi.org/10.1159/000440839.

[102] Yakubenko VP, Byzova TV. Biological and pathophysiological roles of end-products of DHA oxidation. Biochim Biophys Acta Mol Cell Biol Lipids 2017;1862:407–15. https://doi.org/10.1016/j.bbalip.2016.09.022.

[103] Tabas I, Glass CK. Anti-inflammatory therapy in chronic disease: challenges and opportunities. Science 2013;339:166–72. https://doi.org/10.1126/science.1230720.

[104] Perera H, Jeewandara KC, Seneviratne S, Guruge C. Combined ω3 and ω6 supplementation in children with attention-deficit hyperactivity disorder (ADHD) refractory to methylphenidate treatment: a double-blind, placebo-controlled study. J Child Neurol 2012;27:747–53. https://doi.org/10.1177/0883073811435243.

[105] Peng Z, Zhang C, Yan L, Zhang Y, Yang Z, Wang J, Song C. EPA is more effective than DHA to improve depression-like behavior, glia cell dysfunction and hippcampal apoptosis signaling in a chronic stress-induced rat model of depression. Int J Mol Sci 2020;21:1769. https://doi.org/10.3390/ijms21051769.

[106] Veselinović A, Petrović S, Žikić V, Subotić M, Jakovljević V, Jeremić N, Vučić V. Neuroinflammation in autism and supplementation based on omega-3 polyunsaturated fatty acids: a narrative review. Medicina (Kaunas) 2021;57:893. https://doi.org/10.3390/medicina57090893.

[107] De Felice C, Cortelazzo A, Signorini C, Guerranti R, Leoncini S, Pecorelli A, et al. Effects of ω-3 polyunsaturated fatty acids on plasma proteome in Rett syndrome. Mediators Inflamm 2013;2013:723269. https://doi.org/10.1155/2013/723269.

[108] Signorini C, De Felice C, Leoncini S, Giardini A, D'Esposito M, Filosa S, et al. F_4-neuroprostanes mediate neurological severity in Rett syndrome. Clin Chim Acta 2011;412:1399–406. https://doi.org/10.1016/j.cca.2011.04.016.

[109] De Felice C, Signorini C, Durand T, Ciccoli L, Leoncini S, D'Esposito M, et al. Partial rescue of Rett syndrome by ω-3 polyunsaturated fatty acids (PUFAs) oil. Genes Nutr 2012;7:447–58. https://doi.org/10.1007/s12263-012-0285-7.

[110] Ciccoli L, De Felice C, Paccagnini E, Leoncini S, Pecorelli A, Signorini C, et al. Morphological changes and oxidative damage in Rett Syndrome erythrocytes. Biochim Biophys Acta Gen Subj 2012;1820:511–20. https://doi.org/10.1016/j.bbagen.2011.12.002.

[111] Maffei S, De Felice C, Cannarile P, Leoncini S, Signorini C, Pecorelli A, et al. Effects of ω-3 PUFAs supplementation on myocardial function and oxidative stress markers in typical Rett syndrome. Mediat Inflamm 2014;2014:e983178. https://doi.org/10.1155/2014/983178.

[112] Signorini C, De Felice C, Leoncini S, Durand T, Galano J-M, Cortelazzo A, et al. Altered erythrocyte membrane fatty acid profile in typical Rett syndrome: effects of omega-3 polyunsaturated fatty acid supplementation. Prostagl Leukot Essent Fat Acids 2014;91:183–93. https://doi.org/10.1016/j.plefa.2014.08.002.

[113] Dave A, Pillai PP. Docosahexaenoic acid increased MeCP2 mediated mitochondrial respiratory complexes II and III enzyme activities in cortical astrocytes. J Biochem Mol Toxicol 2022:e23002. https://doi.org/10.1002/jbt.23002.

Chapter 16

A glance on antioxidants: The role of sulfur amino acids in retinal disorders

Vanessa Castelli[3,a], Lauren Byrd-Leotis[2,a], Rubina Novelli[2], Laura Brandolini[1], Annamaria Cimini[3,4] and Marcello Allegretti[1]

[1]*R&D, Dompé farmaceutici S.p.A, L'Aquila, Italy;* [2]*R&D, Dompé farmaceutici S.p.A, Milan, Italy;* [3]*Department of Life, Health and Environmental Sciences, University of L'Aquila, L'Aquila, Italy;* [4]*Sbarro Institute for Cancer Research and Molecular Medicine, Center for Biotechnology, Temple University, Philadelphia, PA, United States*

Retina and oxidative stress

The retina is a thin, transparent tissue lining the inner surface of the eye. Its function is to receive light that the eye lens has focused, convert the inputs into neural signals, and send them to the brain for visual processing. The most distal retinal layer is the retinal pigment epithelium (RPE), a quiescent monolayer of nonproliferating cells that provide nutritional support to the photoreceptors [1], which in turn form the underlying receptor layer. The nuclei of the photoreceptor cells, the rods and the cones, are located in the outer nuclear layer (ONL), while in the outer plexiform layer (OPL), both rods and cones make synaptic contact with horizontal cells and bipolar cells. Bipolar cells then transfer the visual message generated in the photoreceptors to the retinal ganglion cells (RGCs), the axons of which collectively form the optic nerve that finally conveys the visual message out of the eye [2] (Fig. 16.1).

The mammalian retina is extremely metabolically active and one of the most highly oxygen-consuming organs of the body [3]. Its energy metabolism is dominated by aerobic glycolysis, but it requires both glycolysis and oxidative phosphorylation to function and initiate the vision process [4]. In addition, the absorption of light by photosensitizer molecules leads to photochemical reactions that further induce the production and accumulation of free radicals and reactive oxygen species (ROS) [5]. As a result of elevated metabolic activity, high oxygen consumption, and prolonged exposure to radiant energy, free radicals are highly and continuously produced in this tissue [6].

In the retina, the level of substrates for oxidative damage is also increased. Components of the retina that are most vulnerable to oxidative stress include, for example, the polyunsaturated fatty acids (PUFA) that constitute the photoreceptors' lipid bilayer determining its grade of fluidity. The high fluidity of this layer is crucial for the good functioning of the visual pigments, which, upon absorption of a photon of light, undergo a conformational change (i.e., cis-to-trans isomerization) that is facilitated when the photoreceptors' lipid bilayer has high fluidity [7]. PUFA are highly prone to oxidation by ROS [8], which can drive lipid peroxidation, a chain reaction, in which one ROS can induce the oxidation of a large number of PUFA [9]. The end-products of lipid peroxidation, e.g., 4-hydroxy-2-nonenal (HNE) and malondialdehyde (MDA), can then react with the chemical groups of amino acids as lysines and histidines, ultimately leading to detrimental effects on photoreceptor function [10] and their elimination from the RPE. About 10% of damaged photoreceptors are engulfed daily by RPE cells by phagocytosis; this is an impressive metabolic task for RPE that, besides providing a means of preventing extensive damage to the photoreceptor layer, also leaves a gap between the photoreceptors and the RPE. Although some of the digested products are recycled back to photoreceptors and other cells of the retina, the synthesis of new photoreceptor membrane is also crucial to maintain the balance in the number of photoreceptor cells, as well as the proper RPE-photoreceptor interaction [11]. In this context, extensive aerobic glycolysis is necessary to cope with the need for new membrane biosynthesis and crucially contributes to the high metabolic rate of this tissue, and ultimately, to the production of ROS [11,12].

[a] These authors contributed equally.

Modulation of Oxidative Stress. https://doi.org/10.1016/B978-0-443-19247-0.00016-3

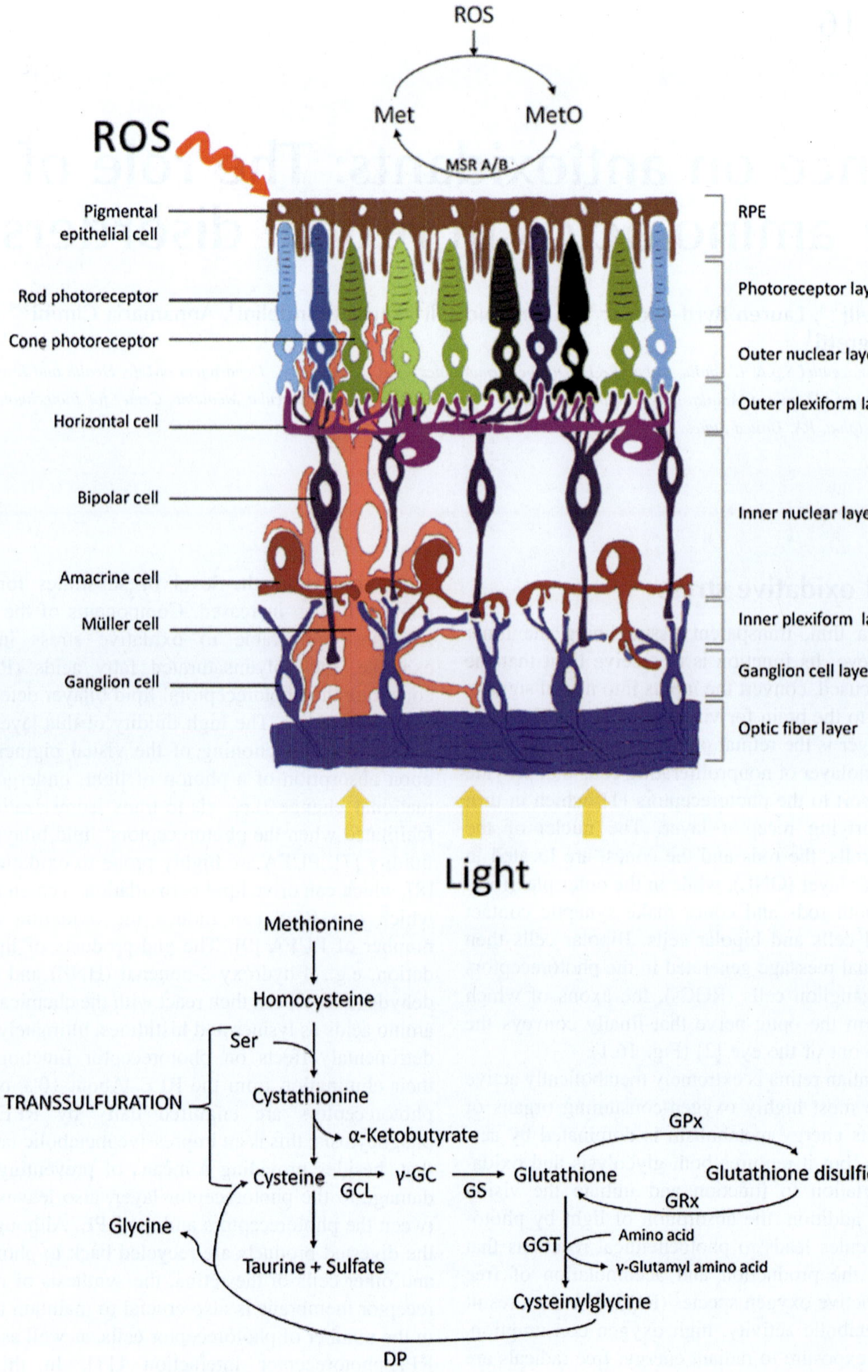

FIGURE 16.1 Structure of the retina and enzymatic pathway of sulfur amino acids. *γ-GC*, γ-glutamylcysteine; *CBS*, cystathionine β-synthase; *DP*, dipeptidase; *GCL*, glutamate cysteine ligase; GGT, γ-glutamyl transpeptidase; *GPx*, glutathione peroxidase; *GRx*, glutathione reductase; *GS*, glutathione synthetase; *Met*, methionine; *MetO*, methionine sulfoxide; *MSR A/B*, methionine sulfoxide reductases; *RPE*, retinal pigment epithelium; *Ser*, serine.

Several factors can contribute to increasing the basal levels of oxidative stress in the retina, but the most important source of ROS generation in the retina is, of course, light. Although it is intrinsic of retinal functions to be exposed to visible light and to convert light inputs into electrical impulses, the damage that prolonged retinal excitation by light can induce, in terms of ROS generation and subsequent photoreceptor death, has been extensively demonstrated [13,14]. Light-induced ROS production appears to be associated both to the physiological exposure of photoreceptors to the light and to the chronic accumulation of the byproducts of photoreceptor turnover. Lipids and proteins resulting from the degradation of photoreceptors can in fact progressively accumulate within the lysosomal compartment of RPE cells as nondegradable clusters of granules, which are collectively named lipofuscin [15]. The precise biochemical composition of lipofuscin is complex and not yet defined, but what is known is that its accumulation is caused by the incomplete degradation of cellular material within the lysosomes due to the oxidation of these byproducts, which contain photo-oxidizable fluorophores highly susceptible to oxidative changes either by normal cell metabolism or oxidative stress [16]. Thus, high levels of light-induced oxidative stress eventually trigger photoreceptor and inner retina apoptosis and severely affect the phagocytic function of the RPE.

Oxidative stress and retinal diseases

ROS production and oxidative stress have been recognized as main contributors to the pathogenesis of several retinal degenerative diseases, including diabetic retinopathy (DR), retinitis pigmentosa (RP), age-related macular degeneration (AMD), and glaucoma [17]. Under pathological conditions, oxidative stress and antioxidative mechanisms are unbalanced, leading to excessive oxidative stress, which in turn promotes inflammatory responses, blood-retinal barrier injury, and retinal tissue damage [18,19]. Thus, especially in their advanced pathological stages, all these retinal diseases involve the same processes of oxidative stress and apoptosis.

Oxidative stress in diabetic retinopathy

Diabetic retinopathy (DR) is a chronic and progressive complication of type 1 and type 2 diabetes. In diabetic patients, chronic hyperglycemia leads to diffuse microvascular damage that especially targets tissues, such as retina, nerve tissues, and kidney, that are more vulnerable to high glucose-induced damage as they cannot change glucose transport rates in case of elevated extracellular glucose concentrations [20]. As a microvascular complication of diabetes, DR is characterized by gradual and progressive alterations in the retinal microvasculature leading to damage of glia and retinal neurons [21].

Oxidative stress plays a key role in the pathogenesis of DR. In addition to a long-term light exposure, chronic hyperglycemia further increases ROS production, thus altering redox homeostasis, and leading to the death of neurons in the retina, followed by the rupture of the blood—retinal barrier and increased vascular permeability [17]. Excessive ROS in retinal cells directly acts on protein and DNA, also affecting mitochondrial function and, in turn, the activity of optic nerve cells, and function of photoreceptors. Besides, mitochondrial dysfunction may reduce mitochondrial energy production, leading to optic nerve degeneration. The accumulation of byproducts caused by metabolic abnormalities induced by hyperglycemia then further stimulates oxidative stress through ROS formation, leading to the death of retinal neurons. Finally, oxygen-derived free radicals participate in lipid peroxidation, critically contributing to the senescence of RPE cells, and leading to the progression of DR.

Oxidative stress in retinitis pigmentosa

Retinitis pigmentosa (RP) is the leading cause of inherited retinal disease worldwide, ultimately affecting millions of people [22,23]. RP collectively refers to a number of degenerative conditions of the retina with causative mutations found in over 50 genes for nonsyndromic RP and 39 genes combined for the RP-associated disorders Usher syndrome and Bardet-Beidl syndrome [22]. Just as the mutations directly responsible for the development of RP are numerous, the presentation of disease is incredibly varied as well, with marked differences in the age of onset, the involvement of particular retinal cells, and the rate of disease progression [22]. In general though, RP is characterized by the progression of vision impairment starting with night blindness, then eventually loss of peripheral vision, and ultimately complete blindness with the loss of central vision [23].

At the cellular level, RP is characterized by the death of photoreceptor cells, first the rods followed by the cones, with oxidative stress playing a significant role in the pathogenesis and progression of cell death. Oxygen levels in the outer retina increase dramatically following the degeneration of the rod cells, provoking further damage to the cone cells, as has been shown by studies linking antioxidants to prolonged maintenance of photoreceptor cells in an RP model [24]. For example, studies on the metabolism of glutathione, a well-known antioxidant peptide, in RP mouse models indicate that the regulation of glutathione production may aid in delaying cone death in RP, as it functions to remove ROS species contributing to further cell damage and death [25].

Oxidative stress in age-related macular degeneration

AMD is a multifactorial disorder that initially affects the RPE and gradually leads to a secondary loss of photoreceptor cells [26–28]. It is characterized by the degeneration of the macula and the loss of a high number of cone photoreceptors, which are responsible for daily visual perception and color vision. A body of evidence indicates that a complex interaction of environmental, genetic, and metabolic factors is responsible for AMD's development and progression, but the exact mechanisms underlying its pathogenesis are still unclear. Among the factors that have been described to be involved in AMD pathogenesis, including apoptosis, the formation of drusen and RPE alterations, immune system activation, senescent failure of homeostatic control, and Bruch's membrane defects, oxidative stress is known to play a crucial role [29]. Elevation of ROS has been associated with the onset and progression of aging, concomitantly with the decrease of antioxidant defenses. With aging, the expression levels of key detoxification enzymes such as glutathione S transferase-1, as well as of nonenzymatic ROS scavengers such as carotenoids and vitamin E, are reduced [30–32]. On the other hand, lipid peroxidation increases and in turn also lipofuscin accumulation, leading to a vicious cycle of lipid peroxidation and glycation-end products [33] production that damages mitochondrial DNA and alters the production/engulfment cycle of photoreceptors [34,35]. Currently, no therapies are available for the "dry type" AMD. In the Age-Related Eye Disease Study (AREDS), administration of nutraceuticals (AREDS and AREDS2), including vitamins C and E, β-carotene, and zinc, has been shown to counteract the disease progression. However, AREDS and AREDS2 supplements were not able to prevent AMD onset. On the other hand, for the "wet-type" AMD, the antivascular endothelial growth factor (VEGF) antibody is used as standard therapy able to rescue visual function [36,37]. However, the use of this therapy is limited by the invasiveness of the administration and its cost. Therefore, it is mandatory to formulate new therapeutic approaches for this pathology, and given the crucial role of oxidative stress in AMD pathogenesis, it has been indicated that antioxidant supplement may counteract cellular damage in the retina, thus reducing the risk and progression of AMD [19].

Oxidative stress in glaucoma

Another disorder that leads to irreversible blindness is glaucoma. Open-angle glaucoma (OAG) is the most common form. OAG is characterized by degeneration of the trabecular meshwork (TM) that rises the intraocular pressure, which in turn, leads to altered axons of RGCs forming the optical nerve, and then progressive concentric damage of the RGCs [38,39]. Degeneration of these cells results in a typical form of the optic disk (cupping) and visual impairment. Furthermore, it is characterized by retinal nerve fiber layer variations and typical visual field defects [40]. The biological mechanism of glaucoma is poorly recognized, and the factors supporting its progress have not been entirely described [41]. One of the leading risk factors for glaucoma advancement, and the only adaptable factor, is elevated intraocular pressure (IOP). Even if the mechanism is still uncertain [42], early neuroinflammation is indicated as an underlying trigger of glaucoma pathology [43,44].

Like AMD, glaucoma is also associated with oxidative stress [45,46]. In fact, it has been reported that the progressive loss of TM cells in glaucoma patients may be attributed to the long-term effects of oxidative injury induced by free radicals [47]. This hypothesis was then supported by in vitro and in vivo studies. Human TM in vitro upon hydrogen peroxide exposure showed a loss of cellular integrity and reduced cell adhesion [48]. Combined treatment with trophic and antioxidant factors was able to prevent the RGCs death in rats with elevated IOP [49]. Also, it has been reported that oxidative damage to DNA is considerably higher in the TM of glaucomatous patients compared to controls [50]. Moreover, in patients, IOP increase and visual impairment are proportional to the amount of oxidative DNA damage affecting TM cells [51]. In addition, the plasma level of glutathione resulted reduced in glaucoma patients [52,53].

Sulfur-containing amino acids and impacts on oxidative stress in the retina

Since the retina is particularly susceptible to oxidative damage and the onset and progression of several retinal diseases have been associated to the generation of ROS and oxidative stress, antioxidant agents and active measures to preserve redox homeostasis have been proposed as potentially effective preventive and/or therapeutic strategies [8]. The sulfur-containing amino acids, methionine, cysteine and their derivatives, exhibit and promote antioxidant properties that aid in preventing and ameliorating oxidative damage in the eye, and their effects have been investigated in the treatment of retinal disorders such as DR, RP, AMD, and glaucoma.

Physiochemical characteristics and metabolism of sulfur amino acids

While the majority of amino acids consist of carbon, hydrogen, oxygen, and nitrogen, there are some, namely methionine and cysteine, in which sulfur replaces oxygen.

In these cases, the lower electronegativity of sulfur related to oxygen leads to significant differences in their physiochemical properties, making these amino acids more hydrophobic and readily oxidized. Thus, methionine and cysteine have very specific functions in cellular proteins and processes [54]. Typically, due to their extremely hydrophobic nature, methionine residues are found in transmembrane domains, in close contact with the lipid bilayer or in the interior core of the protein. Methionine's role in protein translation is also related to its hydrophobicity, as it links the initiator tRNA Met-$tRNA_i^{Met}$ to eIF-2 of the ribosome and the mRNA template [55]. Cysteine, on the other hand, is known for its ability to form disulfide bonds, a nonenzymatic process, stabilizing protein structures. In addition to their roles in protein formation, these amino acids and their catabolism intermediates and products also participate in ROS scavenging and redox homeostasis pathways and are thus considered antioxidants.

The metabolism of both methionine and cysteine leads to the creation of ROS scavenging derivatives. Methionine is a precursor of cysteine, and the conversion pathway produces intermediates such as S-adenosylmethionine (SAM), S-adenosylhomocysteine (SAH), and homocysteine, which are important factors in the redox cell balance maintenance. Transmethylation of methionine, facilitated by the enzymes methionine adenosyltransferase and SAH hydrolase, sequentially generates SAM then SAH and ultimately, homocysteine and adenosine [54]. Homocysteine can be remethylated in a process mediated by methionine synthase or in specific tissues, betaine:homocysteine methyltransferase, and closes the loop of the methionine cycle [56]. This cycle allows for the creation of metabolites that enable methylation in a variety of regulatory pathways. In addition, homocysteine serves as an intermediate in the catabolism of methionine to cysteine. In the liver, kidney, intestine, and pancreas [54], the transsulfuration pathway regulates the transfer of sulfur from homocysteine to cysteine leading to the generation of several sulfur metabolites, which include cysteine and GSH [57] (Fig. 16.1). Cysteine itself is an important ROS scavenger amino acid, but it is also the subject of catabolism to downstream products including taurine and glutathione, a tripeptide with well-documented antioxidant capability [58].

The role of methionine in redox homeostasis in the retina

Methionine readily undergoes oxidation to form methionine sulfoxide (MetO), which is reduced back to methionine in a perpetual oxidation reduction cycle. This capability of methionine to be regularly oxidized allows it to serve as an antioxidant, effectively removing one ROS per cycle iteration [59]. Levine et al. examined the *E. coli* protein glutamine synthetase, where methionine residues surround the active site. Here, they act as a free radical oxygen sink, protecting the active site from H_2O_2-associated ROS by accepting the oxygen atoms to form MetO and H_2O [60]. The enzyme methionine sulfoxide reductase (MSR) then converts MetO back to methionine, completing the redox cycle. The oxidation of methionine results in S and R isomers, as the sulfur becomes a chiral center. Each isomer is acted on by a specific form of MSR, namely methionine sulfoxide reductase A (MSRA) which recognizes the S isomer and methionine sulfoxide reductase B (MSRB) for the R isomer (Fig. 16.1) [61–63]. Both forms of MSR have been found in retinal cells [64,65], and their expression in the eye is high compared to other organ tissues likely due to the high metabolic rate of the mitochondria and the prolonged exposure to oxidative agents [64]. Several studies have compared expression levels of MSRs in retinal tissue, either via knockouts, silencing, or overexpression, in response to oxidative stress, and reached similar conclusions: that MSRs promote resistance to oxidative cytotoxicity [64–67]. Pascual et al. examined the overexpression of MSRB2 in retinal cells and found that under stress caused by three oxidizing agents with different mechanisms, it led to substantial reductions of oxidative cytotoxicity [64], confirming its utility as a general antioxidant. Conversely in *msra−/−* mice, extensive oxidative damage is observed as well as reduced mitochondrial activity [66], in line with reports describing the importance of MSRA in the mitochondria for ATP synthesis in retinal pigment epithelial cells [68]. Taken together, these studies present the importance of methionine and the MSR redox cycle for the maintenance of retinal health upon inevitable exposure to ROS.

Cysteine as a redox sensor and antioxidant precursor

Like methionine, cysteine serves as a source of sulfur and thiol groups for multiple cellular processes. It can be easily oxidized, and its downstream derivatives include glutathione and taurine which are known antioxidants. It is a component of the tripeptide glutathione (GSH, comprised of glutamine, cysteine, and glycine), which is oxidized to the GSSG form by peroxides via the enzymatic actions of glutathione peroxidases. GSSG is then reduced back to GSH by the enzyme glutathione reductase (GR) and is available again to become oxidized by the scavenging of peroxides [69]. Beyond its inclusion in glutathione, cysteine itself serves as a redox sensor contributing to the cell's redox homeostasis [69]. Cysteine is capable of hydrogen peroxide and superoxide anion, DPPH and ABTS radical scavenging [70]. In addition, the oxidation of the cysteine residues in Kelch-like ECH-associating protein 1 (Keap1) causes it to disassociate from Nuclear factor erythroid 2-related factor 2 (Nrf2) which then translocates to the nucleus and promotes expression of antioxidant response genes [71]. The cysteine precursor, N-acetyl-L-cysteine (NAC), directly accepts oxygen free radicals and is used commonly as a therapeutic antioxidant in a wide range of afflictions [58].

Effects of taurine in retinal disorders with oxidative damage

While methionine and cysteine are considered primary amino acids and are incorporated into proteins, other amino acids, though nonproteinogenic, facilitate multiple diverse processes following similar mechanisms. Taurine is one; it is a free sulfur β-amino acid, meaning a sulfonic acid replaces the carboxylic group and the amino-group is located on the beta-carbon unlike the prototypical alpha amino acid structure. Taurine, when not supplied from dietary sources, is a product of methionine and cysteine catabolism. It is formed following a multistep process beginning with a cysteine precursor and the enzymes cysteine deoxygenase (CDO) and cysteine sulfonic decarboxylase (CSAD) [72]. These enzymes have been isolated in the retina [73], in line with the observation that taurine is expressed there in extraordinarily high levels compared to other tissues including the brain and liver [72,73].

As with methionine and cysteine, taurine is expected to have antioxidant properties, though the mechanisms, beyond limited evidence of the sulfur moiety reducing hydrogen peroxide in vitro [74], are not as clearly defined. Taurine has been linked to the amelioration of multiple retinal disorders that are affiliated with or caused by ROS damage and could be acting to counter the cytotoxicity of ROS in place of or in addition to neutralizing them directly. One such example is the taurine-mediated alteration to ratio of phosphotidylethanolamine and phosphatidylcholine in the plasma membrane that reduces susceptibility to oxidative damage [75]. Another is the ability of taurine to upregulate glutathione perioxidase [76], supporting the GSH:GSSG redox cycle, described above. Multiple studies have associated taurine deprivation with retinal cell degeneration [72,77] and with subsequent disorders.

Therapeutic approaches and effects with sulfur amino acids in retinal diseases

Taurine as potential therapy for retinal disorders

Emerging evidence indicates that taurine is essential for photoreceptors' survival, and its deprivation leads to retinal cells loss and, consequently, to retinal disorders [78]. Froger et al. studied the effects of taurine on RGCs degeneration both in vitro and in vivo [79]. Specifically, taurine significantly enhanced the survival of primary RGCs under serum-deprivation conditions and counteracted RGCs loss and N-methyl-D-aspartate (NMDA)-induced RGC excitotoxicity in NMDA-treated retinal explants from adult rats. In vivo, taurine supplementation increased RGC densities in two glaucoma rodent models and in one model of RP with secondary RGC degeneration, suggesting that taurine administration may help in the prevention of oxidative stress and RGC death, thus protecting from retinal degenerative diseases [79].

In line with these data, subsequent studies further confirmed taurine's neuroprotective properties in models of glaucoma. In Sprague–Dawley rats in which endothelin-1 (ET-1) was intravitreally administered to induce retinal and optic nerve injury, taurine was injected as pre-, co-, or post-treatment [80]. Taurine treatment inhibited apoptosis of retinal cells and changes in the morphology of the retina and optic nerve induced by ET-1, especially when given as preventive treatment. Additionally, the protective effect of taurine was associated with decreased retinal oxidative stress, as it improved superoxide dismutase and catalase activities as well as glutathione levels, while decreasing malondialdehyde levels [80].

Additional evidence of the protective effects of taurine in RP was provided using an animal model in which photoreceptor degeneration was induced by an intraperitoneal injection of N-methyl-N-nitrosourea (MNU). Intravenous administration of taurine improved the retinal disorganization characteristic of this model and ameliorated both M-cone and S-cone populations in the degenerative retinas. In addition, vision loss was reduced compared to untreated MNU-injected animals, and such neuroprotective effects were attributed to taurine's ability to reduce photoreceptor apoptosis and oxidative stress in the degenerative retina [81].

Recently, Fan et al. investigated the effects of taurine supplementation (administered intraperitoneally or intragastrically) in early diabetic retinas using a rat model of streptozotocin (STZ)-induced diabetes. Taurine protected retinal cone cells as well as RGCs from diabetes-induced damage by activating retinal taurine transporter, reducing reactive retinal gliosis, enhancing retinal synaptic connections, and reducing retinal cell apoptosis [82]. Another research group used again STZ-diabetic rats to compare the effects of chronic (4 months) taurine treatment with a mixture of vitamin E and selenium. Taurine counteracted oxidative stress in the diabetic retina and improved sodium pump activity in a dose- and time-dependent way, and notably, it sometimes showed better results compared to the mixture of vitamin E and selenium, also suggesting that its effects may not be simply mediated by its antioxidant activity [83]. Finally, the effects of taurine on glutamate uptake and deprivation have been studied in primary Müller cells under diabetic conditions (high glucose), where it was protective against oxidative stress by increasing antioxidant enzymes, thus reinforcing the rational for using taurine as a novel therapeutic approach for DR [84].

Further highlighting taurine's key antioxidant role and its potential as therapy in eye disorders, Ingensiep et al. showed that treatment with taurine increased the response rate of murine RGCs and improved the survival rate of retinal cells under hypoxic stress [85]. In addition, a recent study reported that taurine rescued mitochondria-related metabolic impairment in induced pluripotent stem cells derived from patients with mitochondrial myopathy, encephalopathy, lactic acidosis, and stroke-like episodes (MELAS iPSCs). Notably, taurine also inhibited epithelial mesenchymal transition in RPE differentiated from MELAS iPSCs [86].

Taurine's effects were also investigated clinically in a family with taurine deficiency (altered taurine transport dependent on Solute carrier family member 6, SLC6A6). Authors evaluated taurine levels in the blood and analyzed the fundus and macular with optical coherence tomography after 2 years of taurine supplement, showing, remarkably, that the retinal degeneration was strongly reduced, and the vision was clinically improved particularly in the youngest patients (6 years old) [87].

Cysteine-based supplements as potential therapy for retinal disorders

Excessive light exposure is known to cause damage to photoreceptors and RPE cells and may influence the progression of AMD. Thus, Song et al. studied the effects of N-acetyl-L-cysteine (NAC) treatment in in vitro and in vivo models of light injury. Authors reported that light exposure triggered severe photo-oxidative stress and endoplasmic reticulum stress in photoreceptors and retinas of mice, and that NAC was able to counteract light-induced injury, reducing oxidative stress and endoplasmic reticulum stress-related autophagy [88]. The effect of NAC was evaluated also in primary cultures of RPE from human donors with AMD, in which NAC pretreatment was able to protect RPE cells from oxidative damage, improving cell survival and cellular bioenergetic profile and reducing ATP depletion [89]. Additionally, the potential effects of NAC have been evaluated in ARPE-19 cell line stimulated with all-trans retinoic acid (ATRA), another in vitro model of AMD that is characterized by photoreceptor and RPE degeneration [90]. Also in this model, NAC was able to counteract both oxidative stress (ROS levels reduction) and endoplasmic reticulum stress. In line with these data, NAC pretreatment, other than reducing oxidative stress, was also able to ameliorate the inflammatory conditions in ARPE-19 cells exposed to pro-oxidants [91]. Further sustaining the potential therapeutic usefulness of NAC in AMD, NAC treatment has been recommended for the treatment of AMD for its ability to protect the RPE cells from hydrogen peroxide and super oxide anions generated upon exposure to blue violet light [89,92]. Finally, N-acetylcysteine amide decreases ROS and increases GSH levels in cells exposed to methamphetamine, known to cause several ocular disorders including glaucoma, AMD, and DR [93].

The effects of NAC were evaluated also in a DR model with promising results. In fact in high glucose-exposed RGCs, pretreatment with NAC significantly counteracted ROS production, enhancing the antioxidant defense and ameliorating mitochondrial impairment and inflammatory condition [94]. NAC treatment was proven effective also in a model of RP, in which higher doses of NAC decreased risk of macular loci sensitivity damage and increased reversibility in sensitivity depression in the fovea, thus protecting from irreversible dysfunction in RP [95]. Interestingly, in a phase I clinical study, Campochiaro et al. showed that oral NAC ameliorated sub-optimally functioning macular cones in RP patients (The FIGHT-RP1 Study - Full Text View - ClinicalTrials.gov) [96].

In addition to NAC, S-allyl L-cysteine (SAC), a sulfur-containing amino acid that is a natural constituent of fresh garlic, has shown antioxidant effects against human hydroquinone-induced oxidative damage in RPE cells (AMD model). SAC significantly reduced oxidative stress-induced RPE apoptosis, thus suggesting a potential effect in the treatment of AMD [97]. Notably, SAC potential as a therapeutic approach was confirmed also in retinal ischemia, a medical condition associated with numerous retinal vascular disorders, including AMD, DR, and glaucoma [98].

Conclusions

A crucial role for oxidative stress in eye diseases has been established in the last decade, with preclinical and clinical studies proving more and more the key role of excessive generation of ROS and unbalanced redox mechanisms in the progression of several retinal disorders. Thanks to the peculiar physiochemical characteristics and metabolism of sulfur amino acids, their administration has been considered as a promising approach to prevent or reduce oxidative stress-induced injury in ocular tissues. Their antioxidant properties and their function as ROS scavengers have been proven in several models of retinal disorders, such as DR, RP, AMD, and glaucoma and have assumed therapeutic significance.

References

[1] Travis GH, Golczak M, Moise AR, Palczewski K. Diseases caused by defects in the visual cycle: retinoids as potential therapeutic agents. Annu Rev Pharmacol Toxicol 2007;47:469–512.

[2] Nguyen KH, Patel BC, Tadi P. Anatomy, head and neck, eye retina. In: StatPearls. StatPearls Publishing; 2022.

[3] Hurley JB, Lindsay KJ, Du J. Glucose, lactate, and shuttling of metabolites in vertebrate retinas. J Neurosci Res 2015;93:1079–92.

[4] Ames A, Li YY, Heher EC, Kimble CR. Energy metabolism of rabbit retina as related to function: high cost of Na+ transport. J Neurosci 1992;12:840–53.

[5] van Reyk DM, Gillies MC, Davies MJ. The retina: oxidative stress and diabetes. Redox Rep 2003;8:187–92.

[6] Bokov A, Chaudhuri A, Richardson A. The role of oxidative damage and stress in aging. Mech Ageing Dev 2004;125:811–26.

[7] Giusto NM, et al. Lipid metabolism in vertebrate retinal rod outer segments. Prog Lipid Res 2000;39:315–91.

[8] Léveillard T, Sahel J-A. Metabolic and redox signaling in the retina. Cell Mol Life Sci 2017;74:3649–65.

[9] Catalá A. An overview of lipid peroxidation with emphasis in outer segments of photoreceptors and the chemiluminescence assay. Int J Biochem Cell Biol 2006;38:1482–95.

[10] Kim H-J, Ha S, Lee HY, Lee K-J. ROSics: chemistry and proteomics of cysteine modifications in redox biology. Mass Spectrom Rev 2015;34:184–208.

[11] Punzo C, Xiong W, Cepko CL. Loss of daylight vision in retinal degeneration: are oxidative stress and metabolic dysregulation to blame? J Biol Chem 2012;287:1642–8.

[12] Rajala RVS. Aerobic glycolysis in the retina: functional roles of pyruvate kinase isoforms. Front Cell Dev Biol 2020;8:266.

[13] Grimm C, et al. Rhodopsin-mediated blue-light damage to the rat retina: effect of photoreversal of bleaching. Investig Ophthalmol Vis Sci 2001;42:497–505.

[14] Kuse Y, Ogawa K, Tsuruma K, Shimazawa M, Hara H. Damage of photoreceptor-derived cells in culture induced by light emitting diode-derived blue light. Sci Rep 2014;4:5223.

[15] Sparrow JR, Boulton M. RPE lipofuscin and its role in retinal pathobiology. Exp Eye Res 2005;80:595–606.

[16] Călin EF, et al. Lipofuscin: a key compound in ophthalmic practice. Rom J Ophthalmol 2021;65:109–13.

[17] Wang J, et al. Role of oxidative stress in retinal disease and the early intervention strategies: a review. Oxid Med Cell Longev 2022;2022:e7836828.

[18] Nita M, Grzybowski A. The role of the reactive oxygen species and oxidative stress in the pathomechanism of the age-related ocular diseases and other pathologies of the anterior and posterior eye segments in adults. Oxid Med Cell Longev 2016;2016:e3164734.

[19] Domènech B, Marfany G. The relevance of oxidative stress in the pathogenesis and therapy of retinal dystrophies. Antioxidants 2020;9:347.

[20] Nolan CJ, Damm P, Prentki M. Type 2 diabetes across generations: from pathophysiology to prevention and management. Lancet 2011;378:169–81.

[21] Fletcher EL, Phipps JA, Ward MM, Puthussery T, Wilkinson-Berka JL. Neuronal and glial cell abnormality as predictors of progression of diabetic retinopathy. Curr Pharm Des 2007;13:2699–712.

[22] Daiger S, Sullivan L, Bowne S. Genes and mutations causing retinitis pigmentosa. Clin Genet 2013;84. https://doi.org/10.1111/cge.12203.

[23] Verbakel SK, van Huet R, Boon C, den Hollander A, Collin R, Klaver C, et al. Non-syndromic retinitis pigmentosa. Prog Retin Eye Res 2018;66:157–86. https://doi.org/10.1016/j.preteyeres.2018.03.005.

[24] Komeima K, Rogers BS, Campochiaro PA. Antioxidants slow photoreceptor cell death in mouse models of retinitis pigmentosa. J Cell Physiol 2007;213:809–15.

[25] Sánchez-Vallejo V, et al. Alterations in glutamate cysteine ligase content in the retina of two retinitis pigmentosa animal models. Free Radic Biol Med 2016;96:245–54.

[26] Rein DB, et al. Forecasting age-related macular degeneration through the year 2050: the potential impact of new treatments. Arch Ophthalmol 2009;127:533–40.

[27] Boulton M, Dayhaw-Barker P. The role of the retinal pigment epithelium: topographical variation and ageing changes. Eye 2001;15:384–9.

[28] Gehrs KM, Anderson DH, Johnson LV, Hageman GS. Age-related macular degeneration—emerging pathogenetic and therapeutic concepts. Ann Med 2006;38:450–71.

[29] Michalska-Małecka K, Kabiesz A, Nowak M, Śpiewak D. Age related macular degeneration—challenge for future: pathogenesis and new perspectives for the treatment. Eur Geriatr Med 2015;6:69–75.

[30] Maeda A, Crabb JW, Palczewski K. Microsomal glutathione S-transferase 1 in the retinal pigment epithelium: protection against oxidative stress and a potential role in aging. Biochemistry 2005;44:480–9.

[31] Beatty S, Koh H-H, Phil M, Henson D, Boulton M. The role of oxidative stress in the pathogenesis of age-related macular degeneration. Surv Ophthalmol 2000;45:115–34.

[32] Vitamin E in macular and peripheral tissues of the human eye. Curr Eye Res 14(8). https://www.tandfonline.com/doi/abs/10.3109/02713689508998497.

[33] Glenn JV, Stitt AW. The role of advanced glycation end products in retinal ageing and disease. Biochim Biophys Acta Gen Subj 2009;1790:1109–16.

[34] Lipid peroxidation and antioxidant enzymatic systems in rat retina as a function of age. https://link.springer.com/article/10.1007/BF00968789.

[35] Wolf G. Lipofuscin and macular degeneration. Nutr Rev 2003;61:342–6.

[36] Yang S, Zhao J, Sun X. Resistance to anti-VEGF therapy in neovascular age-related macular degeneration: a comprehensive review. DDDT 2016;10:1857–67.

[37] Boyle J, Vukicevic M, Koklanis K, Itsiopoulos C. Experiences of patients undergoing anti-VEGF treatment for neovascular age-related macular degeneration: a systematic review. Psychol Health Med 2015;20:296–310.

[38] Weinreb RN, Aung T, Medeiros FA. The pathophysiology and treatment of glaucoma: a review. JAMA 2014;311:1901–11.

[39] Mélik Parsadaniantz S, Réaux-le Goazigo A, Sapienza A, Habas C, Baudouin C. Glaucoma: a degenerative optic neuropathy related to neuroinflammation? Cells 2020;9:535.

[40] Costagliola C, et al. Pharmacotherapy of intraocular pressure: part I. Parasympathomimetic, sympathomimetic and sympatholytics. Expert Opin Pharmacother 2009;10:2663–77.

[41] Cherecheanu AP, Garhofer G, Schmidl D, Werkmeister R, Schmetterer L. Ocular perfusion pressure and ocular blood flow in glaucoma. Curr Opin Pharmacol 2013;13:36–42.

[42] Mahabadi N, Foris LA, Tripathy K. Open angle glaucoma. In: StatPearls. StatPearls Publishing; 2022.

[43] Soto I, Howell GR. The complex role of neuroinflammation in glaucoma. Cold Spring Harb Perspect Med 2014;4:a017269.

[44] Williams PA, et al. Neuroinflammation in glaucoma: a new opportunity. Exp Eye Res 2017;157:20–7.

[45] McMonnies C. Reactive oxygen species, oxidative stress, glaucoma and hyperbaric oxygen therapy. J Optom 2018;11:3–9.
[46] The association between oxidative stress and corneal hysteresis in patients with glaucoma. Sci Rep. https://www.nature.com/articles/s41598-020-57520-x.
[47] Alvarado J, Murphy C, Polansky J, Juster R. Age-related changes in trabecular meshwork cellularity. Investig Ophthalmol Vis Sci 1981;21:714–27.
[48] Zhou L, Li Y, Yue BYJT. Oxidative stress affects cytoskeletal structure and cell-matrix interactions in cells from an ocular tissue: the trabecular meshwork. J Cell Physiol 1999;180:182–9.
[49] Ko M, Hu D, Ritch R, Sharma SC. The combined effect of brain-derived neurotrophic factor and a free radical scavenger in experimental glaucoma. Investig Ophthalmol Vis Sci 2000;41:2967–71.
[50] Oxidative deoxyribonucleic acid damage in the eyes of glaucoma patients. Am J Med. https://www.amjmed.com/article/S0002-9343(03)00114-1/fulltext.
[51] Saccà SC, Pascotto A, Camicione P, Capris P, Izzotti A. Oxidative DNA damage in the human trabecular meshwork: clinical correlation in patients with primary open-angle glaucoma. Arch Ophthalmol 2005;123:458–63.
[52] Gherghel D, Griffiths HR, Hilton EJ, Cunliffe IA, Hosking SL. Systemic reduction in glutathione levels occurs in patients with primary open-angle glaucoma. Investig Ophthalmol Vis Sci 2005;46:877–83.
[53] Gherghel D, Mroczkowska S, Qin L. Reduction in blood glutathione levels occurs similarly in patients with primary-open angle or normal tension glaucoma. Investig Ophthalmol Vis Sci 2013;54:3333–9.
[54] Brosnan JT, Brosnan ME. The sulfur-containing amino acids: an overview. J Nutr 2006;136:1636S–40S.
[55] Drabkin HJ, RajBhandary UL. Initiation of protein synthesis in mammalian cells with codons other than AUG and amino acids other than methionine. Mol Cell Biol 1998;18:5140–7.
[56] Parkhitko AA, Jouandin P, Mohr SE, Perrimon N. Methionine metabolism and methyltransferases in the regulation of aging and lifespan extension across species. Aging Cell 2019;18:e13034.
[57] Sbodio JI, Snyder SH, Paul BD. Regulators of the transsulfuration pathway. Br J Pharmacol 2019;176:583–93.
[58] Clemente Plaza N, Reig García-Galbis M, Martínez-Espinosa RM. Effects of the usage of l-cysteine (l-Cys) on human health. Molecules 2018;23:575.
[59] Métayer S, et al. Mechanisms through which sulfur amino acids control protein metabolism and oxidative status. J Nutr Biochem 2008;19:207–15.
[60] Levine RL, Mosoni L, Berlett BS, Stadtman ER. Methionine residues as endogenous antioxidants in proteins. Proc Natl Acad Sci USA 1996;93:15036–40.
[61] Moskovitz J, et al. Purification and characterization of methionine sulfoxide reductases from mouse and *Staphylococcus aureus* and their substrate stereospecificity. Biochem Biophys Res Commun 2002;290:62–5.
[62] Methionine sulfoxide reductase A is a stereospecific methionine oxidase. https://www.pnas.org/doi/10.1073/pnas.1101275108.
[63] Methionine sulfoxide reductase (MsrA) is a regulator of antioxidant defense and lifespan in mammals. https://www.pnas.org/doi/10.1073/pnas.231472998?url_ver=Z39.88-2003&rfr_id=ori%3Arid%3Acrossref.org&rfr_dat=cr_pub++0pubmed.
[64] Pascual I, Larrayoz IM, Campos MM, Rodriguez IR. Methionine sulfoxide reductase B2 is highly expressed in the retina and protects retinal pigmented epithelium cells from oxidative damage. Exp Eye Res 2010;90:420–8.
[65] Lee JW, et al. Gene structure, localization and role in oxidative stress of methionine sulfoxide reductase A (MSRA) in the monkey retina. Exp Eye Res 2006;82:816–27.
[66] Mazzoni F, Dun Y, Vargas JA, Nandrot EF, Finnemann SC. Lack of the antioxidant enzyme methionine sulfoxide reductase A in mice impairs RPE phagocytosis and causes photoreceptor cone dysfunction. Redox Biol 2021;42:101918.
[67] Sreekumar PG, Hinton DR, Kannan R. Methionine sulfoxide reductase A: structure, function and role in ocular pathology. World J Biol Chem 2011;2:184–92.
[68] Independent roles of methionine sulfoxide reductase A in mitochondrial ATP synthesis and as antioxidant in retinal pigment epithelial cells. https://www.ncbi.nlm.nih.gov/pmc/articles/PMC3859712/.
[69] Fra A, Yoboue ED, Sitia R. Cysteines as redox molecular switches and targets of disease. Front Mol Neurosci 2017;10:167.
[70] In vitro antioxidant actions of sulfur-containing amino acids | Elsevier Enhanced Reader. https://reader.elsevier.com/reader/sd/pii/S1878535218300030?token=1005EC00A7CB142201E993D88488E591C1FA10BD8F097B2C56C15DBB74A987A308536612A01D4B1CC89537815B2E637C&originRegion=us-east-1&originCreation=20221202132954.
[71] Dinkova-Kostova AT, et al. Direct evidence that sulfhydryl groups of Keap1 are the sensors regulating induction of phase 2 enzymes that protect against carcinogens and oxidants. Proc Natl Acad Sci USA 2002;99:11908–13.
[72] Froger N, et al. Taurine: the comeback of a neutraceutical in the prevention of retinal degenerations. Prog Retin Eye Res 2014;41:44–63.
[73] Macaione S, Tucci G, Luca GD, Di Giorgio RM. Subcellular distribution of taurine and cysteine sulphinate decarboxylase activity in ox retina. J Neurochem 1976;27:1411–5.
[74] Cozzi R, et al. Taurine and ellagic acid: two differently-acting natural antioxidants. Environ Mol Mutagen 1995. https://onlinelibrary.wiley.com/doi/abs/10.1002/em.2850260310?sid=nlm%3Apubmed.
[75] Hamaguchi T, Azuma J, Schaffer S. Interaction of taurine with methionine: inhibition of myocardial phospholipid methyltransferase. J Cardiovasc Pharmacol 1991;18:224–30.
[76] Flora SJS, Pande M, Bhadauria S, Kannan GM. Combined administration of taurine and meso 2,3-dimercaptosuccinic acid in the treatment of chronic lead intoxication in rats. Hum Exp Toxicol 2004;23:157–66.
[77] Gaucher D, et al. Taurine deficiency damages retinal neurones: cone photoreceptors and retinal ganglion cells. Amino Acids 2012;43:1979–93.
[78] Castelli V, et al. Taurine and oxidative stress in retinal health and disease. CNS Neurosci Ther 2021;27:403–12.
[79] Froger N, et al. Taurine provides neuroprotection against retinal ganglion cell degeneration. PLoS One 2012;7:e42017.
[80] Nor Arfuzir NN, et al. Taurine protects against retinal and optic nerve damage induced by endothelin-1 in rats via antioxidant effects. Neural Regen Res 2018;13:2014–21.
[81] Tao Y, et al. Systemic taurine treatment provides neuroprotection against retinal photoreceptor degeneration and visual function impairments. DDDT 2019;13:2689–702.
[82] Fan Y, et al. Taurine protects retinal cells and improves synaptic connections in early diabetic rats. Curr Eye Res 2020;45:52–63.
[83] Potential therapeutic effect of antioxidants in experimental diabetic retina: a comparison between chronic taurine and vitamin E plus selenium supplementations. Free Radic Res 37(3). https://www.tandfonline.com/doi/abs/10.1080/1071576021000055271.

[84] Zeng K, et al. Effects of taurine on glutamate uptake and degradation in Müller cells under diabetic conditions via antioxidant mechanism. Mol Cell Neurosci 2010;45:192–9.

[85] Ingensiep C, Schaffrath K, Denecke B, Walter P, Johnen S. A multielectrode array-based hypoxia model for the analysis of electrical activity in murine retinae. J Neurosci Res 2021;99:2172–87.

[86] Homma K, et al. Taurine rescues mitochondria-related metabolic impairments in the patient-derived induced pluripotent stem cells and epithelial-mesenchymal transition in the retinal pigment epithelium. Redox Biol 2021;41:101921.

[87] Ansar M, et al. Taurine treatment of retinal degeneration and cardiomyopathy in a consanguineous family with SLC6A6 taurine transporter deficiency. Hum Mol Genet 2020;29:618–23.

[88] Song J-Y, et al. Suppressing endoplasmic reticulum stress-related autophagy attenuates retinal light injury. Aging (Albany NY) 2020;12:16579–96.

[89] Terluk MR, et al. N-acetyl-L-cysteine protects human retinal pigment epithelial cells from oxidative damage: implications for age-related macular degeneration. Oxid Med Cell Longev 2019;2019:5174957.

[90] Wu J, Cui D, Li H, Zeng J. Protective effects of NAC and salubrinal on apoptosis of retinal pigment epithelial cells induced by all-trans retinoic acid. 2022. https://journals.sagepub.com/doi/abs/10.1177/11206721211000674?journalCode=ejoa.

[91] AnandBabu K, Sen P, Angayarkanni N. Oxidized LDL, homocysteine, homocysteine thiolactone and advanced glycation end products act as pro-oxidant metabolites inducing cytokine release, macrophage infiltration and pro-angiogenic effect in ARPE-19 cells. PLoS One 2019;14:e0216899.

[92] Tosi GM, et al. Superior properties of N-acetylcysteine ethyl ester over N-acetyl cysteine to prevent retinal pigment epithelial cells oxidative damage. Int J Mol Sci 2021;22:600.

[93] Ercal N, et al. N-acetyl-L-cysteine amide protects retinal pigment epithelium against methamphetamine-induced oxidative stress. J Biophys Chem 2012. https://doi.org/10.4236/jbpc.2012.32012.

[94] Pal S, Rao GN, Pal A. High glucose-induced ROS accumulation is a critical regulator of ERK1/2-Akt-tuberin-mTOR signalling in RGC-5 cells. Life Sci 2020;256:117914.

[95] Kong X, Hafiz G, Wehling D, Akhlaq A, Campochiaro PA. Locus-level changes in macular sensitivity in patients with retinitis pigmentosa treated with oral N-acetylcysteine. Am J Ophthalmol 2021;221:105–14.

[96] Oral N-acetylcysteine improves cone function in retinitis pigmentosa patients in phase I trial. J Clin Investig. https://www.jci.org/articles/view/132990.

[97] Gianni. S-allyl cysteine protects retinal pigment epithelium cells from hydroquinone-induced apoptosis through mitigating cellular response to oxidative stress. Eur Rev 2020. https://www.europeanreview.org/article/20392.

[98] Fortified S-allyl L-cysteine: animal safety, effect on retinal ischemia, and role of Wnt in the underlying therapeutic mechanism. https://www.hindawi.com/journals/ecam/2020/3025946/.

Chapter 17

Oxidative stress and antioxidant-based therapies in male infertility

Renata Mangione[1], Barbara Tavazzi[2], Giuseppe Lazzarino[3] and Giacomo Lazzarino[2]

[1]*Institute of Biochemistry and Clinical Biochemistry, Catholic University of Rome, Rome, Italy;* [2]*UniCamillus—Saint Camillus International University of Health Sciences, Rome, Italy;* [3]*Department of Biomedical and Biotechnological Sciences, Division of Medical Biochemistry, University of Catania, Catania, Italy*

Introduction

Infertility, defined as the inability to achieve pregnancy after at least 12 months of regular intercourse, is a multifactorial pathological state, and unfortunately affects more than 10% of couples of reproductive ages, approximately 48.5 million, worldwide [1,2], and for long time, females have been considered as the sole ones responsible for pregnancy failures. Over the past decade, it has been shown that at least half of all cases of failure to conceive are attributable to male problems.

Today, among couples with this condition, the male factor is considered the sole cause in ≈20% of all cases, along with a co-contribution of the female factor in the remaining 30% of cases [3,4] (Fig. 17.1).

Many etiological causes of male infertility have also been identified, so much so that it has been termed a multifactorial disease, and these include anatomical abnormalities, genetics, neurological diseases, infections, and a significant contribution of environmental and lifestyle factors [5,6].

Importantly, SARS-Cov-2 viral infection over the past 3 years has also contributed to negatively affect couple fertility [7], as it can increase systemic inflammatory processes, which also lead to increased oxidative/nitrosative stress, a biochemical alteration that is particularly influential in decreasing the fertilization capacity of both individuals in the couple [8].

Regarding morphofunctional abnormalities in spermatozoa, they represent the main causes of male infertility and are distinguished into testicular, extra-testicular, pretesticular, and idiopathic [9], which are the most common and are characterized by a nonmanifest primary cause. Of course, it is also important to consider parameters related to seminal fluid analysis, such as low sperm count, altered sperm quality parameters (concentration, motility, morphology), seminal fluid pH, liquefaction, viscosity, and concentration/ejaculate (normal ≥15 million/ejaculate).

Unfortunately, testicular infertility, primary hypogonadism, is widespread (30%−40% of infertile males), representing a broad profile of acquired pathological conditions, such as genetic or chromosomal abnormalities (Klinefelter syndrome) [10,11], cryptorchidism [12], and Y chromosome microdeletions [13], also acquired conditions such as environmental and lifestyle factors, smoking, drug and alcohol abuse, obesity, testicular tumor occurrence, vascular abnormalities [14−16], and varicocele with altered spermatogenesis [17,18] (Fig. 17.2).

Extratesticular causes are related mainly to altered sperm delivery or ejaculatory dysfunction [19]. The other main family of causes of extratesticular infertility is ejaculatory dysfunction, a heterogeneous group of disorders mainly related to conditions of premature ejaculation, anejaculation, and retrograde ejaculation induced by pharmacological, anatomical, or idiopathic factors [20].

Pathological conditions related to pretesticular causes of infertility affect about 1%−2% of infertile males and are mainly due to deficiency of gonadotropin-releasing hormone, luteinizing hormone, and follicle-stimulating hormone [21,22].

In about 30%−40% of cases, infertile males do not clearly fall into any of the above three groups and are generally classified as idiopathic [9,23,24], that is, the reason for the infertility condition is most likely to go undiagnosed.

As reported earlier, the parameters considered in the evaluation of seminal fluid were defined in the World Health Organization (WHO) guidelines for performing a

Modulation of Oxidative Stress. https://doi.org/10.1016/B978-0-443-19247-0.00010-2

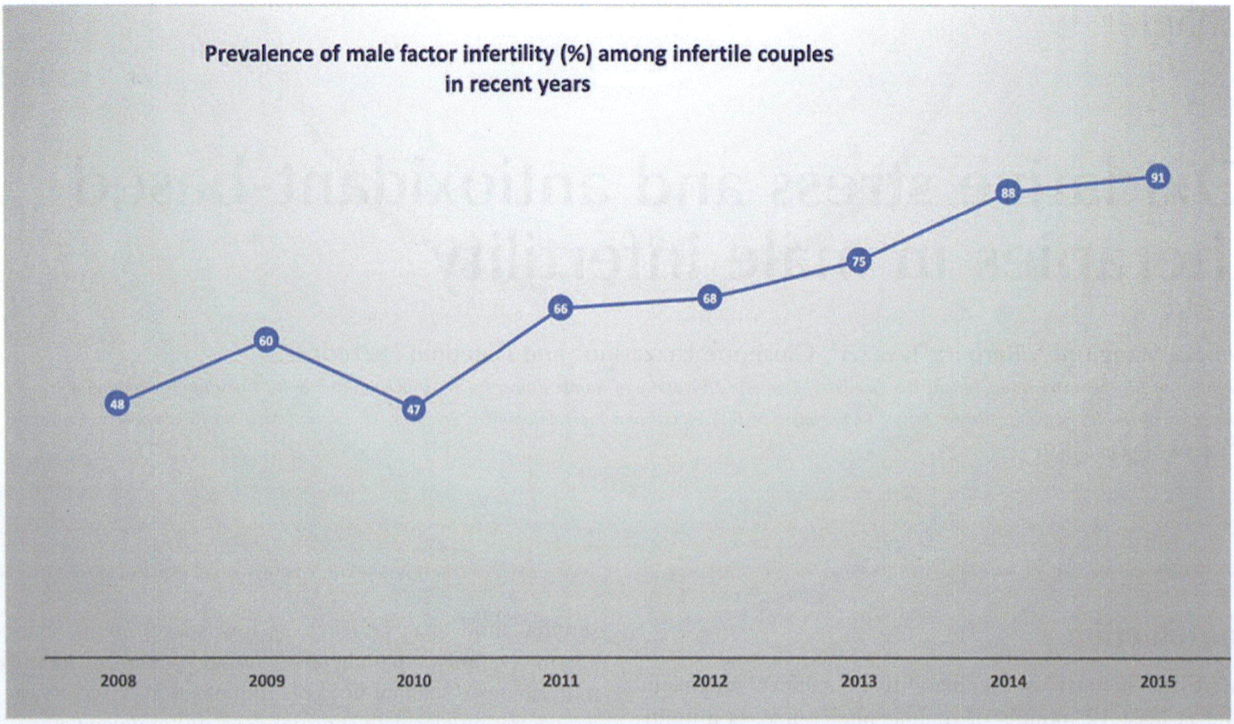

FIGURE 17.1 Couple infertility: it is depending mainly for male factor infertile parameters as reported by the different percentage registered in recent years.

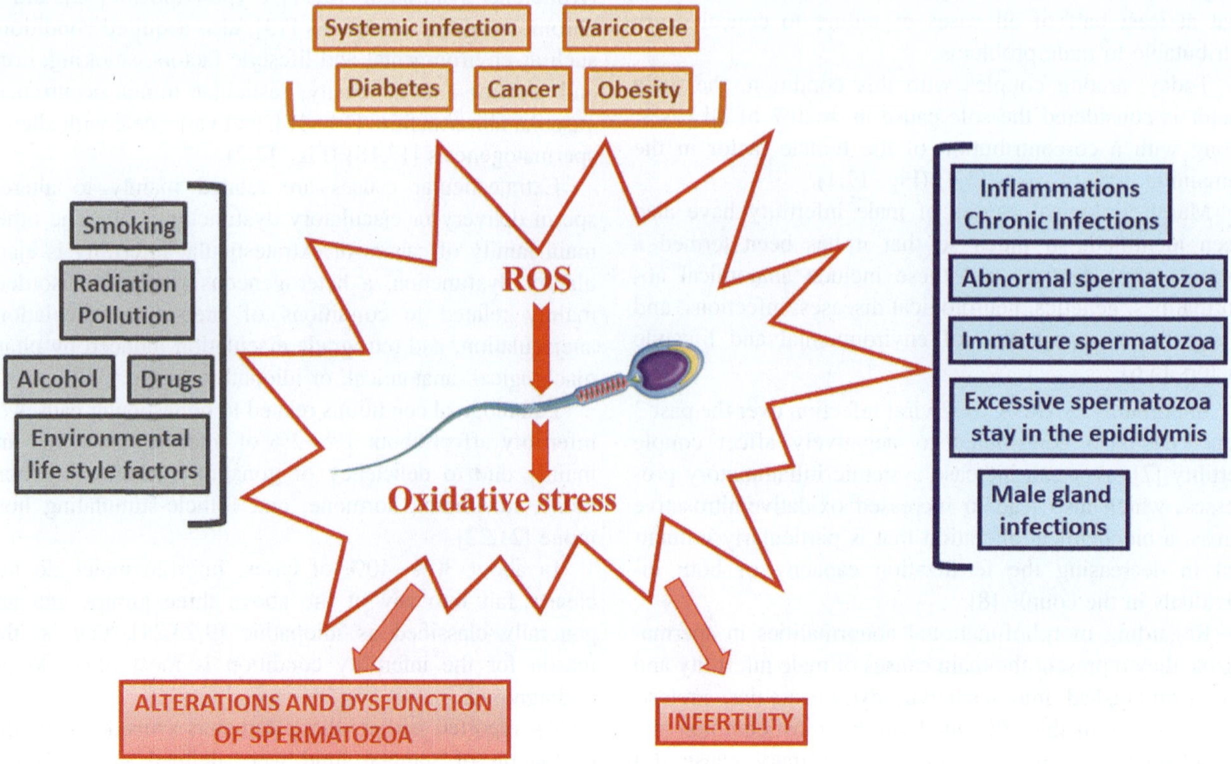

FIGURE 17.2 Principal effectors influencing the male fertility, the systemic pathological diseases, environmental lifestyle factors, and the primary pathologies of male reproductive system.

proper seminal fluid analysis, the latest update of which was published about 10 years ago and introduced many significant changes [25], reiterating that, in cases of infertility, seminal fluid analysis is the first step in the diagnostic.

Based on the results of seminal fluid analysis, several types of conditions can be distinguished, starting with normozoospermia (N), with all values close to normal. Next, one can distinguish: oligozoospermia (O), total number of spermatozoa below the lower reference limit; asthenozoospermia (A), total motility, calculated as progressive and nonprogressive motility, $\leq 40\%$ or progressive motility $\leq 32\%$; teratozoospermia (T), spermatozoa with normal morphology $\leq 4\%$; oligoasthenoteratozoospermia (OAT), abnormality of all three previous variables; asthenoteratozoospermia (AT) and oligoasthenozoospermia (OA) as combination of A + T ad O + A alterations; azoospermia, absence of spermatozoa in the ejaculate and aspermia, total absence of ejaculation [26]. All of them are associated to infertility, but the most present, in the 90% of infertile males, is oligozoospermia.

As mentioned above, semen analysis is important, but unfortunately it does not provide clear and certain indications that any alterations in the morpho-functional parameters of spermatozoa are entirely responsible for the lack of ability to procreate. In fact, the reference values given by WHO are those found in almost all (95%) normal and fertile males, that is, those who have achieved paternity.

Consequently, there is a clear need to search for other analytical tests, particularly with biochemical/molecular techniques, that would allow useful diagnosis and treatment of male infertility and go beyond the morphofunctional assessment of spermatozoa not always associated with male infertility.

Because the molecular mechanisms underlying sperm alterations remain unknown, many scientific studies have focused on gene mutations, post-translational modifications, the role of epigenetics, sperm DNA fragmentation, but especially the role of oxidative/nitrosative stress in men with idiopathic infertility [27].

The role of oxidative/nitrosative stress and the ROS paradox

Under physiological conditions, reactive oxygen species (ROS) play important roles in various processes of human spermatozoa, such as stimulating it to perform the different stages of its maturation [28], capacitation, hyperactivation, acrosome reaction, and sperm-oocyte fusion [29–34].

When there is an imbalance between the production of ROS and the protective action of antioxidant systems responsible for their neutralization and elimination, this is where serious sperm problems can occur. Indeed, overproduction of ROS (singlet oxygen, superoxide anion, and hydroxyl radical) is often present in the sperm of infertile males, adversely affecting sperm function and viability due to severe oxidative damage to various biological macromolecules (proteins, nucleic acids, polyunsaturated fatty acids of biological membrane lipids). These disorders can induce poor fertilization, pregnancy loss, birth defects, and poor embryonic development are related to the high susceptibility of spermatozoa to oxidative insult [35,36]. Also in sperm cells, oxidative stress can be associated with nitrosative stress, due to the uncontrolled production of reactive nitrogen species (RNS), mainly resulting from the spontaneous decomposition of nitric oxide (−NO) and its reaction with superoxide. But it should not be forgotten that the activity of nitric oxide synthase (NOS) isoforms, especially the inducible (iNOS), is generally involved in the excess production of −NO. The special feature of the combination of ROS and RNS is that products with more oxidizing than radicalizing action are formed, such as peroxynitrite ($ONOO^-$), which can then decompose into stable end products such as nitrite and nitrate, used as an indirect measure of nitrosative stress.

The particular association of different radicals involved in oxidative/nitrosative stress provokes defects in sperm stimulation of lipid peroxidation of polyunsaturated fatty acid-rich plasma membranes of spermatozoa [28,37–39] and DNA fragmentation [40,41]. Furthermore, the insurgence of oxidative/nitrosative stress also in spermatozoa is associated with mitochondrial dysfunction.

The damaging activities of ROS and RNS are mainly expressed in altering the expression and catalytic activities of glycolytic enzymes, the Krebs cycle, protein components of the electron transfer chain (ETC), and oxidative phosphorylation (OXPHOS), ultimately leading to reduced efficiency in ATP production, resulting in energy crisis and mitochondrial dysfunction [42–44] (Fig. 17.3).

There is a relevant aspect in the existing relationship between oxidative/nitrosative stress and male infertility, as this stress may originate in cells other than spermatozoa, which, however, are affected by the accumulation in seminal plasma of various toxic compounds resulting from radical activities. For example, the pathological effect of varicocele and increased ROS/RNS concentration has been reported. This pathology is much more prevalent than is generally believed (30%–40% of infertile males), altering testicular hemodynamics and microenvironment (e.g., increased scrotal temperature) [39], not only causes defects in spermatogenesis, but it seems that it may also be responsible for increased production of radicals, perhaps also due to defective activity of antioxidant defenses in sperm [38,39]. It should be pointed out that although several biochemical alterations have been shown in

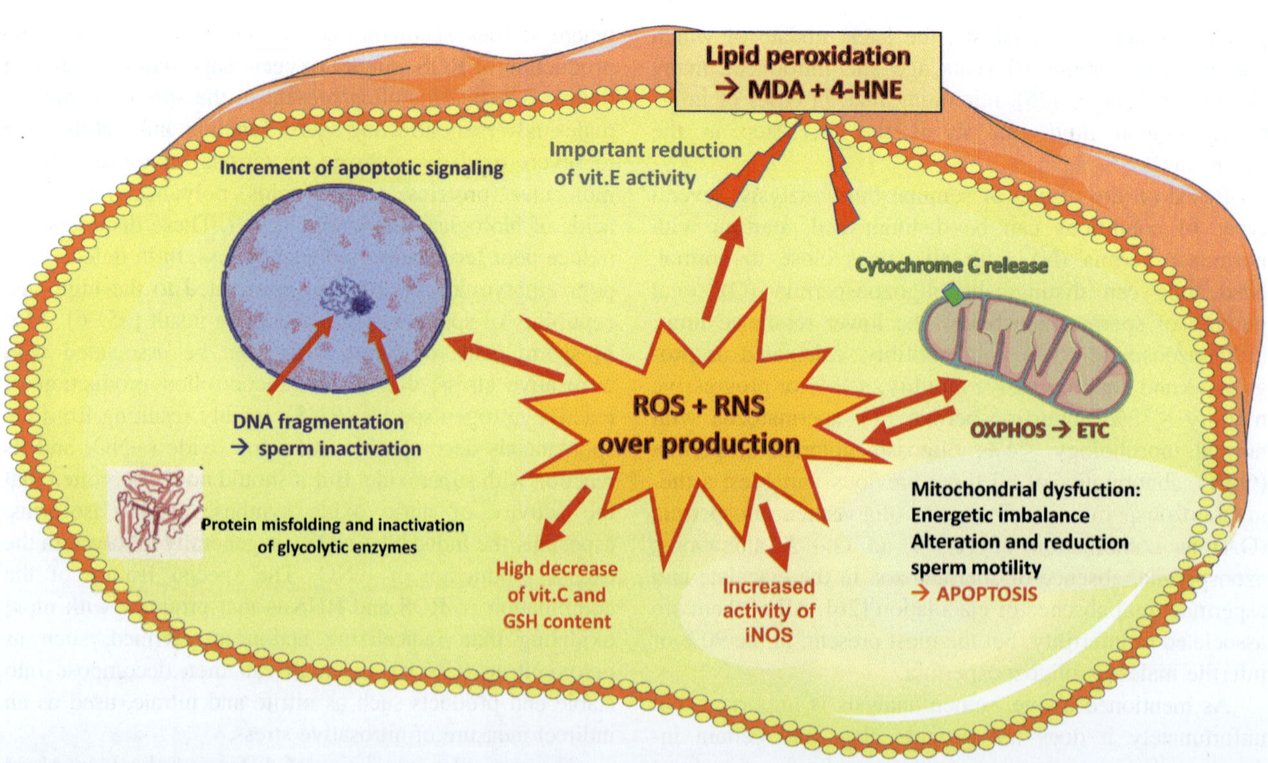

FIGURE 17.3 Exemplification of the principal sources and damaging effects of reactive oxygen species (ROS) and reactive nitrogen species (RNS) overproduction. Mitochondria are both able to produce and the central targets of ROS. Alteration of electron transport by electron transport chain (ETC) impairs mitochondrial ROS generation, inducing a decrease of OXPHOS efficiency and in ATP production. Moreover, it is increased expression of iNOS and the subsequent increase of nitric oxide production. The oxidative/nitrosative stress is not neutralized by vitamin C (VitC) and reduced glutathione (GSH), considerably decreased, as also the membrane α-tocopherol. A cascade of reaction is represented by the induction of the lipid peroxidation of membrane phospholipids the formation of malondialdehyde (MDA) and 4-hydroxynonenale (4-HNE); high rate of protein misfolding and unfolding, leading to the alteration of functional glycolytic enzymes; the DNA oxidation with its fragmentation; and generation of DNA oxidative products such as 8-hydroxy-2′-deoxyguanosine (8-OHdG). At the end, there is the loss of cytochrome *c* from the intermembrane space into the cytoplasm, acting as a signal for triggering apoptosis. All these altered morphofunctional parameters of spermatozoa, deeply affecting male fertility.

varicocele [45,46], a real link between oxidative/nitrosative stress and male infertility is not entirely clear.

In the context of pathological situations, even major infections of the male reproductive tract can induce massive production of radicals due to inflammation and tissue infiltration of leukocytes and leukocytospermia [47]; the pathobiological role of which in the excessive production of ROS and its correlation with male infertility is still debated. In fact, several studies have shown that this parameter is closely correlated with the damage of sperm components, such as membranes and DNA, even when the level of leukocytospermia is below the threshold value ($>1 \times 10^6$ spermatozoa/mL) defined by WHO [25,47].

It cannot be overlooked that in many types of cancer, there is an increase in ROS/RNS and among them is certainly testicular cancer [48,49] that can induce oxidative imbalance and defects in sperm function [49].

Finally, as mentioned earlier, other important sources of ROS and RNS arise from factors related to unhealthy lifestyles, such as smoking, excessive alcohol intake and drug abuse, environmental xenobiotics, heavy metals, and ionizing and nonionizing radiation, as they are capable of greatly increasing ROS and RNS production concomitantly with the decrease of antioxidants in sperm, leading to DNA fragmentation and lipid peroxidation in sperm [50,51].

A unique aspect of mitochondrial metabolism to be highlighted in sperm cells is the so-called ROS paradox. Spermatozoa use oxidative phosphorylation (OXPHOS) as the main source of ATP production, which takes place mainly in the central, very rich mitochondria, while glycolysis takes place in the head and fibrous sheath of the flagellum, where glycolytic enzymes are anchored [52].

At the same time, in mitochondrial metabolism, ROS are produced by the activity of electron transport chain (ETC) complexes, and the concomitant transport of H^+ ions into the intermembrane space of mitochondria, carried out by complexes I, III, and IV, is used to catalyze ATP synthesis and the tetravalent reduction of O_2 to H_2O. Even under physiological conditions, this process produces a significant amount of superoxide and hydroxyl radicals, which account for about 1% of the total oxygen consumed by the cell [53–55].

A very special aspect of ROS and RNS radical production in spermatozoa is related to the presence of unmatured sperm formed during defective spermatogenesis. Indeed, during the last stage of gamete differentiation in the testis, maturation of the spermatids occurs, characterized by remodeling of the nucleus, condensation of chromatin, formation of the acrosome and tail of the spermatozoon, and removal of excess cytoplasm that takes place in the epididymis [56].

Defects in the latter process give rise to immature spermatozoa, characterized by cytoplasmic droplets in the central part [57], and containing the enzyme glucose-6-phosphate dehydrogenase (G6PDH) necessary for the first reaction of the pentose phosphate pathway (PPP). This metabolic pathway is useful for maintaining the reduced form of glutathione (GSH) through the formation of high levels of NADPH and proper glutathione reductase activity.

In immature spermatozoa, high concentrations of NADPH promote ROS production through the activity of the Ca^{++}-dependent, membrane-bound isoform 5 of NADPH oxidase (NOX5) [58–60].

Additional endogenous ROS production comes, albeit with a modest contribution, from peroxisomal β-oxidation, the very long catabolic pathway of fatty acids, and the activity of enzymes of the cytochrome P_{450} family involved in the detoxification of xenobiotics [44,61].

Despite the aforementioned destructive effects that ROS and RNS can induce on sperm function, many studies have clearly demonstrated that controlled levels of ROS and RNS are necessary for spermatozoa to acquire their fertilization capacity during differentiation in the testis, maturation in the epididymis, and capacitation in the female reproductive tract.

In particular, it has been shown that moderate levels of hydrogen peroxide are necessary for proper spermatogenesis in the testis by regulating the number of stem and progenitor cells from which spermatozoa originate, the condensation of chromatin in the nucleus, and the arrangement of mitochondria in the central part of the spermatozoa (Fig. 17.4).

All the reported biochemical indications of ROS/RNS stress on spermatozoa have prompted research to increasingly investigate the correlation between oxidative/nitrosative stress and male infertility, identifying many promising biomarkers in seminal fluid (resulting from the detrimental action of ROS and RNS overproduction on sperm macromolecules) such as malondialdehyde (MDA),

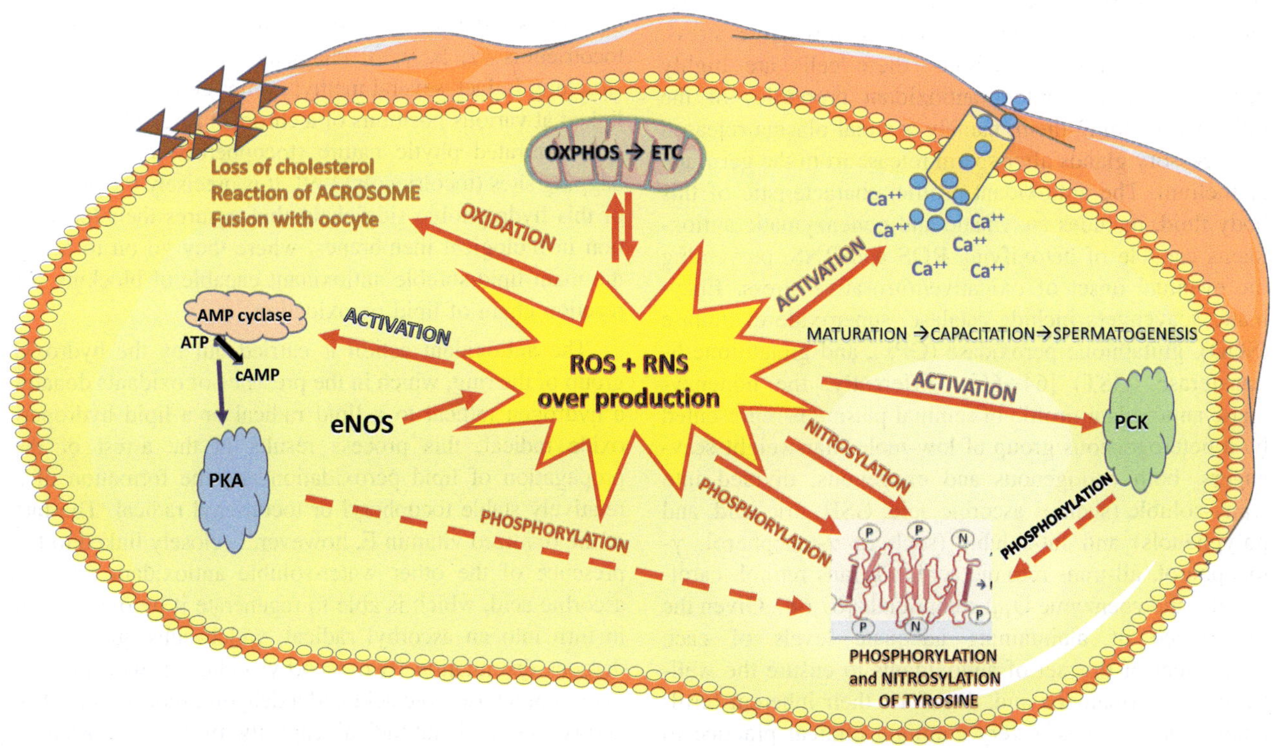

FIGURE 17.4 Involvement of reactive oxygen species (ROS) and reactive nitrogen species (RNS) in the correct development and function of spermatozoa. In functional mitochondria, there is the adequate ATP supply for cell energy demand and a physiological production of ROS, as well as the nitric oxide synthase isoform (eNOS) provides physiological production of RNS. These "normal" quantities of ROS and RNS positively affects numerous intracellular processes of spermatozoa, such as: influx of Ca^{++} triggering the increase in adenylate cyclase activity and the activation of protein kinase A (PKA); the parallel activation of protein kinase C (PKC); the consequent increase in protein phosphorylation; regulation of protein activities through nitrosylation reactions; cholesterol oxidative modification and its ejection from the plasma membrane. Some of these processes are extremely involved during spermatogenesis, maturation and capacitation, as well as in acrosome reaction and fusion with the oocyte.

4-hydroxynonenal (4-HNE), 8-hydroxy-2′-deoxyguanosine (8-OHdG), nitrites and nitrates (NO_2^- and NO_3^-) [44,62,63].

At the same time, efforts were made to understand the role in spermatozoa of scavenger enzymes (SOD, catalase, glutathione peroxidase, heme oxygenase, thioredoxin), and antioxidant molecules (vitamin E and C, GSH, uric acid) that can effectively remove selected ROS (O_2^-, H_2O_2, organic peroxides).

The reducing power of various low-molecular-weight antioxidants [44], which can be classified into hydrophilic (water soluble) and hydrophobic (fat soluble), enables them to exert good protective activity against the activity of various harmful radical species. Their biochemical nature, however, confines them to water-rich (cytoplasm, mitochondrial matrix) and fat-rich (biological membranes) cellular compartments, positively or negatively affecting their ability to scavenge ROS and RNS.

In view of the above-mentioned fundamental beneficial role of ROS and RNS in the differentiation and acquisition of fertilization capacity by spermatozoa, on the one hand, but on the other hand, their detrimental role in the onset of oxidative/nitrosative stress, seminal plasma has evolved as one of the most potent and antioxidant-rich fluids in humans to finely control the amount of ROS and RNS. Although spermatozoa are equipped with endogenous antioxidant defenses against oxidative/nitrosative stress, for obvious structural reasons, these cells are highly dependent on the potent antioxidant properties of the fluids surrounding them, namely seminal plasma released by accessory glands after sperm release from the germinal epithelium. The antioxidant profile, characteristic of this body fluid, includes enzymatic and nonenzymatic antioxidants capable of detoxifying ROS and RNS, preventing the eventual onset of oxidative/nitrosative stress. Enzymatic scavengers include catalase, superoxide dismutase (SOD), glutathione peroxidase (GPx), and glutathione-S-transferase (GST) [64–66]. Differently, the nonenzymatic antioxidant profile of seminal plasma is represented by a heterogeneous group of low-molecular-weight scavengers, both endogenous and exogenous, divided into water-soluble (such as ascorbic acid, GSH, uric acid, and polyphenols) and fat-soluble (such as α-tocopherol, γ-tocopherol, all-trans-retinoic acid, all-trans retinol, carotenoids, and coenzyme Q_{10}) compounds [67,68]. Given the importance of maintaining adequate levels of each component of this set of antioxidants to ensure the well-being of spermatozoa and, therefore, their inherent fertilizing capacity, it is a very common clinical practice to indiscriminately prescribe repeated courses of administration of various types of nutraceuticals/drugs containing antioxidants to infertile males to improve their fertilizing capacity. This treatment approach is generally taken without subjecting patients to preliminary screening to determine the concentration of antioxidants in seminal plasma; in other words, antioxidant treatment is very often administered without knowing the real need for it, caused by a deficiency of one or more low-molecular-weight antioxidants.

Over the past 10 years, a fair number of clinical trials have been conducted to understand the actual efficacy of antioxidant-based therapies in the treatment of male infertility. In these treatments, mainly low-molecular-weight antioxidants with direct and established antioxidant activity against ROS and/or RNS have been used to improve sperm quality and sperm fertilization ability of patients with various infertility conditions.

Treatment of male infertility with antioxidant vitamins

Vitamin E (tocopherol)

The antioxidant vitamins used as therapy to boost endogenous antioxidant defenses and thus counter ROS/RNS stress are vitamin E (tocopherol) and vitamin C (ascorbic acid).

Fat-soluble vitamin E is a term that is used as such, but from a biochemical point of view, it comprises eight different substances, four tocopherols (α, β, γ, δ) and four tocotrienols (α, β, γ, δ) characterized by a very similar structure. In fact, several methyl groups and a side chain are linked at various positions of a chroman ring, which can be of a saturated phytic nature (tocopherols) or with three bagging sites (tocotrienols) [69]. It is precisely the presence of this hydrophobic side chain that ensures their localization in biological membranes, where they go on to act as the main lipid-soluble antioxidant capable of blocking the reaction chain of lipid peroxidation.

The antioxidant action is carried out by the hydroxyl group of the ring, which in the presence of oxidants donates a hydrogen radical to a lipid radical or a lipid hydroperoxide radical; this process results in the arrest of the propagation of lipid peroxidation and the formation of a relatively stable tocopheryl or tocotrienyl radical. The fate of the oxidized vitamin E, however, is closely linked to the presence of the other water-soluble antioxidant vitamin, ascorbic acid, which is able to regenerate it by oxidizing it in turn into an ascorbyl radical, which subsequently undergoes dismutation (two ascorbyl radicals), with the formation of an ascorbic acid and a dehydroascorbic acid. The antioxidant and antiradical capacity of these substances make them considered good scavengers against ROS, although the most effective is α-tocopherol, while γ-tocopherol has been shown to be the most effective tocopherol against RNS, with particular scavenger activity against nitrogen dioxide, with which it forms the stable nitro-adduct 5-nitro-γ-tocopherol [70,71].

It should be considered that vitamin E is normally present in the diet, also depending on the type of dietary habits, such that α-tocopherol is the most abundant in the European diet and γ-tocopherol in the American diet.

The most abundant tocopherol in human tissues and blood plasma is α-tocopherol, whose circulating levels range from 18 to 30 μmol/L [70,71]. Distribution to organs and peripheral tissues is through α-TTP, which incorporates α-tocopherol into lipoproteins and is able to distinguish α-tocopherol from all incoming forms of vitamin E. Although they are effective antioxidants, the concentrations of tocopherols in seminal plasma are about nine times lower (α-tocopherol ~3 μmol/L and γ-tocopherol ~0.06 μmol/L) than those found in blood plasma [70,71], this is because of hydrophobicity and also because of the lack of efficient transport systems that can converse between the two biological fluids.

Moreover, because of their high polyunsaturated fatty acid content, sperm membranes are very sensitive to oxidation caused by high levels of ROS and RNS, and consequently vitamin E for these cells is the most effective fat-soluble antioxidant against oxidative/nitrosative stress-related damage [72], also due to the proper recycling of vitamin E induced by the high levels of ascorbic acid present in seminal plasma.

Several clinical studies have reported that decreased levels of tocopherols in human seminal plasma correlates with increased concentrations of ROS and RNS, markers of lipid peroxidation (MDA), in infertile males [44,71–74], as is also the case with an infrequent genetic disorder known as "isolated vitamin E deficiency" (AVED), although cases of normal spermatogenesis and normal seminal plasma in the presence of significant vitamin E deficiency have also been found [75].

Of note have been several studies evaluating the impact of dietary vitamin E intake, including a case-control study conducted on 32 men with primary infertility due to oligo and/or asthenospermia and/or idiopathic teratozoospermia and 32 age-matched healthy donors [76]; an association between lower intake of vitamin E, zinc, and folate and a negative effect on sperm motility and morphology was demonstrated.

Other studies conducted in a fertile but age-matched male population showed that higher dietary intake of vitamin E, folate, and zinc was positively correlated with less sperm DNA damage. Not only that, but older men who consumed higher levels of the above micronutrients had similar levels of sperm DNA damage as those found in young men, underscoring the importance, regardless of age, of consuming adequate levels of antioxidants to counteract oxidation-mediated damage to sperm DNA [76]. Another important study was conducted on healthy individuals subjected to chronic consumption of foods rich in monounsaturated fatty acids, polyunsaturated fatty acids, and vitamin E to assess their influence on sperm parameters related to male fertility [77].

The result was a significant improvement in the morphofunctional parameters of sperm analysis in these subjects (total sperm count, viability, motility, and morphology), suggesting that these benefits may be due to a reduction in DNA fragmentation mediated by an increased intake of the aforementioned fat-soluble antioxidants [78].

There are conditions in which vitamin E intake does not seem to lead to valid results in male infertility, such as in the case of varicocele and sub-inguinal varicocelectomy; in a study, oral vitamin E was given for 12 months to one group (n = 22), while a placebo to the control group (n = 23) and the results were improvements only related to the surgical technique and not to vitamin E [79].

In addition, the influence of high concentration of α-tocopherol for 3 months to 10 infertile patients selected from a larger cohort of infertile patients with sperm analysis abnormalities and varicocele was checked. Interestingly, after 45 days, an increase in blood α-tocopherol (+88%) was matched by a decrease in γ-tocopherol (−33%), the sperm α-tocopherol increased by 38%, while no changes in γ-tocopherol concentrations were found. This could be caused by hepatic α-TTP activity, which preferentially incorporates α-tocopherol into plasma, as well as to increased hepatic catabolism of γ-tocopherol [70].

There are not many studies conducted in patients with idiopathic oligoasthenozoospermia (OAT) involving the use of vitamin E as an antioxidant, even associated with drug treatment. These include a study of 60 infertile men with this condition who were treated daily for 6 months with vitamin E and the antiestrogen clomiphene citrate, which showed a significant increase in sperm count and progressive sperm motility. Importantly, there was not only an improvement in seminal parameters but also a significant increase in the number of pregnancies achieved at the end of the study (13.3% in the control and 36.7% in the drug-treated group). This led to the conclusion that the combination of antioxidant and antiestrogen therapy is a viable option for the treatment of a selected group of men with oligoasthenozoospermia from uncertain causes [80].

Results on mean sperm concentration and their mean total motility were found, in a second study, also on idiopathic oligoasthenozoospermic patients treated with the same protocol [51].

It should always be remembered that most studies have focused on the efficacy of different mixtures of antioxidants containing vitamin E [81–85], and that this does not make it possible to distinguish the effects of tocopherols from those of the other antioxidants in the mixtures used. In this light, in a study [86] with high numerosity (about 300) subfertile males with at least one recent pathological analysis of the semen, they were daily treated for 3 months with l-carnitine/twice or the combination of l-carnitine and l-arginine plus other antioxidant compounds (zinc, vitamin E, GSH, selenium, coenzyme Q_{10}, and folic acid). The authors reported that both groups, after the administration period, experienced significant improvement in all studied sperm parameters (volume, density, overall progressive motility); however, relative changes in sperm density and overall progressive motility (including fast motility) were higher in the group that received the combined micronutrient treatment.

Other studies report of infertile men with OA treated with a combination of vitamin E combined with vitamin C and other compounds (L-carnitine fumarate and ubiquinol) to see if this type of mix can give better results when combined with tocopherols. In one of them, the results reported a significant increase in total coenzyme Q_{10} (ubiquinone + ubiquinol) and α-tocopherol concentrations in the blood and seminal plasma of treated patients with a significant increase in sperm density, a decrease in sperm abnormalities, and a high pregnancy rate (45%) determined after treatment [87].

Considering at the end a study of a large number of infertile males with idiopathic asthenoteratozoospermia, subjected to a daily oral supplementation of synthetic α-tocopherol (as a protector of cell membranes from oxidative/nitrosative stress) in combination with L-selenomethionine (with the aim of increasing the levels of the Se-dependent enzyme GPx, which eliminates ROS) for 14 weeks. After treatment, there was a 52.6% improvement in sperm analysis parameters (sperm motility and morphology), while the 36.6% of them did not respond to therapy. In particular, in this research was reported that spontaneous pregnancy occurred in 10.8% of patients, allowing to state that the combined administration of vitamin E and Se in asthenoteratozoospermia is a potentially useful therapy not only to improve the quality of seminal parameters but, more importantly, to increase the chances of achieving a normal pregnancy [87] (Table 17.1).

Vitamin C (ascorbic acid)

Ascorbic acid or vitamin C (VitC) is one of the most abundant water-soluble antioxidants within mammalian tissues, acting as a reducing cofactor in several enzymatic reactions [88] and is an essential cellular antioxidant also in conditions of abundance of GSH, protecting tissues, organs, and cells from the harmful effects of ROS and RNS overproduction during oxidative/nitrosative stress [89].

VitC as a fairly good reducing agent, thanks to the standard redox potential of the coupled oxidized/reduced ascorbate, is capable to quickly react with a wide range of radicals, through one or two electrons' reactions generating, respectively, ascorbyl radical or dehydroascorbic acid (DHA) that can be reconverted back to the reduced ascorbic acid form in a direct chemical reaction involving glutathione (GSH) or other scavengers (glutaredoxin, thioredoxin, and GSH reductase).

It is important to consider the critical role of VitC in recycling oxidized α-tocopherol (vitamin E) and maintaining the redox state of α-tocopherol in biological membranes. Because VitC is not synthesized by most mammals (biosynthetic enzyme L-gulono-1,4-lactone oxidase inactive), the human body depends on the ingestion of vitamin C-rich foods to meet its requirements [90], with the recommended daily intake (RDI) ranging from 65 to 90 mg/day. But in VitC metabolism, two types of transporters play a key role on which its cellular uptake depends, depending on the oxidative state of the molecule. Indeed, VitC is transported by high-affinity, low-capacity active sodium-ascorbate transporters (SVCT1 and SVCT2), while DHA internalization is facilitated by hexose transporters (GLUT1, GLUT3, and GLUT4) [91].

It should be mentioned that the ascorbate concentration is relatively low (30–70 μmol/L in the serum of healthy humans) [67] unlike the concentrations of this important antioxidant in peripheral tissues are of interest. Particularly in the brain, ascorbate is highly concentrated, usually reaching concentrations as high as 3000 μmol/L in brain water [92]. In the testis, VitC levels are around 3 mg/100 g wet tissue (about 140 μmol/L tissue water) [93].

The Sertoli cells, forming the blood–testis barrier via tight and adherens junctions, are able to regulate VitC concentrations in the seminiferous epithelium because are rich in ascorbate transporters (SCVT2 and some isoforms of the GLUT transporters) and underlying the key role of VitC in the spermatogenesis [94], playing significant protection against oxidative damage to DNA [95] and prevention of semen agglutination [96].

In seminal plasma, concentration of this abundant water-soluble low-molecular-weight antioxidant has been found up to 10 times higher than those measured in plasma, with values ranging from 200 to 350 μmol/L. Explanations of the mechanisms allowing to reach such abundant vitamin C levels in this peculiar body fluid are still unclear [97]. In general, since VitC concentrations are higher in peripheral tissues than in plasma, the cellular internalization of VitC via SVCT1 and SVCT2 occurs against a concentration gradient; the energy to overcome the electrochemical barrier is provided by the favorable inward gradient for Na^+, which is fostered by the regular extrusion of Na^+ via the Na^+/K^+-ATPase pump.

Furthermore, VitC levels in seminal plasma positively correlate with sperm volume, count, and motility [98] but also with GSH concentration and SOD activity, suggesting a close relationship between different antioxidant defensive mechanisms against ROS-mediated damages [99,100].

Under oxidative stress conditions leading to male infertility, an overall depletion of VitC in the seminal fluid was observed due to the sustained presence of ROS and

TABLE 17.1 Summary of the main results obtained in the studies focusing on the effect of α-tocopherol (vitamin E) administration for the treatment of male infertility.

Authors	Number of patients and type of infertility	Controls (number)	Antioxidant(s) administered (type, doses, and protocol)	Months of treatment	Improvement (sperm parameters and pregnancy rate)
Zerbinati et al. [70]	10 = spermiogram anomalies and varicocele	**No controls**	α-Tocopherol (800 IU)/day	3 months	
Ener et al. [78]	22 = varicocele	23	Vitamin E (2 × 300 mg)/day postvaricocelectomy	12 months	
Ghanem et al. [79]	60 = idiopathic OA	30	Vitamin E (400 mg) and clomiphene citrate (25 mg)/day	6 months	Sperm count, progressive sperm motility and 36.7% pregnancy rate in treated patients versus 13.3% in controls
ElSheikh et al. [80]	60 = idiopathic OA	30	Vitamin E (400 mg) and clomiphene citrate (25 mg)/day	6 months	Mean sperm concentration and mean total sperm motility
Lipovac et al. [86]	143 = at least one recent (1 year) pathological semen analysis result	156	Vitamin E (120 mg), L-carnitine (440 mg), L-arginine (250 mg), zinc (40 mg), GSH (80 mg), selenium (60 μg), CoQ_{10} (15 mg), and folic acid (800 μg)/day	3 months	Volume, density, overall progressive motility (including slow and fast motility) and % of sperm with normal morphology
Moslemi et al. [87]	690 = idiopathic AT	**No controls**	Vitamin E (400 IU) and Se (200 μg)/day	3.5 months	Sperm motility, morphology (52.6% cases) and 10.8% pregnancy rate

A, asthenozoospermia; *AT*, asthenoteratozoospermia; *CoQ_{10}*, oxidized coenzyme Q_{10}; *GSH*, reduced glutathione; *O*, oligozoospermic; *OA*, oligoas-thenozoospermia; *OAT*, oligoasthenoteratozoospermia; *T*, teratozoospermia.

RNS, mainly in patients affected by serious varicocele, by genitourinary infections and by idiopathic infertility, [57,101]. In contrast, with a high dietary intake of several antioxidant nutrients (β-cryptoxanthin, vitamin C, lycopene, and β-carotene), a positive correlation was observed between this and total motile sperm count, showing that an ascorbate intake that met the RDI was positively associated with increased seminal volume [102,103].

The majority of the clinical studies aimed to evaluate the effect of vitamin C supplementation on male infertility were carried out by applying the simultaneous administration of various antioxidants, including ascorbate. Differently, the VitC administration only was conducted in three clinical trials, in which different semen parameters and fertilization capacity of infertile males were evaluated, obtaining contradictory results. In a controlled clinical trial, more than 100 infertile males affected by varicocele and subjected to varicocelectomy were divided into two groups receiving, twice a day, either VitC or placebo (as control group) for the next 3 months after surgery. The VitC-treated patients showed no increase in sperm count and significant amelioration of sperm motility and morphology, suggesting that ascorbate administration positively affected only quality but not the number of spermatozoa [104]. But another clinical study reported that the administration of a high single dose of VitC to 200 subjects with increasing body mass index and ages ranging from 20 to 60 year was able to improve the sperm concentration and motility but not the semen volume and the percentage of normal spermatozoa morphology [105].

As previously affirmed, in most studies, exogenous VitC was administered in combination with other antioxidants (such as vitamin E, carotenoids, and coenzyme Q_{10}), thus rendering it difficult to extrapolate the potential vitamin C beneficial effects on male patients affected by infertility. In a study conducted for 3 months on 20 infertile males with known asthenoteratozoospermia, the combined daily supplementation with VitC, some vitamins of B complex, L-carnitine, CoQ_{10}, and oligoelements was able to induce, a statistical improvement of all semen parameters and DNA integrity, not accompanied by a significant increase in pregnancy rate (5%) [51].

In an infertile male cohort with severe oligoasthenoteratozoospermia, the effects of daily administration of VitC, vitamin E, and L-carnitine as a possible management protocol of clinical utility were monitored [81,82]. After 6 months of treatment, a significant increase in sperm concentration, total sperm count, percentage of sperm with total motility and progressive motility, as well as a significant reduction in sperm with abnormal morphology was observed, although the actual effects of this antioxidant protocol were confounded by the patient's lifestyle change adopted in the study protocol and aimed at minimizing adverse lifestyle factors [82]. In contrast, in a large group of subjects with idiopathic oligoasthenoteratozoospermia, daily supplementation (for 3–6 months) with VitC, coenzyme Q_{10}, and vitamin E was ineffective in changing the number of atypical sperm cells and sperm volume, while it caused significant improvements in sperm cell concentration and sperm motility [92]. It is noteworthy that, after 6 months, this group of patients achieved a total of 48 pregnancies, of which 16 were spontaneous (i.e., occurred without the need for any ART) and 32 required ART, using this treatment protocol [81]. There are several studies that have used on infertile patients with oligozoospermia and/or asthenospermia, prolonged treatments with VitC combined with L-carnitine, coenzyme Q_{10}, antioxidants, selenium, and zinc and have shown a significant improvement only in total motile sperm count, with no effect on other semen parameters [84] or even with a positive effect on various morphofunctional parameters of sperm (concentration, pH, volume, total motility, morphology, count, and progressive motility) [85]. But there were not always positive results; in fact, a randomized, controlled trial of infertile oligozoospermic, asthenospermic, teratozoospermic, and DNA-fragmented patients [63] were randomly divided into a group receiving placebo and a group receiving daily administration of an antioxidant formulation consisting VitC, vitamin D and vitamin E, L-carnitine, zinc and selenium, folic acid, and lycopene (3–6 months).

Compared with the placebo group, this formulation and antioxidant administration protocol did not lead to any statistically significant improvement in semen analysis. More importantly, these results suggested that antioxidant treatment is unable to improve in vivo pregnancy or live birth rates in couples with male factor infertility (Table 17.2).

N-acetylcysteine

Glutathione (GSH) is a tripeptide (γ-L-glutamyl-L-cysteinyl-glycine) is the other most abundant low-molecular-weight hydrophilic antioxidant (1 and 10 mM) that, unlike VitC, mammals are able to synthesize [106].

This tripeptide is localized mainly in the cytoplasm and mitochondria and with different concentrations in different tissues. Although GSH is involved in modulating cell proliferation, apoptosis, inflammatory processes, redox signaling, and xenobiotic detoxification, probably the main function of this hydrophilic compound is to act as an antioxidant [106].

GSH is synthesized through enzymatic reactions that require ATP in two steps: the first is catalyzed by glutamate-cysteine ligase (GCL), which conjugates cysteine to glutamate, producing γ-glutamylcysteine; the second is catalyzed by GSH synthase, which adds glycine to γ-glutamylcysteine, producing GSH as the final product. This hydrophilic compound exists in the thiol-reduced

TABLE 17.2 Summary of the main results obtained in the papers focusing on the effect of vitamin C administration for the treatment of male infertility.

Authors	Number of patients and type of infertility	Controls (number)	Antioxidant(s) administered (type, doses and protocol)	Months of treatment	Improvement (sperm parameters and pregnancy rate)
Abad et al. [51]	20 = AT	**No controls**	VitC (60 mg), L-carnitine (1500 mg), CoQ_{10} (20 mg), vitamin E (10 mg), vitamin B_9 (200 μg), vitamin B_{12} (1 μg), zinc (10 mg), selenium (50 μg)/day	3 months	Sperm concentration, motility, vitality and morphology parameters, DNA integrity, and 5% pregnancy rate
Gual-Frau et al. [81]	20 = grade I varicocele	**No controls**	VitC (60 mg, L-carnitine (1500 mg), CoQ_{10} (20 mg), vitamin E (10 mg), vitamin B_9 (200 μg), vitamin B_{12} (1 μg), zinc (10 mg), selenium (50 μg)/day	3 months	Sperm count and DNA integrity
Magdi et al. [82]	120 = severe OAT	**No controls**	VitC (1 g), vitamin E (400 mg), L-carnitine (2 g)/day	6 months	Sperm concentration, percentage of total motility, and progressive motility
Kobori et al. [83]	169 = idiopathic OAT	**No controls**	VitC (60 mg), CoQ_{10} (120 mg), vitamin E (40 mg)/day	3 and 6 months	Sperm concentration and motility
Cyrus et al. [104]	46 = varicocele	69	VitC 500 mg/day	3 months	Sperm motility and morphology
Rafiee et al. [105]	200 = increasing body mass index	50	VitC 1000 mg/day	6 months	Sperm concentration and motility
Terai et al. [84]	15 = O and/or A	16 = administered with a Chinese herbal medicine	VitC (1000 mg), L-carnitine (750.1 mg), zinc (30 mg), astaxanthin (16.05 mg), Co Q_{10} (90.26 mg), vitamin B_{12} (60.1 μg) and vitamin E (150 mg) 3 times/day	3 months	Total motile sperm count
Sadaghiani et al. [85]	50 = infertile O and A	**No controls**	VitC (100 mg), CoQ_{10} (30 mg), zinc (8 mg), vitamin E (12 mg) and folic acid (400 μg)/day, selenium (200 mg)/other day	3 months	Volume, morphology, motion, count, progressive motility, and pH

A, asthenozoospermia; *AT*, asthenoteratozoospermia; *CoQ_{10}*, oxidized coenzyme Q_{10}; *O*, oligozoospermic; *OA*, oligoasthenozoospermia; *OAT*, oligoasthenoteratozoospermia; *T*, teratozoospermia; *VitC*, ascorbic acid.

(GSH) and disulfide-oxidized (GSSG) forms [107], because of its sulfhydryl group (-SH), which confers active protection against ROS, so much so that GSH is used for the detoxification of hydrogen peroxide and lipid peroxides. These potentially dangerous compounds are reduced through the activity of the two selenium-dependent and selenium-independent forms of the enzyme GPx, in a reaction that oxidizes two molecules of GSH into one molecule of GSSG [108]. The regeneration of GSH is carried out by glutathione reductase (GR), in the presence of reduced NADPH and is thus closely linked to the activity of the PPP enzyme and the malic enzyme, i.e., the two main cellular sites for NADPH generation [109].

It should be mentioned, however, that GSH also acts as a cofactor of the GST family of enzymes, a group of cytosolic and membrane-bound isoenzymes involved in the detoxification of xenobiotics (potentially toxic compounds that often cause increased oxidative/nitrosative stress), achieved through the conjugation of GSH to xenobiotic substrates for their faster extrusion from the cell. In sperm cells, GST is involved not only in the prevention of lipid peroxidation under conditions of elevated ROS and RNS levels but also in the regulation of cell signaling during spermatogenesis, sperm capacitation, and fertilization [110].

But to maintain high levels of GSH, there is a need to also have high amounts of cysteine, which is normally derived from diet, protein breakdown, and methionine trans-sulfuration. Given the critical role of GSH in detoxification reactions, both to eliminate ROS and RNS and to remove xenobiotics, increased cysteine availability is required under oxidative/nitrosative stress conditions. As in the case of VitC, GSH levels in human tissues are significantly higher (2500–4000 μmol/L in tissue water) than its circulating concentrations, which range between 15 and 20 μmol/L [67,111]. Whereas GSH values in seminal plasma have been found equal to or higher than those found in serum, indicating a free distribution of this molecule regulated on its relative concentrations in the two fluids [67,112].

It should be remembered that in male infertility, an important role is exerted by prolonged oxidative/nitrosative stress and is accompanied by data on changes in GSH levels that are somewhat controversial.

In fact, in viable spermatozoa of infertile patients, a study showed increased intracellular levels of total GSH (GSH + GSSG) compared with values found in spermatozoa of fertile control males, and this is probably since the high concentrations of ROS and RNS in spermatozoa of the infertile group increased the demand for antioxidants to counteract oxidative/nitrosative stress, thus leading to increased values of GSH + GSSG [113]. This hypothesized mechanism may have been accomplished by increased GSH transport into the cell through membrane transporters located on the surface of the spermatozoa [113]; the higher concentration of GSH in pathological sperm conditions is related also to an increase of homocysteine, cysteine, cysteinyl-glycine [114].

Unfortunately, not all the work done reports the same results; as in some cases, an opposite condition has been reported, namely an overall depletion of GSH in the seminal plasma of infertile males, caused by increased oxidative/nitrosative stress. For example, in a study of infertile patients with varicocele, genitourinary infection, or idiopathic infertility [115], a significant concomitant decrease of GSH and VitC alone was demonstrated in the seminal plasma of the varicocele group compared with the control group of fertile males. The nonsignificant decrease in GSH in the other two infertility conditions was explained by considering the concomitant oxidative effect exerted by VitC. Compared with control values (fertile males) in another study, a net decrease in the GSH/GSSG ratio was seen in a cohort of infertile patients regardless of the pathology causing infertility, although the most striking differences were seen in the group with varicocele [116].

The results cited so far would lead one to think that supplements administered to increase GSH levels in seminal plasma and spermatozoa may be successful in the treatment of male infertility, but it should be considered that oral administration of GSH is not effective, due to the degradation of the molecule prior to absorption. Therefore, it is thought that the best pharmacological strategy is to stimulate GSH biosynthesis to achieve a net increase in its intracellular concentrations, and this could be achieved by increasing the availability of cysteine to enhance GSH synthesis. In this regard, N-acetylcysteine (NAC) has been widely used as a potential treatment for male infertility (administered alone or in combination with other antioxidants), partly because of its relevant properties of acting as a direct scavenger of ROS and RNS.

This was proven in a randomized, blinded clinical trial conducted on males with asthenoteratozoospermia who were administered NAC orally for 3 months and their semen parameters and DNA fragmentation index were compared with those determined before the start of treatment [117]. The results show that NAC supplementation significantly improved sperm analysis parameters (normal count, motility, and morphology) and greatly reduced DNA fragmentation, indicating that NAC supplementation can protect the morphofunctional characteristics of spermatozoa and reduce ROS- and RNS-mediated DNA damage.

As with the other compounds mentioned so far, NAC in its combination with other antioxidant compounds has also been tested in infertile males, as in the case of an uncontrolled study of males from various couples with at least 2 previous in vitro fertilization (IVF) failures, with no evidence of organic causes of infertility and with measurable DNA fragmentation index (DFI) or nuclear decondensation index (SDI) [118]. Subjects were given a single daily dose of NAC for 2 months, assisted by the presence of other factors (B-complex vitamins, quercetin, betalain, vitamin E, zinc) with the aim of increasing endogenous GSH production by increasing the rate of the so-called one-carbon cycle, a pathway that involves the trans-sulfuration of homocysteine by promoting de novo GSH [118].

At the end of treatment, there was a significant decrease in both DFI and SDI, but no change in total sperm count, fast motility, and normal morphology rates after the administration protocol. Surprisingly, despite these mixed results, there was a significant increase in spontaneous pregnancies and in the success of assisted motherhood techniques [118]. An interesting case of ineffectiveness of NAC administration, but rather of its negative effect, is that of a study conducted in patients with β-thalassemia major, a condition characterized by hypogonadotropic hypogonadism mediated by iron deposition and ROS generation resulting in increased damaged spermatozoa. Combined treatment with L-carnitine and NAC not only proved ineffective in improving fertility, but patients had a significant increase in SDI and teratozoospermia index as the treatment accentuated sperm deformities [119] (Table 17.3).

Coenzyme Q_{10}

Coenzyme Q (ubiquinone) is a fat-soluble compound component of the mitochondrial electron transport chain (ETC) in oxygen-dependent living organisms and is characterized by a redox-active benzoquinone headgroup connected to a side chain of isoprene units, a minimum of 3 to a maximum of 10 units (as is the case in humans). The latter form of coenzyme Q, called coenzyme Q_{10} (CoQ_{10}), is incorporated into the inner membrane of mitochondria, actively participating in ETC. The fully oxidized CoQ_{10} ($CoQ_{10}ox$) accepts a pair of electrons from complex I and complex II and passes them to complex III, where the so-called Q cycle takes place. In this cycle, during which four protons are pumped into the intermembrane space, the reduced ubiquinol ($CoQ_{10}H_2$) is oxidized to ubiquinone ($CoQ_{10}ox$), losing its electrons through two separate one-electron reductions. One of these electrons will serve to reduce the oxidized form of cytochrome *c* (anchored at a specific site in complex III that protrudes into the intermembrane space). The other electron left on the partially reduced semiquinone radical form of ubiquinone (CoQ^-) is transferred internally to cytochromes bL and bH and then used to reduce a $CoQ_{10}ox$ molecule (bound to the so-called Q0 site of complex III) to CoQ^- [120]. The Q cycle, during which a $CoQ_{10}ox$ molecule and a $CoQ_{10}H_2$ molecule are finally obtained from two $CoQ_{10}H_2$ molecules, is a critical process during ETC because electrons can leak out and react with oxygen, forming superoxide and making the Q cycle one of the main sites of mitochondrial ROS production.

Moreover, CoQ_{10} is involved in the protection against lipid peroxidation of low-density lipoproteins (LDL), (where it is oxidized before vitamin E), of mitochondria (where it counteracts the inhibitory effects of ETC substrates) and of plasma membranes (where it acts as an intermediate electron carrier) [121], so the CoQ10 is

TABLE 17.3 Summary of the main results obtained in papers focusing on the effect of N-acetylcysteine (NAC) administration for the treatment of male infertility.

Authors	Number of patients and type of infertility	Controls (number)	Antioxidant(s) administered (type, doses, and protocol)	Months of treatment	Improvement (sperm parameters and pregnancy rate)
Jannatifar et al. [117]	50 = AT	**No controls**	NAC (600 mg)/day	3 months	Sperm count, motility and normal morphology, DNA integrity
Dattilo et al. [118]	84 = ART failures	**No controls**	NAC (250 mg), extract of opuntia fruits (100 mg), quercetin (0.05 mg), betalain (0.001 mg), vitamins B_2 (1.4 mg), B_3 (16 mg), B_6 (1.4 mg), B_9 (400 μg), B_{12} (2.5 μg), zinc (12.5 mg), and vitamin E (12 mg)/day	4 months	DNA integrity, spontaneous pregnancy rate (21%), pregnancy rate (47.6%) and live birth rate (39.3%) after a new ART attempt.
Elsedfy et al. [119]	20 = BTM (hypogonadotropic hypogonadism)	**No controls**	NAC (600 mg) and L-carnitine (2 g)/day	6 months	

A, asthenozoospermia; *AT*, asthenoteratozoospermia; *NAC*, N-acetylcysteine; *O*, oligozoospermic; *OA*, oligoasthenozoospermia; *OAT*, oligoasthenoteratozoospermia; *T*, teratozoospermia.

considered as an endogenous antioxidant compound since its biosynthesis occurs in almost all cell types, and its abundance is not linked on dietary supply.

Due to its main localization, the final steps of CoQ10 biosynthesis are undertaken within the inner mitochondrial membrane and involve many regulatory components such as mitofusin 1 and 2, two proteins implicated in the mitochondrial fusion process [121,122].

The chemical features and the main biological role as a mobile electron transporter in the mitochondrial ETC render CoQ_{10} strictly clustered within mitochondria and poorly abundant in human body fluids, with concentrations ranging between 0.152 and 0.939 μmol/L in human serum [67,123] and between 0.0019 and 0.013 μmol/L in human seminal plasma [67,124].

It is important to recall that since spermatozoa are particularly rich in mitochondria and require a relevant amount of ATP in order to correctly satisfy their energy demand, CoQ_{10} seems to play an important role in the physiology of these germinal cells. Furthermore, the well-established implications of oxidative/nitrosative stress in the insurgence of male infertility render CoQ_{10} potentially involved in the pathophysiology of this condition.

Since in patients affected by varicocele, oligozoospermia, asthenozoospermia, or idiopathic infertility, decreased levels of CoQ_{10} in seminal plasma were measured when compared to control fertile subjects [124–126], the supplementation with exogenous CoQ_{10}, both as a single compound and in combination with other substances, has widely been applied in the treatment of male infertility. The most effective results were obtained when administering $CoQ_{10}H_2$ not only for the improvement of morphofunctional semen parameters but also for decreasing oxidative/nitrosative stress. These results have been obtained in a randomized, double-blind, placebo-controlled trial on high number of men with idiopathic oligoasthenoteratozoospermia, in which 50% of the patients were daily treated for 26 weeks with $CoQ_{10}H_2$ and the remaining 50% with placebo [127]. The authors reported a significant improvement in sperm density, sperm motility and sperm strict morphology in the group treated with $CoQ_{10}H_2$ compared to the placebo group. Interestingly, semen parameters gradually returned to baseline values at 12 weeks after the drug-off period, even though still significant differences in sperm density and motility were recorded [127]. The administration of $CoQ_{10}H_2$ has further been applied (with different dosing period) in other studies for the treatment of the same pathology [128–130].

The overall results showed significant enhancement of the sperm concentration and motility and of semen antioxidant status, progressive motility, and total motility compared to the baseline levels recorded before the beginning of treatment. Additionally, CoQ_{10} supplementation increased the total antioxidant capacity and the glutathione peroxidase levels, with a consequent reduction in ROS levels and in the sperm DNA fragmentation index. Comparing the studies cited above, the beneficial effects of CoQ_{10} supplementation on sperm parameters, and also on the sperm density and motility, seem to be independent of the dosage and the etiology of infertility.

In an important study, conducted on a wide cohort of patients with idiopathic oligoasthenoteratozoospermia has been reported a massive improvement in sperm density, motility, and morphology after 1 year of CoQ_{10} supplementation [131]. Because of the improved semen quality induced by the administration protocol, high pregnancy rates (34.1%) were also observed when the CoQ_{10} administration time was protracted beyond the sixth month, suggesting that oligoasthenoteratozoospermia may effectively be treated by the prolonged use of CoQ_{10} [132]. In addition to the previously mentioned studies reporting the CoQ_{10} supplementation in combination with other compounds [51,83,84,86], has been conducted an observational study on different patients affected by idiopathic asthenozoospermia and daily administered with CoQ_{10} and D-aspartate for 3 months. Notwithstanding no increment of CoQ_{10} in the seminal fluid of treated patients was recorded, it was reported a significant improvement of sperm kinetic parameters and concomitantly decreased levels of ˙NO, peroxynitrites and nitrosative stress-related damages to DNA after 3 months of administration (Table 17.4).

Concluding remarks

In the last 10 years, numerous studies have been performed concerning the effects of the administration of low-molecular-weight antioxidants to contrast male infertility. Surprisingly, only 30 clinical studies tested the effects of the administration of α-tocopherol, ascorbic acid, NAC, and CoQ_{10} (each of them alone or in combination with other antioxidants and/or vitamins and/or micronutrients) to infertile males. It is even more surprising that only 33.3% of these studies (10/30) included, as an outcome measure to determine the effects of the therapy, the pregnancy and/or live birth rates. Of these 10 studies, only 4 were case–control studies, and only 2 of them found improvement of the pregnancy rate in the group of antioxidant-treated patients compared to untreated controls. Additionally, of the 30 studies considered in this review, only 13 on 30 were case–control studies, and 20 enrolled several patients (>40) and 16 carried out the administration of a single antioxidant.

It can be seen from the work presented that it is not easy to determine the true effectiveness of antioxidant-based therapies in improving male infertility due to various factors. For example, studies using the same antioxidant(s) have enrolled infertile males with different pathological conditions, thus making it impossible to compare results,

TABLE 17.4 Summary of the main clinical results obtained in studies focusing on the effect of CoQ_{10} administration for the treatment of male infertility.

Authors	Number of patients and type of infertility	Controls (number)	Antioxidant(s) administered (type, doses, and protocol)	Months of treatment	Improvement (sperm parameters and pregnancy rate)
Safarinejad et al. [127]	114 = idiopathic OAT	114	$CoQ_{10}H_2$ (200 mg)/day	6.5 months	Sperm density, sperm motility, and sperm morphology
Alahmar [128].	65 = idiopathic OAT	**No controls**	$CoQ_{10}H_2$ (200 mg)/day (35 patients) $CoQ_{10}H_2$ (400 mg)/day (30 patients)	3 months	Sperm concentration, progressive motility, and total motility (greater improvement after 400 mg/day dose)
Alahmar et al. [129]	65 = idiopathic OAT	40	CoQ_{10} (unspecified form, 200 mg)/day	3 months	Sperm concentration, progressive motility, total motility, and DNA integrity
Alahmar et al. [130]	35 = idiopathic OAT	35	$CoQ_{10}H_2$ (200 mg)/day	3 months	Sperm concentration and progressive motility
Safarinejad [131].	287 = idiopathic OAT	**No controls**	CoQ_{10} (unspecified form, 300 mg) twice/day	3 months	Sperm concentration, motility percentage, total sperm count, morphology, and 34.1% pregnancy rate
Tirabassi et al. [132]	20 = idiopathic A	**No controls**	CoQ_{10} (unspecified form, 200 mg) and D-aspartate (2660 mg)/day	3 months	Total sperm motility

A, asthenozoospermia; *AT*, asthenoteratozoospermia; *CoQ_{10}*, oxidized coenzyme Q_{10}; *$CoQ_{10}H_2$*, reduced coenzyme Q_{10}; *O*, oligozoospermic; *OA*, oligoasthenozoospermia; *OAT*, oligoasthenoteratozoospermia; *T*, teratozoospermia.

while protocols for administering the same antioxidant have, in most cases, been characterized by different dosages and timing of supplementation. Furthermore, in studies in which antioxidant-based therapies have been tested for the treatment of male infertility, the critical point is that patients enrolled in almost all of these studies were not selected on the basis of a specific deficiency of one or more antioxidants in their seminal fluid. This highlights the fact that before any administration of antioxidants is initiated, care should certainly be taken to determine the complete antioxidant profile in the seminal fluid of infertile patients (using analytical methods that allow quantification of the most important water-soluble and fat-soluble antioxidants and avoiding application of the uninformative measures of so-called "total antioxidant capacity"). Only after obtaining an accurate quantification of the antioxidants in the semen of each individual infertile male will it be possible to accurately select patients and antioxidants to be administered. This type of approach would greatly increase the likelihood of recording benefits in targeted antioxidant treatments, which would replenish the seminal fluid with the missing antioxidants. Importantly, this type of investigation is part of personalized medicine, and should reduce the possible side effects that can arise when indiscriminate supplementation with random antioxidant cocktails is carried out.

It should also be noted that there are no studies to date that consider carotenoids and/or flavonoids as antioxidants to be administered in the treatment of infertile males, although several compounds of these two classes are currently being used as side therapies for the treatment of other disease states characterized by increased oxidative/nitrosative stress. Furthermore, when one considers the central role that mitochondria play in oxidative/nitrosative stress, it is presumable that, for best results, the administration of antioxidants should be accompanied by selected drugs that promote mitochondrial function and energy metabolism.

In conclusion, the results reported in studies using the administration of low-molecular-weight antioxidants to infertile males, in addition to pointing out the above-mentioned shortcomings highlighted in the evaluation of the results, do not allow the following to be established reasonably whether antioxidant-based therapies are effective in treating male infertility, whether there is a better antioxidant to achieve positive results, and which group of infertile males is most likely to have beneficial effects from this therapeutic approach. To clearly define the usefulness of antioxidant administration for the treatment of male infertility, further case-control and longitudinal studies are needed that enroll a larger number of patients, use similar administration protocols (including antioxidant type, dosage, mode, and time of administration), and enroll patients with the same clinical diagnosis of infertility.

References

[1] Inhorn MC, Patrizio P. Infertility around the globe: new thinking on gender, reproductive technologies and global movements in the 21st century. Hum Reprod Update 2015;21:411–26.

[2] Zegers-Hochschild F, Adamson GD, de Mouzon J, Ishihara O, Mansour R, Nygren K, et al. International committee for monitoring assisted reproductive technology; World Health Organization. International committee for monitoring assisted reproductive technology (ICMART) and the World Health Organization (WHO) revised glossary of ART terminology. Fertil Steril 2009;92:1520–4.

[3] Katz DJ, Teloken P, Shoshany O. Male infertility—the other side of the equation. Aust Fam Physician 2017;46:641–6.

[4] Vander Borght M, Wyns C. Fertility and infertility: definition and epidemiology. Clin Biochem 2018;62:2–10.

[5] Anifandis G, Bounartzi T, Messini CI, Dafopoulos K, Sotiriou S, Messinis IE. The impact of cigarette smoking and alcohol consumption on sperm parameters and sperm DNA fragmentation (SDF) measured by Halosperm®. Arch Gynecol Obstet 2014;290:777–82.

[6] Anifandis G, Katsanaki K, Lagodonti G, Messini C, Simopoulou M, Dafopoulos K, Daponte A. The effect of glyphosate on human sperm motility and sperm DNA fragmentation. Int J Environ Res Public Health 2018;15:1117.

[7] Khalili MA, Leisegang K, Majzoub A, Finelli R, Panner Selvam MK, Henkel R, et al. Male fertility and the COVID-19 pandemic: systematic review of the literature. World J Mens Health. 2020;38:506–20.

[8] Dutta S, Sengupta P. SARS-CoV-2 and male infertility: possible multifaceted pathology. Reprod Sci 2020;10:1–4.

[9] Szkodziak P, Wozniak S, Czuczwar P, Wozniakowska E, Milart P, Mroczkowski A, Paszkowski T. Infertility in the light of new scientific reports—focus on male factor. Ann Agric Environ Med 2016;23:227–30.

[10] Hawksworth DJ, Szafran AA, Jordan PW, Dobs AS, Herati AS. Infertility in patients with Klinefelter syndrome: optimal timing for sperm and testicular tissue cryopreservation. Rev Urol 2018;20:56–62.

[11] Kim SY, Lee BY, Oh AR, Park SY, Lee HS, Seo JT. Clinical, hormonal, and genetic evaluation of idiopathic non obstructive azoospermia and Klinefelter syndrome patients. Cytogenet Genome Res 2017;153:190–7.

[12] Docampo MJ, Hadziselimovic F. Molecular pathology of cryptorchidism-induced infertility. Sex Dev 2015;9:269–78.

[13] Kohn TP, Kohn JR, Owen RC, Coward RM. The prevalence of Y-chromosome microdeletions in oligozoospermic men: a systematic review and meta-analysis of European and North American studies. Eur Urol 2019;76:626–36.

[14] Bundhun PK, Janoo G, Bhurtu A, Teeluck AR, Soogund MZS, Pursun M, Huang F. Tobacco smoking and semen quality in infertile males: a systematic review and meta-analysis. BMC Publ Health 2019;19:36.

[15] Sansone A, Di Dato C, de Angelis C, Menafra D, Pozza C, Pivonello R, et al. Smoke, alcohol and drug addiction and male fertility. Reprod Biol Endocrinol 2018;16:3.

[16] Boeri L, Pederzoli F, Capogrosso P, Abbate C, Alfano M, Mancini N, et al. Semen infections in men with primary infertility in the real-life setting. Fertil Steril 2020;113:1174–82.

[17] Jensen CFS, Østergren P, Dupree JM, Ohl DA, Sønksen J, Fode M. Varicocele and male infertility. Nat Rev Urol 2017;14:523–33.

[18] Omar SS, Mahfouz W, Dawood W, Abo El-Wafa RAH, Ghazala RA, Zahran AM. Relation of nitric oxide synthase gene (NOS3) polymorphisms to varicocele risk and post-varicocelectomy seminal oxidative stress reduction. Andrologia 2020;52:e13525.

[19] Ramalingam M, Kini S, Mahmood T. Male fertility and infertility. Obstet Gynaecol Reprod Med 2014;24:326–32.

[20] Hendry WF. Disorders of ejaculation: congenital, acquired and functional. Br J Urol 1998;82:331–41.

[21] Cooper TG, Yeung CH, Nashan D, Nieschlag E. Epididymal markers in human infertility. J Androl 1988;9:91–101.

[22] Lekarev O, Lin-Su K, Vogiatzi MG. Infertility and reproductive function in patients with congenital adrenal hyperplasia: pathophysiology, advances in management, and recent outcomes. Endocrinol Metab Clin N Am 2015;44:705–22.

[23] Ray A, Shah A, Gudi A, Homburg R. Unexplained infertility: an update and review of practice. Reprod Biomed Online 2012;24:591–602.

[24] Kothandaraman N, Agarwal A, Abu-Elmagd M, Al-Qahtani MH. Pathogenic landscape of idiopathic male infertility: new insight towards its regulatory networks. NPJ Genom Med 2016;1:16023.

[25] World Health Organization. WHO laboratory manual for the examination and processing of human semen. 5th ed. Geneva, Switzerland: World Health Organization; 2010. p. 271.

[26] Cooper TG, Noonan E, von Eckardstein S, Auger J, Baker HW, Behre HM, et al. World Health Organization reference values for human semen characteristics. Hum Reprod Update 2010;16:231–45.

[27] Bracke A, Peeters K, Punjabi U, Hoogewijs D, Dewilde S. A search for molecular mechanisms underlying male idiopathic infertility. Reprod Biomed Online 2018;36:327–39.

[28] Aitken RJ, Ryan AL, Baker MA, McLaughlin EA. Redox activity associated with the maturation and capacitation of mammalian spermatozoa. Free Radic Biol Med 2004;36:994–1010.

[29] Baker MA, Aitken RJ. The importance of redox regulated pathways in sperm cell biology. Mol Cell Endocrinol 2004;216:47–54.

[30] Agarwal A, Virk G, Ong C, du Plessis S. Effect of oxidative stress on male reproduction. World J Men's Health 2014;32.

[31] Du Plessis SS, Agarwal A, Halabi J, Tvrda E. Contemporary evidence on the physiological role of reactive oxygen species in human sperm function. J Assist Reprod Genet 2015;32:509–20.

[32] De Lamirande E, Jiang H, Zini A, Kodama H, Gagnon C. Reactive oxygen species and sperm physiology. Rev Reprod 1997;2:48–54.

[33] Sahnoun S, Sellami A, Chakroun N, Mseddi M, Attia H, Rebai T, Lassoued S. Human sperm Toll-like receptor 4 (TLR4) mediates acrosome reaction, oxidative stress markers, and sperm parameters in response to bacterial lipopolysaccharide in infertile men. J Assist Reprod Genet 2017;34:1067–77.

[34] Aitken RJ, Baker HW, Irvine DS. On the nature of semen quality and infertility. Hum Reprod 1995;10:248–9.

[35] Fujii J, Imai H. Redox reactions in mammalian spermatogenesis and the potential targets of reactive oxygen species under oxidative stress. Spermatogenesis 2014;4:e979108.

[36] Azantee YAW, Lokman MI. The future of azoospermic patients: in vitro spermatogenesis. Andrology 2015;4:2.

[37] Oborna I, Wojewodka G, De Sanctis JB, Fingerova H, Svobodova M, et al. Increased lipid peroxidation and abnormal fatty acid profiles in seminal and blood plasma of normozoospermic males from infertile couples. Hum Reprod 2010;25:308–16.

[38] Aitken RJ, Gibb Z, Baker MA, Drevet J, Gharagozloo P. Causes and consequences of oxidative stress in spermatozoa. Reprod Fertil Dev 2016;28:1–10.

[39] Drevet JR, Aitken RJ. Oxidative damage to sperm DNA: attack and defense. Adv Exp Med Biol 2019;1166:107–17.

[40] Homa ST, Vassiliou AM, Stone J, Killeen AP, Dawkins A, Xie J, et al. A comparison between two assays for measuring seminal oxidative stress and their relationship with sperm DNA fragmentation and semen parameters. Genes 2019;10:236.

[41] Bui AD, Sharma R, Henkel R, Agarwal A. Reactive oxygen species impact on sperm DNA and its role in male infertility. Andrologia 2018;50:e13012.

[42] Lazzarino G, Amorini AM, Signoretti S, Musumeci G, Lazzarino G, Caruso G, et al. Pyruvate dehydrogenase and tricarboxylic acid cycle enzymes are sensitive targets of traumatic brain injury induced metabolic derangement. Int J Mol Sci 2019;20:5774.

[43] Tibullo D, Giallongo C, Romano A, Vicario N, Barbato A, Puglisi F, et al. Mitochondrial functions, energy metabolism and protein glycosylation are interconnected processes mediating resistance to bortezomib in multiple myeloma cells. Biomolecules 2020;10:696.

[44] Lazzarino G, Listorti I, Muzii L, Amorini AM, Longo S, Di Stasio E, et al. Low-molecular weight compounds in human seminal plasma as potential biomarkers of male infertility. Hum Reprod 2018;33:1817–28.

[45] Pasqualotto FF, Sundaram A, Sharma RK, Borges Jr E, Pasqualotto EB, Agarwal A. Semen quality and oxidative stress scores in fertile and infertile patients with varicocele. Fertil Steril 2008;89:602–7.

[46] Ferramosca A, Albani D, Coppola L, Zara V. Varicocele negatively affects sperm mitochondrial respiration. Urology 2015;86:735–9.

[47] Fraczek M, Hryhorowicz M, Gill K, Zarzycka M, Gaczarzewicz D, Jedrzejczak P, et al. The effect of bacteriospermia and leukocytospermia on conventional and nonconventional semen parameters in healthy young normozoospermic males. J Reprod Immunol 2016;118:18–27.

[48] Bazalytska SV, Persidsky Y, Romanenko AM. Molecular mechanisms of initiation of carcinogenesis in the testis. Exp Oncol 2019;41:224–34.

[49] Sposito C, Camargo M, Tibaldi DS, Barradas V, Cedenho AP, Nichi M, et al. Antioxidant enzyme profile and lipid peroxidation products in semen samples of testicular germ cell tumor patients submitted to orchiectomy. Int Braz J Urol 2017;43:644–51.

[50] Dorostghoal M, Kazeminejad SR, Shahbazian N, Pourmehdi M, Jabbari A. Oxidative stress status and sperm DNA fragmentation in fertile and infertile men. Andrologia 2017;49.

[51] Abad C, Amengual MJ, Gosálvez J, Coward K, Hannaoui N, Benet J, et al. Effects of oral antioxidant treatment upon the dynamics of human sperm DNA fragmentation and subpopulations of sperm with highly degraded DNA. Andrologia 2013;45:211–6.

[52] Ferramosca A, Zara V. Bioenergetics of mammalian sperm capacitation. BioMed Res Int 2014.

[53] Ribas-Maynou J, Yeste M. Oxidative stress in male infertility: causes, effects in assisted reproductive techniques, and protective support of antioxidants. Biology 2020;9:77.

[54] Baskaran S, Finelli R, Agarwal A, Henkel R. Reactive oxygen species in male reproduction: a boon or a bane? Andrologia 2020.

[55] Gunes S, Metin Mahmutoglu A, Arslan MA, Henkel R. Smoking-induced genetic and epigenetic alterations in infertile men. Andrologia 2018;50:e13124.

[56] Sullivan R, Mieusset R. The human epididymis: its function in sperm maturation. Hum Reprod Update 2016;22:574–87.

[57] Ollero M, Gil-Guzman E, Lopez MC, Sharma RK, Agarwal A, Larson K, et al. Characterization of subsets of human spermatozoa at different stages of maturation: implications in the diagnosis and treatment of male infertility. Hum Reprod 2001;16:1912–21.

[58] Said TM, Agarwal A, Sharma RK, Mascha E, Sikka SC, Thomas Jr AJ. Human sperm superoxide anion generation and correlation with semen quality in patients with male infertility. Fertil Steril 2004;82:871–7.

[59] Barati E, Nikzad H, Karimian M. Oxidative stress and male infertility: current knowledge of pathophysiology and role of antioxidant therapy in disease management. Cell Mol Life Sci 2020;77:93–113.

[60] Aitken J, Krausz C, Buckingham D. Relationships between biochemical markers for residual sperm cytoplasm, reactive oxygen species generation, and the presence of leukocytes and precursor germ cells in human sperm suspensions. Mol Reprod Dev 1994;39:268–79.

[61] Hanukoglu I. Antioxidant protective mechanisms against reactive oxygen species (ROS) generated by mitochondrial P450 systems in steroidogenic cells. Drug Metab Rev 2006;38:171–96.

[62] Vorilhon S, Brugnon F, Kocer A, Dollet S, Bourgne C, Berger M, et al. Accuracy of human sperm DNA oxidation quantification and threshold determination using an 8-OHdG immuno-detection assay. Hum Reprod 2018;33:553–62.

[63] Moazamian R, Polhemus A, Connaughton H, Fraser B, Whiting S, Gharagozloo P, Aitken RJ. Oxidative stress and human spermatozoa: diagnostic and functional significance of aldehydes generated as a result of lipid peroxidation. Mol Hum Reprod 2015;21:502–15.

[64] Kampfer C, Spillner S, Spinnler K, Schwarzer JU, Terradas C, Ponzio R, et al. Evidence for an adaptation in ROS scavenging systems in human testicular peritubular cells from infertility patients. Int J Androl 2012;35:793–801.

[65] Alkan I, Simsek F, Haklar G, Kervanciog lu E, Ozveri H, Yalcin S, Akdas A. Reactive oxygen species production by the spermatozoa of patients with idiopathic infertility: relationship to seminal plasma antioxidants. J Urol 1997;157:140–3.

[66] Otasevic V, Kalezic A, Macanovic B, Jankovic A, Stancic A, Garalejic E, et al. Evaluation of the antioxidative enzymes in the seminal plasma of infertile men: contribution to classic semen quality analysis. Syst Biol Reprod Med 2019;65:343–9.

[67] Lazzarino G, Listorti I, Bilotta G, Capozzolo T, Amorini AM, Longo S, et al. Water- and fat-soluble antioxidants in human seminal plasma and serum of fertile males. Antioxidants 2019;8:96.

[68] Smits RM, Mackenzie-Proctor R, Yazdani A, Stankiewicz MT, Jordan V, Showell MG. Antioxidants for male subfertility. Cochrane Database Syst Rev 2019;3:CD007411.

[69] Comitato R, Ambra R, Virgili F. Tocotrienols: a family of molecules with specific biological activities. Antioxidants 2017;6:93.

[70] Zerbinati C, Caponecchia L, Fiori C, Sebastianelli A, Salacone P, Ciacciarelli M, Iuliano L. Alpha-and gamma-tocopherol levels in human semen and their potential functional implications. Andrologia 2020;52:e13543.

[71] Traber MG. Vitamin E inadequacy in humans: causes and consequences. Adv Nutr 2014;5:503–14.

[72] Morielli T, O'Flaherty C. Oxidative stress impairs function and increases redox protein modifications in human spermatozoa. Reproduction 2015;149:113–23.

[73] Suleiman SA, Ali ME, Zaki ZM, elMalik EM, Nasr MA. Lipid peroxidation and human sperm motility: protective role of vitamin E. J Androl 1996;17:530–7.

[74] Hosomi A, Arita M, Sato Y, Kiyose C, Ueda T, Igarashi O, et al. Affinity for alpha-tocopherol transfer protein as a determinant of the biological activities of vitamin E analogs. FEBS Lett 1997;409:105–8.

[75] Rossato M, Mariotti C. Normal spermatogenesis and sperm function in a subject affected by cerebellar ataxia due to congenital vitamin E deficiency. Andrologia 2014;46:322–4.

[76] Schmid TE, Eskenazi B, Marchetti F, Young S, Weldon RH, Baumgartner A, et al. Micronutrients intake is associated with improved sperm DNA quality in older men. Fertil Steril 2012;98:1130–7.

[77] Salas-Huetos A, Rosique-Esteban N, Becerra-Tomás N, Vizmanos B, Bulló M, Salas-Salvadó J. The effect of nutrients and dietary supplements on sperm quality parameters: a systematic review and meta-analysis of randomized clinical trials. Adv Nutr 2018;9:833–48.

[78] Ener K, Aldemir M, Isik E, Okulu E, Özcan MF, Ugurlu M, et al. The impact of vitamin E supplementation on semen parameters and pregnancy rates after varicocelectomy: a randomised controlled study. Andrologia 2016;48:829–34.

[79] Ghanem H, Shaeer O, El-Segini A. Combination clomiphene citrate andantioxidant therapy for idiopathic male infertility: a randomized controlled trial. Fertil Steril 2010;93:2232–5.

[80] ElSheikh MG, Hosny MB, Elshenoufy A, Elghamrawi H, Fayad A, Abdelrahman S. Combination of vitamin E and clomiphene citrate in treating patients with idiopathic oligoasthenozoospermia: a prospective, randomized trial. Andrology 2015;3:864–7.

[81] Gual-Frau J, Abad C, Amengual MJ, Hannaoui N, Checa MA, Ribas-Maynou J, et al. Oral antioxidant treatment partly improves integrity of human sperm DNA in infertile grade I varicocele patients. Hum Fertil 2015;18:225–9.

[82] Magdi Y, Darwish E, Elbashir S, Majzoub A, Agarwal A. Effect of modifiable lifestyle factors andantioxidant treatment on semen parameters of men with severe oligoasthenoteratozoospermia. Andrologia 2017;49.

[83] Kobori Y, Ota S, Sato R, Yagi H, Soh S, Arai G, Okada H. Antioxidant cosupplementation therapy with vitamin C, vitamin E, and coenzyme Q10 in patients with oligoasthenozoospermia. Arch Ital Urol Androl 2014;86:1–4.

[84] Terai K, Horie S, Fukuhara S, Miyagawa Y, Kobayashi K, Tsujimura A. Combination therapy with antioxidants improves total motile sperm counts: a preliminary study. Reprod Med Biol 2019;19:89–94.

[85] Sadaghiani S, Fallahi S, Heshmati H, Teshnizi SH, Chaijan HA, Ebrahimi FFA, et al. Effect of antioxidant supplements on sperm parameters in infertile male smokers: a single-blinded clinical trial. AIMS Public Health 2020;7:92–9.

[86] Lipovac M, Bodner F, Imhof M, Chedraui P. Comparison of the effect of a combination of eight micronutrients versus a standard mono preparation on sperm parameters. Reprod Biol Endocrinol 2016;14:84.

[87] Moslemi MK, Tavanbakhsh S. Selenium-vitamin E supplementation in infertile men: effects on semen parameters and pregnancy rate. Int J Gen Med 2011;4:99–104.

[88] Lykkesfeldt J, Michels AJ, Frei B. Vitamin C. Adv Nutr 2014;5:16–8.

[89] Getoff N. Vitamin C: electron emission, free radicals and biological versatility. In Vivo 2013;27:565–70.

[90] Nishikimi M, Yagi K. Molecular basis for the deficiency in humans of gulonolactone oxidase, a key enzyme for ascorbic acid biosynthesis. Am J Clin Nutr 1991;54:1203S–8S.

[91] Savini I, Rossi A, Pierro C, Avigliano L, Catani MV. SVCT1 and SVCT2: key proteins for vitamin C uptake. AminoAcids 2008;34:347–55.

[92] Di Pietro V, Lazzarino G, Amorini AM, Tavazzi B, D'Urso S, Longo S, et al. Neuroglobin expression and oxidant/antioxidant balance after graded traumatic brain injury in the rat. Free Radic Biol Med 2014;69:258–64.

[93] Hornig D. Distribution of ascorbic acid, metabolites and analogues in man and animals. Ann N Y Acad Sci 1975;258:103–18.

[94] Angulo C, Maldonado R, Pulgar E, Mancilla H, Córdova A, Villarroel F, et al. Vitamin C andoxidative stress in the seminiferous epithelium. Biol Res 2011;44:169–80.

[95] Guz J, Gackowski D, Foksinski M, Rozalski R, Zarakowska E, Siomek A, et al. Comparison of oxidative stress/DNA damage in semen and blood of fertile and infertile men. PLoS One 2013;8:e68490.

[96] Berger GK, Smith-Harrison LI, Sandlow JI. Sperm agglutination: prevalence and contributory factors. Andrologia 2019;51:e13254.

[97] Kand'ár R, Drábková P, Hampl R. The determination of ascorbic acid and uric acid in human seminal plasma using an HPLC with UV detection. J Chromatogr B Analyt Technol Biomed Life Sci 2011;879:2834–9.

[98] Nsonwu-Anyanwu CA, Ekong RE, Offor JS, Awusha FO, Orji CO, Umoh IE, et al. Heavy metals, biomarkers of oxidative stress and changes in sperm function: a case-control study. Int J Reprod Biomed 2019;17:163–74.

[99] Yan L, Liu J, Wu S, Zhang S, Ji G, Gu A. Seminal superoxide dismutase activity and its relationship with semen quality and SOD gene polymorphism. J Assist Reprod Genet 2014;31:549–54.

[100] Abd-Elmoaty MA, Saleh R, Sharma R, Agarwal A. Increased levels of oxidants and reduced antioxidants in semen of infertile men with varicocele. Fertil Steril 2010;94:1531–4.

[101] Tawadrous GA, Aziz AA, Mostafa T. Seminal soluble fats relationship with oxidative stress in infertile men with varicocele. Urology 2013;82:820–3.

[102] Mínguez-Alarcón L, Mendiola J, López-Espín JJ, Sarabia-Cos L, Vivero-Salmerón G, Vioque J, et al. Dietary intake of antioxidant nutrients is associated with semen quality in young university students. Hum Reprod 2012;27:2807–14.

[103] Mendiola J, Torres-Cantero AM, Vioque J, Moreno-Grau JM, Ten J, Roca M, et al. A low intake of antioxidant nutrients is associated with poor semen quality in patients attending fertility clinics. Fertil Steril 2010;93:1128–33.

[104] Cyrus A, Kabir A, Goodarzi D, Moghimi M. The effect of adjuvant vitamin C after varicocele surgery on sperm quality and quantity in infertile men: a double-blind placebo controlled clinical trial. Int Braz J Urol 2015;41:230–8.

[105] Rafiee B, Morowvat MH, Rahimi-Ghalati N. Comparing the effectiveness of dietary vitamin C and exercise interventions on fertility parameters in normal obese men. Urol J 2016;13:2635–9.

[106] Lu SC. Glutathione synthesis. Biochim Biophys Acta 2013;1830:3143–53.

[107] Flohé L. The fairy tale of the GSSG/GSH redox potential. Biochim Biophys Acta 2013;1830:3139–42.

[108] Brigelius-Flohé R, Maiorino M. Glutathione peroxidases. Biochim Biophys Acta 2013;1830:3289–303.

[109] Couto N, Wood J, Barber J. The role of glutathione reductase and related enzymes on cellular redox homoeostasis network. Free Radic Biol Med 2016;95:27–42.

[110] Llavanera M, Mateo-Otero Y, Bonet S, Barranco I, Fernández-Fuertes B, Yeste M. The triple role of glutathione S-transferases in mammalian male fertility. Cell Mol Life Sci 2020;77:2331–42.

[111] Look MP, Rockstroh JK, Rao GS, Kreuzer KA, Barton S, Lemoch H, et al. Serum selenium, plasma glutathione (GSH) and erythrocyte glutathione peroxidase (GSH-Px)-levels in asymptomatic versus symptomatic human immunodeficiency virus-1 (HIV-1)-infection. Eur J Clin Nutr 1997;51:266–72.

[112] Atig F, Raffa M, Habib BA, Kerkeni A, Saad A, Ajina M. Impact of seminal trace element and glutathione levels on semen quality of Tunisian infertile men. BMC Urol 2012;12:6.

[113] Moretti E, Collodel G, Fiaschi AI, Micheli L, Iacoponi F, Cerretani D. Nitric oxide, malondialdheyde and non-enzymatic antioxidants assessed in viable spermatozoa from selected infertile men. Reprod Biol 2017;17:370–5.

[114] Kralikova M, Crha I, Huser M, Melounova J, Zakova J, Matejovicova M, Ventruba P. The intracellular concentration of homocysteine and related thiols is negatively correlated to sperm quality after highly effective method of sperm lysis. Andrologia 2017;49.

[115] Micheli L, Cerretani D, Collodel G, Menchiari A, Moltoni L, Fiaschi AI, Moretti E. Evaluation of enzymatic and non-enzymatic antioxidants in seminal plasma of men with genitourinary infections, varicocele, and idiopathic infertility. Andrology 2016;4:456–64.

[116] Moretti E, Micheli L, Noto D, Fiaschi AI, Menchiari A, Cerretani D. Resistin in human seminal plasma: relationship with lipid peroxidation, CAT activity, GSH/GSSG ratio, and semen parameters. Oxid Med Cell Longev 2019:2192093.

[117] Jannatifar R, Parivar K, Roodbari NH, Nasr-Esfahani MH. Effects of N-acetyl-cysteine supplementation on sperm quality, chromatin integrity and level of oxidative stress in infertile men. Reprod Biol Endocrinol 2019;17:24.

[118] Dattilo M, Cornet D, Amar E, Cohen M, Menezo Y. The importance of the one carbon cycle nutritional support in human male fertility: a preliminary clinical report. Reprod Biol Endocrinol 2014;12:71.

[119] Elsedfy H, De Sanctis V, Ahmed AY, Mohamed NR, Arafa M, Elalfy MS. A pilot study on sperm DNA damage in β-thalassemia major: is there a role for antioxidants? Acta Biomed 2018;89:47–54.

[120] Liu SS. Mitochondrial Q cycle-derived superoxide and chemiosmotic bioenergetics. Ann N Y Acad Sci 2010;1201:84–95.

[121] Wang Y, Hekimi S. Understanding ubiquinone. Trends Cell Biol 2016;26:367–78.

[122] Di Pietro V, Lazzarino G, Amorini AM, Signoretti S, Hill LJ, Porto E, et al. Fusion or fission: the destiny of mitochondria in traumatic brain injury of different severities. Sci Rep 2017;7:9189.

[123] Niklowitz P, Onur S, Fischer A, Laudes M, Palussen M, Menke T, Döring F. Coenzyme Q_{10} serum concentration and redox status in European adults: influence of age, sex, and lipoprotein concentration. J Clin Biochem Nutr 2016;58:240–5.

[124] Abdul-Rasheed OF, Farid YY, Al-Nasiri US. Coenzyme Q_{10} andoxidative stress markers in seminal plasma of Iraqi patients with male infertility. Saudi Med J 2010;31:501–6.

[125] Mancini A, Balercia G. Coenzyme $Q_{(10)}$ in male infertility: physiopathology and therapy. Biofactors 2011;37:374–80.

[126] Eroglu M, Sahin S, Durukan B, Ozakpinar OB, Erdinc N, Turkgeldi L, et al. Blood serum and seminal plasma selenium, total antioxidant capacity and coenzyme Q10 levels in relation to semen parameters in men with idiopathic infertility. Biol Trace Elem Res 2014;159:46–51.

[127] Safarinejad MR, Safarinejad S, Shafiei N, Safarinejad S. Effects of the reduced form of coenzyme Q_{10} (ubiquinol) on semen parameters in men with idiopathic infertility: a double-blind, placebo controlled, randomized study. J Urol 2012;188:526–31.

[128] Alahmar AT. The impact of two doses of coenzyme Q_{10} on semen parameters andantioxidant status in men with idiopathic oligoasthenoteratozoospermia. Clin Exp Reprod Med 2019;46:112–8.

[129] Alahmar AT, Calogero AE, Sengupta P, Qutta S. Coenzyme Q_{10} improves sperm parameters, oxidative stress markers and sperm DNA fragmentation in infertile patients with idiopathic oligoasthenozoospermia. World J Mens Health 2020;39:346–51.

[130] Alahmar AT, Sengupta P. Impact of coenzyme Q_{10} and selenium on seminal fluid parameters and antioxidant status in men with idiopathic infertility. Biol Trace Elem Res 2021;199:1246–52.

[131] Safarinejad MR. The effect of coenzyme Q_{10} supplementation on partner pregnancy rate in infertile men with idiopathic oligoasthenoteratozoospermia: an open-label prospective study. Int Urol Nephrol 2012;44:689–700.

[132] Tirabassi G, Vignini A, Tiano L, Buldreghini E, Brugè F, Silvestri S, et al. Protective effects of coenzyme Q_{10} and aspartic acid on oxidative stress and DNA damage in subjects affected by idiopathic asthenozoospermia. Endocrine 2015;49:549–52.

Further reading

[1] Zhang G, Jiang F, Chen Q, Yang H, Zhou N, Sun L, et al. Associations of ambient air pollutant exposure with seminal plasma MDA, sperm mtDNA copy number, and mtDNA integrity. Environ Int 2020;136:105483.

Chapter 18

Modulation of oxidative stress in psoriasis: Pathophysiology and therapy

P. Wójcik[1], W. Łuczaj[1], N. Zarkovic[2] and E. Skrzydlewska[1]

[1]*Department of Analytical Chemistry, Medical University of Bialystok, Bialystok, Poland;* [2]*LabOS, Division of Molecular Medicine, Rudjer Boskovic Institute, Zagreb, Croatia*

Psoriasis is a chronic, immune-mediated inflammatory skin disease that affects approximately 2%−8% of the Western population (USA and Europe). As frequency of psoriasis is much lower in Asian population, even in highly developed countries, this suggests that Caucasian race is more prone to develop psoriasis than others, independently on the standard of living [1]. The most common form of psoriasis is psoriasis vulgaris, when the symptoms of psoriasis affect only the skin, including even its entire surface. Nevertheless the lesions may also extend to other parts of the body, leading to psoriatic arthritis or erythroderma, and indirectly cause/exacerbate cardiovascular or depressive diseases [2−4].

The development of psoriasis is associated with genetic and environmental factors causing increased activation of the immune system and chronic inflammation both in skin cells and in blood [5]. It has therefore been observed that lymphocytes and their cytokines, especially interferon (IFNγ) and interleukin 17 (IL-17), affect other cells, leading to chronic inflammation and characteristic symptoms such as skin plaques in psoriasis or arthrosis and loss of movement in psoriatic arthritis. Moreover, the proinflammatory phenotype of lymphocytes and other cells of the immune system are observed both locally in the skin or joints, but also in blood cells, which confirms the occurrence of general inflammation in psoriasis. Therefore, psoriasis is often accompanying with other diseases, like atherosclerosis, hypertension, ischemic heart disease, and myocardial infarction [6−8].

In addition to the overall proinflammatory phenotype and activation in psoriasis, different lymphocyte subpopulations play a different role. It is well known that in psoriasis, there is an imbalance between Th1 and Th2 lymphocytes with Th1 dominance. The level of Th17 and Th22 lymphocytes and the cytokines produced by them also increases. This leads to the activation of the so-called cellular response instead of humoral response [9]. Therefore, factors that aggravate this imbalance are believed to be promoting psoriasis and factors that activate Th2 cells to be antipsoriatic. The cause of this imbalance is unknown but is very often associated with a malfunction of dendritic cells, which is also shown by the fact that activation of Toll-like receptors on dendritic cells leads to the development of psoriasis in animal models [10,11]. Nevertheless, since psoriasis is not fully understood, it is also possible that changes in lymphocytes and dendritic cells are secondary to changes in keratinocytes. On the other hand, the participation of different subpopulations of lymphocytes playing different roles, and moreover, of dendritic cells indicates their importance in the pathophysiology of psoriasis, which is still difficult to define.

As a result, however, infiltration of skin by immune cells and activation of dendritic cells are observed [12]. As a consequence, epidermal keratinocytes are constantly stimulated to proliferate, which leads to their accumulation, which leads to skin lesions, characteristic symptom of psoriasis [13]. Moreover, keratinocytes metabolism is dysregulated in several ways. For example, keratinocytes in psoriatic lesions produce a number of proteins, including the S100 proteins, which attract leukocytes [14,15]. Changes in the signaling pathways in the skin tissue affected by psoriasis are then observed, including activation of mitogen-activated kinases (e.g., p38, ERK1/2, JNK) [16,17], and transcription factors involved in the inflammatory response (e.g., NFkB, Foxp3, HIF-1a) cause cell proliferation (STAT3) [18−20]. In some patients, psoriasis is characterized by a more severe clinical course, leading to the development of psoriatic arthritis [21,22].

Consequently, taking into account not fully defined etiology, especially in terms of metabolic changes resulting

Modulation of Oxidative Stress. https://doi.org/10.1016/B978-0-443-19247-0.00014-X

from the influence of inflammation, e.g., on the local and systemic redox balance and the resulting oxidative stress and its consequences for the human body, including comorbidities, psoriasis is a serious medical challenge.

Inflammation and redox balance/ imbalance

Psoriasis as a chronic inflammatory disease is characterized by systemic abnormalities such as increased activation of leukocytes, especially neutrophils, which in turn results in overproduction of reactive oxygen and nitrogen species (ROS and RNS), including superoxide anion radical and hydrogen peroxide, observed in the blood of patients with psoriasis [23,24]. Since the inflammation is also accompanied by hypoxia, with elevated VEGF level and angiogenesis, an additional ROS generation occurs, which has also been observed in psoriatic patients [23,24]. The main source of ROS in cells is usually mitochondria, the respiratory chain of which can be disrupted by a variety of factors including phospholipid metabolites such as endocannabinoids, which level is elevated in mononuclear cells of psoriatic patients [25–27]. Endocannabinoids (mainly AEA and 2-AG) can stimulate the work of mitochondria, including the production of hydrogen peroxide by increasing the penetration of calcium ions into the cells [26]. Moreover, activation of cannabinoid receptors (CB1) by endocannabinoids, observed in mononuclear cells of psoriasis patients, leads to the enhanced generation of ROS and by stimulation of NOS leading to increased production of superoxide and nitric oxide [27]. Increased generation of ROS also results from the increased activity of NADPH and xanthine oxidases in granulocytes and plasma of patients with psoriasis, especially psoriatic arthritis [28]. Increased ROS production is usually accompanied by disturbances in the antioxidant system, which has also been observed in patients with psoriasis.

It has been shown that an increase in ROS levels in patients with psoriasis is accompanied by a decrease in total antioxidant capacity in blood cells such as granulocytes, lymphocytes, and monocytes [29]. Moreover in blood of patients with psoriasis, increased ROS generation is accompanied by decreased antioxidant abilities manifested by a diminishing of vitamin C, E, β-carotene levels, and paraoxonase and superoxide dismutase activity as well as decreased efficiency of glutathione and thioredoxin systems and by high catalase activity in plasma and circulating immune cells [27,28,30]. It has also been shown that certain mutations in the gene encoding glutathione S-transferase are responsible for an increased incidence of psoriasis [30]. Moreover, the levels of both catalase and glutathione reductase are also reduced in RBC [29].

The decrease in the level/activity of protein antioxidants does not correspond to the increased level of the Nrf2 transcription factor responsible for the biosynthesis of cellular cytoprotective proteins, including antioxidants. However, the biological activity of this transcription factor is modulated by specific activators and inhibitors, in particular cytosol Nrf2 inhibitor—Keap1 protein, which, by forming an adduct with Nrf2, directs it to ubiquitination and consequent proteasomal degradation. However, both ROS and electrophilic lipid peroxidation products, including 4-HNE, which levels are elevated in psoriasis to form adducts with Keap1, counteract the formation of Keap1–Nrf2 complexes. Moreover, in the development of psoriasis vulgaris, the level of the nuclear Nrf2 inhibitor—Bach1 protein—is increased [28]. On the other hand, many proteins acting as Nrf2 activators, such as KAP1, p62, and p21, are elevated in psoriasis vulgaris (PsV), while their levels are lowered in psoriatic arthritis (PsA) [28]. As a consequence, the resultant of the above changes is the increase in the transcriptional activity of Nrf2, as evidenced by the increased level of the main product of its activity, heme oxygenase 1 (HO-1), especially in patients with psoriatic arthritis. On the other hand, it has been shown that increased expression of HO-1, especially high in lymphocytes of PsA patients, leads to activation of ERK5, which consequently lowers the transcriptional activity of NFκB [28], confirmed by the reduction of TNFα expression in lymphocytes of these patients. A differentiated metabolic response depending on the type of psoriasis was also observed at the p62 protein level, which is an activator of both transcription factors Nrf2 and NFκB. In vitro studies have shown that the level of p62 is regulated by the AP1S3 protein, and mutations in the AP1S3 gene are observed in psoriasis [31]. The increased level of p62 in psoriasis vulgaris may suggest that it promotes NFκB activation, which is confirmed by the increased level of the p52 subunit of this transcription factor [32]. It is known that p62 directly influences the expression of NFκB but also activates IKK, a factor responsible for the phosphorylation of NFκB and the inhibition of the NFκB inhibitor IkB [33]. As a consequence, increased expression of p62 in psoriasis vulgaris patients' lymphocytes may be responsible for the increased level and transcriptional activity of NFκB [32]. However, the product of the transcriptional activity of NFκB, the cytokine TNFα, by activating the death receptors (TNFR1 and TNFR2) intensifies the receptor-dependent proapoptotic pathway, leading to caspase 8 activation [34,35].

On the other hand, ROS can activate the intrinsic apoptotic pathway with increased expression of caspase 9 [36]. Increased levels of caspases 8 and 9 initiate ER and mitochondrial apoptotic pathways of lymphocytes, resulting in high caspase 3 levels. It was found that the proapoptotic activity of TNFα is supported by the level of the p53 transcription factor, which is expressed more than twice as high in PsV patients' lymphocytes. This is due to the fact that the p53 regulator is the MDM2 protein, the structure of which is modified by electrophiles, including both ROS and lipid peroxidation products, leading to the breakdown of the p53-MDM2 complex and activation of p53 protein [37]. On the other hand, activated p53 may be responsible for the reduction of Bcl2 levels in the lymphocytes of both PsV and PsA patients [9]. In contrast, p53 can increase the expression of the Bax protein, which is responsible for the formation of pores in the mitochondrial membrane and the release of cytochrome *c* in psoriasis vulgaris patients. The differentiating situation was observed in the lymphocytes of PsA patients [9]. This suggests that a decreased level of p62 protein was associated with a decrease in NFκB levels and a decrease in the onset of lymphocyte apoptosis. Additionally, higher rates of apoptosis are found in PsV despite the higher transcriptional activity of Nrf2. This may indicate that regulation of p53 by ROS is more important than Nrf2 in regulating of lymphocyte death. It also confirms that the compensatory mechanisms in psoriasis are ineffective compared to pro-oxidative or proinflammatory factors [9,38,39]. Increased levels of NFκB and TNFα were also visible in the plasma of patients with psoriasis, while the degree of expression of these proteins in the plasma of psoriasis patients does not depend on the type of psoriasis, but the increase in the expression of both NFκB and TNFα in lymphocytes is significantly higher in patients with PsV and PsA [9,28]. It is also suggested that the differences in the levels of NFκB and TNFα as well as the activation of proapoptotic pathways between psoriasis vulgaris and psoriatic arthritis patients may be related to the endocannabinoid system. It was shown that the level of endocannabinoids in the lymphocytes of psoriatic arthritis patients may be lowered by decreased expression of endocannabinoid receptors, while in PsV patients, both the level of endocannabinoids and the expression of their receptors are increased [27].

Thus, inflammation and the cells of the immune system are largely responsible for the development of oxidative stress in psoriasis. Among immune cells, granulocytes and especially neutrophils are a potent cause of oxidative stress for several main reasons. First, they are the main and most numerous cells of the immune system. Moreover, they react strongly to pro-inflammatory stimuli and are able to migrate and penetrate the skin, and skin infiltration by neutrophils has been observed in psoriasis. Neutrophils play a major role in fighting bacteria, and they do so in three basic ways. First, they can phagocytose the bacteria. Then, the pathogen is killed, usually with the participation of ROS-dependent mechanism. Second, neutrophils can degranulate, thereby releasing the contents of their granules to the outside of the cell, what is especially used when the pathogen is too large for phagocytosis. However, it is also very detrimental to the host, as the neutrophil granules contain large amounts of pro-oxidative enzymes, which leads to a significant increase in the ROS level in the neutrophil environment. Accordingly, evolutionarily neutrophils are able to perform NETosis, a type of programmed death in which the cytotoxic and pro-oxidative contents of a granule are attached to DNA and released, leading to the formation of networks known as NETs. As in this case, the content of the granule is attached to the DNA and directly adheres to the pathogens, and the damage is less than with degranulation, but still a large amount of ROS is released and may interact with other host cells. In the case of psoriasis, an increase in the activity of prooxidative enzymes in neutrophils as well as an increase in the tendency to create a network of NETs by these cells has been observed. This confirms that they play an important role in the development of oxidative stress in psoriasis. Moreover, neutrophils also produce a number of cytokines, thus contributing to the overall severity of inflammation and, consequently, oxidative stress. Levels of TNF-α, IL-1, and IFN-γ are increased in psoriasis which activate inducible nitric oxide synthase (iNOS). Also, the level of iNOS mRNA is significantly increased in psoriasis [40,41]. Nitric oxide (NO) synthesized by iNOS has a vasodilating effect, and NO levels in psoriasis were also elevated [42].

Still, immune cells are not only a source of ROS but are also strongly modulated by them. Oxidative stress increases inflammation and production of proinflammatory cytokines and activates leukocytes. In psoriasis, its effect is especially visible, as oxidative stress modulates not only the functioning of lymphocytes but also their differentiation, which is critical for the pathophysiology of psoriasis. In vitro studies have shown that oxidative stress increases the activation of dendritic cells [43], the production of IL-8 and TNF-α by these cells, as well as TLR expression, which may play an important role in their abnormal responses to autoantigens [44]. Therefore, on the other hand, increased ROS levels lead to increased activation of lymphocytes by dendritic cells [45]. It has been shown that the activation of dendritic cells is weaker, and that lower amounts of cytokines such as IL-1β, IL-12, TNF-α, and IFN-γ are formed in vitro in the presence of antioxidative vitamins [46]. Moreover, a study showed that lymphocytes co-cultured with dendritic cells previously treated with these vitamins are characterized by reduced proliferation and a shifted response toward Th2, i.e., production of IL-10, IL-4, and IL-5. Other antioxidant (bursopentine) suppresses the LPS-induced dendritic cells activation, observed as a decrease in the production of TNF-α as well as inhibition of the maturation of these cells [47]. Since activation of dendritic cells and interactions between dendritic cells and lymphocytes appears to be key in the development of autoimmune diseases, oxidative stress may be associated with the development of autoimmune diseases through action on dendritic cells [47]. Oxidative stress not only induces T lymphocyte polarization by enhancing their interaction with dendritic cells but may also directly increase Th17 development via the mTOR pathway [10,11]. Antioxidants like resveratrol, which can inhibit the mTOR pathway, are known to have a positive effect in mice models of immunologic diseases [48]. In the case of B lymphocytes [49], their increased activation may be caused by the increased activity of T lymphocytes, higher cytokine levels, or the direct influence of ROS. Oxidative stress caused by hydrogen peroxide has been shown to result in higher activation and maturation of B lymphocytes, and thus they may also contribute to the development of diseases in which the pathophysiology of B cells leads to production of autoantibodies. In the presence of the antioxidants, the phosphorylation of the p38 MAPK kinase also decreases, indicating inhibition of the p38 MAPK pathway [46].

Despite the fact that most of abovementioned changes are observed in peripheral blood leukocytes, skin-infiltrating leukocytes probably react in similar way, as some of abovementioned parameters were also confirmed in skin infiltrating leukocytes. Among them, increased amount of neutrophil extracellular traps is observed in biopsies of psoriatic skin. Since the formation of extracellular traps results in the activation of oxidative burst and generation of huge amounts of ROS in neutrophils, it proves that both peripheral blood and skin-infiltrating neutrophils are affected by pro-oxidative conditions [50]. Moreover, as during NETosis, all molecules and proteins contained within cells, including various cytokines, NETosis may be a strong inducer of a proinflammatory response in autoimmune diseases. In psoriasis, neutrophils are observed to be the most IL-17 positive skin infiltrating cells, indicating they can be an important source of this and other cytokines [51]. Still, also lymphocytes are present in skin in higher amount and are overactivated. Nevertheless, it has not been measured, if they are as strongly affected by oxidative stress as peripheral blood cells, but it is very likely, especially as in general in skin of psoriatic patients higher generation of ROS and NOS has been observed [52].

Still, all abovementioned changes in immune cells also influence not only other leukocytes but also fibroblasts and keratinocytes. It has been found, inter alia, that the antioxidant astilbin reduces both the production of ROS and the proliferation of keratinocytes, suggesting an important role for ROS-induced changes not only in immune cells but also in keratinocytes [53]. It is well known that oxidative stress activates protective mechanisms, such as Nrf2. Nevertheless, in psoriatic keratinocytes, it has been observed that Nrf2 activation leads to higher expression of the keratins K6, K16, and K17, which enhance the proliferation of keratinocytes [54]. Therefore, in this case, Nrf2 activation may not be beneficial for patients. Also in psoriatic fibroblasts, increased ROS generation, 8-isoprostanes levels, and protein carboxylation are observed as well as lower total antioxidant capacity. These changes may lead to increased MAPKs activation and therefore increased proliferation of these cells. Additionally, this may promote the production of proinflammatory cytokines, such as Il-6 and Il-8 by fibroblasts, which lead to further proliferation of keratinocytes.

Lipid mediators in psoriasis

A consequence of the disturbed redox balance observed in the development of psoriasis is oxidative stress, leading to metabolic changes that exacerbate the development of the disease. Such a situation is related to the reactions of ROS unbalanced by antioxidants with lipids, proteins, and nucleic acids, which consequently modifies their structure and functions [16]. Such changes have also been observed in psoriasis [28].

ROS reacting with lipids act as short-term signaling molecules and stimulate the production of lipid mediators through direct reactions of ROS-dependent peroxidation and oxidation by lipid oxidizing enzymes, activated under oxidative stress conditions (Fig. 18.1). In the case of lipid peroxidation, the molecules of these compounds are oxidized after the formation of lipid radicals. The initiators of nonenzymatic lipid peroxidation are mainly hydroxyl and hydroperoxyl radicals, which initiate oxidative chain reactions. The most susceptible to peroxidation are membrane phospholipids containing polyunsaturated fatty acids (PUFAs), including arachidonic, linoleic, linolenic, eicosapentaenoic, and docosahexaenoic acids [55]. As a consequence, studies on phospholipid profile of psoriatic patients revealed differential expression of several phospholipid classes. It has been reported that phosphatidylcholines and phosphatidyl inositols containing the above PUFAs were reduced in mononuclear cells of psoriasis patients [27]. In addition, a significant elevation of sphingomyelins content and reduced levels of phosphatidylcholines, phosphatidyl inositols, phosphatidyl serines, and ether-linked phosphatidylethanolamines, have been associated with transepidermal barrier impairment and apoptosis in the keratinocytes of patients with PsV [56].

Arachidonic and linoleic acids are the main PUFAs that undergo oxidation in ROS-dependent reactions with the formation of lipid hydroperoxides, which, through oxidative fragmentation, are then converted into biologically active lipid mediators, such as extremely reactive, α,β-unsaturated aldehydes, including 4-hydroxynonenal (4-HNE), malondialdehyde (MDA) and other small molecular electrophilic aldehydes, elevated levels of which were observed in cells of the psoriatic skin but also in cells and blood plasma of PsV and PsA patients [28,57]. On the other hand, phospholipid PUFAs undergo oxidative cyclization leading to the formation of F2-isoprostanes (F2-IsoP) and neuroprostanes, which are released from the phospholipid

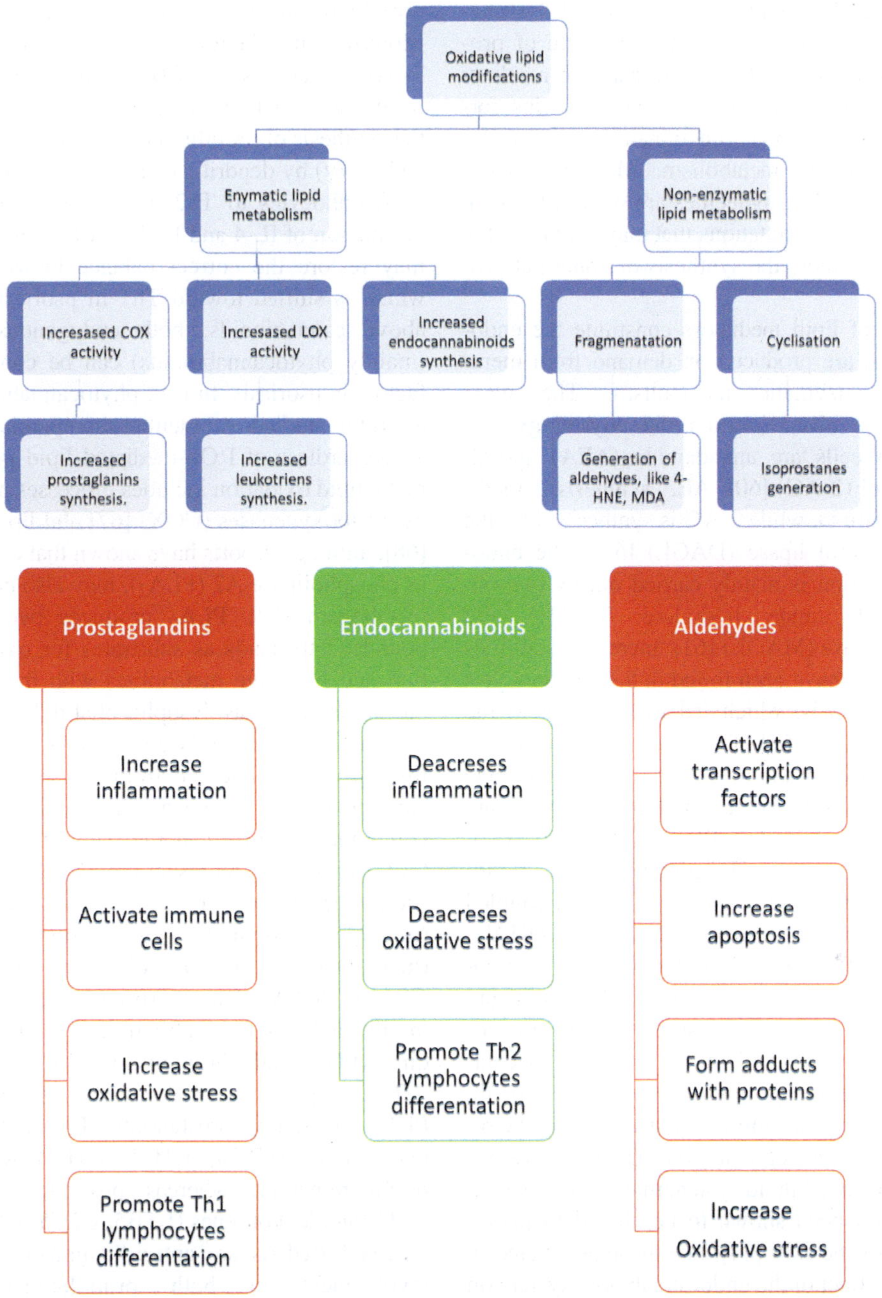

FIGURE 18.1 Oxidative lipid modifications and their impact on psoriasis pathophysiology.

structure by PLA2. Increased levels of free F2-IsoP and neuroprostanes have also been reported in the skin cells of the blood of psoriasis patients [28].

The formation of lipid peroxidation products directly affects the physical properties and functioning of cell membranes, in which, by disturbing the asymmetry of lipids, the hydrophobicity is reduced, resulting in their depolarization and disruption of integrity [58]. The products of oxidative modification of phospholipids further promote oxidative damages by changing the function of immunocompetent cells [59]. Such a mechanism in the case of 8-isoPGF2 has been shown to be based on the activation of TNFα [28]. Regardless of the above, the products of lipid peroxidation, due to their chemical structure (presence of carbonyl groups and carbon-carbon double bonds) and electrophilic properties, are chemically highly reactive molecules that can easily form adducts with most of the nucleophilic components of the cell, including DNA, lipids, peptides, and proteins, leading to disturbances of cellular metabolism [59]. It was shown that these reactions reduce the level of reactive lipid peroxidation products, while increasing the formation of adducts with proteins that promote disturbed cell signaling, leading to cell dysfunction and apoptosis [59]. Changes in the structure of proteins, regardless of direct oxidation, are also the result of adducts of lipid peroxidation products with proteins formation, which modifies their functionality and, consequently, cellular/systemic metabolism. Moreover under oxidative stress, even DNA molecules are oxidized, which promotes the formation of mutations that may aggravate the disease process or promote the synthesis of abnormal proteins [59].

Another group of lipid mediators constitute the endocannabinoids which are produced on demand from membrane lipid by enzymatic metabolism. The main endocannabinoids involved in both the physiology and pathology of skin cells are anandamide (AEA) and 2-arachidonyloglicerol (2-AG) [60]. AEA synthesis is mediated by phospholipase D, while 2-AG is synthesized by the action of diacylglycerol lipase (DAGL) [61]. The endocannabinoid degradation is mainly carried out by two enzymes, fatty acid amide hydrolase (FAAH) and monoacylglycerol lipase (MAGL) [61]. Increased activities of FAAH and MAGL have been found in the keratinocytes of patients with psoriasis, which led to reduction in the level of AEA and 2-AG [57]. The level of endocannabinoids is also regulated by the activity of ABC membrane transporters (multidrug resistance protein 1-MDR1 and breast cancer resistance protein-BCRP), the activity of which is elevated in psoriasis keratinocytes [57]. Endocannabinoids are endogenous ligands G protein-coupled membrane cannabinoid receptors (CB1, CB2, TRPV1, and GPR55) [61]. All of the above are part of the endocannabinoid system that has been identified in skin and having an important role in many aspects of skin homeostasis [62]. Endocannabinoid system is involved in cutaneous function by regulating, among others, cell growth, differentiation and survival, immune and inflammatory responses, and sensory phenomena [63]. Therefore, dysregulation of the endocannabinoid system may be involved in skin disease and has been shown to be altered in pathological conditions of the skin [64], like those associated to psoriasis [28]. The effect of the endocannabinoid system on human keratinocyte growth and differentiation includes mechanisms of CB1 and CB2 receptors-dependent and independent as well as connected with activation of TRPV1 and PPARγ receptors [64]. Activation of CB1/2, TRPVs, and PPARs in keratinocytes from psoriatic patients was observed [57]. However, receptors ability to target inflammation and angiogenesis support a potential role for cannabinoids in the treatment of psoriasis [63]. It has been shown that activation of the CB1 promotes the increase, while the activation of the CB2 receptor and the vanilloid receptor 1 (TRPV1) promotes the reduction of ROS and inflammatory mediators [65]. Thus, CB2 receptor agonists and CB1 receptor antagonists reduce the level of proinflammatory cytokines and oxidative stress [65]. Moreover, it is believed that endocannabinoids, especially 2-AG, are agonists of CB2 in immune cells and therefore have immunosuppressive effects. Moreover, by inhibiting the synthesis of proinflammatory cytokines (e.g., IL6, IL12, and IFNγ) by dendritic cells, they promote the polarization of lymphocytes to Th2 instead of Th1, by inducing the production of IL-4 and IL-10 [66]. Therefore, cannabinoids may restore the correct balance between Th1 and Th2, which is shifted toward Th1 in psoriasis [66]. Given the above cannabinoids, both endogenous and exogenous (mainly phytocannabinoids) can be considered protective factors in psoriasis. In fact, phytocannabinoids in particular are often studied as potential therapeutic agents [57].

Regardless of ROS-mediated lipid peroxidation, enzymatic lipid oxidation includes processes primarily catalyzed by cyclooxygenases (COX) [67] and lipoxygenases (LOX) [68], although reports have shown that other enzymes, such as phospholipase A2 (PLA_2), may also be involved in lipid metabolism [69]. PLA_2 produces two classes of compounds: fatty acids as substrates for oxidative fragmentation and bioactive metabolites with the phosphoglyceride backbone, such as lysophosphatidylcholines or platelet-activating factors, as well as oxygenated derivatives of free fatty acids released from the sn-2 position including eicosanoids, which are another large group of bio-active compounds involved in the pathophysiology of psoriasis [70]. Eicosanoids represent large group of lipid metabolites (lipid species) derived from peroxidation of both ω-6 (mainly arachidonic (AA) and linoleic acid (LA)) and ω-3 (mainly eicosapentaenoic (EPA) and docosahexaenoic acid (DHA)) PUFAs. Due to structural differences eicosanoid family includes two subfamilies, prostanoids [prostaglandins (PGs) and thromboxanes (TXs)] and leukotriens (LTx). Importantly, eicosanoids derived from omega-6 PUFAs including prostanoids (TXA2, PGE2, PGI2) and leukotrienes (LTB4, LTC4, LTE4) were identified as proinflammatory, whereas prostanoids (TXA3, PGE3, PGI3) and leukotrienes (LTB5, LTC5, LTE5) derived from omega-3 PUFAs are anti-inflammatory [71]. Due to the involvement in both proinflammatory and anti-inflammatory processes, eicosanoids play a key role in inflammatory signaling and may modulate skin diseases, especially psoriasis [72,73]. Both proinflammatory and anti-inflammatory eicosanoids were suggested as potential biomarkers of PsA, since have been positively correlated with joint disease score [74]. Increased levels of proinflammatory eicosanoids including the oxidized lipid mediators of AA and LA, namely, 8-, 12-, 15-hydroxyeicosatetraenoic acid (8-, 12-, 15-HETE) and 13-hydroxyoctadecadienoic acid (13-HODE) have been also found in skin biopsies and peripheral blood from psoriasis patients [75]. Moreover, enhanced activities of COX-1 and COX-2 in mononuclear cells of patients with PsV and PsA accompanied by significant increase in the level of TxB2 have been also reported [76]. Importantly, TXB2 as a stable metabolite derived from TxA2, which have been shown to promotion of the development of psoriatic dermatitis [76]. In addition to the above, promotion of skin inflammation through NFκB-mediated metabolic pathways by inhibiting IκB kinase (IKK) activity was previously suggested, since elevated levels of LTB4 and PGJ2 have been found in mononuclear cells of patients with PsV [77].

It should be emphasized that although some prostanoids and leukotrienes have been found at higher levels in human psoriatic skin, the importance of these eicosanoids and especially their role in the pathophysiology of psoriasis remains unclear and requires further research. Nevertheless, among other eicosanoids prostaglandin PGE2, which has been shown to promote the development of psoriatic dermatitis through the regulation of IL-23/IL-17 pathways, seems to be the most important in psoriasis [78]. Furthermore, quite recent study on psoriasis mouse model in vivo revealed that the regulation of PGE2-EP2/EP4 signaling could lead to the reduction in Th17 cells in patients with psoriasis and thus become a new target in the pharmacotherapy of psoriasis [79]. Considering that activation of Th17 cells play an important role in stimulation of keratinocyte proliferation and the secretion of inflammatory cytokines, future research on the therapy of psoriasis should focus on the relationship between phospholipid metabolism and Th17 cell activation [80,81].

Nevertheless altered lipid metabolism not only concern intracellular lipid modifications. Also lipoproteins and apolipoproteins are changed in psoriasis. Proteins involved in lipid metabolism are also disturbed in psoriasis, especially changes in the expression of apolipoprotein E or A (ApoE, ApoA) [82] but also a significant decrease in the level of apolipoprotein M (ApoM), which is mainly enriched with high-density lipoprotein (HDL) and in smaller amounts of low- and very-low-density lipoprotein (LDL and VLDL) was observed [83,84]. ApoM is known to reduce the migration and proliferation of vascular endothelial cells, thereby inhibiting T cell activation and proliferation and lipid oxidation [85,86], so ApoM deficiency can significantly contribute to inflammation and psoriatic lesions. In addition, the expression of lipoprotein lipase (LPL) has been shown to decrease, which affects the hydrolyzation of the triglycerides in lipoproteins into free fatty acids and glycerol, and consequently the conversion of VLDL into IDL and then to LDL, thereby resulting in an imbalance in the ratio of VLDL/LDL in psoriatic patients [86]. LPL deficiency also leads to an elevated level of triglycerides in the bloodstream, which further enhances the inflammatory reactions [86]. Moreover, a reduced level of sulfated glycoprotein 2 in patients with psoriasis indicates impairment of the hydrolysis of some glycolipids [87,88]. There is therefore a strong similarity of action between apolipoproteins and lipopolysaccharide binding protein (LBP). These small molecules have been suggested to control the response to LPS under physiological conditions by forming LPS complexes that bind monocytes and macrophages [89]. Thus, the lower levels of LBP observed in psoriasis patients may interfere with the body's response to LPS, and levels of which in the serum and keratinocytes of psoriasis patients have been described as overexpressed [90,91].

Protein modifications and their consequences in psoriasis

Under oxidative conditions associated with the development of psoriasis, proteins undergo post-translational modifications through oxidation or adduct formation, which cause changes in the structure and function of proteins, often with significant effects on downstream cells. During the reaction of proteins with sugars/oxidized sugars, advanced glycation products are formed—AGEs, which contribute to the development of disease [92]. Observed in psoriasis is increased proliferation of keratinocytes, which results in greater demand and higher degradation of glucose by these cells. Therefore, it has been suggested that AGES also play role in the pathogenesis of psoriasis [93]. The skin is sensitive to changes caused by the accumulation of AGEs in the skin, which promotes increased production of ROS, which consequently increases the generation of oxidized LDL and peroxidation products in the skin [93]. AGEs may favor chronic inflammation with the activation of monocytes, macrophages, neutrophils, and endothelial cells; these cells, once activated, produce proinflammatory cytokines and other reactive oxygen forms, resulting in molecular modifications and additional production of AGE, with further amplification of the inflammatory response [94,95]. The formation of AGEs occurs in the body in a physiological state but is greatly exacerbated not only in oxidative stress, but also in hyperglycemia and hyperlipidemia. The most frequently observed AGEs are: carboxymethyl lysine (CML) is formed by the reaction of lysine side chains with glyoxal as well as carboxyethyl lysine (CEL). However AGEs react with RAGE receptors, which are found, inter alia, on the surface of keratinocytes, epithelial cells, dendritic cells, monocytes, and macrophages [93]. RAGE, on the other hand, acts through the NF-κβ factor and tyrosine kinase [96]. In addition to AGEs, RAGE is also stimulated by psoriasin and HMGB1, among others. Increased levels of HMGB1 have been shown both in the serum of patients suffering from psoriasis and another autoimmune disease—rheumatoid arthritis. However, psoriasin is also elevated in psoriasis. In vitro studies have shown that HMGB1 determines the differentiation of Th17 helper lymphocytes [97]. Moreover, glycated proteins can become antigens and thus intensify the immune reaction [98].

Proteins are also modified by the reaction of lipid peroxidation products, which levels are also enhanced in psoriasis (acrolein, MDA, 4-HNE, 15-deoxy-Δ12,14-prostaglandin J2, and isoprostanes) with the amino acid residues of proteins, mainly histidine, cysteine, and lysine to form advanced lip(id)oxidation end products (ALEs) [99]. ALEs can modify the functions of proteins by covalently modifying them, which may result in the loss of their biological functions [100].

Significantly increased lipid peroxidation in psoriasis promotes interactions of electrophilic reactive aldehydes, e.g., 4-HNE with proteins and adducts formation. The levels of 4-HNE-protein adducts have been shown to be approximately 2.5-fold higher in the plasma of psoriasis patients compared to healthy controls [82]. This suggests the influence of these modifications on the activity and proteins functions. It has been indicated that in the plasma of psoriasis patients, 4-HNE forms adducts with the Rho GTPase activating protein 12, adenylate kinase 7, which is mainly involved in catalytic activity that is not observed in the plasma of healthy individuals. It has been suggested that 4-HNE-Rho GTPase activating protein adduct also triggers Rho GTPase activity and inhibits apoptosis. Moreover, Rho GTPase triggers a cascade of Rho kinase activity, leading to the migration of neutrophils and disruption of intercellular connections between skin cells [101,102]. As a result, excessive keratinocytes exfoliation was observed in the patients with psoriasis.

In the keratinocytes of patients with psoriasis, a threefold increase in the level of 4-HNE-protein adducts formed on cysteine and histidine residues, and not lysine, which is the main amino acid forming connections with 4-HNE in keratinocytes of healthy people, was found [57]. Moreover, 4-HNE-protein adducts in the keratinocytes of patients mainly concern proteins with antioxidant and antiapoptotic properties, while in the case of healthy people, the adducts created concern structural proteins. These changes are believed to be particularly important in the case of the transcription factor Nrf2, which has been found to be highly active, which is believed to be a key factor in promoting the proliferation of keratinocytes in psoriasis [38]. The activity of Nrf2 depends on the level and structure of its cytosolic inhibitor Keap1, in which critical cysteine is predisposed to form 4-HNE-Cys adducts [103,104]. Therefore, the formation of 4-HNE-Keap1 adducts may further exacerbate exfoliation. Moreover, these changes, which are of a similar size in the case of lymphocytes, indicate the existence of an interaction of lymphocytes with keratinocytes and suggest an amplification of the proliferation signal and a direct link between the processes occurring in both types of cells.

4-HNE also interacts with His196, His267, Cys311, or Ser473 residues of AKT kinase results in a reduction of AKT sensitivity to phosphorylation, while modifications of Ser473, considered to be the main AKT regulatory site, lead to a decrease in the activity of this protein [103,104]. As AKT promotes cell survival, decrease in its activity may be an antiapoptotic factor in case of psoriatic cells, especially in cells which have been subjected to stressors such as UV, which in the case of keratinocytes results in the intensification of apoptosis, and decreased level of p-AKT [38].

As mentioned above, some residues are more sensitive to oxidation than other. Therefore, proteins that contain cysteine, lysine, or histidine residues very often are involved in signal transmission. It is a regulatory mechanism for both protein kinases, proteolytic proteins, and transcription factors. On the one hand, it allows you to counteract the effects of oxidative stress; on the other hand, it intensifies the inflammatory process, depending on which protein is oxidized. It is proved that ROS-dependent signaling plays an important role in regulation of different proteins in psoriasis. At first, oxidation of cysteine residues in tyrosine kinases, observed in psoriasis, reduce the biological activity of these enzymes. Consequently, they cannot fulfill their biological role—dephosphorylation of protein kinases, which, in consequence, remains in the active form. This situation applies to the following enzymes: phosphoinositol 3-kinase (PI3K), protein kinase C (PKC), AMP-dependent cyclic protein kinase (PKA), and GMP-dependent cyclic kinase (PKG), which participate in development of psoriasis [105]. As all of them are involved in inflammation regulation; they may play important role in psoriasis pathophysiology. It has been proved on mice model. It is known that IMQ induce psoriasis like changes in mice through activation of TLR-7 and TLR-9 receptors on dendritic cells. Nevertheless, in PI3K-knockout mice, response to IMQ is much less intense, which leads to leads to a much lower intensity of skin lesions and lower production of Il-17 [106]. In humans, the situation is similar, as activation of TLR-7 or TLR-9 receptors in human dendritic cells results in the activation of PI3K. It has also been shown that activation of PI3K is necessary for the production of IFN but not of the other factors produced by dendritic cells [107]. As IFN plays an important role both in initiation of psoriasis and its further development, it may be one of the reasons why PI3K activation is important in psoriasis pathophysiology, other one is that it inhibits apoptosis of keratinocytes [108]. Nevertheless, PI3K is not the only kinase which takes part in dendritic cells functioning, as PKC is important in activation of T-cells by dendritic cells. PKCθ isoform is transferred to T cell during contact with dendritic cells [107]. PKC in T cells is required for proliferation and IFN-γ production [109]. Furthermore, its action is crucial for production of IL-2, which increases proliferation of T cells [108]. Moreover, in PKCθ-deficient mice, NF-κB activation is disrupted, as well as production of IFN-γ and IL-17 [108]. As PKC is involved in regulation of cells involved in psoriasis development as well as synthesis important molecules in psoriasis pathophysiology, PKC inhibitors are considered and tested as potential therapeutic factors in psoriasis, and preclinical trials shows that after their administration clinical symptoms are ameliorated [110,111]. On the other hand, activation of the cyclic AMP-dependent kinase paradoxically causes an anti-inflammatory effects [112].

Another group of proteins that are activated during oxidative conditions are transcription factors. Still, in their case, situation is more complicated and usually is not related to direct interaction between ROS and transcription factor, rather on modification of their activators\inhibitors or corresponding sequences on DNA, as even DNA can be modified by ROS. Therefore, an increased level of 8-hydroxy guanosine, which is consider as a good marker of oxidative DNA damage, is observed in psoriasis [113]. This can interact with gene activation by transcription factors. For example, substitution of guanosine by 8-oxodG in the binding sequence of the transcription factor AP-1 or Sp1 reduces the binding of these factors to DNA and, consequently, disrupts their function. AP-1 is essential for fibroblast differentiation and is involved in the process of apoptosis. Sp1 is also involved in the process of apoptosis, which in addition increases the transcription of ubiquitin C and CD39, which is considered to be a suppressor of excessive immune response [114–117].

Different mechanisms of ROS action take place in case of Nrf2. In this case, its inhibitor Keap1 protein is prone to oxidative modifications. This process is similar to activation of Nrf2 by 4-HNE, as normally, Keap1 is in complex with Nrf2, but during oxidative conditions interaction between ROS and cysteine residues in Keap1 leads to complex breakdown and release of Nrf2, which then activate transcription on different, mostly cytoprotective genes.

More complicated situation is in the case of NFκB, as in these cases, oxidative conditions leads to increased proteolysis of its inhibitor. ROS actions lead to different modifications of the structure of proteins, which usually lead to changes in their functionality. Therefore, in order to avoid metabolic changes, the modified proteins should be degraded. Still, increased proteolysis and increased protein carbonylation are observed in the dermis of psoriasis skin biopsies, isolated psoriatic fibroblasts, and serum obtained from psoriatic patients [118,119]. Moreover, it has been shown that the increase in the level of proinflammatory factors in psoriatic fibroblasts is accompanied by increased expression of proteins involved in proteolytic processes, such as proteasomes, particularly the 26S and S100A8/A9 proteasome components. The ubiquitin-proteasome pathway, activated during the development of psoriasis, also plays a key role in the selective degradation of intracellular proteins, including those involved in the control of inflammatory processes [120]. It is noted that the increase in the level of 26S proteasome subunits may contribute to the increased degradation of IκB, which is a cytosolic inhibitor of the NFκB transcription factor [121–123]. As a result, NFκB, by improving the inflammatory response, promotes T cell responses in psoriasis [124]. In vitro and in vivo examinations have shown that 26S proteasome inhibitors inhibit cell proliferation and migration under inflammatory conditions [124], highlighting the potential for the inhibition of the proteasome as a treatment option for inflammatory disorders such as psoriasis [120]. IκB can be also degraded by calpain, which also leads to activation of NFκB and increased inflammation [125]. Another protein with proteolytic activity associated with inflammation is calpain, calcium-dependent neutral protease, which main role is the regulation of various fundamental cellular functions, such as cell cycle and apoptosis, but it is also involved in the initiation of inflammation by the degradation of IκB and the activation of NFκB [125]. An increase in the level of calpain has already been identified in the skin tissue of psoriatic patients [126,127]. However, calpain also stimulates the migration of fibroblasts and myoblasts, which are necessary for the treatment of damaged skin [128] (Fig. 18.2).

On the other hand, abovementioned protein S100A8/A9 in the psoriatic epidermis is to activate the complement component 3 protein (C3) in keratinocytes. After activation, C3 is translocated to the dermis, where it stimulates immune cells to produce cytokines, interleukins, and growth factors, thereby contributing to the development of psoriasis [129–131]. Still it is known that of fibroblasts play important role in this intercellular communication. Fibroblasts in psoriatic skin display the upregulation of 14-3-3 sigma (σ) and zeta/delta (ζ/δ) protein isoforms. Other studies showed that 14-3-3 protein levels in psoriatic skin biopsies are changed in various ways, depending on the isoform; 14-3-3τ and σ are upregulated [132–134], while 14-3-3β and 14-3-3ζ are downregulated [135] in psoriatic fibroblasts is observed, as well as in phagocytes [135]. 14-3-3 is involved in the regulation of transcription and translation through its interaction with DNA/mRNA-binding proteins, such as tris-tetraprolin (TTP), which induces the destabilization and degradation of cytokine mRNA (including TNFα mRNA). After phosphorylation, TTP can bind to 14-3-3, which inhibits the mRNA-degrading capabilities of TTP. Therefore, in several skin diseases characterized by hyperproliferative keratinocytes, increased levels of 14-3-3 result in the overexpression of cytokines [132]. These changes are accompanied by the upregulation of kinases [136]. Conversely, in the case of DNA-damage or the overexpression of dysregulated genes, 14-3-3σ is upregulated by a p53-dependent pathway and partially prevents cells from entering mitosis [137].

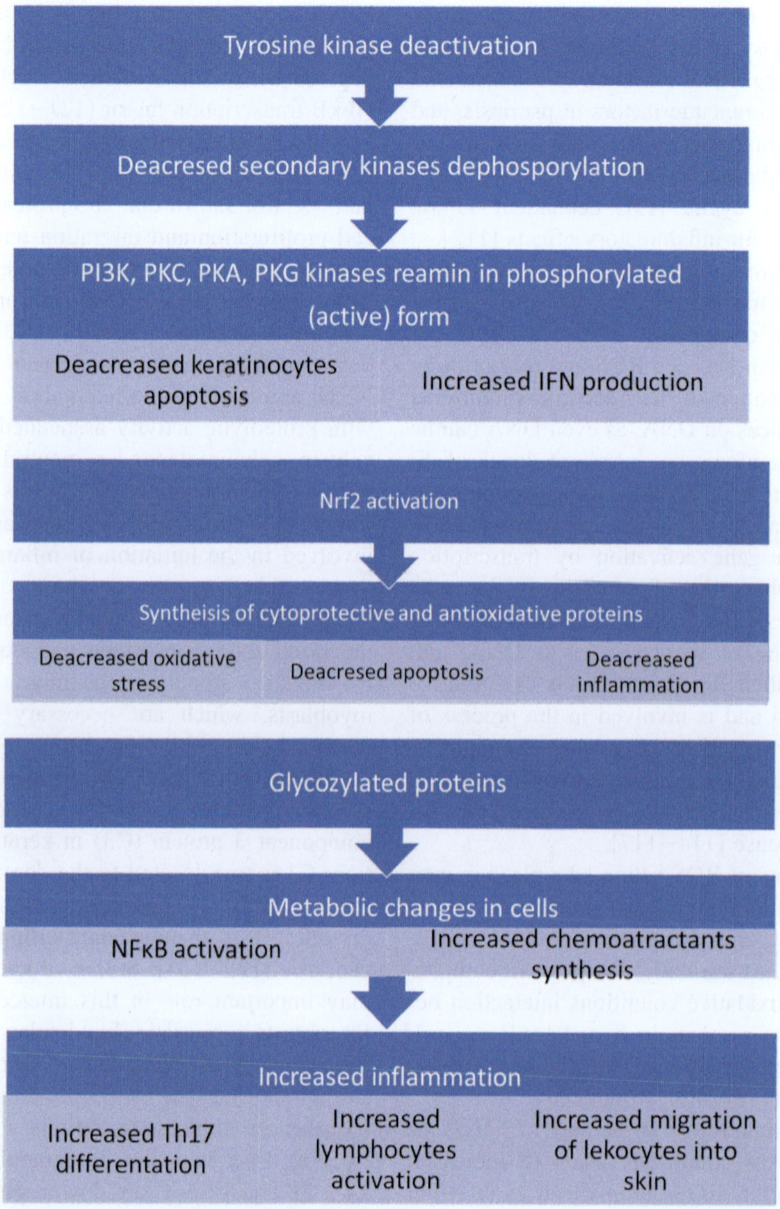

FIGURE 18.2 Oxidative modifications that alter protein functions and their impact on psoriasis.

Medical and experimental treatment of psoriasis

Not fully understood etiology of psoriasis limits current therapies to only alleviate symptoms by extinguishing inflammation, inhibiting skin cell proliferation or activating apoptosis of skin infiltrating lymphocytes. Because the development of psoriasis is associated with inflammation and oxidative stress, the primary severity of oxidative stress and lipid peroxidation causes the NFκB activation with cytokines and chemokines causing inflammation development, which in turn results in increased oxidative stress and its consequences. However, when inflammation is the primary event, it leads to oxidative stress and increased lipid peroxidation, which intensifies inflammation [23,24]. Moreover, ROS and lipid peroxidation products are important immune cell regulators. In case of neutrophils, they are necessary for the functioning, when in lymphocytes, they regulate differentiation into Th1 or Th2 subpopulations. As typical therapies which target only inflammatory pathways were unable to get a long-time recovery, in order to increase the effectiveness of pharmacotherapy of psoriasis, for many years, different compounds have been sought for simultaneously targeting oxidative stress and inflammation aiming to block their vicious circle. Some compounds are also being investigated to see if they can be used in addition to conventional antipsoriasis therapies.

Nevertheless, as oxidative stress and inflammation are interacting with each other, and most drugs affected different metabolic pathways; it is very difficult to determine exact mechanism of action of particular drug. This situation take place in most therapies used in psoriasis treatment, like anti-inflammatory drugs (both corticosteroids, and nonsteroidal anti-inflammatory drugs), natural products or TNFα inhibitors. Even though the goal of these therapies is to decrease inflammation and PASI, they also reduce the level of oxidative stress by decreasing the onset of ROS/lipid peroxidation and/or by increasing the antioxidant capacity of the affected skin and immune cells. These may be caused by reduction of the biological activity of NFκB and/or direct modification of the level of TNFα [138]. For example, infliximab—TNFα inhibitor not only improved PASI score but also decreased ROS levels and NADPH oxidase activity in leukocytes as well as thiobarbituric acid reactive substances (TBARS) compared to untreated psoriatic patients. Nevertheless, these parameters do not reach the values observed in completely healthy subjects [29,139].

The other drugs based on anti-inflammatory signaling, but affecting oxidative stress, are PPARγ modulators. These drugs use their immunomodulatory and antiproliferative effects [140]. In transgenic mouse model, activation of PPARβ/δ triggers inflammation [141]; when PPARγ ligands reduced epidermal hyperplasia, it may suggest that PPARγ activation may contribute to the prevention of psoriatic lesions [141]. On the other hand, activation of PPARγ exerts antiproliferative effects using cultures of normal human keratinocytes and lymphocytes in which the PPARγ agonist—GED-0507-34 effects and suppresses the inflammatory signal by inhibiting NFκB, and consequently reduced expression of proinflammatory cytokines such as IL6, IL8, IL12, IL21, IL23, TNFα, and COX-2 [142], thereby reducing generation of 4-HNE.

However, the action of many drugs used to treat psoriasis shows an unexpected effect on the lipid peroxidation process (including 4-HNE generation). Commonly used cyclosporin that acts by inhibition of membrane transport proteins has been found to act also as factor enhancing 4-HNE level in plasma [143]. Similarly, even topically used dithranol (anthralin) by its prooxidative effects causes formation of superoxide anion and hydrogen peroxide, which stimulate proinflammatory cytokines following NFκB activation [144].

Still in some therapies, their impact on ROS level is direct, because they act as antioxidants, or they directly induce anti-inflammatory pathways, including Nrf2. Therefore, it can be assumed that alleviating of oxidative stress is their primary mechanism of action, so we focus on them in this chapter. Among them, there are physical factors, like UV radiation, which paradoxically further enhances ROS generation, but also chemical drugs, that are suggested for their antioxidative properties. Finally, as psoriasis is at least partially dependent on exogenous factors as well as lifestyle, the impact of lifestyle changes on prevention and treatment of psoriasis is discussed in the end of this chapter.

As abovementioned, the physical factor which is most frequently used in the treatment of psoriasis is UV phototherapy (both UVA and UVB light), aiming to increase the effectiveness of pharmacotherapy of psoriasis vulgaris, which, in turn, may be destructive for the skin, even leading to cancer [145]. Both of these types of irradiation produce different biological effects including ROS (mainly superoxide anion and hydrogen peroxide) and 4-HNE enhanced generation [145,146]. On the other hand, UVA and UVB irradiation have been shown to decrease presentation of antigens, resulting in diminished T-cell responses and inflammatory suppression [147].

Antioxidants usually prove as beneficial in the treatment of psoriasis because cell signaling pathways such as MAPK or JAK/STAT are sensitive to redox conditions and have been shown to be involved in the progression of psoriasis [148]. As an example of topical or orally used natural substances are vitamin D analogs (calcipotriol, tacalcitol, calcitriol) [149]. Vitamin D, as a fatty soluble antioxidant molecule, is known as a lipid protector and is used in therapies for a number of diseases [150]. It has been shown that vitamin D protects against oxidative stress [149,150] and prevents lipid peroxidation [151], effectively lowering the 4-HNE level in cells under both physiological and oxidative conditions [151]. Antioxidants such as SOD and NAC have been shown to inhibit oxidative stress and 4-HNE levels in synoviocytes, acting as ROS scavengers, while NAC-induced NFκB reduction is associated with reduced proinflammatory cytokine release and angiogenesis [152]. The therapeutic potential of other medically used compounds such as dimethyl fumarate is associated with the induction of several antioxidant pathways increasing the levels of GSH, NAD(P)H quinone oxidoreductase 1, Nrf2, as well as acting anti-inflammatory by lowering the levels of cytokines and adhesive molecules [153].

Unfortunately, antipsoriatic therapies with synthetic drugs are often characterized by side effects, while biological drugs treatments are expensive. To minimize these problems, herbal preparations, nutraceuticals, or dietary supplements are increasingly used as alternative or complementary therapy. Currently, approximately 80% of people around the world use preventive and therapeutic natural products because of their relative safety, effectiveness, and low cost, if matching the integrative biomedicine approach.

The most frequently studied and used to treat psoriasis natural antioxidants are polyphenols such as flavonoids, lignans, floroglucynols, quinones, stilbenes, phenylpropanoids, and diarylheptanoids, which can all modulate the inflammatory pathways. Among them, quercetin, apigenin, luteolin, and baicalein showed anti-inflammatory activity in vitro and in animal models [154–157]. One of such polyphenols that interacts with multiple pathophysiological targets that can safely and inexpensively reduce inflammatory processes is curcumin, which significantly reduces 4-HNE levels as well 4-HNE-mediated oxidative modifications of proteins even by 80% [158]. Moreover, the polyphenol-rich extract from green alga Codium fragile applied topically on skin in therapy against psoriasis decreased 4-HNE levels and protein oxidation protecting skin against proinflammatory and oxidative damages induced by UVB [159].

Other natural compounds used as oral or topical medications for the treatment of psoriasis include omega-3 fatty acids such as eicosapentaenoic acid, due to their anti-inflammatory properties, which are particularly manifested by reduced levels of TNFα and 4-HNE-protein adducts (even by 30%) in the blood, especially if used by long-term administration [160,161]. However, recent research results show that supplementing the diet with eicosapentaenoic acid only affects lipid metabolism, reducing the level of eicosanoids that are a potential source of itching [162].

An important element in therapy with natural preparations, including antioxidants, is that, when accompanied by other antioxidant compounds, they show synergy of action. Therefore, it is believed that the most effective form of therapy is currently the use of a mixture of natural antioxidants, which are usually plant extracts. Since different components generally modify different metabolic pathways, this usually results in differing pharmacological effects. However, regardless of the type of therapy used, a balanced diet also plays an important role in improving metabolic disorders. Namely, it was found, among others, that regular consumption of fresh fruit, vegetables, and spices rich in different phytochemicals can reduce oxidative stress and inflammation and may relieve symptoms of psoriasis [163].

Therefore, we may conclude that until the exact and detailed etiopathogenesis of psoriasis is determined, we could rely mostly on nutritional approach and anti-inflammatory medicaments aiming to prevent or control at least some aspects of psoriasis, like any other chronic inflammatory disorder. However, assessing the level of 4-HNE, acting as a signaling molecule to regulate proliferation, differentiation, and apoptosis, might help to make major progress in these areas, especially if we keep in mind that complex, often contradictory effects of 4-HNE are not only concentration-dependent but also dependent on its ability to modify various enzymes, cytokines and their receptors, and even regulate the activity of antioxidants (enzymatic and nonenzymatic, especially GSH). This might be crucial not only for the metabolic, degenerative, and inflammatory aspects of stress-related diseases but especially for the onset of the most dangerous of them all—cancer.

UV phototherapy

One of the most commonly used therapy in psoriasis is UV phototherapy. The most important difference between UV therapy and others presented in this chapter is the fact that UV, as the only therapeutic agent, acts pro-oxidative and proinflammatory, but alleviates skin lesions. What is more, UV radiation is known trigger factor that may cause the appearance of symptoms of psoriasis as well as other skin diseases. This effect is probably caused by the fact that during therapy intensity of UV is very high; therefore, the proapoptotic effect, dependent on ROS, becomes the dominant mechanism of UV action, instead of its proinflammatory actions. Therefore, intensification of apoptosis of both psoriatic and of healthy keratinocytes prevents accumulation of cells in skin. Among three main pathways of apoptosis, UV radiation is known as the activator of two of them in psoriatic keratinocytes. The UV irradiation enhances ROS generation; this way enhancing TNFα production, which activates the extrinsic pathway of apoptosis. Extrinsic pathway involves caspase-8, which is the initiator of caspases cascade, and further activates caspase-3 [164]. Caspase-8 and -3 levels are increased in keratinocytes after exposure to UV radiation and play important role in cells apoptosis [165,166]. Still, UV radiation may lead to damages in macromolecules, directly, or by ROS. ROS or lipid peroxidation products and consequently modified proteins may activate the ER stress-initiated apoptotic pathway, which initiator is caspase-2, with also increased level in UV-radiated keratinocytes [167]. Therefore, UV ameliorates keratinocytes accumulation and in this way, relieves the symptoms of the disease. Still, UV radiation may interact with both keratinocytes, and skin infiltrating leukocytes [168,169]. Some authors suggest, that UV impact on leukocytes, which decreases their number is more important than their impact on keratinocytes and is responsible for its positive impact on condition of psoriatic patients [170,171] (Table 18.1).

Still, UV therapy has also a lot of disadvantages as UV radiation is in fact a harmful factor, which positive impact is caused by its ability to kill cells. Nevertheless, of course not every pathologic cell is killed, and it is impossible to target only psoriatic cells, without influencing healthy. Therefore, UV radiation has some side effects. It is known that UV irradiation used in psoriasis phototherapy increases the level of proinflammatory cytokines and biomarkers of oxidative stress in keratinocytes [172–174]. It may be caused by the fact that UV also increases the

TABLE 18.1 Physical and chemical factor in treatment of psoriasis.

Physical or chemical factor	Affected cells	Effects	Clinical results
UV radiation	Skin infiltrating leukocytes	Increased apoptosis	Improvement of the patient's condition Decreased PASI score
	Keratinocytes	Increased apoptosis Increased ROS generation	
Cannabidiol	Keratinocytes	Increased apoptosis Decreased inflammation Decreased oxidative stress	Decreased PASI score.
	Neutrophils	Decreased oxidative stress Decreased migration Decreased NETosis	
	Lymphocytes	Decreased activation Shifting differentiation toward TH2	
Dimethyl fumarate	Keratinocytes	Reduced hyperproliferation	Improvement of the patient's condition Decreased PASI score Improved epidermal thickness Decreased lymphocytes infiltration Higher Nrf2 pathway activity in skin biopsies
Propylthiouracil	Keratinocytes	Increased differentiation	Decreased PASI score
	Lymphocytes	Decreased activation	
Curcumin	Lymphocytes	Decreased activation Decreased IFNγ production Decreased proliferation	Decreased PASI score
	Keratinocytes	Increased apoptosis	
Luteolin	Keratinocytes	Decreased inflammation	Decreased expression of proinflammatory cytokines in skin and plasma Lessons amelioration Restoration Th1/Th2 cells balance
	Lymphocytes	Promotion of Th2 differentiation	
	Macrophages	Decreased activation Decreased cytokines synthesis	

phosphorylation of the p38 MAPK kinases, which suggest activation of p38 MAPK pathway [46]. This pathway activation leads to overproduction of TNFα and IL1, which on one hand enhances apoptosis, but on other hand, this cytokines has proinflammatory impact [175,176]. It is known the glutathione S-transferase (GST) isoforms (GSTK1, GSTM1, and GSTT1) from the skin of psoriatic patients are significantly higher compared to control group, and their expression levels are not changed after treatment with narrowband ultraviolet B phototherapy [177]. Even the levels of CYP1A1 and CYP2E1 are significantly higher in pre- and post-treatment in the psoriatic tissues than in control ones. Only CYP1B1 level is similar to that of the control group before treatment, while after treatment, the level increased [177].

Therefore, as UV is pretty effective, but have a lot of side effects. Research is currently underway to find compounds that, in combination with UV, could mitigate its negative effects and increase its effectiveness, while reducing side effects. As its negative effects are caused mainly by its proinflammatory and pro-oxidative properties, compounds which are anti-inflammatory and antioxidants may be excellent candidates for that purpose. In particular, they may prevent nonaffected cells against negative effects of UV radiation. And due to anti-inflammatory and antioxidative properties, it is believed that phytocannabinoid–cannabidiol may be such compounds.

Cannabidiol

Cannabinoid is a phytocannabinoid, which is obtained from *Cannabis Sativa*. Similar to other cannabinoids, it has anti-inflammatory and antioxidative properties [178]. Nevertheless as in opposite to other phytocannabinoids, it has no psychoactive properties; it is believed to be very promising compound in therapy of various diseases. It acts mainly through the activation of G protein-bound receptors. Among them, the most important are the cannabinoid receptors (CB1 and CB2), which have opposing effects relative to each other [179,180]. Activation of CB1 has pro-oxidative and proinflammatory effects, while CB2 activation is believed to trigger antioxidant and anti-inflammatory reactions [179,180]. As CB2 receptors is predominates in immune cells, cannabidiol is considered to be the negative regulator of inflammation, and the increased activation of cannabinoid receptors in autoimmune diseases is very often viewed as a protective mechanism [181]. This is supported by the fact that mutations in the CB2 receptor lead to higher lymphocyte activity. Moreover, other receptors like peroxisome proliferator-activated receptor (PPAR), particularly PPAR-δ and PPAR-γ, are also activated by CBD and act in an immunosuppressive manner [182].

In fact, in psoriasis vulgaris, expression of CB2 receptors is enhanced in granulocytes and peripheral blood mononuclear cells (PBMC), while in psoriatic arthritis, expression of CB2 receptors is decreased despite an elevation of endocannabinoids [27,28]. Therefore, exacerbation of psoriasis vulgaris to psoriatic arthritis may be caused by disturbances in the endocannabinoid system. In vitro studies have shown that CBD reduces inflammation and oxidative stress in keratinocytes in both healthy individuals and patients with psoriasis vulgaris, which may indicate its therapeutic properties [57]. Moreover, CBD inhibits neutrophil migration and ROS production, as well as reduces the formation of a NETotic network in neutrophils [32,183]. In case of lymphocytes, CBD decreases their activation and production of IL17 [184]. Animal studies show that mice treated orally with cannabidiol shows lower production of TNFα and IFNγ, which are markers of Th1 response and higher of IL4 and IL10, characteristic for Th2 response. Therefore, CBD probably promote differentiation of lymphocytes into Th1, similarly as endocannabinoids [185]. However, topical application of CBD-containing oil decreases the PASI score in patients with psoriasis vulgaris [186].

Cannabidiol is also considered as a compound which may be used in combination with other therapies, such as abovementioned UVB irradiation as it can protect both diseased and healthy cells from the negative effects of UV irradiation. Furthermore, each of apoptotic pathways can be modulated by CBD as well as by UV irradiations [34,187]. Moreover, CBD acts as an activator of the Nrf2 transcription factor, which may further induce the transcription of the antiapoptotic protein Bcl2 [188–190]. On the other hand, CBD may also induce apoptosis by inhibition of expression of antiapoptotic proteins, such as protein kinase B (AKT) and increasing the release of cytochrome *c* from mitochondria, which enhances apoptosis [191]. According to current studies, CBD protects both psoriatic and healthy keratinocytes against UVB-induced apoptosis, but differences in expression of p53, p38, and caspase 8 observed between healthy and psoriatic keratinocytes after combined CBD and UVB treatment indicate that CBD protects healthy keratinocytes against apoptosis more than psoriatic cells. Given its anti-inflammatory and antioxidant effects, CBD may be considered a potentially adjuvant option in the integrated biomedical treatment of psoriasis.

Dimethyl fumarate

Dimethyl fumarate is used in therapies of many diseases. Its mechanism of action is not fully understood, still it is known, that it increases Nrf2 activity and transcription of antioxidative proteins, therefore acting cytoprotectively, and anti-inflammatory. It may also influence proinflammatory signal pathways through modulation of other transcription factor-NFkB, which leads to decrease in its translocation to cell nucleus, leading to transcription of proinflammatory cytokines like TNFα, IL8, and IL1FB.

Therefore, 50%–70% of psoriasis vulgaris patients treated with oral dimethyl fumarate show a clinical improvement of their condition after 16 weeks of treatment. Moreover, this treatment is safe and shows no serious side effects [153]. In six patients with moderate-to-severe psoriasis treated with DMF 720 mg daily for 16 weeks, the mean PASI, superficial microcirculation and clinical local scores (SUM scores) were reduced by about 50%. Additionally hyperproliferation of keratinocytes was reduced, and therefore, epidermal thickness was significantly improved. Moreover, skin infiltration by T lymphocytes was much decreased [192]. Importantly, gene expression profiling performed on RNA derived from biopsies of psoriatic plaques taken before and after 12 weeks of dimethyl fumarate treatment revealed that this therapy specifically induces activation of the Nrf2 and GSH pathways in psoriatic skin. This suggests that the antioxidant efficacy of FAE may be the mechanism explaining the beneficial clinical effects of FAE in patients with psoriasis, rather than its effect on other metabolic pathways [193].

Propylthiouracil

Propylthiouracil is another antioxidant which is consider as potential medicine against psoriasis [194] as it has resulted in significant clinical improvement and reduced PASI scores in all patients, as well as a significant reduction in epidermal thickness [195,196]. This leads to better quality of life of psoriatic patients [197]. The results of this trial also showed that SOD, and GSH-Px in plasma, erythrocytes, and skin biopsies were increased after treatment, while MDA level was decreased [198]. Propylthiouracil acts both on keratinocytes, increasing their differentiation, and on lymphocytes, the activation of which is lower after treatment [199,200].

Curcumin

Curcumin is a plant-derived compound that has anti-inflammatory and antioxidant properties. Few of the patients respond to oral curcumin. However, in patients who respond to curcumin, it has a strong effect as PASI is significantly reduced [201]. Nevertheless, oral curcumin in the lecithin system and in combination with a topical steroid showed higher efficacy because the PASI was significantly lower in the group treated with steroids and curcumin than in the group treated with curcumin alone. This therapy also significantly decreased the level of IL22 [202]. Moreover, curcumin reduces the activation and proliferation of lymphocytes and the production of various cytokines by them, including IFNγ, which is crucial for the development of psoriasis [203]. Curcumin also has the ability to activate the transcription factor Nrf2 [204]. This has resulted in the activation of apoptosis in the mitochondrial pathway, despite the fact that Nrf2 increases the transcription of Bcl2, which is an inhibitor of this pathway [205,206]. Overall, curcumin is probably not potent enough to be an effective antipsoriasis drug when used on its own, but it may support other pharmacological treatments.

Quercetin

Quercetin is a flavonoid abundant in many plants, including *Ginkgo biloba, Hypericum perforatum,* and *Houttuynia cordata Thunb* [207–209]. By modulating MAPK signaling and the NF-κB and Nrf-2 pathways, quercetin alleviates the symptoms of inflammatory diseases, including psoriasis [156,210]. In a mouse model of IMQ-induced psoriasis, quercetin lowers the PASI score and reduces epidermal thickness and parakeratosis found in skin from animals with induced psoriasis compared to controls. Treatment of quercetin also increases level of antioxidants, such as SOD, GSH, and CAT, while it reduces the lipid peroxidation assessed by the level of MDA [156].

Apigenin

Apigenin is a biologically active flavonoid found in large amounts in chrysanthemum extracts and has healing properties in inflammatory diseases. Apigenin has been shown to prevent the UVB-induced increase in cyclooxygenase-2 (COX-2) expression in keratinocyte cultures [211,212]. In a mouse model, apigenin-enriched diets have been shown to attenuate the development of atopic dermatitis-like lesions [213]. Moreover, apigenin prevents chronic inflammation and therefore can be used in protective preparations in psoriasis [214].

Luteolin

In case of this flavonoid, animal experiments indicated high efficacy. It action leads to amelioration of skin lesions. Additionally it decreases infiltration of skin by macrophages, lymphocytes, and neutrophils. Moreover, it downregulated the expression of cytokines like IL6, IL1β, TNFα, IL17A, and IL23 in both skin lesions and plasma. It may be caused by the fact that luteolin is a compound that has significant influence on macrophages. I mice macrophages cell line RAW 264.7 luteolin decreases expression of proinflammatory cytokines, like IL17, IL6, TNFα, and IL23.

In the case of this flavonoid, animal experiments have shown high efficacy in soothing skin lesions. It has been found to reduce the infiltration of the skin by macrophages, lymphocytes, and neutrophils and to lower the expression of cytokines such as IL6, IL1β, TNFα, IL17A, and IL23, both in skin lesions and in plasma [155]. This was confirmed by studies on macrophages of the RAW 264.7 mouse cell line, in which luteolin reduces the expression of proinflammatory cytokines such as IL17, IL6, TNFα, and IL23. Additionally, in the same cells, luteolin decreases level of prooxidative enzymes like inducible nitric oxide synthase (iNOS), which leads to lower level of nitric oxide as well as COX-2, which suggest lower generation of prostaglandins [155]. Luteolin also affects mouse lymphocytes in the IMQ-induced psoriasis model. Administration of this flavonoid leads to at least partial restoration of Th1/Th2 balance and also reduces the level of Th17 cells [154]. Nevertheless, luteolin not only affects the immune cells but also directly modifies the metabolism of keratinocytes. It reduces the production of Il6, Il8, and VEGF by human keratinocytes previously treated with TNFα. This flavonoid also reduces TNF induced mRNA expression of NFκB confirming its anti-inflammatory properties.

Lifestyle in psoriasis prevention

The oxidative-reductive as well as pro-/anti-inflammatory balance in the human body is regulated not only by genes, proteins, and other endogenous factors but also by various environmental stimuli. In the case of the skin, this is especially important because the skin is the outer shell of the body, which is influenced by all exogenous factors. The skin is also well supplied with tissue, so substances of both endogenous origin and those administered orally can easily penetrate the skin cells. The human environment contains many pro-oxidative and proinflammatory factors. Also, some components of the diet are anti- or pro-oxidative in nature. Regardless of exogenous factors, the redox balance is also determined by the state of our body. Therefore, both environmental factors and lifestyle can influence the development of psoriasis. It is therefore very likely that a change in diet or lifestyle can prevent the development and/or alleviate the symptoms of psoriasis.

Among the environmental factors, cigarette smoke is a known trigger of psoriasis. It has been shown that heavy smokers are more likely to suffer from psoriasis than non-smokers. In addition, psoriasis is more common in smokers than in those who have never smoked or never smoked [215,216], suggesting that quitting smoking may improve the effectiveness of antipsoriasis therapies. It is known that cigarette smoke is a source of ROS and other pro-oxidative factors; therefore, smoking may not only increase the risk of psoriasis but also reduce the effectiveness of therapy, as most of them are associated with the reduction of oxidative stress, and cigarette smoke acts as a stimulant.

On the other hand, the influence of overconsumption of alcohol on the development of psoriasis is less obvious. Beer consumption is known to increase the psoriasis disability index (PDI), and moderate amounts of wine, on the other hand, lower both PDI and Psoriasis Life Stress Inventory (PLSI) [217]. And people who regularly consume high doses of alcohol are more likely to suffer from psoriasis than people who consume less. On the other hand, people who do not drink alcohol at all are more likely to develop psoriasis than those who drink low amounts of alcohol [215]. This may be related to the pro-oxidative effect of ethanol. On the other hand, wines containing antioxidants, potentially up to certain limits, can protect against oxidative stress and the development of psoriasis.

The likelihood of developing psoriasis should be reduced by a diet rich in fruit and vegetables containing high amounts of natural antioxidants. For example, it has been shown that a high rate of β-carotene consumption correlates with a lower likelihood of developing psoriasis [218,219]. On the other hand, it was found in in vitro studies that a high concentration of β-carotene has a pro-oxidative effect on keratinocytes [220].

However, not only diet but also physical activity contributes to the development of psoriasis. It has been shown that patients who exercise regularly have less skin involvement than those who do not exercise [221]. Exercise has been shown to reduce the secretion of TNFα, a cytokine important in the pathophysiology of psoriasis [222]. In addition, obese people have elevated levels of Il6, also involved in the development of psoriasis [223]. Therefore, the influence of physical activity on the pro-/antioxidant balance also seems to be significant. Physical activity increases the activity of glutathione peroxidase in the blood and superoxide dismutase in erythrocytes [224]. Moreover, physical activity lowers the level of oxidized LDL and increases the resistance of LDL to oxidation [225]. Moreover, the reduction of TNFα levels may indirectly reduce the amount of ROS produced by neutrophils.

Therefore, it seems that an important element in alleviating the symptoms of psoriasis should be maintaining a healthy lifestyle by patients, including an appropriate diet, body weight, quitting smoking, and physical activity. Although the mechanisms responsible for the effects of the above-mentioned factors on psoriasis are unknown, their contribution to the pathogenesis of psoriasis appears to be well understood. While the results regarding the effects of alcohol on psoriasis are inconclusive, it appears that alcohol abuse may also be a trigger for psoriasis.

References

[1] Parisi R, Symmons DPM, Griffiths CEM, Ashcroft DM. Identification and management of psoriasis and associated comorbidity (IMPACT) project team global epidemiology of psoriasis: a systematic review of incidence and prevalence. J Invest Dermatol 2013;133:377–85. https://doi.org/10.1038/jid.2012.339.

[2] Mease PJ, Armstrong AW. Managing patients with psoriatic disease: the diagnosis and pharmacologic treatment of psoriatic arthritis in patients with psoriasis. Drugs 2014;74:423–41. https://doi.org/10.1007/s40265-014-0191-y.

[3] Hawkes JE, Chan TC, Krueger JG. Psoriasis pathogenesis and the development of novel targeted immune therapies. J Allergy Clin Immunol 2017;140:645–53. https://doi.org/10.1016/j.jaci.2017.07.004.

[4] Dowlatshahi EA, Wakkee M, Arends LR, Nijsten T. The prevalence and odds of depressive symptoms and clinical depression in psoriasis patients: a systematic review and meta-analysis. J Invest Dermatol 2014;134:1542–51. https://doi.org/10.1038/jid.2013.508.

[5] Gonçalves RSG, Pereira GA, de Andrade Lima E, Martins THF, Junior JOA, Carvalho JB, et al. Validation of the toronto psoriatic arthritis screen II (ToPAS II) questionnaire in a Brazilian population. Clin Rheumatol 2020. https://doi.org/10.1007/s10067-020-05509-2.

[6] Langley RGB, Krueger GG, Griffiths CEM. Psoriasis: epidemiology, clinical features, and quality of life. Ann Rheum Dis 2005;64:ii18–23. https://doi.org/10.1136/ard.2004.033217.

[7] Gelfand JM, Neimann AL, Shin DB, Wang X, Margolis DJ, Troxel AB. Risk of myocardial infarction in patients with psoriasis. JAMA 2006;296:1735–41. https://doi.org/10.1001/jama.296.14.1735.

[8] Miller IM, Ellervik C, Yazdanyar S, Jemec GBE. Meta-analysis of psoriasis, cardiovascular disease, and associated risk factors. J Am Acad Dermatol 2013;69:1014–24. https://doi.org/10.1016/j.jaad.2013.06.053.

[9] Wójcik P, Gegotek A, Wroński A, Jastrząb A, Żebrowska A, Skrzydlewska E. Effect of redox imbalance on protein modifications in lymphocytes of psoriatic patients. J Biochem 2020;167:323–31. https://doi.org/10.1093/jb/mvz096.

[10] Yang J, Yang X, Zou H, Li M. Oxidative stress and Treg and Th17 dysfunction in systemic lupus erythematosus. Oxid Med Cell Longev 2016;2016:2526174. https://doi.org/10.1155/2016/2526174.

[11] Delgoffe GM, Pollizzi KN, Waickman AT, Heikamp E, Meyers DJ, Horton MR, et al. The kinase MTOR regulates the differentiation of helper T cells through the selective activation of signaling by MTORC1 and MTORC2. Nat Immunol 2011;12:295–303. https://doi.org/10.1038/ni.2005.

[12] Zaba LC, Fuentes-Duculan J, Eungdamrong NJ, Abello MV, Novitskaya I, Pierson KC, et al. Psoriasis is characterized by accumulation of immunostimulatory and Th1/Th17 cell-polarizing myeloid dendritic cells. J Invest Dermatol 2009;129:79–88. https://doi.org/10.1038/jid.2008.194.

[13] Goodfield M. Skin lesions in psoriasis. Bailliere's Clin Rheumatol 1994;8:295–316. https://doi.org/10.1016/s0950-3579(94)80020-0.

[14] Nograles KE, Zaba LC, Guttman E, Fuentes-Duculan J, Suarez-Farinas M, Cardinale I, et al. Th17 cytokines interleukin (IL)-17 and IL-22 modulate distinct inflammatory and keratinocyte-response pathways. Br J Dermatol 2008;159:1092–102. https://doi.org/10.1111/j.1365-2133.2008.08769.x.

[15] Liang SC, Tan X-Y, Luxenberg DP, Karim R, Dunussi-Joannopoulos K, Collins M, Fouser LA. Interleukin (IL)-22 and IL-17 are coexpressed by Th17 cells and cooperatively enhance expression of antimicrobial peptides. J Exp Med 2006;203:2271–9. https://doi.org/10.1084/jem.20061308.

[16] Zhou Q, Mrowietz U, Rostami-Yazdi M. Oxidative stress in the pathogenesis of psoriasis. Free Radic Biol Med 2009;47:891–905. https://doi.org/10.1016/j.freeradbiomed.2009.06.033.

[17] Mavropoulos A, Rigopoulou EI, Liaskos C, Bogdanos DP, Sakkas LI. The role of P38 MAPK in the aetiopathogenesis of psoriasis and psoriatic arthritis. Clin Dev Immunol 2013;2013. https://doi.org/10.1155/2013/569751.

[18] Onderdijk AJ, Balak DMW, Baerveldt EM, Florencia EF, Kant M, Laman JD, et al. Regulated genes in psoriatic skin during treatment with fumaric acid esters. Br J Dermatol 2014;171:732–41. https://doi.org/10.1111/bjd.13128.

[19] Lowes MA, Bowcock AM, Krueger JG. Pathogenesis and therapy of psoriasis. Nature 2007;445:866–73. https://doi.org/10.1038/nature05663.

[20] Miraglia E, Nylén F, Johansson K, Arnér E, Cebula M, Farmand S, et al. Entinostat up-regulates the *CAMP* gene encoding LL-37 via activation of STAT3 and HIF-1α transcription factors. Sci Rep 2016;6:33274. https://doi.org/10.1038/srep33274.

[21] Świerkot J, Chlebicki A, Nowak B, Sokolik R, Wiland P, Szechiński J. Original paper the safety and efficacy of adalimumab for the treatment of ankylosing spondylitis (AS) and active psoriatic arthritis (PsA) in patients in a 16-week study. Reumatologia/Rheumatology 2007;45:248–57.

[22] FitzGerald O., Ogdie A., Chandran V., Coates L.C., Kavanaugh A., Tillett W., Leung Y.Y., deWit M., Scher J.U., Mease P.J. Psoriatic arthritis. Nat Rev Dis Primers 2021;7(1):59. https://doi.org/10.1038/s41572-021-00293-y. PMID: 34385474.

[23] Rosenberger C, Solovan C, Rosenberger AD, Jinping L, Treudler R, Frei U, et al. Upregulation of hypoxia-inducible factors in normal and psoriatic skin. J Invest Dermatol 2007;127:2445–52. https://doi.org/10.1038/sj.jid.5700874.

[24] McGarry T, Biniecka M, Veale DJ, Fearon U. Hypoxia, oxidative stress and inflammation. Free Radic Biol Med 2018;125:15–24. https://doi.org/10.1016/j.freeradbiomed.2018.03.042.

[25] Lipina C, Irving AJ, Hundal HS. Mitochondria: a possible nexus for the regulation of energy homeostasis by the endocannabinoid system? Am J Physiol Endocrinol Metab 2014;307:E1–13. https://doi.org/10.1152/ajpendo.00100.2014.

[26] Dan Dunn J, Alvarez LA, Zhang X, Soldati T. Reactive oxygen species and mitochondria: a nexus of cellular homeostasis. Redox Biol 2015;6:472–85. https://doi.org/10.1016/j.redox.2015.09.005.

[27] Wójcik P, Biernacki M, Wroński A, Łuczaj W, Waeg G, Žarković N, Skrzydlewska E. Altered lipid metabolism in blood mononuclear cells of psoriatic patients indicates differential changes in psoriasis vulgaris and psoriatic arthritis. Int J Mol Sci 2019;20:4249. https://doi.org/10.3390/ijms20174249.

[28] Ambrożewicz E, Wójcik P, Wroński A, Łuczaj W, Jastrząb A, Žarković N, Skrzydlewska E. Pathophysiological alterations of redox signaling and endocannabinoid system in granulocytes and plasma of psoriatic patients. Cells 2018;7. https://doi.org/10.3390/cells7100159.

[29] Barygina VV, Becatti M, Soldi G, Prignano F, Lotti T, Nassi P, et al. Altered redox status in the blood of psoriatic patients: involvement of NADPH oxidase and role of anti-TNF-α therapy. Redox Rep 2013;18:100–6. https://doi.org/10.1179/1351000213Y.0000000045.

[30] Ferretti G, Bacchetti T, Campanati A, Simonetti O, Liberati G, Offidani A. Correlation between lipoprotein(a) and lipid

peroxidation in psoriasis: role of the enzyme paraoxonase-1. Br J Dermatol 2012;166:204–7. https://doi.org/10.1111/j.1365-2133.2011.10539.x.

[31] Setta-Kaffetzi N, Simpson MA, Navarini AA, Patel VM, Lu H-C, Allen MH, et al. AP1S3 mutations are associated with pustular psoriasis and impaired toll-like receptor 3 trafficking. Am J Hum Genet 2014;94:790–7. https://doi.org/10.1016/j.ajhg.2014.04.005.

[32] Wójcik P, Garley M, Wroński A, Jabłońska E, Skrzydlewska E. Cannabidiol modifies the formation of NETs in neutrophils of psoriatic patients. Int J Mol Sci 2020;21:6795. https://doi.org/10.3390/ijms21186795.

[33] Milne GL, Yin H, Hardy KD, Davies SS, Roberts LJ. Isoprostane generation and function. Chem Rev 2011;111:5973–96. https://doi.org/10.1021/cr200160h.

[34] Dondelinger Y, Aguileta MA, Goossens V, Dubuisson C, Grootjans S, Dejardin E, et al. RIPK3 contributes to TNFR1-mediated RIPK1 kinase-dependent apoptosis in conditions of CIAP1/2 depletion or TAK1 kinase inhibition. Cell Death Differ 2013;20:1381–92. https://doi.org/10.1038/cdd.2013.94.

[35] Jiang Y, Yu M, Hu X, Han L, Yang K, Ba H, et al. STAT1 mediates transmembrane TNF-alpha-induced formation of death-inducing signaling complex and apoptotic signaling via TNFR1. Cell Death Differ 2017;24:660–71. https://doi.org/10.1038/cdd.2016.162.

[36] Kim J-Y, Park J-H. ROS-dependent caspase-9 activation in hypoxic cell death. FEBS Lett 2003;549:94–8. https://doi.org/10.1016/s0014-5793(03)00795-6.

[37] Greijer AE, van der Wall E. The role of hypoxia inducible factor 1 (HIF-1) in hypoxia induced apoptosis. J Clin Pathol 2004;57:1009–14. https://doi.org/10.1136/jcp.2003.015032.

[38] Wójcik P, Gegotek A, Žarković N, Skrzydlewska E. Disease-dependent antiapoptotic effects of cannabidiol for keratinocytes observed upon UV irradiation. Int J Mol Sci 2021;22:9956. https://doi.org/10.3390/ijms22189956.

[39] Wójcik P, Žarković N, Gegotek A, Skrzydlewska E. Involvement of metabolic lipid mediators in the regulation of apoptosis. Biomolecules 2020;10. https://doi.org/10.3390/biom10030402.

[40] Reuter S, Gupta SC, Chaturvedi MM, Aggarwal BB. Oxidative stress, inflammation, and cancer: how are they linked? Free Radic Biol Med 2010;49:1603–16. https://doi.org/10.1016/j.freeradbiomed.2010.09.006.

[41] Lowes MA, Chamian F, Abello MV, Fuentes-Duculan J, Lin S-L, Nussbaum R, et al. Increase in TNF-alpha and inducible nitric oxide synthase-expressing dendritic cells in psoriasis and reduction with efalizumab (anti-CD11a). Proc Natl Acad Sci USA 2005;102:19057–62. https://doi.org/10.1073/pnas.0509736102.

[42] Gokhale NR, Belgaumkar VA, Pandit DP, Deshpande S, Damle DK. A study of serum nitric oxide levels in psoriasis. Indian J Dermatol Venereol Leprol 2005;71:175. https://doi.org/10.4103/0378-6323.16232.

[43] Pazmandi K, Magyarics Z, Boldogh I, Csillag A, Rajnavolgyi E, Bacsi A. Modulatory effects of low-dose hydrogen peroxide on the function of human plasmacytoid dendritic cells. Free Radic Biol Med 2012;52:635–45. https://doi.org/10.1016/j.freeradbiomed.2011.11.022.

[44] Akhter N, Madhoun A, Arefanian H, Wilson A, Kochumon S, Thomas R, et al. Oxidative stress induces expression of the toll-like receptors (TLRs) 2 and 4 in the human peripheral blood mononuclear cells: implications for metabolic inflammation. Cell Physiol Biochem 2019;53:1–18.

[45] Rutault K, Alderman C, Chain BM, Katz DR. Reactive oxygen species activate human peripheral blood dendritic cells. Free Radic Biol Med 1999;26:232–8. https://doi.org/10.1016/s0891-5849(98)00194-4.

[46] Tan PH, Sagoo P, Chan C, Yates JB, Campbell J, Beutelspacher SC, et al. Inhibition of NF-KB and oxidative pathways in human dendritic cells by antioxidative vitamins generates regulatory T cells. J Immunol Res 2005;174:7633–44. https://doi.org/10.4049/jimmunol.174.12.7633.

[47] Qin T, Yin Y, Yu Q, Yang Q. Bursopentin (BP5) protects dendritic cells from lipopolysaccharide-induced oxidative stress for immunosuppression. PLoS One 2015;10. https://doi.org/10.1371/journal.pone.0117477.

[48] Park D, Jeong H, Lee MN, Koh A, Kwon O, Yang YR, et al. Resveratrol induces autophagy by directly inhibiting MTOR through ATP competition. Sci Rep 2016;6:21772. https://doi.org/10.1038/srep21772.

[49] Sizzano F, Collino S, Cominetti O, Monti D, Garagnani P, Ostan R, et al. Evaluation of lymphocyte response to the induced oxidative stress in a cohort of ageing subjects, including semi-supercentenarians and their offspring. Mediators Inflamm 2018;2018:7109312. https://doi.org/10.1155/2018/7109312.

[50] Lambert S, Hambro CA, Johnston A, Stuart PE, Tsoi LC, Nair RP, Elder JT. Neutrophil extracellular traps induce human Th17 cells: effect of psoriasis-associated TRAF3IP2 genotype. J Invest Dermatol 2019;139:1245–53. https://doi.org/10.1016/j.jid.2018.11.021.

[51] Lin AM, Rubin CJ, Khandpur R, Wang JY, Riblett M, Yalavarthi S, et al. Mast cells and neutrophils release IL-17 through extracellular trap formation in psoriasis. J Immunol 2011;187:490–500. https://doi.org/10.4049/jimmunol.1100123.

[52] Sirsjö A, Karlsson M, Gidlöf A, Rollman O, Törmä H. Increased expression of inducible nitric oxide synthase in psoriatic skin and cytokine-stimulated cultured keratinocytes. Br J Dermatol 1996;134:643–8. https://doi.org/10.1111/j.1365-2133.1996.tb06963.x.

[53] Wang W, Yuhai, Wang H, Chasuna, Bagenna. Astilbin reduces ROS accumulation and VEGF expression through Nrf2 in psoriasis-like skin disease. Biol Res 2019;52. https://doi.org/10.1186/s40659-019-0255-2.

[54] Yang L, Fan X, Cui T, Dang E, Wang G. Nrf2 promotes keratinocyte proliferation in psoriasis through up-regulation of keratin 6, keratin 16, and keratin 17. J Invest Dermatol 2017;137:2168–76. https://doi.org/10.1016/j.jid.2017.05.015.

[55] Halliwell B, Chirico S. Lipid peroxidation: its mechanism, measurement, and significance. Am J Clin Nutr 1993;57:715S–25S. https://doi.org/10.1093/ajcn/57.5.715S.

[56] Łuczaj W, Dobrzyńska I, Wroński A, Domingues MR, Domingues P, Skrzydlewska E. Cannabidiol-mediated changes to the phospholipid profile of UVB-irradiated keratinocytes from psoriatic patients. Int J Mol Sci 2020;21:6592.

[57] Jarocka-Karpowicz I, Biernacki M, Wroński A, Gegotek A, Skrzydlewska E. Cannabidiol effects on phospholipid metabolism in keratinocytes from patients with psoriasis vulgaris. Biomolecules 2020;10. https://doi.org/10.3390/biom10030367.

[58] Sen T, Sen N, Tripathi G, Chatterjee U, Chakrabarti S. Lipid peroxidation associated cardiolipin loss and membrane depolarization

in rat brain mitochondria. Neurochem Int 2006;49:20–7. https://doi.org/10.1016/j.neuint.2005.12.018.

[59] Ayala A, Muñoz MF, Argüelles S. Lipid peroxidation: production, metabolism, and signaling mechanisms of malondialdehyde and 4-hydroxy-2-nonenal. Oxid Med Cell Longev 2014;2014:360438. https://doi.org/10.1155/2014/360438.

[60] Río CD, Millán E, García V, Appendino G, DeMesa J, Muñoz E. The endocannabinoid system of the skin. A potential approach for the treatment of skin disorders. Biochem Pharmacol 2018;157:122–33. https://doi.org/10.1016/j.bcp.2018.08.022.

[61] Di Marzo V. Endocannabinoids: synthesis and degradation. Rev Physiol Biochem Pharmacol 2008;160:1–24. https://doi.org/10.1007/112_0505.

[62] Sheriff T, Lin MJ, Dubin D, Khorasani H. The potential role of cannabinoids in dermatology. J Dermatol Treat 2019:1–7. https://doi.org/10.1080/09546634.2019.1675854.

[63] Bíró T, Tóth BI, Haskó G, Paus R, Pacher P. The endocannabinoid system of the skin in health and disease: novel perspectives and therapeutic opportunities. Trends Pharmacol Sci 2009;30:411–20.

[64] Tóth KF, Ádám D, Bíró T, Oláh A. Cannabinoid signaling in the skin: therapeutic potential of the "C(Ut)Annabinoid" system. Molecules 2019;24. https://doi.org/10.3390/molecules24050918.

[65] Han KH, Lim S, Ryu J, Lee C-W, Kim Y, Kang J-H, et al. CB1 and CB2 cannabinoid receptors differentially regulate the production of reactive oxygen species by macrophages. Cardiovasc Res 2009;84:378–86. https://doi.org/10.1093/cvr/cvp240.

[66] Chiurchiù V, Cencioni MT, Bisicchia E, Bardi MD, Gasperini C, Borsellino G, et al. Distinct modulation of human myeloid and plasmacytoid dendritic cells by anandamide in multiple sclerosis. Ann Neurol 2013;73:626–36. https://doi.org/10.1002/ana.23875.

[67] Liu B, Qu L, Yan S. Cyclooxygenase-2 promotes tumor growth and suppresses tumor immunity. Cancer Cell Int 2015;15:106. https://doi.org/10.1186/s12935-015-0260-7.

[68] Brash AR. Lipoxygenases: a chronological perspective on the synthesis of S and R fatty acid hydroperoxides. In: Yokomizo T, Murakami M, editors. Bioactive lipid mediators: current reviews and protocols. Tokyo: Springer Japan; 2015, ISBN 978-4-431-55669-5. p. 69–84.

[69] Muralikrishna Adibhatla R, Hatcher JF. Phospholipase A2, reactive oxygen species, and lipid peroxidation in cerebral ischemia. Free Radic Biol Med 2006;40:376–87. https://doi.org/10.1016/j.freeradbiomed.2005.08.044.

[70] Caslake MJ, Packard CJ, Suckling KE, Holmes SD, Chamberlain P, Macphee CH. Lipoprotein-associated phospholipase A2, platelet-activating factor acetylhydrolase: a potential new risk factor for coronary artery disease. Atherosclerosis 2000;150:413–9. https://doi.org/10.1016/S0021-9150(99)00406-2.

[71] Christie PE, Henderson WR. Lipid inflammatory mediators: leukotrienes, prostaglandins, platelet-activating factor. Clin Allergy Immunol 2002;16:233–54.

[72] Lone AM, Taskén K. Proinflammatory and immunoregulatory roles of eicosanoids in T cells. Front Immunol 2013;4. https://doi.org/10.3389/fimmu.2013.00130.

[73] Tilley SL, Coffman TM, Koller BH. Mixed messages: modulation of inflammation and immune responses by prostaglandins and thromboxanes. J Clin Invest 2001;108:15–23. https://doi.org/10.1172/JCI13416.

[74] Coras R, Kavanaugh A, Boyd T, Huynh Q, Pedersen B, Armando AM, et al. Pro- and anti-inflammatory eicosanoids in psoriatic arthritis. Metabolomics 2019;15:65. https://doi.org/10.1007/s11306-019-1527-0.

[75] Sorokin AV, Domenichiello AF, Dey AK, Yuan Z-X, Goyal A, Rose SM, et al. Bioactive lipid mediator profiles in human psoriasis skin and blood. J Invest Dermatol 2018;138:1518–28. https://doi.org/10.1016/j.jid.2018.02.003.

[76] Ueharaguchi Y, Honda T, Kusuba N, Hanakawa S, Adachi A, Sawada Y, et al. Thromboxane A2 facilitates IL-17A production from Vγ4+ Γδ T cells and promotes psoriatic dermatitis in mice. J Allergy Clin Immunol 2018;142:680–683.e2. https://doi.org/10.1016/j.jaci.2018.01.054.

[77] Paul S, Traver MK, Kashyap AK, Washington MA, Latoche JR, Schaefer BC. T cell receptor signals to NF-KB are transmitted by a cytosolic p62-Bcl10-Malt1-IKK signalosome. Sci Signal 2014;7:ra45. https://doi.org/10.1126/scisignal.2004882.

[78] Honda T, Kabashima K. Prostanoids and leukotrienes in the pathophysiology of atopic dermatitis and psoriasis. Int Immunol 2019;31:589–95. https://doi.org/10.1093/intimm/dxy087.

[79] Lee J, Aoki T, Thumkeo D, Siriwach R, Yao C, Narumiya S. T cell-intrinsic prostaglandin E2-EP2/EP4 signaling is critical in pathogenic TH17 cell-driven inflammation. J Allergy Clin Immunol 2019;143:631–43. https://doi.org/10.1016/j.jaci.2018.05.036.

[80] Lowes MA, Suarez-Farinas M, Krueger JG. Immunology of psoriasis. Annu Rev Immunol 2014;32:227–55.

[81] Zeichner JA, Armstrong A. The role of IL-17 in the pathogenesis and treatment of psoriasis. J Clin Aesthet Dermatol 2016;9:S3–6.

[82] Gegotek A, Domingues P, Wroński A, Wójcik P, Skrzydlewska E. Proteomic plasma profile of psoriatic patients. J Pharm Biomed Anal 2018;155:185–93. https://doi.org/10.1016/j.jpba.2018.03.068.

[83] Christoffersen C, Jauhiainen M, Moser M, Porse B, Ehnholm C, Boesl M, et al. Effect of apolipoprotein M on high density lipoprotein metabolism and atherosclerosis in low density lipoprotein receptor knock-out mice. J Biol Chem 2008;283:1839–47. https://doi.org/10.1074/jbc.M704576200.

[84] Campalani E, Allen MH, Fairhurst D, Young HS, Mendonca CO, Burden AD, et al. Apolipoprotein E gene polymorphisms are associated with psoriasis but do not determine disease response to acitretin. Br J Dermatol 2006;154:345–52. https://doi.org/10.1111/j.1365-2133.2005.06950.x.

[85] Christoffersen C, Nielsen LB. Apolipoprotein M: bridging HDL and endothelial function. Curr Opin Lipidol 2013;24:295–300. https://doi.org/10.1097/MOL.0b013e328361f6ad.

[86] Mallbris L, Granath F, Hamsten A, Ståhle M. Psoriasis is associated with lipid abnormalities at the onset of skin disease. J Am Acad Dermatol 2006;54:614–21. https://doi.org/10.1016/j.jaad.2005.11.1079.

[87] Maley F, Trimble RB, Tarentino AL, Plummer TH. Characterization of glycoproteins and their associated oligosaccharides through the use of endoglycosidases. Anal Biochem 1989;180:195–204.

[88] Reindl J, Pesek J, Krüger T, Wendler S, Nemitz S, Muckova P, et al. Proteomic biomarkers for psoriasis and psoriasis arthritis. J Proteonomics 2016;140:55–61. https://doi.org/10.1016/j.jprot.2016.03.040.

[89] Hailman E, Lichenstein HS, Wurfel MM, Miller DS, Johnson DA, Kelley M, et al. Lipopolysaccharide (LPS)-binding protein accelerates the binding of LPS to CD14. J Exp Med 1994;179:269–77.

[90] de Jongh GJ, Zeeuwen PLJM, Kucharekova M, Pfundt R, van der Valk PG, Blokx W, et al. High expression levels of keratinocyte antimicrobial proteins in psoriasis compared with atopic dermatitis. J Invest Dermatol 2005;125:1163–73. https://doi.org/10.1111/j.0022-202X.2005.23935.x.

[91] Romaní J, Caixàs A, Escoté X, Carrascosa JM, Ribera M, Rigla M, et al. Lipopolysaccharide-binding protein is increased in patients with psoriasis with metabolic syndrome, and correlates with C-reactive protein. Clin Exp Dermatol 2013;38:81–4. https://doi.org/10.1111/ced.12007.

[92] Prasad C, Davis KE, Imrhan V, Juma S, Vijayagopal P. Advanced glycation end products and risks for chronic diseases: intervening through lifestyle modification. Am J Lifestyle Med 2017;13:384–404. https://doi.org/10.1177/1559827617708991.

[93] Papagrigoraki A, Maurelli M, del Giglio M, Gisondi P, Girolomoni G. Advanced glycation end products in the pathogenesis of psoriasis. Int J Mol Sci 2017;18:2471. https://doi.org/10.3390/ijms18112471.

[94] Teodorowicz M, Hendriks WH, Wichers HJ, Savelkoul HFJ. Immunomodulation by processed animal feed: the role of maillard reaction products and advanced glycation end-products (AGEs). Front Immunol 2018;9:2088. https://doi.org/10.3389/fimmu.2018.02088.

[95] Ott C, Jacobs K, Haucke E, Navarrete Santos A, Grune T, Simm A. Role of advanced glycation end products in cellular signaling. Redox Biol 2014;2:411–29. https://doi.org/10.1016/j.redox.2013.12.016.

[96] Sparvero LJ, Asafu-Adjei D, Kang R, Tang D, Amin N, Im J, et al. RAGE (receptor for advanced glycation endproducts), RAGE ligands, and their role in cancer and inflammation. J Transl Med 2009;7:17. https://doi.org/10.1186/1479-5876-7-17.

[97] Shi Y, Sandoghchian Shotorbani S, Su Z, Liu Y, Tong J, Zheng D, et al. Enhanced HMGB1 expression may contribute to Th17 cells activation in rheumatoid arthritis. Clin Dev Immunol 2012;2012. https://doi.org/10.1155/2012/295081.

[98] Damasiewicz-Bodzek A, Wielkoszyński T. Advanced protein glycation in psoriasis. J Eur Acad Dermatol Venereol 2012;26:172–9. https://doi.org/10.1111/j.1468-3083.2011.04024.x.

[99] Moldogazieva NT, Mokhosoev IM, Mel'nikova TI, Porozov YB, Terentiev AA. Oxidative stress and advanced lipoxidation and glycation end products (ALEs and AGEs) in aging and age-related diseases. Oxid Med Cell Longev 2019;2019:3085756. https://doi.org/10.1155/2019/3085756.

[100] Vistoli G, De Maddis D, Cipak A, Zarkovic N, Carini M, Aldini G. Advanced glycoxidation and lipoxidation end products (AGEs and ALEs): an overview of their mechanisms of formation. Free Radic Res 2013;47(1):3–27. https://doi.org/10.3109/10715762.2013.815348.

[101] Popoff MR, Geny B. Multifaceted role of Rho, Rac, Cdc42 and Ras in intercellular junctions, lessons from toxins. Biochim Biophys Acta Biomembr 2009;1788:797–812. https://doi.org/10.1016/j.bbamem.2009.01.011.

[102] Biro M, Munoz MA, Weninger W. Targeting Rho-GTPases in immune cell migration and inflammation. Br J Pharmacol 2014;171:5491–506. https://doi.org/10.1111/bph.12658.

[103] Shearn CT, Fritz KS, Reigan P, Petersen DR. Modification of Akt2 by 4-hydroxynonenal inhibits insulin-dependent Akt signaling in HepG2 cells. Biochemistry 2011;50:3984–96. https://doi.org/10.1021/bi200029w.

[104] Ji G, Yu N, Xue X, Li Z. 4-Hydroxy-2-nonenal induces apoptosis by inhibiting AKT signaling in human osteosarcoma cells. Sci World J 2014. Available online: https://www.hindawi.com/journals/tswj/2014/873525/. [Accessed 29 November 2018].

[105] 196029.Pdf.

[106] Roller A, Perino A, Dapavo P, Soro E, Okkenhaug K, Hirsch E, Ji H. Blockade of phosphatidylinositol 3-kinase (PI3K)δ or PI3Kγ reduces IL-17 and ameliorates imiquimod-induced psoriasis-like dermatitis. J Immunol 2012;189:4612–20. https://doi.org/10.4049/jimmunol.1103173. Epub 2012 Sep 28. PMID: 23024273.

[107] Guiducci C, Ghirelli C, Marloie-Provost M-A, Matray T, Coffman RL, Liu Y-J, et al. PI3K is critical for the nuclear translocation of IRF-7 and type I IFN production by human plasmacytoid predendritic cells in response to TLR activation. J Exp Med 2008;205:315–22. https://doi.org/10.1084/jem.20070763.

[108] Calautti E, Li J, Saoncella S, Brissette JL, Goetinck PF. Phosphoinositide 3-kinase signaling to Akt promotes keratinocyte differentiation versus death. J Biol Chem 2005;280:32856–65. https://doi.org/10.1074/jbc.M506119200.

[109] Monks CR, Kupfer H, Tamir I, Barlow A, Kupfer A. Selective modulation of protein kinase C-theta during T-cell activation. Nature 1997;385:83–6. https://doi.org/10.1038/385083a0.

[110] Bauer B, Krumböck N, Ghaffari-Tabrizi N, Kampfer S, Villunger A, Wilda M, et al. T cell expressed PKCtheta demonstrates cell-type selective function. Eur J Immunol 2000;30:3645–54. https://doi.org/10.1002/1521-4141(200012)30:12<3645::AID-IMMU3645>3.0.CO;2-#.

[111] Skvara H, Dawid M, Kleyn E, Wolff B, Meingassner JG, Knight H, et al. The PKC inhibitor AEB071 may be a therapeutic option for psoriasis. J Clin Invest 2008;118:3151–9. https://doi.org/10.1172/JCI35636.

[112] Manicassamy S, Gupta S, Sun Z. Selective function of PKC-theta in T cells. Cell Mol Immunol 2006;3:263–70.

[113] Basavaraj Kh, Vasu Devaraju P, Rao Ks. Studies on serum 8-hydroxy guanosine (8-OHdG) as reliable biomarker for psoriasis. J Eur Acad Dermatol Venereol 2013;27:655–7. https://doi.org/10.1111/j.1468-3083.2011.04441.x.

[114] Ghosh R, Mitchell DL. Effect of oxidative DNA damage in promoter elements on transcription factor binding. Nucleic Acids Res 1999;27:3213–8. https://doi.org/10.1093/nar/27.15.3213.

[115] Karin M, Liu ZG, Zandi E. AP-1 function and regulation. Curr Opin Cell Biol 1997;9:240–6.

[116] Beishline K, Azizkhan-Clifford J. Sp1 and the "hallmarks of cancer.". FEBS J 2015;282:224–58. https://doi.org/10.1111/febs.13148.

[117] Dwyer KM, Deaglio S, Gao W, Friedman D, Strom TB, Robson SC. CD39 and control of cellular immune responses. Purinergic Signal 2007;3:171–80. https://doi.org/10.1007/s11302-006-9050-y.

[118] Dimon-Gadal S, Gerbaud P, Guibourdenche J, Evain-Brion D, Raynaud F, Thérond P, Anderson WB. Increased oxidative damage to fibroblasts in skin with and without lesions in psoriasis. J Invest Dermatol 2000;114:984–9. https://doi.org/10.1046/j.1523-1747.2000.00962.x.

[119] Yazici C, Köse K, Utaş S, Tanrikulu E, Taşlidere N. A novel approach in psoriasis: first usage of known protein oxidation markers to prove oxidative stress. Arch Dermatol Res 2016;308:207–12. https://doi.org/10.1007/s00403-016-1624-0.

[120] Elliott PJ, Zollner TM, Boehncke W-H. Proteasome inhibition: a new anti-inflammatory strategy. J Mol Med 2003;81:235–45. https://doi.org/10.1007/s00109-003-0422-2.

[121] Kwak M-K, Wakabayashi N, Greenlaw JL, Yamamoto M, Kensler TW. Antioxidants enhance mammalian proteasome expression through the Keap1-Nrf2 signaling pathway. Mol Cell Biol 2003;23:8786–94. https://doi.org/10.1128/MCB.23.23.8786-8794.2003.

[122] Weiss YG, Bromberg Z, Raj N, Raphael J, Goloubinoff P, Ben-Neriah Y, Deutschman CS. Enhanced heat shock protein 70 expression alters proteasomal degradation of IkappaB kinase in experimental acute respiratory distress syndrome. Crit Care Med 2007;35:2128–38. https://doi.org/10.1097/01.ccm.0000278915.78030.74.

[123] Gegotek A, Domingues P, Wroński A, Skrzydlewska E. Changes in proteome of fibroblasts isolated from psoriatic skin lesions. Int J Mol Sci 2020;21:5363. https://doi.org/10.3390/ijms21155363.

[124] Zollner TM, Podda M, Pien C, Elliott PJ, Kaufmann R, Boehncke W-H. Proteasome inhibition reduces superantigen-mediated T cell activation and the severity of psoriasis in a SCID-hu model. J Clin Invest 2002;109:671–9. https://doi.org/10.1172/JCI12736.

[125] Cuzzocrea S, McDonald MC, Mazzon E, Siriwardena D, Serraino I, Dugo L, et al. Calpain inhibitor I reduces the development of acute and chronic inflammation. Am J Pathol 2000;157:2065–79. https://doi.org/10.1016/S0002-9440(10)64845-6.

[126] Matsushita Y, Shimada Y, Kawara S, Takehara K, Sato S. Autoantibodies directed against the protease inhibitor calpastatin in psoriasis. Clin Exp Immunol 2005;139:355–62. https://doi.org/10.1111/j.1365-2249.2005.02701.x.

[127] Lei H, Li X, Jing B, Xu H, Wu Y. Human S100A7 induces mature interleukin1α expression by RAGE-P38 MAPK-calpain1 pathway in psoriasis. PLoS One 2017;12:e0169788. https://doi.org/10.1371/journal.pone.0169788.

[128] Leloup L, Mazères G, Daury L, Cottin P, Brustis J-J. Involvement of calpains in growth factor-mediated migration. Int J Biochem Cell Biol 2006;38:2049–63. https://doi.org/10.1016/j.biocel.2006.04.012.

[129] Ekman A-K, Vegfors J, Eding CB, Enerbäck C. Overexpression of psoriasin (S100A7) contributes to dysregulated differentiation in psoriasis. Acta Derm Venereol 2017;97:441–8. https://doi.org/10.2340/00015555-2596.

[130] Schonthaler HB, Guinea-Viniegra J, Wculek SK, Ruppen I, Ximénez-Embún P, Guío-Carrión A, et al. S100A8-S100A9 protein complex mediates psoriasis by regulating the expression of complement factor C3. Immunity 2013;39:1171–81. https://doi.org/10.1016/j.immuni.2013.11.011.

[131] Kerkhoff C, Voss A, Scholzen TE, Averill MM, Zänker KS, Bornfeldt KE. Novel insights into the role of S100A8/A9 in skin biology. Exp Dermatol 2012;21:822–6. https://doi.org/10.1111/j.1600-0625.2012.01571.x.

[132] Raaby L, Otkjær K, Salvskov-Iversen ML, Johansen C, Iversen L. A characterization of the expression of 14-3-3 isoforms in psoriasis, basal cell carcinoma, atopic dermatitis and contact dermatitis. Dermatol Rep 2010;2:e14. https://doi.org/10.4081/dr.2010.e14.

[133] Lodygin D, Yazdi AS, Sander CA, Herzinger T, Hermeking H. Analysis of 14-3-3sigma expression in hyperproliferative skin diseases reveals selective loss associated with CpG-methylation in basal cell carcinoma. Oncogene 2003;22:5519–24. https://doi.org/10.1038/sj.onc.1206854.

[134] Carlén LM, Sánchez F, Bergman A-C, Becker S, Hirschberg D, Franzén B, et al. Proteome analysis of skin distinguishes acute guttate from chronic plaque psoriasis. J Invest Dermatol 2005;124:63–9. https://doi.org/10.1111/j.0022-202X.2004.23501.x.

[135] Man X, Zhang X, Tang J, Chen Y, Li H, Xu B, Pan L. Down-regulation of 14-3-3β and 14-3-3ζ in lesions of psoriasis vulgaris. Clin Exp Dermatol 2013;38:390–5. https://doi.org/10.1111/ced.12014.

[136] Chamcheu JC, Chaves-Rodriquez M-I, Adhami VM, Siddiqui IA, Wood GS, Longley BJ, Mukhtar H. Upregulation of PI3K/AKT/MTOR, FABP5 and PPARβ/δ in human psoriasis and imiquimod-induced murine psoriasiform dermatitis model. Acta Derm Venereol 2016;96:854–6. https://doi.org/10.2340/00015555-2359.

[137] Fu H, Subramanian RR, Masters SC. 14-3-3 proteins: structure, function, and regulation. Annu Rev Pharmacol Toxicol 2000;40:617–47. https://doi.org/10.1146/annurev.pharmtox.40.1.617.

[138] Rendon A, Schäkel K. Psoriasis pathogenesis and treatment. Int J Mol Sci 2019;20. https://doi.org/10.3390/ijms20061475.

[139] Elango T, Dayalan H, Gnanaraj P, Malligarjunan H, Subramanian S. Impact of methotrexate on oxidative stress and apoptosis markers in psoriatic patients. Clin Exp Med 2014;14:431–7. https://doi.org/10.1007/s10238-013-0252-7.

[140] Gross B, Staels B. PPAR agonists: multimodal drugs for the treatment of type-2 diabetes. Best Pract Res Clin Endocrinol Metab 2007;21:687–710. https://doi.org/10.1016/j.beem.2007.09.004.

[141] Sertznig P, Reichrath J. Peroxisome proliferator-activated receptors (PPARs) in dermatology. Dermatoendocrinol 2011;3:130–5. https://doi.org/10.4161/derm.3.3.15025.

[142] Mastrofrancesco A, Kovacs D, Sarra M, Bastonini E, Cardinali G, Aspite N, et al. Preclinical studies of a specific PPARγ modulator in the control of skin inflammation. J Invest Dermatol 2014;134:1001–11. https://doi.org/10.1038/jid.2013.448.

[143] Colombo MD, Cassano N, Bellia G, Vena GA. Cyclosporine regimens in plaque psoriasis: an overview with special emphasis on dose, duration, and old and new treatment approaches. Sci World J 2013;2013:805705. https://doi.org/10.1155/2013/805705.

[144] Schmidt KN, Podda M, Packer L, Baeuerle PA. Anti-psoriatic drug anthralin activates transcription factor NF-kappa B in murine keratinocytes. J Immunol 1996;156:4514–9.

[145] Narayanan DL, Saladi RN, Fox JL. Ultraviolet radiation and skin cancer. Int J Dermatol 2010;49:978–86. https://doi.org/10.1111/j.1365-4632.2010.04474.x.

[146] Larroque-Cardoso P, Camaré C, Nadal-Wollbold F, Grazide M-H, Pucelle M, Garoby-Salom S, et al. Elastin modification by 4-hydroxynonenal in hairless mice exposed to UV-A. Role in photoaging and actinic elastosis. J Invest Dermatol 2015;135:1873–81. https://doi.org/10.1038/jid.2015.84.

[147] Abo Elnazar SY, Ghazy AA, Ghoneim HE, Taha A-RM, Abouelella AM. Effect of ultraviolet irradiation on the interplay

between Th1 and Th2 lymphocytes. Front Pharmacol 2015;6:56. https://doi.org/10.3389/fphar.2015.00056.

[148] Jasek-Gajda E, Jurkowska H, Jasińska M, Lis GJ. Targeting the MAPK/ERK and PI3K/AKT signaling pathways affects NRF2, Trx and GSH antioxidant systems in leukemia cells. Antioxidants 2020;9:633. https://doi.org/10.3390/antiox9070633.

[149] Yin K, Agrawal DK. Vitamin D and inflammatory diseases. J Inflamm Res 2014;7:69−87. https://doi.org/10.2147/JIR.S63898.

[150] Mousa A, Misso M, Teede H, Scragg R, Courten B. de Effect of vitamin D supplementation on inflammation: protocol for a systematic review. BMJ Open 2016;6:e010804. https://doi.org/10.1136/bmjopen-2015-010804.

[151] Ke C-Y, Yang F-L, Wu W-T, Chung C-H, Lee R-P, Yang W-T, et al. Vitamin D3 reduces tissue damage and oxidative stress caused by exhaustive exercise. Int J Med Sci 2016;13:147−53. https://doi.org/10.7150/ijms.13746.

[152] Tsuji F, Miyake Y, Aono H, Kawashima Y, Mita S. Effects of bucillamine and N-acetyl-l-cysteine on cytokine production and collagen-induced arthritis (CIA). Clin Exp Immunol 1999;115:26−31. https://doi.org/10.1046/j.1365-2249.1999.00749.x.

[153] Pathirana D, Ormerod AD, Saiag P, Smith C, Spuls PI, Nast A, et al. European S3-guidelines on the systemic treatment of psoriasis vulgaris. J Eur Acad Dermatol Venereol 2009;23(2):1−70. https://doi.org/10.1111/j.1468-3083.2009.03389.x.

[154] Lv J, Zhou D, Wang Y, Sun W, Zhang C, Xu J, et al. Effects of luteolin on treatment of psoriasis by repressing HSP90. Int Immunopharmacol 2020;79:106070. https://doi.org/10.1016/j.intimp.2019.106070.

[155] Zhou W, Hu M, Zang X, Liu Q, Du J, Hu J, et al. Luteolin attenuates imiquimod-induced psoriasis-like skin lesions in BALB/c mice via suppression of inflammation response. Biomed Pharmacother 2020;131:110696. https://doi.org/10.1016/j.biopha.2020.110696.

[156] Chen H, Lu C, Liu H, Wang M, Zhao H, Yan Y, Han L. Quercetin ameliorates imiquimod-induced psoriasis-like skin inflammation in mice via the NF-KB pathway. Int Immunopharmacol 2017;48:110−7. https://doi.org/10.1016/j.intimp.2017.04.022.

[157] Man M-Q, Hupe M, Sun R, Man G, Mauro TM, Elias PM. Topical apigenin alleviates cutaneous inflammation in murine models. Evid Based Complement Altern Med 2012;2012:912028. https://doi.org/10.1155/2012/912028.

[158] Ooko E, Kadioglu O, Greten HJ, Efferth T. Pharmacogenomic characterization and isobologram analysis of the combination of ascorbic acid and curcumin—two main metabolites of Curcuma longa—in cancer cells. Front Pharmacol 2017;8:38. https://doi.org/10.3389/fphar.2017.00038.

[159] Lee C, Park GH, Ahn E, Kim B-A, Park C-I, Jang J-H. Protective effect of *Codium fragile* against UVB-induced pro-inflammatory and oxidative damages in HaCaT cells and BALB/c mice. Fitoterapia 2013;86. https://doi.org/10.1016/j.fitote.2013.01.020.

[160] Fogagnolo Mauricio A, Minatel E, Santo Neto H, Marques MJ. Effects of fish oil containing eicosapentaenoic acid and docosahexaenoic acid on dystrophic mdx mice. Clin Nutr 2013;32:636−42. https://doi.org/10.1016/j.clnu.2012.11.013.

[161] Zhao Y, Joshi-Barve S, Barve S, Chen LH. Eicosapentaenoic acid prevents LPS-induced TNF-alpha expression by preventing NF-kappaB activation. J Am Coll Nutr 2004;23:71−8. https://doi.org/10.1080/07315724.2004.10719345.

[162] Moreno JJ. Differential effects of arachidonic and eicosapentaenoic acid-derived eicosanoids on polymorphonuclear transmigration across endothelial cell cultures. J Pharmacol Exp Ther 2009;331:1111−7. https://doi.org/10.1124/jpet.109.157891.

[163] Zuccotti E, Oliveri M, Girometta C, Ratto D, Di Iorio C, Occhinegro A, Rossi P. Nutritional strategies for psoriasis: current scientific evidence in clinical trials. Eur Rev Med Pharmacol Sci 2018;22:8537−51. https://doi.org/10.26355/eurrev_201812_16554.

[164] Wu Y, Zhao D, Zhuang J, Zhang F, Xu C. Caspase-8 and caspase-9 functioned differently at different stages of the cyclic stretch-induced apoptosis in human periodontal ligament cells. PLoS One 2016;11:e0168268. https://doi.org/10.1371/journal.pone.0168268.

[165] Deshmukh J, Pofahl R, Haase I. Epidermal Rac1 regulates the DNA damage response and protects from UV-light-induced keratinocyte apoptosis and skin carcinogenesis. Cell Death Dis 2017;8:e2664. https://doi.org/10.1038/cddis.2017.63.

[166] Noh D, Choi JG, Huh E, Oh MS. Tectorigenin, a flavonoid-based compound of leopard lily rhizome, attenuates UV-B-induced apoptosis and collagen degradation by inhibiting oxidative stress in human keratinocytes. Nutrients 2018;10. https://doi.org/10.3390/nu10121998.

[167] Rasheva VI, Domingos PM. Cellular responses to endoplasmic reticulum stress and apoptosis. Apoptosis 2009;14:996−1007. https://doi.org/10.1007/s10495-009-0341-y.

[168] Soonthornchai W, Tangtanatakul P, Meephansan J, Ruchusatsawat K, Reantragoon R, Hirankarn N, Wongpiyabovorn J. Down-regulation of MiR-155 after treatment with narrow-band UVB and methotrexate associates with apoptosis of keratinocytes in psoriasis. Asian Pac J Allergy Immunol 2019. https://doi.org/10.12932/AP-031218-0451.

[169] Morita A. Current developments in phototherapy for psoriasis. J Dermatol 2018;45:287−92. https://doi.org/10.1111/1346-8138.14213.

[170] Fattouh M, El-Din AN, El-Hamd MA. Role of lymphocyte subpopulations in the immunopathogenesis of psoriasis and the effect of narrow band UVB phototherapy on the immunological profile of psoriasis patients. Egypt J Immunol 2017;24:105−17.

[171] Tobin AM, Maguire B, Enright H, Kirby B. The effects of phototherapy on the numbers of circulating natural killer cells and T lymphocytes in psoriasis. Photodermatol Photoimmunol Photomed 2009;25:109−10. https://doi.org/10.1111/j.1600-0781.2009.00409.x.

[172] Zhang P, Wu MXA. Clinical review of phototherapy for psoriasis. Lasers Med Sci 2018;33:173−80. https://doi.org/10.1007/s10103-017-2360-1.

[173] Dobrzyńska I, Szachowicz-Petelska B, Skrzydlewska E, Figaszewski ZA. Effects of UVB radiation on the physicochemical properties of fibroblasts and keratinocytes. J Membr Biol 2016;249:319−25. https://doi.org/10.1007/s00232-016-9870-9.

[174] Kim KM, Im A-R, Park SK, Shin HS, Chae S-W. Protective effects of timosaponin AIII against UVB-radiation induced inflammation and DNA injury in human epidermal keratinocytes. Biol Pharm Bull 2019;42:1524−31. https://doi.org/10.1248/bpb.b19-00222.

[175] Koga Y, Tsurumaki H, Aoki-Saito H, Sato M, Yatomi M, Takehara K, Hisada T. Roles of cyclic AMP response element binding activation in the ERK1/2 and P38 MAPK signalling pathway in central nervous system, cardiovascular system, osteoclast differentiation and mucin and cytokine production. Int J Mol Sci 2019;20. https://doi.org/10.3390/ijms20061346.

[176] Cuadrado A, Nebreda AR. Mechanisms and functions of P38 MAPK signalling. Biochem J 2010;429:403–17. https://doi.org/10.1042/BJ20100323.

[177] Karadag AS, Uzunçakmak TK, Ozkanli S, Oguztuzun S, Moran B, Akbulak O, et al. An investigation of cytochrome P450 (CYP) and glutathione S-transferase (GST) isoenzyme protein expression and related interactions with phototherapy in patients with psoriasis vulgaris. Int J Dermatol 2017;56. https://doi.org/10.1111/ijd.13343.

[178] Atalay S, Jarocka-Karpowicz I, Skrzydlewska E. Antioxidative and anti-inflammatory properties of cannabidiol. Antioxidants 2019;9. https://doi.org/10.3390/antiox9010021.

[179] Tsuboi K, Uyama T, Okamoto Y, Ueda N. Endocannabinoids and related N-acylethanolamines: biological activities and metabolism. Inflamm Regen 2018;38:28. https://doi.org/10.1186/s41232-018-0086-5.

[180] Matthews AT, Lee JH, Borazjani A, Mangum LC, Hou X, Ross MK. Oxyradical stress increases the biosynthesis of 2-arachidonoylglycerol: involvement of NADPH oxidase. Am J Physiol Cell Physiol 2016;311:C960–74. https://doi.org/10.1152/ajpcell.00251.2015.

[181] Turcotte C, Blanchet M-R, Laviolette M, Flamand N. The CB2 receptor and its role as a regulator of inflammation. Cell Mol Life Sci 2016;73:4449–70. https://doi.org/10.1007/s00018-016-2300-4.

[182] Hohmann U, Pelzer M, Kleine J, Hohmann T, Ghadban C, Dehghani F. Opposite effects of neuroprotective cannabinoids, palmitoylethanolamide, and 2-arachidonoylglycerol on function and morphology of microglia. Front Neurosci 2019;13:1180. https://doi.org/10.3389/fnins.2019.01180.

[183] Souza MC, Rosas EC. Cannabinoid receptors as regulators of neutrophil activity in inflammatory diseases. Neutrophils 2018. https://doi.org/10.5772/intechopen.81995.

[184] Khuja I, Yekhtin Z, Or R, Almogi-Hazan O. Cannabinoids reduce inflammation but inhibit lymphocyte recovery in murine models of bone marrow transplantation. Int J Mol Sci 2019;20:668. https://doi.org/10.3390/ijms20030668.

[185] Peyravian N, Deo S, Daunert S, Jimenez JJ. Cannabidiol as a novel therapeutic for immune modulation. ITT 2020;9:131–40. https://doi.org/10.2147/ITT.S263690.

[186] Palmieri B, Laurino C, Vadalà M. A therapeutic effect of cbd-enriched ointment in inflammatory skin diseases and cutaneous scars. Clin Ter 2019;170:e93–9. https://doi.org/10.7417/CT.2019.2116.

[187] Elmore S. Apoptosis: a review of programmed cell death. Toxicol Pathol 2007;35:495–516. https://doi.org/10.1080/01926230701320337.

[188] Atalay S, Gegotek A, Wroński A, Domigues P, Skrzydlewska E. Therapeutic application of cannabidiol on UVA and UVB irradiated rat skin. A proteomic study. J Pharm Biomed Anal 2021;192:113656. https://doi.org/10.1016/j.jpba.2020.113656.

[189] Atalay S, Dobrzyńska I, Gegotek A, Skrzydlewska E. Cannabidiol protects keratinocyte cell membranes following exposure to UVB and hydrogen peroxide. Redox Biol 2020;36:101613. https://doi.org/10.1016/j.redox.2020.101613.

[190] Siddiqui WA, Ahad A, Ahsan H. The mystery of BCL2 family: Bcl-2 proteins and apoptosis: an update. Arch Toxicol 2015;89:289–317. https://doi.org/10.1007/s00204-014-1448-7.

[191] Shrivastava A, Kuzontkoski PM, Groopman JE, Prasad A. Cannabidiol induces programmed cell death in breast cancer cells by coordinating the cross-talk between apoptosis and autophagy. Mol Cancer Ther 2011;10:1161–72. https://doi.org/10.1158/1535-7163.MCT-10-1100.

[192] Bovenschen HJ, Langewouters AMG, van de Kerkhof PCM. Dimethylfumarate for psoriasis: pronounced effects on lesional T-cell subsets, epidermal proliferation and differentiation, but not on natural killer T cells in immunohistochemical study. Am J Clin Dermatol 2010;11:343–50. https://doi.org/10.2165/11533240-000000000-00000.

[193] Roll A, Reich K, Boer A. Use of fumaric acid esters in psoriasis. Indian J Dermatol Venereol Leprol 2007;73:133–7. https://doi.org/10.4103/0378-6323.31908.

[194] Elias AN, Goodman MM, Liem WH, Barr RJ. Propylthiouracil in psoriasis: results of an open trial. J Am Acad Dermatol 1993;29:78–81. https://doi.org/10.1016/0190-9622(93)70156-n.

[195] Utaş S, Köse K, Yazici C, Akdaş A, Keleştimur F. Antioxidant potential of propylthiouracil in patients with psoriasis. Clin Biochem 2002;35:241–6. https://doi.org/10.1016/s0009-9120(02)00294-1.

[196] Elias AN, Nanda VS, Barr RJ. CD1a expression in psoriatic skin following treatment with propylthiouracil, an antithyroid thioureylene. BMC Dermatol 2003;3:3. https://doi.org/10.1186/1471-5945-3-3.

[197] Malligarjunan H, Dayalan H, Gnanaraj P, Elango T, Subramanian S. Impact of propylthiouracil on quality of life in psoriasis patients. Indian J Med Sci 2011;65:331–6. https://doi.org/10.4103/0019-5359.107769.

[198] Gnanaraj P, Dayalan H, Elango T, Malligarjunan H, Raghavan V, Rao R. Downregulation of involucrin in psoriatic lesions following therapy with propylthiouracil, an anti-thyroid thioureylene: immunohistochemistry and gene expression analysis. Int J Dermatol 2015;54:302–6. https://doi.org/10.1111/ijd.12565.

[199] Arul S, Dayalan H, Jegadeesan M, Damodharan P. Induction of differentiation in psoriatic keratinocytes by propylthiouracil and fructose. BBA Clin 2016;6:82–6. https://doi.org/10.1016/j.bbacli.2016.06.002.

[200] Hallengren B, Forsgren A, Melander A. Effects of antithyroid drugs on lymphocyte function in vitro. J Clin Endocrinol Metab 1980;51:298–301. https://doi.org/10.1210/jcem-51-2-298.

[201] Kurd SK, Smith N, VanVoorhees A, Troxel AB, Badmaev V, Seykora JT, Gelfand JM. Oral curcumin in the treatment of moderate to severe psoriasis vulgaris: a prospective clinical trial. J Am Acad Dermatol 2008;58:625–31. https://doi.org/10.1016/j.jaad.2007.12.035.

[202] Antiga E, Bonciolini V, Volpi W, Del Bianco E, Caproni M. Oral curcumin (Meriva) is effective as an adjuvant treatment and is able to reduce IL-22 serum levels in patients with psoriasis vulgaris. BioMed Res Int 2015;2015:283634. https://doi.org/10.1155/2015/283634.

[203] Gao X, Kuo J, Jiang H, Deeb D, Liu Y, Divine G, et al. Immunomodulatory activity of curcumin: suppression of lymphocyte proliferation, development of cell-mediated cytotoxicity, and cytokine production in vitro. Biochem Pharmacol 2004;68:51–61. https://doi.org/10.1016/j.bcp.2004.03.015.

[204] Ashrafizadeh M, Ahmadi Z, Mohammadinejad R, Farkhondeh T, Samarghandian S. Curcumin activates the Nrf2 pathway and induces cellular protection against oxidative injury. Curr Mol Med 2020;20. https://doi.org/10.2174/1566524019666191016150757.

[205] Zhao R, Yang B, Wang L, Xue P, Deng B, Zhang G, et al. Curcumin protects human keratinocytes against inorganic arsenite-

induced acute cytotoxicity through an NRF2-dependent mechanism. Oxid Med Cell Longev 2013;2013:412576. https://doi.org/10.1155/2013/412576.

[206] Song W, Ren Y-J, Liu L-L, Zhao Y-Y, Li Q-F, Yang H-B. Curcumin induced the cell death of immortalized human keratinocytes (HaCaT) through caspase-independent and caspase-dependent pathways. Food Funct 2021;12:8669–80. https://doi.org/10.1039/d1fo01560e.

[207] Koyu H, Haznedaroglu MZ. Investigation of impact of storage conditions on *Hypericum perforatum* L. dried total extract. J Food Drug Anal 2015;23:545–51. https://doi.org/10.1016/j.jfda.2015.04.002.

[208] Xu X, Ye H, Wang W, Yu L, Chen G. Determination of flavonoids in *Houttuynia cordata* Thunb. and *Saururus chinensis* (Lour.) Bail. by capillary electrophoresis with electrochemical detection. Talanta 2006;68:759–64. https://doi.org/10.1016/j.talanta.2005.05.027.

[209] Ma Y-C, Mani A, Cai Y, Thomson J, Ma J, Peudru F, et al. An effective identification and quantification method for *Ginkgo biloba* flavonol glycosides with targeted evaluation of adulterated products. Phytomedicine 2016;23:377–87. https://doi.org/10.1016/j.phymed.2016.02.003.

[210] Shen P, Lin W, Deng X, Ba X, Han L, Chen Z, et al. Potential implications of quercetin in autoimmune diseases. Front Immunol 2021;12.

[211] Van Dross RT, Hong X, Essengue S, Fischer SM, Pelling JC. Modulation of UVB-induced and basal cyclooxygenase-2 (COX-2) expression by apigenin in mouse keratinocytes: role of USF transcription factors. Mol Carcinog 2007;46:303–14. https://doi.org/10.1002/mc.20281.

[212] Tong X, Van Dross RT, Abu-Yousif A, Morrison AR, Pelling JC. Apigenin prevents UVB-induced cyclooxygenase 2 expression: coupled MRNA stabilization and translational inhibition. Mol Cell Biol 2007;27:283–96. https://doi.org/10.1128/MCB.01282-06.

[213] Yano S, Umeda D, Yamashita S, Yamada K, Tachibana H. Dietary apigenin attenuates the development of atopic dermatitis-like skin lesions in NC/Nga mice. J Nutr Biochem 2009;20:876–81. https://doi.org/10.1016/j.jnutbio.2008.08.002.

[214] Arsić I, Tadić V, Vlaović D, Homšek I, Vesić S, Isailović G, Vuleta G. Preparation of novel apigenin-enriched, liposomal and non-liposomal, antiinflammatory topical formulations as substitutes for corticosteroid therapy. Phytother Res 2011;25:228–33. https://doi.org/10.1002/ptr.3245.

[215] Schäfer T. Epidemiology of psoriasis. DRM 2006;212:327–37. https://doi.org/10.1159/000092283.

[216] Bø K, Thoresen M, Dalgard F. Smokers report more psoriasis, but not atopic dermatitis or hand eczema: results from a Norwegian population survey among adults. Dermatology (Basel) 2008;216:40–5. https://doi.org/10.1159/000109357.

[217] Davidsson S, Blomqvist K, Molin L, Mørk C, Sigurgeirsson B, Zachariae H, Zachariae R. Lifestyle of Nordic people with psoriasis. Int J Dermatol 2005;44:378–83. https://doi.org/10.1111/j.1365-4632.2005.01925.x.

[218] Naldi L, Parazzini F, Peli L, Chatenoud L, Cainelli T. The psoriasis study group of the Italian group for epidemiologic research in dermatology dietary factors and the risk of psoriasis. Results of an Italian case–control study. Br J Dermatol 1996;134:101–6. https://doi.org/10.1046/j.1365-2133.1996.d01-734.x.

[219] Kavli G, Førde OH, Arnesen E, Stenvold SE. Psoriasis: familial predisposition and environmental factors. Br Med J 1985;291:999–1000.

[220] Lohan SB, Vitt K, Scholz P, Keck CM, Meinke MC. ROS production and glutathione response in keratinocytes after application of β-carotene and VIS/NIR irradiation. Chem Biol Interact 2018;280:1–7. https://doi.org/10.1016/j.cbi.2017.12.002.

[221] Raychaudhuri SP, Gross J. Psoriasis risk factors: role of lifestyle practices. Cutis 2000;66:348–52.

[222] Keylock KT, Vieira VJ, Wallig MA, DiPietro LA, Schrementi M, Woods JA. Exercise accelerates cutaneous wound healing and decreases wound inflammation in aged mice. Am J Physiol Regul Integr Comp Physiol 2008;294:R179–84. https://doi.org/10.1152/ajpregu.00177.2007.

[223] Fantuzzi G. Adipose tissue, adipokines, and inflammation. J Allergy Clin Immunol 2005;115:911–9. https://doi.org/10.1016/j.jaci.2005.02.023.

[224] Covas M, Elosua R, Fitó M, Alcántara M, Coca L, Marrugat J. Relationship between physical activity and oxidative stress biomarkers in women. Med Sci Sports Exerc 2002;34:814–9.

[225] Elosua R, Molina L, Fito M, Arquer A, Sanchez-Quesada JL, Covas MI, et al. Response of oxidative stress biomarkers to a 16-week aerobic physical activity program, and to acute physical activity, in healthy young men and women. Atherosclerosis 2003;167:327–34. https://doi.org/10.1016/S0021-9150(03)00018-2.

Index

'*Note:* Page numbers followed by "f" indicate figures, "t" indicate tables.'

K

L

M

N

O

P

Q

R

S